NANOMEDICINE FOR NEURODEGENERATIVE DISORDERS

Selective Treatment Strategies

NANOMEDICINE FOR NEURODEGENERATIVE DISORDERS

Selective Treatment Strategies

Edited by

Rishabha Malviya, PhD

Kamla Pathak, PhD

Swati Verma, MPharm

AAP | APPLE ACADEMIC PRESS

First edition published 2025

Apple Academic Press Inc.
1265 Goldenrod Circle, NE,
Palm Bay, FL 32905 USA

760 Laurentian Drive, Unit 19,
Burlington, ON L7N 0A4, CANADA

CRC Press
2385 NW Executive Center Drive,
Suite 320, Boca Raton FL 33431

4 Park Square, Milton Park,
Abingdon, Oxon, OX14 4RN UK

Library and Archives Canada Cataloguing in Publication

Title: Nanomedicine for neurodegenerative disorders : selective treatment strategies / edited by Rishabha Malviya, PhD, Kamla Pathak, PhD, Swati Verma, MPharm.
Names: Malviya, Rishabha, editor. | Pathak, Kamla, 1963- editor. | Verma, Swati, 1994- editor.
Description: First edition. | Includes bibliographical references and index.
Identifiers: Canadiana (print) 20240487583 | Canadiana (ebook) 20240486978 | ISBN 9781774916124 (hardcover) | ISBN 9781774916131 (softcover) | ISBN 9781003486565 (ebook)
Subjects: LCSH: Nervous system—Degeneration—Treatment. | LCSH: Drug carriers (Pharmacy) | LCSH: Drug delivery systems. | LCSH: Nanomedicine.
Classification: LCC RC349.8 .N36 2025 | DDC 616.8/0461—dc23

Library of Congress Cataloging-in-Publication Data

CIP data on file with US Library of Congress

ISBN: 978-1-77491-612-4 (hbk)
ISBN: 978-1-77491-613-1 (pbk)
ISBN: 978-1-00348-656-5 (ebk)

About the Editors

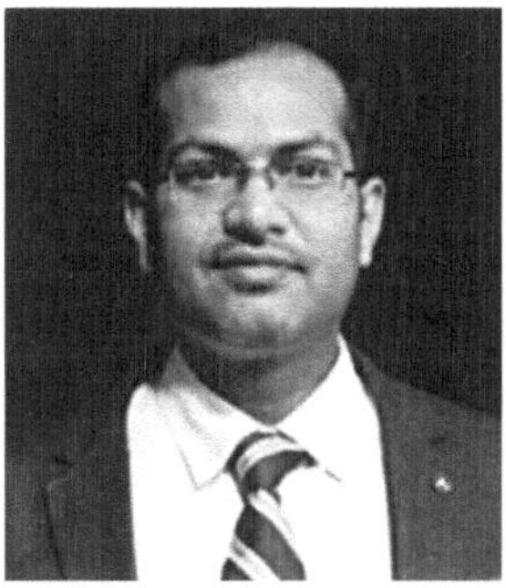

Rishabha Malviya, PhD

Associate Professor, Department of Pharmacy, School of Medical and Allied Sciences, Galgotias University, Greater Noida, Uttar Pradesh, India

Rishabha Malviya, PhD, has 11 years of research experience and is presently working as Associate Professor in the Department of Pharmacy, School of Medical and Allied Sciences, Galgotias University, Greater Noida, Uttar Pradesh, India. His areas of interest include formulation optimization, nanoformulation, targeted drug delivery, localized drug delivery, and characterization of natural polymers as pharmaceutical excipients. He has authored more than 150 research and review papers for national and international journals of repute. He holds over 50 patents and has published many papers in reputed national and international journals, for which he received an outstanding reviewer award from Elsevier. He has edited 13 books (Wiley, Springer Nature, CRC Press/Taylor and Francis, Apple Academic Press, River Publisher, Lambert, and OMICS Publishing Group) and authored 15 book chapters. His name has been included in the *World's Top 2% Scientists* list by Elsevier BV and Stanford University. He is reviewer, editor, and editorial board member of more than 50 national and international journals. He was an invited author for the magazine *Atlas of Science* as well as a pharma magazine dealing with B2B industry, Ingredient South Asia. He completed a BPharm from Uttar Pradesh Technical University and MPharm (Pharmaceutics) from Gautam Buddha Technical University, Lucknow Uttar Pradesh. His PhD (Pharmacy) work was in novel formulation development techniques.

Kamla Pathak, PhD

Dean and Professor, Faculty of Pharmacy, Uttar Pradesh University of Medical Sciences, Etawah, India

Kamla Pathak, PhD, is Dean and Professor, Faculty of Pharmacy, Uttar Pradesh University of Medical Sciences, Etawah, India. With teaching and research experience of more than 30 years, she is actively engaged in research on oral controlled, modulated, and targeted and topical drug delivery systems, and has received many awards for her work. She has over 270 publications in journals of international and national repute. She also holds three patents and has authored four books and more than 20 book chapters. She has also written many abstracts in various scientific forums and has been a reviewer for national and international journals in pharmaceutics. Professor Pathak has served as a member of the editorial advisory board of AAPS Pharm Sci Tech and is also a member of various professional bodies. She has guided more than 120 PhD and postgraduate students. She is also associated with the Indian pharmaceutical industry in the capacity of a scientific consultant. She is credited as reviewer of several scientific projects including Knowledge Foundation, Sweden, and Israel Science Foundation. She has participated at national and international seminars and conferences as organizer, invited speaker, and chairperson of scientific sessions. She has been listed in the top 2% Indian scientists in the subsection Pharmacology and Pharmacy, in the *World's Top 2% Scientists* list released by Stanford University in 2020 and 2021. She graduated (Pharmaceutics) from the University Institute of Pharmaceutical Sciences, Panjab University, Chandigarh, India, earning her doctorate in Pharmacy in 1991 from the same institute.

Swati Verma, MPharm

Department of Pharmacy, School of Medical and Allied Sciences, Galgotias University, Greater Noida, Uttar Pradesh, India

Swati Verma, MPharm, is currently working in the Department of Pharmacy, School of Medical and Allied Sciences, Galgotias University, Greater Noida, Uttar Pradesh, India. Her areas of interest are in computer-aided drug design, analytical chemistry, targeted drug delivery, and nanoformulation. She has authored four book chapters, edited two books, and many review papers published in international journals. She completed a BPharm at Dr. A.P.J. Abdul Kalam Technical University and MPharm (Pharmaceutical Chemistry) at Banasthali Vidyapith, Rajasthan, India. Her PhD work is in neurodisorders.

Contents

Contributors

Suryawanshi Ajay
Department of Pharmaceutics, National Institute of Pharmaceutical Education and Research, Raebareli, Uttar Pradesh, India

Anubhav Ananad
Department of Pharmaceutics, Hygia Institute of Pharmaceutical Education and Research, Lucknow, Uttar Pradesh, India

Isaac O. Babatunde
Phytomedicine and Toxicology Laboratories, Department of Biochemistry, Faculty of Basic and Applied Sciences, Osun State University, Osogbo, Nigeria

Soubhik Bhattacharyya
Department of Pharmacy, Arka Jain University, Tata Jamshedpur, Jharkhand, India

Bhavna Bohra
Department of Pharmacology, Institute of Pharmacy, Nirma University, S.G. Highway, Ahmedabad, Gujarat, India

Hina Chadha
Department of Pharmacy, Vishveshwarya Group of Institutions, Greater Noida, Uttar Pradesh, India

Vijay R. Chidrawar
Department of Pharmacology, Raghavendra Institute of Pharmaceutical Education and Research, Andhra Pradesh, India

Shibu Das
School of Pharmaceutical Sciences, Maharishi University of Information Technology, Lucknow, Uttar Pradesh, India

Shraddha Dwivedi
Department of Zoology, Government Degree College, Haripur, Nihastha, Raibareliy Uttar Pradesh, India

Obiora Reginald Ejinaka
Federal School of Medical Laboratory Science, Jos-Nigeria

Nkereuwem Sunday Etukudoh
Federal School of Medical Laboratory Science, Jos-Nigeria

Mahesh Gaikwad
Department of Pharmaceutics, National Institute of Pharmaceutical Education and Research (NIPER)-Raebareli, Bijnor, Lucknow, Uttar Pradesh, India

Ujjwal Gupta
Department of Pharmaceutics, National Institute of Pharmaceutical Education and Research, Raebareli, Uttar Pradesh, India

Dignesh Khunt
Graduate School of Pharmacy, Gujarat Technological University, Gandhinagar, Gujarat, India

Girish Kumar
Amity Institute of Pharmacy, Amity University, Greater Noida Campus, Uttar Pradesh, India

Chandana Majee
Department of Pharmaceutical Chemistry, Noida Institute of Engineering and Technology (Pharmacy Institute), Greater Noida, Uttar Pradesh, India

Rishabha Malviya
Department of Pharmacy, School of Medical and Allied Sciences, Galgotias University, Greater Noida, Gautam Buddha Nagar, Uttar Pradesh, India

Farhan Mazahir
Department of Pharmaceutics, National Institute of Pharmaceutical Education and Research, Raebareli, Uttar Pradesh, India

Rupa Mazumder
Department of Pharmaceutical Chemistry, Noida Institute of Engineering and Technology (Pharmacy Institute), Greater Noida, Uttar Pradesh, India

Dhanalekshmi Unnikrishnan Meenakshi
College of Pharmacy, National University of Science and Technology, Muscat, Oman

Sudhanshu Mishra
Department of Pharmaceutical Science and Technology, Madan Mohan Malviya University of Technology, Gorakhpur, Uttar Pradesh, India

Ankita Moharana
Department of Pharmacy, Arka Jain University, Tata Jamshedpur, Jharkhand, India

Smit Nayi
Graduate School of Pharmacy, Gujarat Technological University, Gandhinagar, Gujarat, India

Uchejeso Mark Obeta
Federal School of Medical Laboratory Science, Jos-Nigeria

Amaechi Eze Odono
Federal School of Medical Laboratory Science, Jos-Nigeria

Smriti Ojha
Department of Pharmaceutical Science and Technology, Madan Mohan Malviya University of Technology, Gorakhpur, Uttar Pradesh, India

Johnson O. Oladele
Department of Chemical Sciences, Faculty of Science, Kings University, Ode-Omu, Osun State, Nigeria

Oluwaseun T. Oladele
Phytomedicine and Toxicology Laboratories, Department of Biochemistry, Faculty of Basic and Applied Sciences, Osun State University, Osogbo, Nigeria

Himanshu Paliwal
Marwadi University Research Center Department of Pharmaceutics, Faculty of Pharmacy, Marwadi University, Rajkot, Gujarat, India

Bhawani Pantela
Department of Pharmaceutical Chemistry, Noida Institute of Engineering and Technology (Pharmacy Institute), Greater Noida, Uttar Pradesh, India

Akshay Parihar
Faculty of Pharmaceutical Sciences, The ICFAI university, Himachal Pradesh

Fagun Pathak
Department of Pharmacology, Institute of Pharmacy, Nirma University, Ahmedabad, Gujarat, India

Kamla Pathak
Faculty of Pharmacy, Uttar Pradesh University of Medical Sciences, Saifai, Etawah, Uttar Pradesh, India

Gajanan Paul
Department of Pharmaceutics, National Institute of Pharmaceutical Education and Research (NIPER)-Raebareli, Bijnor, Lucknow, Uttar Pradesh, India

Prashant L. Pingale
GES's Sir Dr. M. S. Gosavi College of Pharmaceutical Education and Research, Nashik, Maharashtra, India

Bhupendra G. Prajapati
Shree S.K. Patel College of Pharmaceutical Education and Research, Ganpat University, Mehsana, Gujarat, India
Faculty of Pharmacy, Silpakorn University, Nakhon Pathom, Thailand

Bhagawati Saxena
Department of Pharmacology, Institute of Pharmacy, Nirma University, S.G. Highway, Ahmedabad, Gujarat, India

Viral Shah
Department of Pharmaceutics, Sal Institute of Pharmacy, Sola, Ahmedabad, Gujarat, India

Brijesh Shah
Postdoctoral Scholar at Anodyne Nanotech-Tufts University, Faculty of Technology, University College of Technology, Boston, Massachusetts, United States

Sunny R. Shah
B. K. Mody Government Pharmacy College, Gujarat Technological University, Rajkot, India

Akanksha Sharma
Monad College of Pharmacy, Monad University, Kastla, Kasmabad, Pilkhuwa, Uttar Pradesh, India

Anjali Sharma
Central Drugs Standard Control Organisation (CDSCO), FDA Bhawan, Kotla Road, New Delhi, India

Ashwani Sharma
Delhi Pharmaceutical Sciences and Research University (DPSRU), New Delhi, India

Pankaj Sharma
Department of Pharmaceutics, ShriRam College of Pharmacy, Morena, Madhya Pradesh, India

Devang Sheth
L. M. College of Pharmacy, Gujarat Technological University, Ahmedabad, India

Padmini Shukla
Faculty of Pharmacy, Uttar Pradesh University of Medical Sciences, Saifai, Etawah, Uttar Pradesh, India

Prabodh Shukla
Faculty of Pharmacy, Uttar Pradesh University of Medical Sciences, Saifai, Etawah, Uttar Pradesh, India

Aditi Singh
Ashoka Institute of Pharmacy, Ashoka Engineering Chauraha, Sarnath, Varanasi, Uttar Pradesh, India

Ruchi Singh
Swaminarayan University, Shree Swaminarayan College of Pharmacy, Saij Kalol, Gandhinagar, Gujarat, India

Sudarshan Singh
Faculty of Pharmacy, Chiang Mai University, Chiang Mai, Thailand

Teerapol Srichana
Marwadi University Research Center Department of Pharmaceutics, Faculty of Pharmacy, Marwadi University, Rajkot, Gujarat, India

Alka Srivastava
School of Pharmaceutical Sciences, Maharishi University of Information Technology, Lucknow, Uttar Pradesh, India

Noopur Srivastava
School of Pharmaceutical Sciences, Maharishi University of Information Technology, Lucknow, Uttar Pradesh, India

Srishti Tiwari
Narayan Institute of Pharmacy, Jamuhar, Sasaram, Bihar, India

Garima Tripathi
Narayan Institute of Pharmacy, Jamuhar, Sasaram, Bihar, India

Pawan Upadhyay
School of Pharmaceutical Sciences, Maharishi University of Information Technology, Lucknow, Uttar Pradesh, India

Ashish Verma
Accurate College of Pharmacy, Knowledge Park III, Greater Noida, Uttar Pradesh, India

Shilpa Verma
Department of Pharmaceutics, National Institute of Pharmaceutical Education and Research (NIPER)-Raebareli, Bijnor, Lucknow, Uttar Pradesh, India

Tarun Virmani
Amity Institute of Pharmacy, Amity University, Greater Noida Campus, Uttar Pradesh, India

Awesh K. Yadav
Department of Pharmaceutics, National Institute of Pharmaceutical Education and Research (NIPER)-Raebareli, Bijnor, Lucknow, Uttar Pradesh, India

Abbreviations

AA	arachidonic acid
ABC	ATP-binding cassette
AChE	acetylcholinesterase
AD	Alzheimer's disease
ADA	adenosine deaminase
AGE	advanced glycation end
AgNP	silver nanoparticles
AGP	alpha(1)-acid glycoprotein
AHP	analytical hierarchy process
AJ	adherent junctions
ALA	alpha-linolenic acid
ALS	amyotrophic lateral sclerosis
AMT	adsorptive-mediated transcytosis
ANG1	angiopoietin 1
API	active pharmaceutical ingredient
APP	amyloid precursor protein
APS	atypical Parkinsonian syndromes
APTI	Association of Pharmaceutical Teachers in India
ARE	antioxidant response element
ASK1	apoptosis signal-regulating kinase 1
ATP	adenosine triphosphate
AUC	area under the curve
AuNP	gold nanoparticles
AZT	azidothymidine
BBB	blood–brain barrier
BCFB	blood-cerebrospinal fluid barrier
BCEC	brain capillary endothelial cells
BCRP	breast cancer resistance protein
BDNF	brain-derived neurotrophic factor
bFGF	basic fibroblast growth factor
BIT	Birla Institute of Technology
BK	bradykinin
BM	basement membrane
BSCB	blood-spinal cord barrier

BTB	blood tumor barrier
CAPE	caffeic acid phenethyl ester
CAPP	cerebral and peripheral perfusion
CBD	corticobasal degeneration
CIRI	cerebral ischemia-reperfusion damage
CJD	Creutzfeldt–Jakob disease
CMC	critical micelle concentration
CMT	carrier-mediated transcytosis
CNF	carbon nanofibers
CNS	central nervous system
CNT	carbon nanotubes
CoX-2	cyclooxygenase 2
CP	choroid plexus
CPP	cell-penetrating peptide
CRD	carbohydrate recognition domains
CSF	cerebrospinal fluid
CSI	chemical shift imaging
CSLN	cationic solid lipid nanoparticles
CT	computed tomography
CVD	chemical vapor deposition
DA	dopamine
DAMP	damage-associated molecular patterns
DAT	dopamine transporter
DDS	drug delivery system
DHA	docosahexaenoic acid
DHDP	dihexadecyl phosphate
DLS	dynamic light scattering
DMEM	Dulbecco's modified eagle medium
DND	detonated nanodiamonds
DNP	DNA nanoparticles
DTI	diffusion tensor imaging
EC	endothelial cells
ECG	epicatechin-3-gallate
ECGC	epigallocatechin gallate
EEG	electroencephalography
EGC	epigallocatechin
ELISA	enzyme-linked immunosorbent assay
EMA	European Medicine Agency
EPA	eicosapentaenoic acid

EPK	extracellular controlled protein kinase
EPR	enhanced permeability and retention
ERK	extracellular signal-regulated kinases
EV	extracellular vesicles
FDA	Food and Drug Administration
FTIR	Fourier transform infrared spectroscopy
GBM	graphene-based materials
GDNF	glial cell line-derived neurotrophic factor
GFAP	glial fibrillary acidic protein
GFP	mice with green fluorescent protein
GLUT1	glucose transport receptor
GLX	glycocalyx
GNP	gold nanoparticles
GO	graphene oxide
GOQD	GO quantum dots
GPA	geniposidic acid
GRAS	generally recognized as safe
GSH	glutathione
GSK3	glucose synthase kinase 3
HA	hyaluronic acid
HAND	human immunodeficiency virus associated neurodegenerative disorders
HBMEC	human brain microvascular endothelial cells
HD	Huntington's disease
HIF-1	hypoxia-inducible factor 1
hNSC	human neuronal stem cells
HPHT	high pressure high temperature
HPLC	high performance liquid chromatography
HRP	horseradish peroxidase
HRTEM	high-resolution transmission electron microscopy
HSA	human serum albumin
HVA	homovanillic acid
IAN	Indian Academy of Neuroscience
ICV	intra-cerbroventricular
IFN	interferon
IGF	insulin-like growth factor
IJBMI	International Journal of Business and Management Invention
IND	investigational new drug
IPGA	Indian Pharmacy Graduate Association

IPS	Indian Pharmacological Society
ISF	interstitial fluid
JAM	junctional adhesion molecules
JEV	Japanese encephalitis virus
JNK	Jun N-terminal kinases
LAM	leukocyte adhesion molecules
LDC	lipid drug conjugates
LDL	low-density lipoprotein
LDLR	low-density lipoprotein receptors
LIF	leukemia inhibitory factor
LMN	lower motor neuron
LN	laminin
LNP	lipid nanoparticles
LPS	lipopolysaccharide
LRP	lipoprotein receptor-related protein
LRRK2	leucine-rich repeat kinase 2
LSPR	localized surface plasmon resonance
LSR	lipolysis-stimulated receptor
LT	leukotrienes
LUMO	lowest unoccupied molecular orbital
LUV	large unilamellar vesicles
M6P	mannose 6-phosphate
MAGI	membrane-associated guanylate kinase
MAO-B	monoamine oxidase type b
MAPK	mitogen-activated protein kinase
MCAO	middle cerebral artery occlusion
MCDM	multicriteria decision making
MCI	moderate cognitive impairment
MCP-1	monocyte chemotactic protein-1
MDA	malondialdehyde
MDM-2	murine double-minute 2
MDR	multidrug resistance
MLV	multilamellar vesicles
MMP	matrix metalloproteinases
MNP	metal nanoparticles
MR	magnetic resonance
MRI	magnetic resonance imaging
MRP	multiresistant proteins
MRP-1	multidrug resistant protein-1

MS	multiple sclerosis
NAA	N-acetyl aspartate levels
ND	neurodegenerative disease
NDD	drug for neurodegenerative diseases
NFB	nuclear factor kappa b
NFHS	neurofilament-heavy subunit
NFL	neurofilament light chains
NFT	neurofibrillary tangles
NGB	new generation of biomarkers
NIH	National Institutes of Health
NIPER	National Institute of Pharmaceutical Education and Research
NLC	nanostructured lipid carriers
NLC-CEF	ceftriaxone-loaded nanostructured lipid carriers
NO	nitric oxide
NP	nanoparticles
NSC	neural stem cells
NSE	neuronal-specific enolase
NV	nitrogen vacancy
OAT	organic anion transporters
OCB	oligoclonal bands
ORN	olfactory receptors neurons
PACA	poly-alkyl-cyanoacrylate
PBCA	poly(butyl cyanoacrylate
PBMC	peripheral blood mononuclear cells
PCL	polycaprolactone
PD	Parkinson's Disease
PDE	phosphodiesterases
PDI	polydispersity index
PEG	polyethylene glycol
PEI	polyethyleneimine
PET	positron emission tomography
PF	protein folding
PG	prostaglandin
PHF	paired helical filaments
PLA	polylactic acid
PLGA	polylactic-co-glycolic acid
PLS	primary lateral sclerosis
PLVAP	plasmalemma vesicle-associated protein
PMA	progressive muscular atrophy

PMCA	protein misfolding cyclic amplification
PNP	polymeric nanoparticles
PS1	presenilin 1
PS2	presenilin 2
PSP	progressive supranuclear palsy
PUFA	polyunsaturated fatty acids
PVA	polyvinyl alcohol
PVP	poly(vinylpyrrolidone)
QbD	quality by design
QNP	quercetin nanoparticles
QTF	quetiapine fumarate
RA	rosmarinus acid
RC	reliability coefficient
RES	reticuloendothelial system
RI	random consistency index
RL	rivastigmine liposomes
RMT	receptor-mediated transcytosis
RNAi	RNA interference
RNS	reactive nitrogen species
ROS	reactive oxygen species
RVG	rabies virus glycoprotein
SAH	subarachnoid hemorrhage
SASP	senescence-associated secretory phenotype
SCID	several combined immunodeficiency
SLNP	solid lipid nanoparticles
SMA	spinal muscular atrophy
SOD	superoxide dismutase
SOD1	endogenous gene superoxide dismutase 1
SPECT	single-photon emission tomography
SUV	small unilamellar vesicles
SWCNT	single-wall carbon nanotubes
SXR	steroid and xenobiotic receptor
TAM	tumor-associated macrophages
TAT	trans-activating transcriptor
TEM	transmission electron microscopy
TH	tyrosine hydroxylase
TLR	toll-like receptors
TM	thrombomodulin
TMC	N-trimethyl chitosan

tPA	tissue plasminogen activator
TRBP	TAR-RNA binding protein
TRH	thyrotropin-releasing hormone
TSE	transmissible spongiform encephalopathies
UMN	upper motor neuron
UPS	ubiquitin-proteasome system
VEGF	vascular endothelial growth factor
WGA	wheat germ agglutinin
WHO	World Health Organization
XRD	X-ray diffraction
ZO	zonulae occludens

Foreword

I feel extremely happy and privileged to write a foreword for this book edited by Prof. Kamala Pathak and Dr. Rishabha Malviya, who are well known to me through their research outcomes.

This is a wonderful book on one of the topics which is directly related to the health of the people. The title of the book is self-explanatory: *Nanomedicine for Neurodegenerative Disorders: Selective Treatment Strategies.* Neuron-related illnesses have a significant impact on our society. These diseases cover a large range of pathologies with neuronal disruption pathologies, such as neurodegenerative disorders (e.g., Alzheimer's and Parkinson's) and metabolic diseases that are rigorously controlled by neural connections.

Patients suffering from these illnesses suffer from substantial medical bills and interruptions to their regular life. Current therapies used to treat these illnesses are considered as supportive. Therefore, a treatment strategy that targets the disease's root cause rather than merely its symptoms is desired. The much-needed drive in the battle against these diseases may emerge from the use of nanomedicine to successfully target the contributing factors in the development of CNS disorders. Nanomedicines have the capacity to adequately deliver therapeutics to the brain, indicating promising results in the treatment of neuron-related diseases.

However, it is also essential to acknowledge the enormous gap between the bench and the bedside and to identify the limitations of the current strategies. The technical depth and information in this book will, in my belief, be helpful for healthcare professionals in treating neurodegenerative disorders. This book will give readers profound insights into the recent uses of several cutting-edge nanocarriers that contain active pharmaceutical ingredients for the effective treatment of illnesses connected to neurons.

I am very sure that readers of this book will receive insight in identifying new targets in specific brain cells by studying mechanisms underlying neurodegenerative disorders and will use this knowledge with nanotechnology research to formulate optimized nanotherapeutics toward effective treatments of brain-related diseases.

—**Dr. Brahmeshwar Mishra**
Professor (HAG Scale) and Former Head
Department of Pharmaceutical Engineering and Technology
IIT(BHU), Varanasi, Uttar Pradesh, India

Preface

The demand for the development of therapeutic techniques toward a cure for neurodegenerative diseases (NDs) has increased in recent years reasoned by the fact that the population is getting older. Diseases like ND, which cause a gradual decline in neuronal structure and function, are frequently linked to actual neuronal death. Many medications have been tested, but as of yet, no one treatment can either stop the course of these diseases or make patients healthier again. NDs include devastating conditions from dementia, such as Alzheimer's, Parkinson's, amyotrophic lateral sclerosis, frontotemporal degeneration, Huntington's disease (HD), and prion disorders. P-glycoproteins, blood-cerebrospinal fluid barrier, and blood–brain barrier (BBB) are all major potential reasons for therapy failure caused by neurological diseases.

Recently developed nanotechnology allows for the possibility of employing nanotechnology and developing nanomaterials to enhance the distribution of potential drug treatments, hence overcoming in accordance with the aforementioned limits. This book will discuss some of the most fundamental and ever-evolving approaches to overcoming obstacles in drug distribution including local drug administration; receptor-mediated transcytosis; physicochemical BBB rupture; cell-penetrating peptides; and magnetic BBB breakdown. Pharmaceutical delivery has improved with nanoparticles becoming significantly more efficient. BBB breaching and reduced invasiveness are both benefits of using nanoengineered particles as nanodrugs. Numerous types of nanoparticles have been created to enhance drug delivery effectiveness, including those that are inorganic, magnetic, polymeric, and carbon-based. Although there have been many books written about neurodegenerative illnesses, there are still certain questions that need answers before they can be effectively treated.

Covering the most essential advancements in drug nanoformulation directed to the brain, this volume will be beneficial for new graduates as well as for pharmaceutical scientists, clinical researchers, and others seeking to overcome the obstacles in nanotechnology-technology-based medication delivery to treat NDs.

CHAPTER 1

Neurodegenerative Disorders: Concepts, Types, and Treatment Strategies

CHANDANA MAJEE, RUPA MAZUMDER, and BHAWANI PANTELA

Department of Pharmaceutical Chemistry, Noida Institute of Engineering and Technology (Pharmacy Institute), Gr. Noida, Uttar Pradesh, India

ABSTRACT

The number of neurodegenerative patients are increasing gradually with the population size and life expectancy trends. Globally, 50 million people are affected with neurodegenerative diseases (NDD), and by 2050, about 115 million people may be affected. In this disease, the central nervous system (CNS) progressively deteriorated and neurons' structure or function was lost. Such neuronal damage may eventually involve cell death. Alterations in axonal transport, neoinflammatory, proteolytic stress, oxidative stress, dysregulated RNA processing, mitochondrial dysfunction, glutamate toxicity calcium load, and aging are some of the molecular and cellular causes of neurogenerative diseases. Significant obstacles arise from the lack of knowledge about a potential root cause that underlies the pathogenesis of this disease.

New quantitative imaging methods have largely been replaced by structural–neuroimaging methods in the majority of neurodegenerative conditions. The creation of brain imaging biomarkers is crucial for making advancements in the diagnosis, characterization, and monitoring of neurodegenerative disorders (NDDs).

Amyloid-β, tau, BACE1, γ-secretase, repeat-associated non-ATG (RAN) peptides, etc. are the primary therapeutic targets of the majority of NDDs. Cyclic nucleotide phosphodiesterases are a frequent target for various neurogenerative disorders.

Nanomedicine for Neurodegenerative Disorders: Selective Treatment Strategies. Rishabha Malviya, Kamla Pathak, & Swati Verma (Eds.)

The majority of medications only have a limited potential to reduce symptoms, due to their poor ability to penetrate the blood–brain barrier (BBB) and reach the CNS. Based on these presumptions, it can be seen that designed nanocarriers, such as lipid-nanocarriers, are suitable tools to improve the absorption of medications into the CNS. Liposomal delivery technologies are thought to be the best vehicles for conventional medications as well as neuroprotective small molecules and compounds from green extraction.

1.1 INTRODUCTION

The term "neurodegeneration" is frequently used and is thought to have a common understanding of what it means. Finding a clear definition of neurodegeneration is much harder than we may assume. Frequently, neurodegeneration is even incompletely described in the most inclusive dictionaries. The word "degeneration" refers to a process wherein tissues or organs lose structure or function, while the lipid nanocarriers identify nerve cells (i.e., neurons), according to its etymology. In the healthcare setting, neurodegenerative diseases (NDDs) are defined by a significant number of neurological problems with a variety of medical and pathological manifestations that target specific components of neurons in important functional anatomical systems; they are created for unknown reasons and progress adamantly.[1–5] Conversely, neoplasm, edema, hemorrhage, and trauma of the nervous system, which are now not predominant neuronal diseases, are now not measured to be neurodegenerative disorders (NDDs). In addition to the gradual loss of neurons that results from NDDs, the brain, and other peripheral organs accumulate proteins with altered physicochemical characteristics. Neurodegenerative illnesses are categorized using protein-based methods. This demonstrates how protein–processing systems contribute to the onset of illness.[6–8]

1.2 PATHOGENESIS OF NEURODEGENERATIVE DISEASES

Genetic alterations that are inherited can cause some neurological issues. These problems run in families because fathers and mothers pass the incorrect gene to their offspring. The maximum neurodegenerative problems are related to environmental and genetic factors.[9,10] This makes it hard to predict who will increase disease. Some neurological problems may be brought on by inherited genetic changes. Fathers and mothers convey the wrong genes to their children, which causes these issues to run in families. For instance, Alzheimer's disease (AD), rare forms of motor neuron disease, and Huntington's disease. Environmental factors also have a role in NDDs. Parkinson's disease (PD) is linked to continuous exposure to poisons, hazardous chemicals, and pesticides. The biggest recognized hazard issue for many neurodegenerative issues is age. More than 350,000 people in Australia have dementia, while there are about 80,000 people who have PD. 5.4 million Americans suffered from AD in 2016. In 2020, the numbers of PD patients were 930,000 in the United States. Although precise protein accumulation/deposition and anatomic vulnerability are typically used to describe NDDs, these conditions also contribute to a number of crucial processes that result in progressive neuronal dysfunction and death, including oxidative stress, proteotoxic stress, neuroedema, cell death with its associated irregularities in the autophagosomal/lysosomal and ubiquitin-proteasomal systems.[11–15] Furthermore, it is challenging to understand that the protein irregularities that characterize NDDs can exist prior to the onset of clinical indications and that a character may exhibit more than one NDD method. At present, diagnostic biomarkers are now not available, except in uncommon instances in which a causative genetic mutation can be proven to be the purpose of the sickness Hence, precise in vivo biomarkers, which include molecular imaging and biofluid markers are the most important to investigate priority. The pathogenic features of NDDs that are typically acknowledged include metabolic alteration, energy and ion homeostasis disruption, and molecular damage. The unfolded protein response and protein elimination routes such as the ubiquitin-proteasome system and the autophagy-lysosome pathway are significant pathogenesis features that are highlighted by the proteinopathy hypothesis. According to a recent theory known as "prion-like spreading," the proteins linked to NDDs move throughout the nervous system and affect anatomical regions in a sequential/hierarchical manner. This theory, which is based on research into prion diseases, suggests that pathogenic NDD-associated proteins spread from cell to cell and undergo template-directed protein misfolding. It has been suggested that cerebral NDDs and systemic amyloidosis, which are sometimes known as "inducible proteinopathies" can be treated by exposing susceptible hosts to homologous molecular templates. 11 Indeed, research from cell culture and animal experimental models has shown that cells may take up pathogenic proteins and spread disease to other cells for the majority of the proteins indicated above.[16,17]

1.3 CLASSIFICATION OF NEURODEGENERATIVE DISEASES

The following criteria are used to classify NDDs:

1. Basic clinical traits, such as those of motor neuron disease, parkinsonism, dementia, or AD.
2., Neurodegenerative sites in the body's anatomy (e.g., extrapyramidal disorders, frontotemporal degenerations, or spinocerebellar degenerations).
3. The main molecular abnormality (TDP-43 tauopathies, amyloidosis, and synucleinopathies).

The classification of neurodegeneration diseases is given in Figure 1.1.

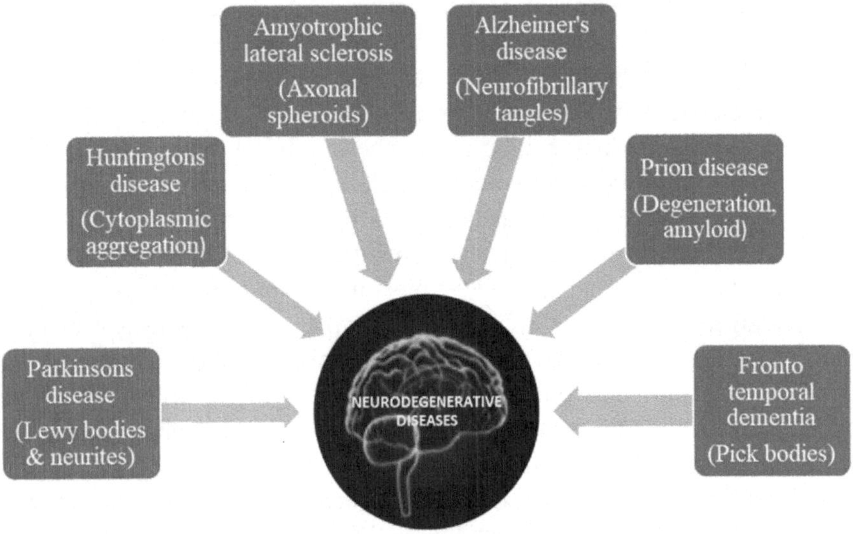

FIGURE 1.1 The classification of neurodegenerative diseases.

1.3.1 ALZHEIMER'S DISEASE

Alzheimer's disease is a NDD that slowly erodes mental capacity. Brain regions linked to memory and language gradually lose nerve cells. The ability to memorize events, identify things and people, remember the meaning of words, and use judgment becomes increasingly challenging with time.[19,20] Typically, symptoms start to show up after age 65, and the prevalence dramatically rises with age. AD must be separated from other systems of dementia, such as frontotemporal dementia, vascular dementia, dementia related to Lewy bodies, and dementia with reversible dementias.

However, contrary to popular belief, this disease is not usually associated with aging. About 65% of dementia cases are caused by AD, which is the most communal kind in old persons. This is due to gene alterations that, in some belongings of early-onset AD, can be handed down from parent to child. This kind of illness can be brought on by changes in the *APP, PSE N1&N2* genes, according to research. Intracellular neurofibrillary tangles, which are visible in senile plaques, and extracellular β-amyloid deposits are the primary two pathology indicators of AD and synapses led on by neurofibrillary tangles, and β-amyloid deposition which often starts in the mesial temporal lobe. The effects of β-neurofibrillary tangles and amyloid peptides on the brain are not entirely understood. For the correct reason, there are a number of theories that were considered. The amyloid hypothesis clarifies the slow development of β-amyloid in the brain AND the gathering of β-amyloids in the brain that result in neuronal synapse loss, cell death, and neurotransmitter shortages, which are variables in the clinical symptoms of dementia.[21–24]

1.3.2 PARKINSON'S DISEASE

Parkinson's disease is the utmost common neurodegenerative condition, often affecting 2–3% of adults under the age of 65. Parkinson's disease often causes symptoms in the central, peripheral, and gut nervous systems. The underlying pathogenic process involves numerous neural systems and advances slowly yet relentlessly. Only a small subset of fragile nerve cells reveals the disease-causing changes to the neuronal cytoskeleton. Lewy neurites and Lewy bodies are eventually produced by affected neurons in their perikaryal and neuronal developments. The finding of PD is still primarily clinical, thus it is critical to detect the early symptoms as well as those that point to additional causes of parkinsonism.[25,26] Tremor, stiffness, and bradykinesia are characteristics of PD, and as the health deteriorates, some patients may have postural variability. Loss of nigrostriatal dopaminergic innervation is a pathological indicator of this disease and additional cells in the neural network are also damaged by neurodegeneration, which is not just affecting nigral dopaminergic neurons. The clinical history of PD, in nonmotor symptoms, including sleep issues, and loss of smell, may manifest years before motor symptoms. Both idiopathic and familial PD are thought to have a pathogenic role in mitochondrial malfunction. For the past 40 years, peripheral decarboxylase inhibitors and levodopa have been observed as the gold standard for the treatment of PD. In many respects, it is still the most effective pharmaceutical treatment. Numerous studies that showed the effect of caffeine on the start of the disease have found that coffee drinkers had a decreased chance of getting PD.[27–30]

1.3.3 FRONTOTEMPORAL DEMENTIA

Frontotemporal dementia is generally clinically and pathologically distinct from other types of dementia.[31] Frontotemporal dementia, which causes up to 20% of episodes of presenile dementia, is the most commonly affected degenerative dementia in middle age after AD. The key clinical feature is a significant change in personality and social biobehavioral coexists with relatively intact instrumental functions of partial cognition, perception, memory, and praxis.[31,32] The capacity to understand the meaning of words, objects, faces, nonverbal ambient noises, smells, tastes, and tactile inputs is impacted by one kind of dementia. A gradual loss of ideas is a hallmark of semantic dementia. The capacity to comprehend the meaning of words, faces, objects, tastes, smells, nonverbal environmental sounds, and tactile stimuli is impaired by dementia. For frontotemporal dementia, few effective therapies are presently available. Because neurochemical testing harvest revealed any abnormalities of the cholinergic system, pharmaceutical medications meant to treat AD are unlikely to benefit persons with frontotemporal dementia. Extrapyramidal indications develop in a limited percentage of patients, leading to a different class of dementia with parkinsonism. The pattern of histological alteration is also uneven, being identified by microvacuolation, which is often linked to histopathological changes of motor neuron disease or severe gliosis.[33–35]

1.3.4 PRION DISEASES

The normal prion protein, which typically has a helical structure, undergoes a modification that results in an irregular form of the protein, which is what causes a group of neurodegenerative illnesses known as prion diseases. One potential mechanism by which the development of PrPSc could lead to neurodegeneration is the loss of a crucial biological function of PrPC.[36–38] The direct toxicity of the misfolded protein may be another way that PrPSc production is linked to the disease. The three possible pathways through which prion diseases might develop are sporadic (spontaneous), genetic (familial), and acquired (infectious/transmitted). Nerve cell loss, gliosis, vacuolation, and PrPSc deposit were observed in prion disease. These diseases can be classified as Gerstmann–Straussler–Scheinker syndrome, Kuru, Creutzfeldt–Jakob disease, and fatal familial insomnia.[39,40]

1.3.5 HUNTINGTON'S DISEASE

The nervous system is impacted by Huntington's disease. This disease is mainly a genetic disorder caused by a changed gene. Neurological problems are caused by the brain being damaged by toxic protein buildup. The diagnosis of Huntington's disease can take some time. Initial warning signs and symptoms are slight, irregular movements, minute emotional and mood swings, stumbling, short-term memory problems, irritability, and depression. Numerous pathways are involved in the malfunction and death of neurons caused by mutant Huntingtin.[41,42] These include the exon 1 mHTT fragment's direct effects, the protein's propensity to aggregate abnormally, and its belongings on cellular axonal transport, transcription, proteostasis, translation, and synaptic function. With Huntington's disease, mouth and throat muscles can become very difficult to control. The person finds it challenging to speak, swallow, and consume as a result.[43,44]

1.3.6 AMYOTROPHIC LATERAL SCLEROSIS

Amyotrophic lateral sclerosis (ALS), a deadly NDD, affects the human motor system (ALS). Epidemiological studies in ALS have been hampered by the difficulty of pinpointing the moment at which the illness first manifested as well as the potentially long delay between the onset of pathological changes and the manifestation of clinical disease. A complicated interaction between genetic and molecular pathways seems to be one of the pathophysiological mechanisms behind the development of ALS, and this interaction appears to involve multiple factors. Autophagy, dysfunction of the sodium/potassium ion pump, structural abnormalities of mitochondria, and altered axonal transport networks have all been the etiology of ALS in addition to glutamate-induced excitotoxicity.[46–48]

Some polymorphisms found in ALS patients do not completely segregate with disease and may perhaps represent genetic risk factors rather than causal mutations. This disease includes mutations in the ciliary vascular endothelial growth factor (VEGF), neurofilament-heavy subunit (NFHS), and neurotrophic factor (CNTF) According to studies, the heavy metals in cigarettes promote oxidative stress, inflammation, and neurotoxicity, which raise the risk of ALS. Athletes are more prone to developing ALS as compared to the general population, however, participating in various physical activities has not been connected to a higher risk of raising the illness.[49,50]

1.4 MODERN TOOLS FOR DETECTING NEURODEGENERATIVE DISEASES

Traditional MR imaging is limited in its ability to diagnose NDDs. In the early, diagnostic period of NDDs, magnetic resonance imaging (MRI) is frequently employed, largely to rule out the alternate diagnosis. Quantitative MRI techniques such as voxel-based morphometry and surface-based morphometry are better at spotting disease-specific atrophy patterns than age-matched comparisons.

Clinical MRI pulse sequences are sensibly diagnosed to capture entire brain imaging information in a short-lived amount of time, usually using slice gaps and having a comparatively low three-dimensional tenacity. On the other way, high-resolution, high-quality, three-dimensional data sets without slice gaps are needed for quantifiable imaging systems.[51,52] The two most used methods for determining group-level grey matter modification are SBM and VBM. The first step in the typical VBM pipeline is the tissue-type division of three-D structural data into the components of cerebrospinal fluid (CSF) gray matter, and grey–white matter.[53] The following methods are generally used to account for the post of cortical different thickness in SBM motion corrections such as removal of nonbrain tissues, fragmentation of the thalamic deep grey matter volume structures, intensity normalization, the geometry of the grey/white matter borderline, and fully automated topology alterations.[54,55]

Since it is based on anisotropic water diffusion which occurs in neural fibers such as spinal cord, nerve, or brain white matter, diffusion tensor imaging (DTI) is used to trace neural fiber pathways. The basis of DTI is the idea that water molecules flow "isotropically"—randomly, and freely in any route—in an open medium. However, in a biological context, different membranes, fibers, and macromolecules impede such mobility. To define white matter veracity at the voxel level, a variety of DTI-derived metrics are used, including mean axial diffusivity, fractional anisotropy, and so on. Functional magnetic resonance imaging (fMRI) is a noninvasive functional imaging technique that was originally developed as a tool for experimental physiology and psychology but is now frequently utilized in the planning of epilepsy surgery and studies on neurodegeneration.[56,57]

Using near-infrared spectroscopy, adult human brain performance in a variety of activities has been noninvasively examined. The blood oxygen-related indication in the brain tissue is measured with the help of fMRI to analyze regions of metabolic action, either when doing a particular activity or at rest.[58,59]

The most widely used use of the noninvasive detection method that functionally maps the water protons is known as magnetic resonance (MR), sometimes known as nuclear MR or nuclear magnetic resonance (NMR). By using MR spectroscopy (MRS), tissue chemicals instead of water, naturally occurring metabolites that contain phosphorus, potassium, carbon, sodium, nitrogen, and fluorine, have their protons identified (MRS). The metabolic status of certain brain regions can be revealed via spectroscopy. MRS frequently relies on sodium- or phosphorus-based proton nuclei. Proton spectroscopy has a very good signal-to-noise ratio; as a result, it accurately measures brain metabolites. Researchers make use of a single-voxel approach in magnetic resonance spectroscopy (MRS). This method allows for a precise and extensive investigation of a specific area of the brain. When metabolic changes are mainly observed in the broader regions of the brain, in this time multivoxel techniques such as chemical shift imaging (CSI) are employed.[60,61] At least 20 different methods can be used for this. However, more sophisticated localization methods are used in the therapeutic context of neurospectroscopic spectroscopy single-voxel or CSI approaches for localized MRS most typically using ISIS STEAM or PRESS sequences.[62]

1.5 BRAIN TARGETING SITE FOR THE NEUROGENERATIVE DISEASES

The biggest and most intricate organ in the human body, the brain, matures properly throughout time. However, this normal aging might be further accelerated by pathological aging and the formation of NDs. The brain is safeguarded by the blood–brain barrier (BBB), which has two primary cell types: Neurons and glia. The BBB and a number of cytochrome-450 enzymes, such as alkaline phosphatase, γ-glutamyl transpeptidase, aromatic acid decarboxylase, and others, control the entry of substances required to preserve the brain's internal environment. Although BBB dysfunction has long been thought to be merely a ramification of clinical events, new research is beginning to suggest its crucial involvement in the pathogenesis of a number of disorders. Increased BBB permeability also increases the risk of natural seizures in epilepsy. Furthermore, healthy aging enhanced BBB permeability significantly correlates with enhanced immune responses. The reduction of neuron function and neuronal cell death is associated with the occurrence of ND. One of the most dangerous and difficult issues in contemporary new neuromedicine is the investigation and development of effective therapeutic techniques for the treatment of neurodegenerative illnesses. At the same time, any potential dangers and development costs are outweighed by the social and economic significance of solving these issues, at least in part. Nowadays, a lot of scientists are very interested in finding the precise proteins that cause neurodegeneration. Additionally, a new area of focus for targeting damaged neurons is nanotechnology-based methods. Different types of nanostructures have been created with the intention of treating neurodegeneration, and electrospun nanofibers appear to play a significant role as biomedical products for both disease detection and treatment.[63–65]

Neurodegenerative disorders may be slowed or prevented from progressing with the help of medications that modulate unexplored targets. The dark kinome, which includes uncharacterized human kinases, has a number of potential proteins. In the human brain, kinases are widely expressed and control important pathways. It offers enormous promise to target kinases to slow or stop neurodegeneration. High-caliber tiny molecules can shed light on how kinases work in the brain.[66,67]

Due to the similarity of the pathological and clinical etiologies of AD and PD, it may be possible to develop new therapeutic targets by analyzing issues affected by both diseases. Brodmann area 9 plays a very important role in NDDs such as PD and AD recognition, reasoning skills, and motor behavior. Additionally, these patients exhibit decreased BA9 neuronal activity. We have chosen this tissue because BA9 has an impact on both disorders. High-throughput BA9-RNA sequencing data are used to find the tissue-specific network and differentially expressed genes that help with the various treatments.[68,69]

Instead of its creation, the breakdown of cGMP and cAMP into the consistent inactive counterparts, 50 GMP and AMP play a very important role in the regulator of cyclic nucleotides. The enzymes in charge of this process are these phophosphodiesterases (PDEs). Primarily, based on their sequence homology, the PDE family includes 11 subfamilies, which are encoded by 21 known genes. Additionally, there may be several splice variants for each gene product (such as PDE4D1-PDE4D9), having approximately 100 dissimilar PDE-proteins. Different subtypes can be distinguished by their localization, subcellular dispersion, regulatory mechanisms, and enzymatic and kinetic properties, among other traits. The majority of these subtypes have multiple gene products. The differential in affinity for the two different cyclic nucleotides is used to make a basic differentiation between subfamilies. PDEs are broken down by enzymes called cyclic nucleotide PDEs (cGMP). As a result, they play a key role in controlling the amount of cyclic nucleotide-mediated signaling. PDE(4,7 and 8) alterations in the brain are linked to AD. Major depressive illness is connected with PDE4 and PDE11 dysfunction. Due to their widespread presence in striatal neurons, PDE1B and PDE10 have been the subject of the common studies into PD. Genetic abnormalities In the PDE8B gene are likely to be the cause of the neurodegenerative processes of autosomal-dominant striatal degeneration, another uncommon neurodegenerative striatal motor condition. NRF2 has been demonstrated to exert anti-inflammatory effects, influence both mitochondrial function and biogenesis, and regulate the expression of antioxidant genes. This is due to the fact that NRF2 has emerged as a viable therapeutic target and that mitochondrial failure and neuroinflammation are traits of many NDDs.[70–73]

1.6 BIOMARKERS FOR NEUROGENERATIVE DISEASES

The use of biomarkers as indications of both normal and pathological biological processes is very important. Pathologies, biochemistries, and genetic alterations that are specific to a disease can provide detailed information about its nature. A good biomarker should be accurate and trustworthy, able to differentiate between health conditions and serious illnesses, and discriminate between various diseases. In recent years, significant attempts have been made to recognize the neuropathological, genetic biomarkers, and biochemical of the disorders to diagnose diseases at an earlier stage. Biological compounds known as biomarkers can be utilized to detect the presence or beginning of many disorders. The current gold standard is a neuropathologic diagnosis, which is often only possible through an autopsy after the patient has died away.[76,77]

The biomarkers of the NDDs are discussed in the following subsections.

1.6.1 ALZHEIMER'S DISEASE (AD) BIOMARKER

Biological biomarkers suggested genetic markers and biochemical markers of AD are discussed in the following subsections.

1.6.1.1 GENETIC MARKERS: THE GENETIC MARKERS OF ALZHEIMER'S DISEASE

βAPP gene mutations: The first AD defenselessness gene identified has 770 amino acids and is the longest isoform of the transmembrane protein produced by the *APP* gene. The first genetic variant associated with this condition was located in the *APP* gene present in chromosome 21.[78]

Presenilin gene mutations: Presenilin 1 (*PS1*) and presenilin 2 (*PS2*) present in the chromosome are two homologous presenilin genes that have been associated with AD cases. There are now more than 120 unique mutations known to exist in the *PS1* gene. The bulk of these mutation-caused changes involve the substitution of just one amino acid. However, the *PS1* and *PS2* presenilin genes appear to have overlapping or comparable roles. This hypothesis was supported by the fact that *PS2* mutations, such as *PS1* mutations, might increase the synthesis of long-tailed A peptides.[79]

Apo-E polymorphisms: The apolipoprotein, a plasma protein, facilitates the transfer of cholesterol (ApoE). ApoE is connected to the creation and repair of the central nervous system (CNS) both during development and after injury. The apoE gene present in chromosome 19 contains 3 alleles. The delayed sporadic form of AD is linked to a somewhat earlier familial variant by the *ApoE 4* gene.[80]

1.6.1.2 BIOCHEMICAL MARKERS

Through the study of spinal fluid, the maximum potential biochemical indicators of AD have been discovered CSF.

CSF total tau: According to numerous research, AD patients have considerably greater total tau protein levels in their CSF fluid. The CSF-tau appears to be particularly sensitive to detecting AD but less specific for other dementias.[81]

Combination of CSF-Aβ42 and CSF-tau markers: Researchers have shown that combining the CSF indicators rather than utilizing them individually may greatly boost their efficacy, raising both their specificity and sensitivity for detecting AD patients. In reality, by combining a number of CSF biomarkers with other investigative methods, it is feasible to ensure the accuracy of the clinical analysis.[82]

CSF Phospho-tau (P-tau): Biomarkers for blood investigation indicating the pathology of AD, phosphorylated tau, and amyloid-have the potential to be utilized as scalable testing for clinical and different diagnoses of dementia. The typical increase level of AD-related with controls is around 250%, and P-ability tau's to distinguish between person aging has a mean sensitivity of up to 70%, and specificity of around 94%. Furthermore, a recent study revealed that when Mtf levels in serum were evaluated among healthy individuals and AD patients withheld-to-moderate phases, they did not significantly fluctuate when evaluated by SDS-PAGE under nonreducing environments.[83]

1.6.2 PARKINSON'S DISEASE BIOMARKER

The various genetic biomarkers related to PD are described below.

1.6.2.1 GENETIC MARKERS FOR PARKINSON'S DISEASE

Through genetic linkage and positional cloning research, a number of harmful single-gene mutations have been identified in several of these families. Following is a discussion on the most important of these genes.

***Parkin* gene:** The *parkin* gene is present in chromosome 6q25.2–27, has approximately 1.5 megabytes, and contains 12 exons, and was discovered. The discovery of 465 amino acid parkin protein plays a significant role in the pathogenesis of idiopathic PD. In conclusion, because mutations in the *parkin* gene typically produce familial early-onset and isolated juvenile Parkinsonism, it is one of the best genetic indications of familial early-onset PD that is currently available. In conclusion, because mutations in the parkin gene usually result in familial early-onset and isolated juvenile Parkinsonism, it is one of the best genetic predictors of PD that is currently known.[84]

***α-synuclein* gene:** The rare early onset familial type of PD is characterized by mutations in the synuclein gene, which is found on chromosome 4. Another mutation in the synuclein gene, this time an alanine to proline substitution at position 30 of the -synuclein protein induced by a single base-pair change from C to G at position 88, was discovered in a German family.[85]

***UCH-L1* gene:** According to a current proteomic investigation, the extremely prevalent protein, ubiquitin C-terminal hydrolase-L1 (UCH-L1), has been identified as a possible biomarker. The ubiquitin carboxy-terminal-hydrolase-L1 gene on chromosome 4 encodes a protein that belongs to the family of deubiquitinating enzymes. It is tempting to speculate that the enzyme modifies aggregated or damaged proteins, which would otherwise accumulate in the cell in dangerous quantities. The relationship of the neuronal enzyme UCH-L1 with PD puts into doubt the idea that each enzyme expresses a single enzymatic activity *in vivo* (PD). Unable to be explained by its known hydrolase activity, UCH-L1, particularly those variations linked to increased vulnerability to PD, causes the accumulation of -synuclein in cultured cells.[86]

***PINK1* gene:** The 581 amino acid protein is encoded by the PTEN-induced putative kinase 1 (*PINK1*) gene, which has 8 exons and widths around 1.8 kb. Recently, two homozygous *PINK1* gene mutations linked to PD were discovered. A Spanish family had G309D, and two Italian families had W437OPA substitutions. Recently, two homozygous *PINK1* gene mutations linked to PD were discovered.[87]

***DJ-1* gene:** A highly preserved protein that is ubiquitous is encoded by the *DJ-1* gene. It has been established that PARK7, a monogenic variant of human parkinsonism, and *DJ-1* mutations are related to diseases. Although the *DJ-1* protein's exact role in the body is uncertain, evidence points to its participation in the response to oxidative stress. Understanding the physiological function of *DJ-1* may help us better comprehend how brain neuronal maintenance mechanisms work.[88]

1.6.2.2 BIOCHEMICAL MARKERS FOR PARKINSON'S DISEASE

Two important biochemical markers that have proven very useful in determining the onset of the disease are the loss of the dopamine transporter (DAT), which has been identified by PET imaging, and the presence of the -synuclein protein, which is found in the Lewy body lesions, which are the characteristics of PD.

DAT: A Na^+ and Cl-the transport-coupled electrogenic process are used by the DAT to mediate the absorption of dopamine (DA) into dopaminergic neurons. The uptake of poisons that cause Parkinson's syndrome is facilitated by the DAT. When the neuronal depopulation exceeds 50%, the concentration of DAT starts to decline, which also explains why neurological deficiency symptoms manifest. Because of this, striatal DAT concentration—and specifically putamen DAT concentration—is a highly sensitive indicator for detecting the early stages of PD.[89]

Lewy bodies: These are shown to be a -synuclein-containing PD. The brain encompasses large amounts of human–synuclein protein, which is mostly expressed in presynaptic nerve terminals. This protein was originally associated with the etiology of a neurodegenerative illness as an innovative peptide distinct from an amyloid peptide. Lewy bodies are revealed to be a -synuclein-containing PD symptom. The brain contains large amounts of human–synuclein protein, which is mostly synthesized in presynaptic nerve terminals. As a new peptide that was unrelated to the amyloid peptide, the protein was initially connected to the etiology of NDD.[90]

1.6.3 BIOMARKER FOR AMYOTROPHIC LATERAL SCLEROSIS (ALS)

Researchers are mostly seeking direct indications for the motor neuronal degeneration in the spinal cord and when it comes to ALS biomarkers. A specific phenotype is related to the recessive D90A-SOD1 mutation. One of the rare mutations with a consistent phenotype, this one is still a mystery. Thus, a reasonably definite genetic molecular diagnosis may be drawn from the clinical analysis. Several biomarkers have been postulated as possible substitute indicators for the finding of ALS, including elevated glutamate levels in the blood and CSF, oxidative products in the blood, aberrant EAAT2 (GLT1) mRNA splicing variants in the CSF, and alterations in 1 H-MRS N-acetyl aspartate levels (NAA). Regarding how glutamate is presented There may be two more genetic markers for ALS because the genes *ALS2* and *NEFH* have also been connected to the disease. Due to the lack of concrete evidence linking the LMN and UMN to multilevel damage, early-stage ALS is extremely difficult to detect. LMN denervation on electromyography may aid in the confirmation of the diagnosis when a patient solely displays UMN-specific clinical indicators of ALS.[91]

1.7 BARRIERS TO DRUG DELIVERY TO THE CNS

The CNS is protected from medicines by a number of barriers, including the BBB, blood-CSF barrier (BCB), and blood tumor barrier (BTB).

The blood-brain barrier (BBB): Endothelial cells, brain capillaries, which are mostly made up of pericytes and astrocytes, and the BBB are what make up the brain. The permeable BBB allows for the passage of nutrients, proteins, and enzymes but not of water-soluble drugs. As a result, it makes it difficult for drugs and other therapeutic and diagnostic agents to be used in the treatment of ND diseases.[92]

Blood-cerebrospinal fluid barrier (BCSFB): Between the CSF space and the circulating blood, the BCB serves as a barrier. Prior to entering the

CNS, the CSF barrier (BCB) undergoes systemically operated therapeutic medication. Cerebrospinal fluid (CSF) can exchange molecules with the brain parenchyma's interstitial fluid and precisely control the entry of blood-borne compounds into the CSF. The BCB passes the molecules in both active and passive transfer modes.

Blood–tumor barrier: Administering medications intracranially becomes more difficult when there are CNS tumors. The physiological barriers in CNS malignancies prohibit medicines from being transported by the circulatory system. Some techniques to facilitate drug passage across TJs include inhibiting efflux drug transporters, opening TJs using a mannitol hyperosmotic solution, and receptor-mediated drug delivery systems.[93]

1.8 DRUG DELIVERY SYSTEM IN NEURODEGENERATIVE DISEASES

Several drug delivery techniques have been developed for actual drug distribution without any boundaries, as illustrated in

a) BBB disruption
b) Biotechnology-based delivery
c) Chemistry-based delivery
d) Intracerebral delivery
e) Intrathecal delivery
f) Intranasal delivery

The various approaches of drug delivery are pictorially described in Figure 1.2.

1.8.1 INVASIVE APPROACH

Rare peptides with low molecular weight compounds and lipid-soluble nutrients can effectively cross the barrier when using the invasive technique, either by active diffusion or particular transport mechanisms. Direct implies intrathecal and intracerebral administration invasive procedure to take a craniotomy and administer the medication to the brain. Both of them have a wide range of small- and big-molecule delivery. Through this intranasal route, a number of substances, including infections, toxic agents, and viruses, among many others, can be transported to the CNS. The two main drawbacks are the accidental release of anticancer drugs into healthy brain tissues and physiological stress.[94]

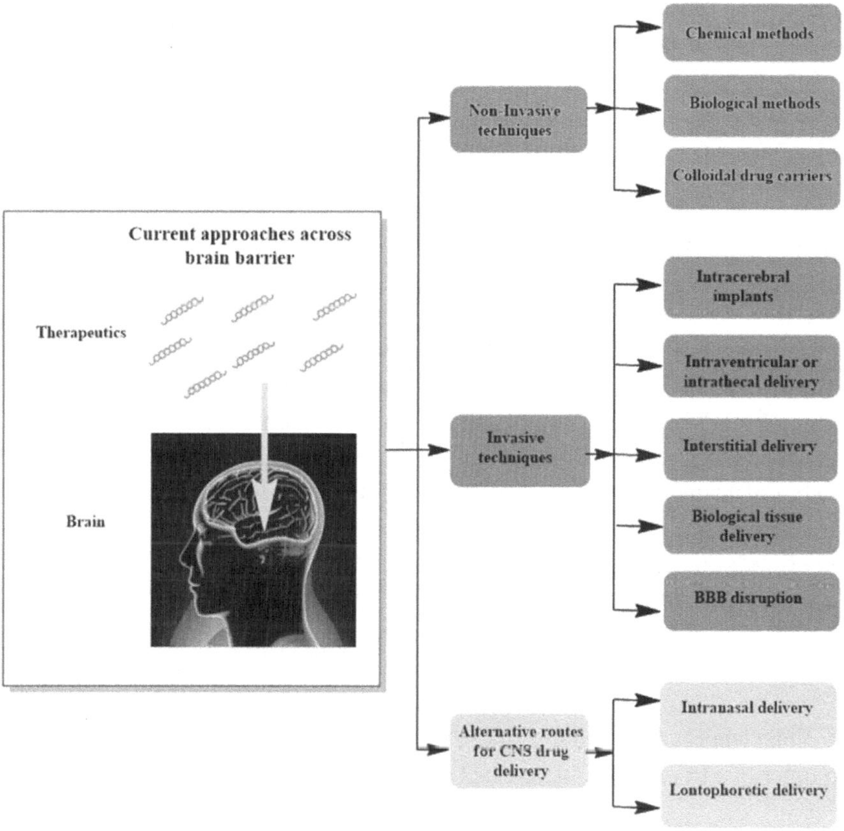

FIGURE 1.2 Current methods for delivering drugs to the brain.

1.8.2 INTRACEREBRAL DELIVER

Direct injections or implants into the defined area are introduced utilizing stereotactic coordinates, and/or continuous intraventricular infusion of the drug into the brain tissue, to create a more concentrated and effective pharmaceutical release to select regions of the brain. Clinical trials using this approach for PD were successful. Chemicals in the brain travel slowly because of the closely organized cells in the grey and white matter microenvironments. As a result, a higher dosage is required to reach the correct drug concentration.

The intended implanted devices are based on polymeric matrixes with pharmaceuticals encapsulated inside that are biodegradable and biocompatible. At the intended delivery site, where the reservoir is to be placed, the skull is opened. The drug's physicochemical behavior has a significant impact on how well it penetrates the body, and in most cases, only a small amount of the molecule is given. For instance, better outcomes were seen when a brain implant containing nerve growth factor was used to treat paraplegic individuals.[95]

1.8.3 BBB DISRUPTION

The observation that systemically injected dyes are barred from the growing mammalian brain led Lina Stern, a professor and the director of the Department of Physiological Chemistry at the University of Geneva, to coin the name "blood–brain barrier" (BBB). The BBB membrane is biochemically disturbed to increase the positive effects of drugs and their directed release to the brain. Therefore, this method needs to deliver the medication compounds directly to the CNS with the use of energy or certain molecules. The main benefit of this strategy is that it can target a specific part of the brain. Two methods are used to preproof the phenomenon of BBB disruption; To increase the release of chemotherapeutic medications to brain tumors, several chemical compounds with higher osmotic pressure, such as mannitol hyperosmotic solution, are frequently used. Endothelial cells are impacted by this, whereas ultrasound and electromagnetic radiation cause the tight connections to extend and contract.[96]

1.8.4 NONINVASIVE

The wide drug distribution throughout the brain blood vascular network is made possible by a number of noninvasive brain drug delivery techniques. Using this method, which increases BBTB permeability, drugs can pass through the BBTB more easily. Occluding, claudins and junctional adhesion molecules are the main proteins in tight junctions (TJs) in the BBB (JAMs). The production of these TJ proteins might be reduced using microbubbles and ultrasonic irradiation, which momentarily opens the BBB without having a negative impact on healthy brain tissue. The expression of these TJ proteins can be decreased using ultrasound irradiation and microbubbles, which momentarily open the BBB without having a negative impact on healthy brain tissue. These techniques, which include prodrugs, receptor-mediated drug delivery, carrier-mediated drug delivery, chemical drug delivery, and lipophilic analogs, typically rely on drug modifications. However, noninvasive systemic medicine delivery to the brain has proven challenging, which has sped up the development of novel drug-targeting strategies.[97]

1.8.5 CHEMISTRY-BASED APPROACH

The right chemicals are considered in this method while distributing medication material via BBB. The drug can be lapidated in two distinct ways using this technique. First, by conjugating the drug's water-soluble molecules with molecules that are lipid soluble, the polar functional groups on those molecules can be obscured. Second, a medicine that is water soluble can be conjugated with a drug carrier that is lipid soluble. Despite the fact that a number of delivery techniques for neurotherapeutics have been created, these strategies have been the focus of intensive study over the past 20 years. Examples include chimeric peptides and cationic proteins.

1.8.6 BIOTECHNOLOGY-BASED APPROACH

The field of biotechnology has garnered a lot of interest from scientists in a variety of different disciplines. This method, which is frequently used in recombinant DNA and polymerase chain reaction protein engineering, entails implanting embryonic neural grafts into the dysfunctional area of the brain. The delivery of medications to brain tumors and neuropharmaceuticals to the brain is made possible through biotechnology. This approach can also be used to successfully treat PD. These grafts do not, however, last for a longer time without becoming neovascular in

1.8.7 INTRANASAL DELIVERY

For systemic pharmacological action, the intranasal route has been used to deliver drugs directly into the bloodstream through the nasal mucosa. This uses a modest dose, is self-administered, and avoids sterile ways to consume the trigeminal nerves that connect the nasal mucosa and trigeminal nerves to the brain. This allows for quick absorption and beginning of the action, the lack of hepatic, uncomplicated administration, and other advantages by avoiding gastrointestinal degradation and protein binding in the emulation. In turn, this enhances medication absorption and lessens systemic side effects. Intranasal administration can be used to administer cytokines, neurotrophins, neuropeptides, genes, and chemotherapeutics, to name a few. The main drawbacks of this approach include the mucosal enzymes that degrade drugs, the lack of professional administration, the little time spent in the nasal cavity, and the restrictions imposed by nasal anatomy.[98,99]

1.9 FORMULATIONS FOR NEURODEGENERATIVE DISEASES

By controlling a material's size and shape in the nanoscale range, nanotechnology allows for the design, characterization, formulation, and applications of materials (1–100 nm). Nanosystems range in size from micro- to nanometers and are manufactured utilizing top–down lithographic and nonlithographic fabrication techniques. Over time, nanotechnology has developed in several ways. Nanomedicine is used to treat and prevent a variety of illnesses. Due to their large surface-to-volume ratio, nanoparticles exhibit a variety of optical, magnetic, and physiological features inside the human body. The two types of nanoparticles are inorganic (such as gold nanoparticles) and organic (such as liposomes). Polymeric nanoparticles can shield a medicine from degradation because they are constructed of biocompatible and biodegradable polymers.

Liposomes are nanocarriers made up of an aqueous core and phospholipid bilayer. Both hydrophilic and hydrophobic medicinal substances can be encapsulated by them. Small unilamellar vesicles (SUVs), large unilamellar vesicles (LUVs), or multilamellar vesicles (MLVs) are the three types that can exist. Liposomes are, biocompatible have little toxicity, and degrade naturally. They may also prevent the medicine from degrading, increasing the drug's bioavailability. They are capable of crossing the BBB through transcytosis or active transport by binding to a particular receptor. The intranasal pathway, which can access the brain via the olfactory and trigeminal nerves, is another way to get over the BBB. The intranasal distribution of liposomes has various benefits, including quick transport to the brain, avoiding systemic side effects, and passing first-pass metabolism.[100,101]

1.10 ROLE OF AYURVEDA IN NEURODEGENERATIVE DISEASES

The history of using herbal remedies dates back to the dawn of written history. There is proof that almost all ancient civilizations, including Indian, Egyptian, Chinese, Greek, and Roman, used plants to heal ailments and revive biological systems.

According to Ayurvedic medicine, the majority of NDDs are brought on by severe Vata (the humor of space and air) imbalance in the body and mind, particularly in the brain and one of the seven tissues of the body known as majja, or marrow, which is one of the seven tissues. The ways and intensities in which imbalance may happen are numerous. Depending on how it presents, each NDD varies from one another and from person to person.[102]

Ayurveda has found several plants with medicinal benefits for treating neurological illnesses and antioxidant characteristics. The four important Ayurvedic medicinal plants *Bacopa monnieri* (Brahmi), *Withania somnifera* (ashwagandha), *Centella asiatica* (gotu kola), and *Mucuna pruriens* (velvet bean) are explored in length in this chapter along with their role in neurological ailments.[103]

Hippocampal CA3 neurons were found to benefit from the dendritic development-promoting effects of fresh *C. asiatica* leaf extracts. The active ingredients of *C. asiatica*, asiatic acid, asiaticoside, and SM2, displayed neuroprotective effects and reduced amyloid and free radical-induced cell death in B103 cell cultures and hippocampus slices.[104]

Ayurveda has emerged as the most successful treatment for PD when compared to contemporary medical research. For a long-lasting solution, this comprehensive therapeutic approach addresses both the internal elements of the body and the internal causes of disease. A potential treatment strategy for PD prevention is to stop -synuclein from aggregating. In research by Ruben et al., amyloid-(A) levels in the brain and A aggregation were investigated in an aqueous leaf extract of *C. asiatica* (2014). This in vitro study showed that *C. asiatica* extract can cure PD by inhibiting the formation of oligomers to aggregates and -synuclein aggregation. Parkinson's disease Ayurvedic treatment stimulates brain function.

Parkinson's disease treatment in Ayurveda mainly aims to strengthen the nervous system and rejuvenate tissues of the brain. Ayurvedic home remedies work well in this problem as it has a personalized and natural treatment approach. If you choose the best Ayurvedic treatment for PD, you can better control your movement and do your routine tasks smoothly.[105,106]

1.11 ALTERNATIVE TRIAL DESIGNS FOR NDDS

All efforts to date have been fruitless in finding disease-modifying medicines. All the drugs that showed promise in preclinical animals did not produce the same results in people. It must be mentioned that the failure rate when producing symptomatic medications is also very high, which serves to emphasize the difficulty of doing research in this area even more. Another unsolved issue is how to distinguish between symptomatic and disease-modifying effects. Two recommendations for the development of medications for PD and AD were released by the European Medicine Agency (EMA) in 2008; these guidelines give regulatory indications to differentiate between effects on symptoms and effects on disease progression.

Drug therapy is said to have a disease-modifying impact when it slows the progression of underlying pathological or pathophysiological disease processes and is followed by an improvement in clinical signs and symptoms. As a result, a true disease-modifying effect cannot be proved with absolute certainty using only clinical outcome data; it also requires strong supporting data from a biomarker program. For the assertion of a symptomatic effect, the proof of clinical improvement alone will be adequate. Although these suggestions appear fair, it is unlikely that the complete claim of disease modulator will be realized soon based on these criteria given there are yet no verified biomarkers.[107]

There isn't a universal trial design that is expressly advised for any particular study type. The typical placebo-controlled single-period studies have significant limitations in separating the effects of study medication due to symptom relief from true effects on disease progression. In these trials, patients are randomly assigned to receive one or more doses of the active medicine or a placebo, and differences in various functional scores between the groups' baseline and last visit are compared. As a result, alternative designs have been posted. Delayed start and rerandomize withdrawal designs are two examples of so-called two-period designs, in which some or all patients change treatments over the course of the study.

Drug development for NDDs is a time-consuming, difficult, and costly process. It is necessary to find ways to improve drug development for NDDs. Basket trials are frequently employed in cancer, and the Food and Medication Administration has advocated them as a way to improve the effectiveness of drug development. It is difficult to determine if a difference between groups at the conclusion of the first period is due to impacts on symptoms, disease-modifying effects, or both since one group is receiving active medication while the control is receiving a placebo. Both groups receive the therapy during the second session. If at the conclusion of this time span there are still disparities between the two groups, it may be possible to infer a disease-modifying effect.

Similar to this, in a random randomized drawl design, individuals are randomly assigned to either an active therapy followed by a placo (A/P) or a placebo followed by a placo (P/P). Differences in period 1 should indicate the overall treatment effect, and period 2 should estimate the components that affect symptoms and the course of the disease. The so-called ADAGIO research is an example of a two-period design from recent times. The study's goal was to determine whether rasagiline, an inhibitor of monoamine oxidase type B (MAO-B), had a disease-modifying effect on PD motor impairment throughout an 18-month observation period. Three hierarchical endpoints are required to be reached as a result of the application of a delayed start design.[108]

The three primary objectives were met, and the study drug was declared to have a potential disease-modifying effect at the dose of 1 mg (but not 2 mg). At the end of the observation period, a major motor characteristic on the outcome scale [total unified Parkinson's disease rating scale (UPDRS) score] showed only a change of 1.68 points over a baseline total score of 20.6; this difference reflects an improvement of just 8% with the research treatment. Perhaps a more noticeable difference would have been anticipated in the presence of a disease-modifying therapy after an 18-month timeframe. Despite the trial's positive conclusion (in terms of statistical significance), more research is still required to determine its clinical benefit. The PROUD research, which examined the DA–agonist medication pramipexole as a potential disease modulator in PD, did not produce encouraging findings. Only 2.7% of active clinical studies include results based on technology.[109,110]

1.12 CLINICAL TRIAL ON NEURODEGENERATIVE DISORDERS

We are open to and supportive of initiatives to further advance the methods used to evaluate medications to treat various NDDs, even though our earlier experiences in trials for some NDDs have resulted in helpful, standard trial endpoints and study designs. It may be possible to hasten the development of treatments for neurodegenerative illnesses by using creative clinical trial designs. Drug developers are investigating and putting in practice cutting-edge approaches to clinical trial design, such as platform and adaptive designs, to maximize the statistical power of studies and reduce study length, participant risk, and the overall number of participants needed for trial conduct—often with the help of the U.S. Food and Drug Administration (FDA) guidance. Additionally, they continue to look for novel ways to collect and include patient-reported outcomes in studies, as well as to manage and make use of shared data.[110]

Drug companies are also taking steps to increase access to clinical trials for all types of patients and volunteers, including those who are members of racial and ethnic minorities and those who reside in remote areas. Decentralized trials—designs that effectively bring the trial to the participant—are one of these strategies to boost access and enrolment for people who do not live close to a research facility or for those who are traveling to an investigational site might be highly taxing; people with reduced mobility can travel; thanks to remote monitoring and digital tools; the creation of trial randomization plans that will enable more individuals to receive an experimental therapy during the study; and open-label extension studies to give people randomly assigned to a placebo comparator in the placebo-controlled phase of a clinical trial quick access to the trial medicine. We are completely aware of the worries that participants in clinical trials express to us regarding the use of placebo-controlled studies, and we share their annoyance with such approaches. However, the history of new pharmaceuticals reveals that for every effective treatment, roughly 40 treatments—many of which were hailed as extremely promising—failed. Even if we passionately seek a curative cure, we would nevertheless choose a procedure that offers a significant incremental benefit. Without a comparison, a medicine with a large effect size may be evaluated adequately, but only a controlled study will be able to find a smaller but still significant benefit and can be used to compare a candidate to a placebo. It is also crucial to remember that patients in these studies get standard-of-care therapy in addition to the experimental medication or a placebo (where it is offered). Even though we are aware that such trial designs are necessary, we collaborate with sponsors to reduce the use of placebo by using unequal randomization (more participants receive the study drug), as well as by keeping the length of the placebo-controlled period as short as is necessary to evaluate the drug's response. Additionally, after completing the placebo-controlled phase, participants are given the option to enroll in open-label treatment phases with the study medicine The FDA and researchers are collaborating to support and promote these developments.[111,112]

Basket studies are a particular type of master protocol developed to evaluate a single investigational drug or treatment combination in diverse populations based on disease stage, histology, number of prior therapies, genetic or other biomarkers, or demographic factors, according to the FDA. Although originally developed for the study of cancer therapy, basket trials can also be used to test drugs for other diseases, such as NDDs. According to FDA regulations, each subpopulation in a basket trial comprises of a sub-study Each disease-defined sub-study should have specific goals, a rationale supporting the inclusion of each population, and a complete statistical analysis plan that includes explanations for sample size and stopping criteria for futility. The adoption of master protocols, such as basket trials, is encouraged by the FDA. They point out that these protocols are adaptable and can include methods that focus on efficiency, like a shared placebo control arm and centralized data collection. Basket studies, which allow patients with a variety of NDD types to be treated in clinics to be referred, can hasten the recruitment of participants in trials. By using basket trials instead of individual trials for each NDD, costs and logistical difficulties are avoided. The usage of basket trials in cancer medication development programs has significantly increased, with phase 1b/2 being their main application. NDD basket trials have been used in all stages of development, with phase 2 accounting for 46% of all NDD basket trials.[114,115]

Characteristics of basket trials for symptomatic agents in NDDs are listed in Table 1.1.

TABLE 1.1 Basket Trials of Drugs on Various Neurodegenerative Diseases.[116–118]

Neurodegenerative disorders	Drug	Objective of treatment	Number of basket trials
Huntington's disease, AD	Alprazolam	Decreased anxiety	1
Corticobasal degeneration, progressive supranuclear palsy	Apomorphine	Reduces Pain	1
PD, multiple system atrophy	Ampreloxetine	Orthostatic hypotension management	1
Dementia with Lewy bodies, AD, progressive supranuclear palsy, Huntington's disease	Avp-786	Decrease in disinhibition	1
PD, dementia with Lewy bodies	Armodafinil	Enhanced cognition and enhanced attention	1
Huntington's disease, dementia with Lewy bodies, PD	Ramelteon	Better sleep efficiency	1
Multiple system atrophy, PD	Carbidopa	Motor performance is enhanced	1
PD, multiple system atrophy, progressive supranuclear palsy	Droxidopa	Symptoms, both motor and nonmotor, are better, and blood pressure is higher	7
AD, PD, dementia with Lewy bodies	Pimavanserin	Reduction of hallucinations and delusions in dementia-related psychosis	2
Multiple system atrophy, PD	Entacapone	Enhanced motor performance	1

1.12.1 ROLE OF STATINS IN NEURODEGENERATIVE DISORDER

Statins, which have already been authorized as anti-hyperlipidemic pharmaceuticals, are the main topic of research into repurposed drugs. Statins have been demonstrated to have neuroprotective effects in a variety of brain diseases because they are anti-inflammatory and antioxidant. Furthermore, they lessen protein aggregation and amyloid plaques, which are, respectively, the origins of AD and PD. As neuroprotective medications, they promote remyelination and assist in lowering the psychomotor symptoms of Huntington's disease and multiple sclerosis.

The reductase enzyme that is crucial for the conversion of 3-hydroxy-3-methylglutaryl-coenzyme A (HMG CoA) to mevalonate—a crucial step in the cholesterol production pathway—controls the quantity of cholesterol in the body and the emergence of cardiac issues. Drugs that target the HMG CoA reductase specifically would prevent the creation of cholesterol.

The HMG CoA reductase enzyme is competitively and irreversibly inhibited by statins, which lowers serum cholesterol levels and stimulates the expression of the gene that regulates low-density lipoprotein (LDL) receptors. Hepatocytes' enhanced LDL receptors absorb free LDL and its precursors (such as IDLP and VLDLP). Statins also prevent the synthesis of Apolipoprotein B-100 and significantly lessen the creation of triglyceride-rich lipoproteins. They essentially do this by raising the serum level of HDL while decreasing levels of LDL and triglycerides. To treat hypercholesterolemia, dyslipidemia, hyperlipidemia, etc., they are therefore recommended widely. They can be obtained as fungi-derived compounds or generated synthetically (such as atorvastatin, fluvastatin, pitavastatin, and rosuvastatin) (such as lovastatin, and pravastatin simvastatin). All the clinical trials were data obtained from Clinicaltrials.gov.it. In this study record, we have obtained number of clinical trials of different statin drugs that are completed, active, and recruiting.[119,120]

1.13 CONCLUSION

Millions of individuals worldwide are affected by NDDs. The two most prevalent neurodegenerative illnesses are AD and PD. The main features of NDs, include AD and Parkinson's neuronal death. Thus, neurogenesis is the most frequently expected therapeutic approach for these conditions. Research has identified several core functions by which neurodegeneration occurs, including the formation of insoluble protein deposition, necrosis,

TABLE 1.2 Overall Status of Statin Group of 'Drug's Clinical Trials.[121–123]

Trial no	Drug	Status of the trial	Details of the research study	Result
NCT00486044	Simvastatin	Completed	Analyzing simvastatin's possible place in medical treatment	1. Changes in beta-amyloid-42, CSF, and regional cerebral blood flow on MRI were seen 2. Less inflammatory indicators are present 3. The cognitive Performance has changed
NCT00053599	Simvastatin	Completed	Cholesterol-lowering drugs' role in AD progression	No study findings are published
NCT01142336	Simvastatin	Completed	Analyzing how simvastatin affects biomarkers.	1. CSF change from baseline in Aβ42 was identified at 1 year 2. A 1-year change from baseline was found in CSF total tau and CSF ptau181
NCT00939822	Simvastatin	Completed	Statins' effects on β-amyloid and cerebral blood flow are being studied in relation to AD.	1. A compound called β-amyloid-42 has been identified in the CSF and the plaques in the brains of AD patients. 2. Compared to β-amyloid forms, β-amyloid-42 has stronger effects on the cerebrovascular system of AD patients
NCT02787590	Simvastatin	Active	Simvastatin research for the neuroprotective treatment of mild PD	There was a change in the MDS-UPDRS (information on the patient's state of mind and mood)
NCT00647348	Simvastatin	Recruiting	Simvastatin in secondary multiple sclerosis: Investigation	1. Whole brain volume percentage change was noted 2. Better condition advancement and less disability were noted
NCT00492765	Simvastatin	Completed	In addition to Interferon-1a, Simvastatin is used to treat relapsing-remitting multiple sclerosis	No study findings are published

TABLE 1.2 *(Continued)*

Trial no	Drug	Status of the trial	Details of the research study	Result
NCT03896217	Simvastatin	Recruiting	Simvastatin research for treating secondary multiple sclerosis	Using the MRI technology, the effect on cerebral blood flow and glutamate level was seen
NCT03242499	Lovastatin	Recruiting	Early Stage PD: Lovastatin-based neuroprotective therapy	There was a change in the MDS-UPDRS (information on the patient's state of mind and mood)
NCT00046358	Lovastatin	Completed	Short-term statin and NSAID effects on A-level in AD are evaluated	No study findings have been published
NCT00151502	Atorvastatin	Completed	A cholinesterase inhibitor combined with atorvastatin was studied for safety and effectiveness in AD patients	No study findings have been published
NCT00024531	Atorvastatin	Competed	Using Lipitor to treat AD	No study findings have been published
NCT00751907	Atorvastatin	Competed	pilot investigation on cerebral and peripheral perfusion (CAPP).	Alter in regional cerebral flow and endothelial function was seen
NCT03411291	Atorvastatin	Competed	A preliminary investigation on the effects of statins on cerebral blood flow and neural activity	Changes in the brain's metabolite concentration and rate of perfusion were noticed
NCT00303277	Pravastatin	Competed	Inhibitors of HMG CoA reductase: Do they affect A levels?	Alteration in the levels of CSF-beta and other biomarkers were observed
NCT00200655	Pravastatin	Competed	Pravastatin's effectiveness and safety in relapsing-remitting disease are evaluated	Gadolinium-positive lesions numbers changed significantly (at 6 months in each group) as was evident

excitotoxicity, apoptosis, and neuroinflammation, despite the fact that there are several causes of neurodegenerative illnesses. The majority of the present generation of therapeutic targets are based on known disease gene products and the enzymes that regulate their metabolism. Targeting proteins for neurogenerative diseases are Amyloid-β (Aβ), tau, α-synuclein, TDP-43, SOD1, FUS, Ataxin-1, ataxin-2 ataxin-3, and ataxin-7. Drug transport to the brain is still difficult, nevertheless, because of many important parameters such as the drug's molecular weight, BBB, and lipophilicity. Due to these considerations, treating NDs is more difficult and limits the therapeutic effectiveness of medications. Thus, targeted medication delivery to the brain using nanoparticles has been investigated in recent years for neurogenesis, and it offers a viable framework for enhancing therapeutic approaches. The amazing progress in our understanding of the processes behind NDDs is heralding a new era in which neurologists would be pioneers of regenerative therapy rather than chroniclers of decline.

KEYWORDS

- **neurodegenerative diseases**
- **biomarker**
- **clinical trial**
- **MRI**
- **drug delivery**
- **statin**

REFERENCES

1. Kovacs, G. G. Concepts and Classification of Neurodegenerative Diseases. In *Handbook of Clinical Neurology*; Elsevier, 2018, Vol. 145; pp 301–307.
2. Checkoway, H.; Lundin, J. I.; Kelada, S. N. Neurodegenerative Diseases. *IARC Sci. Publ.* **2011,** *163* 407–419.
3. Amor, S.; Puentes, F.; Baker, D.; Valk, P. V. D. Inflammation in Neurodegenerative Diseases. *Immunology* **2010,** *129* (2), 154–169.
4. Voet, S.; Srinivasan, S.; Lamkanfi, M.; Van Loo, G. Inflammasomes in Neuroinflammatory and Neurodegenerative Diseases. *EMBO Mol. Med.* **2019,** *11* (6), E10248.
5. Gao, H.-M.; Hong, J.-S. Why Neurodegenerative Diseases are Progressive: Uncontrolled Inflammation Drives Disease Progression. *Trends Immunol.* **2008,** *29* (8), 357–365.

6. Kovacs, G. G. Concepts and Classification of Neurodegenerative Diseases. In *Handbook of Clinical Neurology*; Elsevier, 2018; Vol. 145, pp 301–307.
7. Kovacs, G. G.; Lee, V. M.; Trojanowski, J. Q. Protein Astrogliopathies in Human Neurodegenerative Diseases and Aging. *Brain Pathol.* **2017,** *27* (5), 675–690.
8. Collinge, J. Mammalian Prions and Their Wider Relevance in Neurodegenerative Diseases. *Nature* **2016,** *539* (7628), 217–226.
9. Suter, U.; Scherer, S. S. Disease Mechanisms in Inherited Neuropathies. *Nat. Rev. Neurosci.* **2003,** *4* (9), 714–726.
10. Klein, C.; Schlossmacher, M. G. The Genetics of Parkinson Disease: Implications for Neurological Care. *Nat. Clin. Pract. Neurol.* **2006,** *2* (3), 136–146.
11. Neary, D.; Snowden, J. Frontal Lobe Dementia, Motor Neuron Disease, and Clinical and Neuropathological Criteria. *J. Neurol. Neurosurg. Psychiatry* **2013,** *84* (7), 713–714.
12. Ibrahim, J. E. Long-Term Care Homes as Hot Spots in Australia. In *Outsmarting the Next Pandemic: What Covid-19 Can Teach Us*; 2021.
13. Barchet, T. M.; Amiji, M. M. Challenges and Opportunities in CNS Delivery of Therapeutics for Neurodegenerative Diseases. *Expert Opin. Drug Deliv.* **2009,** *6* (3), 211–225.
14. Vegeto, E.; Villa, A.; Torre, S. D.; Crippa, V.; Rusmini, P.; Cristofani, R.; Galbiati, M.; Maggi, A.; Poletti, A. The Role of Sex and Sex Hormones in Neurodegenerative Diseases. *Endocr. Rev.* **2020,** *41* (2), 273–319.
15. Burghaus, L.; Eggers, C.; Timmermann, L.; Fink, G. R.; Diederich, N. J. Hallucinations in Neurodegenerative Diseases. *CNS Neurosci. Ther.* **2012,** *18* (2), 149–159.
16. Terwel, D.; Dewachter, I.; Van Leuven, F. Axonal Transport, Tau Protein, and Neurodegeneration in Alzheimer's Disease. *Neuromol. Med.* **2002,** *2* (2), 151–165.
17. Spires-Jones, T. L.; Attems, J.; Thal, D. R. Interactions of Pathological Proteins in Neurodegenerative Diseases. *Acta Neuropathol.* **2017,** *134* (2), 187–205.
18. Zeng, W.; Wang, C. Classification of Neurodegenerative Diseases using Gait Dynamics via Deterministic Learning. *Inform. Sci.* **2015,** *317,* 246–258.
19. Yankner, B. A. Mechanisms of Neuronal Degeneration in Alzheimer's Disease. *Neuron* **1996,** *16* (5), 921–932.
20. Lanoiselée, H.-M.; Nicolas, G.; Wallon, D.; Rovelet-Lecrux, A.; Lacour, M.; Rousseau, S.; Richard, A.-C.; et al. APP, PSEN1, and PSEN2 Mutations in Early-Onset Alzheimer Disease: A Genetic Screening Study of Familial and Sporadic Cases. *PLoS Med.* **2017,** *14* (3), E1002270.
21. Reddy, P. H.; Manczak, M.; Mao, P.; Calkins, M. J.; Reddy, A. P.; Shirendeb, U. Amyloid-B and Mitochondria in Aging and Alzheimer's Disease: Implications for Synaptic Damage and Cognitive Decline. *J. Alzheimers Dis.* **2010,** *20* (S2), S499–S512.
22. Goedert, M. Neurofibrillary Pathology of Alzheimer's Disease and other Tauopathies. *Prog. Brain Res.* **1998,** *117,* 287–306.
23. Dunckley, T.; Beach, T. G.; Ramsey, K. E.; Grover, A.; Mastroeni, D.; Walker, D. G.; Lafleur, B. J.; et al. Gene Expression Correlates of Neurofibrillary Tangles in Alzheimer's Disease. *Neurobiol. Aging* **2006,** *27* (10), 1359–1371.
24. Kovacech, B.; Novak, M. Tau Truncation is a Productive Posttranslational Modification of Neurofibrillary Degeneration in Alzheimer's Disease. *Curr. Alzheimer Res.* **2010,** *7* (8), 708–716.
25. Burke, R. E.; O'Malley, K. Axon Degeneration in Parkinson's Disease. *Exp. Neurol.* **2013,** *246* 72–83.

26. Nuber, S.; Rajsombath, M.; Minakaki, G.; Winkler, J.; Müller, C. P.; Ericsson, M.; Caldarone, B.; Dettmer, U.; Selkoe, D. J. Abrogating Native A-Synuclein Tetramers in Mice Causes A L-DOPA-Responsive Motor Syndrome Closely Resembling Parkinson's Disease. *Neuron* **2018,** *100* (1), 75–90.
27. Beitz, J. M. Parkinson's Disease: A Review. *Front. Biosci. (Schol Ed)* **2014,** *6* (1), 65–74.
28. Shukla, V.; Mishra, S. K.; Pant, H. C. Oxidative Stress in Neurodegeneration. *Adv. Pharmacol. Sci.* **2011** (2011).
29. Brooks, D. J. Optimizing Levodopa Therapy for Parkinson's Disease with Levodopa/Carbidopa/Entacapone: Implications from a Clinical and Patient Perspective. *Neuropsychiatr. Dis. Treat.* **2008,** *4* (1), 39.
30. Hong, C. T.; Chan, L.; Bai, C.-H. The Effect of Caffeine on the Risk and Progression of Parkinson's Disease: A Meta-Analysis. *Nutrients* **2020,** *12* (6), 1860.
31. Vermeiren, Y.; Janssens, J.; Aerts, T.; Martin, J.-J.; Sieben, A.; Van Dam, D.; De Deyn, P. P. Brain Serotonergic and Noradrenergic Deficiencies in Behavioral Variant Frontotemporal Dementia Compared to Early-Onset Alzheimer's Disease. *J. Alzheimers Dis.* **2016,** *53* (3), 1079–1096.
32. Tsai, R. M.; Boxer, A. L. Therapy and Clinical Trials in Frontotemporal Dementia: Past, Present, and Future. *J. Neurochem.* 138 211–221.
33. Laakso, M. P.; Frisoni, G. B.; Könönen, M.; Mikkonen, M.; Beltramello, A.; Geroldi, C.; Bianchetti, A.; Trabucchi, M.; Soininen, H.; Aronen, H. J. Hippocampus and Entorhinal Cortex in Frontotemporal Dementia and Alzheimer's Disease: A Morphometric MRI Study. *Biol. Psychiatry* **2016,** *47* (12), (2000): 1056–1063.
34. Reilly, J.; Peelle, J. E. Effects of Semantic Impairment on Language Processing in Semantic Dementia. In *Seminars in Speech and Language*; © Thieme Medical Publishers, 2008; Vol. *29* (01), pp 32–43.
35. Rabins, P. V.; Rovner, B. W.; Rummans, T.; Schneider, L. S.; Tariot, P. N. Guideline Watch (October 2014): Practice Guideline for the Treatment of Patients With Alzheimer's Disease and other Dementias. *Focus* **2017,** *15* (1), 110–128.
36. Westergard, L.; Christensen, H. M.; Harris, D. A. The Cellular Prion Protein (PrPC): Its Physiological Function and Role in Disease. *Biochim. Biophys. Acta* **2007,** *1772* (6), 629–644.
37. Harris, D. A. Cellular Biology of Prion Diseases. *Clin. Microbiol. Rev.* **1999,** *12* (3), 429–444.
38. Spinner, D. S.; Cho, In, S, Park, S. Y.; Kim, J. I.; Meeker, H. C.; Ye, X.; Lafauci, G.; et al. Accelerated Prion Disease Pathogenesis in Toll-Like Receptor 4 Signaling-Mutant Mice. *J. Virol.* **2008,** *82* (21), 10701–10708.
39. Glatzel, M.; Stoeck, K.; Seeger, H.; Lührs, T.; Aguzzi, A. Human Prion Diseases: Molecular and Clinical Aspects. *Arch. Neurol.* **2005,** *62* (4), 545–552.
40. Collinge, J. Prion Diseases of Humans and Animals: Their Causes and Molecular Basis. *Annu. Rev. Neurosci.* **2001,** *24* (1), 519–550.
41. Mccolgan, P.; Tabrizi, S. J. Huntington's Disease: A Clinical Review. *Eur. J. Neurol.* **2018,** *25* (1), 24–34.
42. Chiang, M.-C.; Chen, C.-M.; Lee, M.-R.; Chen, H.-W.; Chen, H.-M.; Wu, Yu-S, Hung, C.-H.; et al. Modulation of Energy Deficiency in Huntington's Disease via Activation of the Peroxisome Proliferator-Activated Receptor Gamma. *Hum. Mol. Genet.* **2010,** *19* (20), 4043–4058.
43. Ghosh, R.; Tabrizi, S. J. Clinical Features of Huntington's Disease. *Adv. Exp. Med. Biol.* **2018,** *1049,* 1–28.

44. Ghosh, R.; Tabrizi, S. J. Clinical Aspects of Huntington's Disease. In *Behavioral Neurobiology of Huntington's Disease and Parkinson's Disease*; 2013, pp 3–31.
45. Mulligan, V. K.; Chakrabartty, A. Protein Misfolding in the Late-Onset Neurodegenerative Diseases: Common Themes and the Unique Case of Amyotrophic Lateral Sclerosis. *Proteins Struct. Funct. Bioinf.* **2013,** *81* (8), 1285–1303.
46. Vucic, S.; Rothstein, J. D.; Kiernan, M. C. Advances in Treating Amyotrophic Lateral Sclerosis: Insights from Pathophysiological Studies. *Trends Neurosci.* **2014,** *37* (8), 433–442.
47. Wang, W.; Zhang, F.; Li, L.; Tang, F.; Siedlak, S. L.; Fujioka, H.; et al. MFN2 Couples Glutamate Excitotoxicity and Mitochondrial Dysfunction in Motor Neurons. *J. Biol. Chem.* **2015,** *290,* 168–182.
48. Chia, R.; Chiò, A.; Traynor, B. J. Novel Genes Associated with Amyotrophic Lateral Sclerosis: Diagnostic and Clinical Implications. *Lancet Neurol.* **2018,** *17* (1), 94–102.
49. Fernandez-Santiago, R.; Sharma, M.; Mueller, J. C.; Gohlke, H.; Illig, T.; Anneser, J.; Münch, C.; Ludolph, A.; Kamm, C.; Gasser, T. Possible Gender-Dependent Association of Vascular Endothelial Growth Factor (VEGF) Gene and ALS. *Neurology* **2006,** *66* (12), 1929–1931.
50. Jawaid, A.; Murthy, S. B.; Wilson, A. M.; Qureshi, S. U.; Amro, M. J.; Wheaton, M.; Simpson, E.; et al. A Decrease in Body Mass Index is Associated with Faster Progression of Motor Symptoms and Shorter Survival in ALS. *Amyotroph. Lateral Scler.* **2010,** *11* (6), 542–548.
51. Hauser, R. A.; Olanow, C. W. Magnetic Resonance Imaging of Neurodegenerative Diseases. *J. Neuroimaging* **1994,** *4* (3), 146–158.
52. Iyer, P. M.; Doherty, C. P.; Bede, P. Imaging Biomarkers in Neurodegenerative Conditions. In *Neurodegenerative Disorders*; Springer: Cham, 2016; pp 13–27.
53. Jónsson, B. A.; Bjornsdottir, G.; Thorgeirsson, T. E.; Ellingsen, L. M.; Bragi Walters, G.; Gudbjartsson, D. F.; Stefansson, H.; Stefansson, K.; Ulfarsson, M. O. Brain Age Prediction Using Deep Learning Uncovers Associated Sequence Variants. *Nat. Commun.* **2019,** *10* (1), 1–10.
54. Beaulieu, C. The Basis of Anisotropic Water Diffusion in the Nervous System–A Technical Review. *NMR Biomed.* **2002,** *15* (7 and 8), 435–455.
55. Helms, G. Segmentation of Human Brain Using Structural MRI. *MAGMA* **2016,** *29* (2), 111–124.
56. Bertholdo, D.; Watcharakorn, A.; Castillo, M. Brain Proton Magnetic Resonance Spectroscopy: Introduction and Overview. *Neuroimaging Clin.* **2013,** *23* (3), 359–380.
57. Landman, B. A.; Farrell, J. A.D.; Jones, C. K.; Smith, S. A.; Prince, J. L.; Mori, S. Effects of Diffusion Weighting Schemes on the Reproducibility of DTI-Derived Fractional Anisotropy, Mean Diffusivity, and Principal Eigenvector Measurements at 1.5 T. *Neuroimage* **2007,** *36* (4), 1123–1138.
58. Lee, S.-P.; Silva, A. C.; Ugurbil, K.; Kim, S.-G. Diffusion-Weighted Spin-Echo fMRI at 9.4 T: Microvascular/Tissue Contribution to BOLD Signal Changes. *Magn. Reson. Med.* **1999,** *42* (5), 919–928.
59. Strangman, G.; Culver, J. P.; Thompson, J. H.; Boas, D. A. A Quantitative Comparison of Simultaneous BOLD fMRI and NIRS Recordings during Functional Brain Activation. *Neuroimage* **2002,** *17* (2), 719–731.
60. Di Costanzo, A.; Trojsi, F.; Tosetti, M.; Giannatempo, G. M.; Nemore, F.; Piccirillo, M.; Bonavita, S.; Tedeschi, G.; Scarabino, T. High-Field Proton MRS of Human Brain. *Eur. J. Radiol.* **2003,** *48* (2), 146–153.

61. Ross, B.; Bluml, S. Magnetic Resonance Spectroscopy of the Human Brain. *Anat. Rec.* **2001,** *265* (2), 54–84.
62. Rosen, Y.; Lenkinski, R. E. Recent Advances in Magnetic Resonance Neurospectroscopy. *Neurotherapeutics* **2007,** *4* (3), 330–345.
63. Gupta, M.; Lee, H. J.; Barden, C. J.; Weaver, D. F. The Blood–Brain Barrier (BBB) Score. *J. Med. Chem.* **2019,** *62* (21), 9824–9836.
64. Stolp, H. B.; Dziegielewska, K. M. Role of Developmental Inflammation and Blood–Brain Barrier Dysfunction in Neurodevelopmental and Neurodegenerative Diseases. *Neuropathol. Appl. Neurobiol.* **2009,** *35* (2), 132–146.
65. Kaindl, A. M.; Degos, V.; Peineau, S.; Gouadon, E.; Chhor, V.; Loron, G.; Le Charpentier, T.; et al. Activation of Microglial N-Methyl-D-Aspartate Receptors Triggers Inflammation and Neuronal Cell Death in the Developing and Mature Brain. *Ann. Neurol.* **2012,** *72* (4), 536–549.
66. Neurodegenerative Disorders may be Slowed or Prevented from Progressing with the Help of Medications that Modulate Unexplored Targets.
67. Premont, R. T.; Gainetdinov, R. R. Physiological Roles of G Protein-Coupled Receptor Kinases and Arrestins. *Annu. Rev. Physiol.* **2007,** *69* (1), 511–534.
68. Reilly, J.; Rodriguez, A. D.; Lamy, M.; Neils-Strunjas, J. Cognition, Language, and Clinical Pathological Features of Non-Alzheimer's Dementias: An Overview. *J. Commun. Disord.* **2010,** *43* (5), 438–452.
69. Sala-Llonch, R.; Pena-Gomez, C.; Arenaza-Urquijo, E. M.; Vidal-Piñeiro, D.; Bargallo, N.; Junque, C.; Bartres-Faz, D. Brain Connectivity During Resting State and Subsequent Working Memory Task Predicts Behavioural Performance. *Cortex* **2012,** *48* (9), 1187–1196.
70. Savai, R.; Pullamsetti, S. S.; Banat, G.-A.; Weissmann, N.; Ghofrani, H. A.; Grimminger, F.; Schermuly, R. T. Targeting Cancer with Phosphodiesterase Inhibitors. *Expert Opin Investig. Drugs* **2010,** *19* (1), 117–131.
71. Terasaki, W. L.; Appleman, M. M. The Role of Cyclic GMP in the Regulation of Cyclic AMP Hydrolysis. *Metabolism* **1975,** *24* (3), 311–319.
72. Vila, M.; Przedborski, S. Targeting Programmed Cell Death in Neurodegenerative Diseases. *Nat. Rev. Neurosci.* **2003,** *4* (5), 365–375.
73. Brandes, M. S.; Gray, N. E. NRF2 as a Therapeutic Target in Neurodegenerative Diseases. *ASN Neuro* **2020,** *12*, 1759091419899782.
74. Vidal, R. L.; Matus, S.; Bargsted, L.; Hetz, C. Targeting Autophagy in Neurodegenerative Diseases. *Trends Pharmacol. Sci.* **2014,** *35* (11), 583–591.
75. Kim, H.-R.; Lee, P.; Seo, S. W.; Roh, J. H.; Oh, M.; Oh, J. S.; Oh, S. J.; Kim, J. S.; Jeong, Y. Comparison of Amyloid β and tau Spread Models in Alzheimer's Disease. *Cereb. Cortex* **2019,** *29* (10), 4291–4302.
76. Toledo, J. B.; Cairns, N. J.; Da, X.; Chen, K.; Carter, D.; Fleisher, A.; Householder, E.; et al. Clinical and Multimodal Biomarker Correlates of ADNI Neuropathological Findings. *Acta Neuropathol. Commun.* **2013,** *1* (1), 1–13.
77. Uitti, R. J.; Calne, D. B.; Dickson, D. W.; Wszolek, Z. K. Is the Neuropathological 'Gold Standard' Diagnosis Dead? Implications of Clinicopathological Findings in an Autosomal Dominant Neurodegenerative Disorder. *Parkinsonism Relat. Disord.* **2004,** *10* (8), 461–463.
78. Steiner, H.; Capell, A.; Leimer, U.; Haass, C. Genes and Mechanisms Involved in the -Amyloid Generation and Alzheimer's Disease. *Eur. Arch. Psychiatr. Clin. Neurosci.* **1999,** *249* (6), 266–270.

79. Larner, A. J.; Doran, M. Clinical Phenotypic Heterogeneity of Alzheimer's Disease Associated with Mutations of the Presenilin–1 Gene. *J. Neurol.* **2006,** *253* (2), 139–158.
80. Ramassamy, C.; Averill, D.; Beffert, U.; Bastianetto, S.; Theroux, L.; Lussier-Cacan, S.; Cohn, J. S.; et al. Oxidative Damage and Protection by Antioxidants in the Frontal Cortex of Alzheimer's Disease is Related to the Apolipoprotein E Genotype. *Free Rad. Biol. Med.* **1999,** *27* (5 and 6), 544–553.
81. Hampel, H.; Goernitz, A.; Buerger, K. Advances in the Development of Biomarkers for Alzheimer's Disease: from CSF Total tau and Aβ1–42 Proteins to Phosphorylated Tau Protein. *Brain Res. Bull.* **2003,** *61* (3), 243–253.
82. Andreasen, N.; Minthon, L.; Davidsson, P.; Vanmechelen, E.; Vanderstichele, H.; Winblad, B.; Blennow, K. Evaluation of CSF-tau and CSF-Aβ42 As Diagnostic Markers for Alzheimer Disease in Clinical Practice. *Arch. Neurol.* **2001,** *58* (3), 373–379.
83. Andreasen, N.; Sjögren, M.; Blennow, K. CSF Markers for Alzheimer's Disease: Total Tau, Phospho-Tau and Aβ42. *World J. Biol. Psychiatry* **2003,** *4* (4), 147–155.
84. Farrer, M.; Maraganore, D. M.; Lockhart, P.; Singleton, A.; Lesnick, T. G.; De Andrade, M.; West, A.; De Silva, R.; Hardy, J.; Hernandez, D. alpha-Synuclein Gene Haplotypes are Associated with Parkinson's Disease. *Hum. Mol. Genet.* **2001,** *10* (17), 1847–1851.
85. Farrer, M.; Maraganore, D. M.; Lockhart, P.; Singleton, A.; Lesnick, T. G.; De Andrade, M.; West, A.; De Silva, R.; Hardy, J.; Hernandez, D. alpha-Synuclein Gene Haplotypes are Associated With Parkinson's Disease. Hum. Mol. Genet. **2001,** *10* (17), 1847–1851.
86. Setsuie, R.; Wada, K. The Functions of UCH-L1 and Its Relation to Neurodegenerative Diseases. *Neurochem. Int.* **2007,** *51* (2–4), 105–111.
87. Hernandez, D. G.; Reed, X.; Singleton, A. B. Genetics in Parkinson Disease: Mendelian Versus Non-Mendelian Inheritance. *J. Neurochem.* **2016,** *139,* 59–74.
88. Ariga, H.; Takahashi-Niki, K.; Kato, I.; Maita, H.; Niki, T.; Iguchi-Ariga, S. M. M. Neuroprotective Function of DJ-1 in Parkinson's Disease. *Oxid. Med. Cell. Long.* **2013** (2013).
89. Tolosa, E.; Coelho, M.; Gallardo, M. DAT Imaging in Drug-Induced and Psychogenic Parkinsonism. *Mov. Disord.* **2003,** *18* (S7), S28-S33.
90. Gibb, W. R. G.; Lees, A. J. The Significance of the Lewy Body in the Diagnosis of Idiopathic Parkinson's Disease. *Neuropathol. Appl. Neurobiol.* **1989,** *15* (1), 27–44.
91. Turner, M. R.; Grosskreutz, J.; Kassubek, J.; Abrahams, S.; Agosta, F.; Benatar, M.; Filippi, M.; et al. Towards a Neuroimaging Biomarker for Amyotrophic Lateral Sclerosis. *Lancet Neurol.* **2011,** *10* (5), 400–403.
92. Misra, A.; Ganesh, S.; Shahiwala, A.; Shah, S. P. Drug Delivery to the Central Nervous System: A Review. *J. Pharm. Pharm. Sci.* **2003,** *6* (2), 252–273.
93. Stolp, H. B.; Dziegielewska, K. M. Role of Developmental Inflammation and Blood–Brain Barrier Dysfunction in Neurodevelopmental and Neurodegenerative Diseases. *Neuropathol. Appl. Neurobiol.* **2009,** *35* (2), 132–146.
94. Kumar, A.; Zhou, L.; Zhi, K.; Raji, B.; Pernell, S.; Tadrous, E.; Kodidela, S.; Nookala, A.; Kochat, H.; Kumar, S. Challenges in Biomaterial-Based Drug Delivery Approach for the Treatment of Neurodegenerative Diseases: Opportunities for Extracellular Vesicles. *Int. J. Mol. Sci.* **2020,** *22* (1), 138.
95. Begley, D. J. Delivery of Therapeutic Agents to the Central Nervous System: The Problems and the Possibilities. *Pharmacol. Ther.* **2004,** *104* (1), 29–45.
96. Sanches, C.; Stengel, C.; Godard, J.; Mertz, J.; Teichmann, M.; Migliaccio, R.; Valero-Cabré, A. Past, Present, and Future of Non-Invasive Brain Stimulation Approaches to

Treat Cognitive Impairment in Neurodegenerative Diseases: Time for a Comprehensive Critical Review. *Front. Aging Neurosci.* **2021,** *12* (578339.

97. Luissint, A.-C.; Artus, C.; Glacial, F.; Ganeshamoorthy, K.; Couraud, P.-O. Tight Junctions at the Blood–Brain Barrier: Physiological Architecture and Disease-Associated Dysregulation. *Fluids Barriers CNS* **2012,** *9* (1), 1–12.
98. Farr, A. C.; Xiong, M. P. Challenges and Opportunities of Deferoxamine Delivery for Treatment of Alzheimer's Disease, Parkinson's Disease, and Intracerebral Hemorrhage. *Mol. Pharm.* **2020,** *18* (2), 593–609.
99. Navarro, G.; Morales, P.; Rodríguez-Cueto, C.; Fernández-Ruiz, J.; Jagerovic, N.; Franco, R. Targeting Cannabinoid CB2 Receptors in the Central Nervous System. Medicinal Chemistry Approaches with Focus on Neurodegenerative Disorders. *Front. Neurosci.* **2016,** *10*, 406.
100. Tomoshige, S.; Ishikawa, M. Protacs and other Chemical Protein Degradation Technologies for the Treatment of Neurodegenerative Disorders. *Angew. Chem. Int. Ed.* **2021,** *60* (7), 3346–3354.
101. Cacciatore, I.; Ciulla, M.; Fornasari, E.; Marinelli, L.; Di Stefano, A. Solid Lipid Nanoparticles as a Drug Delivery System for the Treatment of Neurodegenerative Diseases. *Expert Opin. Drug Deliv.* **2016,** *13* (8), 1121–1131.
102. Teixeira, M. I.; Lopes, C. M.; Helena Amaral, M.; Costa, P. C. Current Insights on Lipid Nanocarrier-Assisted Drug Delivery in the Treatment of Neurodegenerative Diseases. *Eur. J. Pharm. Biopharm.* **2020**, *149,* 192–217.
103. Prasad, N. A. Parkinsonism in Ayurvedic Perspective, a Bird's Eye. *Glob. J. Res. Med. Plants Indig. Med.* **2012,** *1* (11), 629.
104. Mannangatti, P.; Naidu, K. N. Indian Herbs for the Treatment of Neurodegenerative Disease. In *The Benefits of Natural Products for Neurodegenerative Diseases*; Springer: Cham, 2016; pp 323–336.
105. Pathak-Gandhi, N.; Vaidya, A. D. B. Management of Parkinson's Disease in Ayurveda: Medicinal Plants and Adjuvant Measures. *J. Ethnopharmacol.* **2017,** *197,* 46–51.
106. Farooqui, A. A.; Farooqui, T.; Madan, A.; Ong, J. H.-J.; Ong, W. Y.. Ayurvedic Medicine for the Treatment of Dementia: Mechanistic Aspects. *Evid.-Based Complement. Altern. Med.* **2018** (2018).
107. van Andel, D. M. Crossing Borders in Neurodevelopmental Disorders: Towards Rational Treatments and Stratified Trial Designs. Ph.D. Dissertation, Utrecht University, 2021.
108. Santen, G. W.; Cohen, A. F. Rare Disease Specialists and Clinical Pharmacologists Unite: Increase Collection of Longitudinal Data!. *Br. J. Clin. Pharmacol.* **2019,** *85* (11), 2457.
109. Moreno, L.; Barone, G.; Dubois, S. G.; Molenaar, J.; Fischer, M.; Schulte, J.; Eggert, A.; et al. Accelerating Drug Development for Neuroblastoma: Summary of the Second Neuroblastoma Drug Development Strategy Forum from Innovative Therapies for Children with Cancer and International Society of Paediatric Oncology Europe Neuroblastoma. *Eur. J. Cancer* **2020,** *136,* 52–68.
110. Schapira, A.; Albrecht, S.; Barone, P.; Comella, C.; Hsu, H.; Massey, D.; Mcdermott, M.; et al. P1. 203 Immediate vs. Delayed-Start Pramipexole in Early Parkinson's Disease: the PROUD Study. *Parkinsonism Relat. Disord.* **2009,** *15,* S81.
111. Olanow, C. W.; Rascol, O.; Hauser, R.; Feigin, P. D.; Jankovic, J.; Lang, A.; Langston, W.; et al. A Double-Blind, Delayed-Start Trial of Rasagiline in Parkinson's Disease. *N. Engl. J. Med.* **2009,** *361* (13), 1268–1278.

112. Woolfall, K.; Shilling, V.; Hickey, H.; Smyth, R. L.; Sowden, E.; Williamson, P. R.; Young, B. Parents' Agendas in Paediatric Clinical Trial Recruitment are Different Froresearchers' and Often Remain Unvoiced: A Qualitative Study. *PLoS One* **2013,** *8* (7), E67352.
113. Mitsikostas, D. D.; Chalarakis, N. G.; Mantonakis, L. I.; Delicha, E.-M.; Sfikakis, P. P. Nocebo in Fibromyalgia: Meta-Analysis of Placebo-Controlled Clinical Trials and Implications for Practice. *Eur. J. Neurol.* **2012,** *19* (5), 672–680.
114. Lavori, P. W. Placebo Control Groups in Randomized Treatment Trials: a Statistician's Perspective. *Biol. Psychiatry* **2000,** *47* (8), 717–723.
115. Park, J. J. H.; Harari, O.; Dron, L.; Lester, R. T.; Thorlund, K.; Mills, E. J. An Overview of Platform Trials with a Checklist for Clinical Readers. *J. Clin. Epidemiol.* **2020,** *125,* 1–8.
116. Mehta, A. R.; Chataway, J.; Pal, S.; Parmar, M. K. B.; Chandran, S. Trials for Neurodegenerative Diseases: Time to Innovate. *Lancet Neurol.* **2021,** *20* (12), 984.
117. Stanford, P. D. Research Summary: Basket Trials and Neurodegenerative Disease.
118. Katsuno, M.; Tanaka, F.; Sobue, G. Perspectives on Molecular Targeted Therapies and Clinical Trials for Neurodegenerative Diseases. *J. Neurol. Neurosurg. Psychiatry* **2012,** *83* (3), 329–335.
119. Lieberman, A.; Lyons, K.; Levine, J.; Myerburg, R. Statins, Cholesterol, Co-enzyme Q10, and Parkinson's Disease. *Parkinsonism Relat. Disord.* **2005,** *11* (2), 81–84.
120. Q10, and Parkinson's Disease. *Parkinsonism Relat. Disord.* **2005,** *11* (2), 81–84.
121. Griffin, E. F.; Yan, X.; Caldwell, K. A.; Caldwell, G. A. Distinct Functional Roles of Vps41-Mediated Neuroprotection in Alzheimer's and Parkinson's Disease Models of Neurodegeneration. *Hum. Mol. Genet.* **2018,** *27* (24), 4176–4193.
122. Saravi, S.; Soheil, S.; Seyed Sobhan Saeedi Saravi, Alireza Arefidoust, and Ahmad Reza Dehpour. The Beneficial Effects of HMG-CoA Reductase Inhibitors in the Processes of Neurodegeneration. *Metab. Brain Dis.* **2017,** *32* (4), 949–965.
123. Wang, Q.; Yan, J.; Chen, X.; Li, J.; Yang, Yu, Weng, J. P.; Deng, C.; Yenari, M. A. Statins: Multiple Neuroprotective Mechanisms in Neurodegenerative Diseases. *Exp. Neurol.* **2011,** *230* (1), 27–3

CHAPTER 2

Overview of the Blood-Brain Barrier (BBB) Transport Mechanisms

SHILPA VERMA, MAHESH GAIKWAD, GAJANAN PAUL, and A. K. YADAV

Department of Pharmaceutics, National Institute of Pharmaceutical Education and Research, Raebareli, Uttar Pradesh, India

ABSTRACT

The blood–brain barrier (BBB) has a dynamic structure that functions as a gatekeeper and is formed by the tight junction (TJ) between the microvascular endothelial (MVE) cells (ECs). The interaction of several transmembrane proteins (occludin and claudin) seals the paracellular pathway and restricts the entry of foreign substances/molecules into the brain. The cellular constituents are responsible for maintaining brain homeostasis, regulating influx and efflux, and protecting the neural network from injury. The selective permeation of BBB prevents the movement of larger molecules. Generally, drugs or proteins that are less than 400 Da, and lipophilic molecules are easily transported to the BBB. Unfortunately, less than 5% of the active pharmaceutical ingredient can pass through the BBB. Many therapeutic molecules that are difficult to transport across BBB challenge the treatment of many neurological disorders. The receptors and transport proteins expressed on the luminal surface of brain capillary endothelial cells (BCECs) may be useful to traverse various molecules across the BBB. Moreover, the presence of several transporters on the endothelial surface of BBB has been reported. The different mechanisms to transport the molecules or substances to the brain are paracellular, transcellular pathway, adsorptive mediated transcytosis, receptor-mediated transcytosis (RMT), and carrier-mediated transcytosis. RMT includes nonstereoselective vesicular

Nanomedicine for Neurodegenerative Disorders: Selective Treatment Strategies. Rishabha Malviya, Kamla Pathak, & Swati Verma (Eds.)

transportation and has been exploited widely for transporting both large and tiny therapeutic molecules by researchers. The uptake of solute is due to the presence of a special transporter on the surface of apical luminal and abluminal membranes. The blood-to-brain influx transport systems at the BBB can be utilized to deliver the drug to the brain. However, the penetration of the drug into the brain may be hindered by the brain-to-blood efflux transport systems, that is, which include adenosine triphosphate (ATP)-binding cassette transporters. The cerebral clearance of endogenous neurotoxic chemicals linked with central nervous system (CNS) diseases is also facilitated by the efflux transport systems present. Transcytosis of the vesicular process is efficient in carrying several bigger molecules. In this chapter, we present an overview of the various transport mechanisms to deliver the substances/molecules/biomedical agents to the brain.

2.1 INTRODUCTION

The normal brain of an adult human weighs 2% compared to the body's total mass yet uses 20% of the body's total resting energy. As the brain lacks a pool for storing fuel, so it relies on a constant source of energy substrates (chiefly glucose) and other nutrients (amino acids, monocarboxylates such as lactate minerals and vitamins) via its complex vascular system. The blood vessels in the brain have a total length of about 650 km, with capillaries making up about 85% of this length. Since neurons are just 8–20 μM from blood arteries due to an intercapillary distance of 40 μM, practically every neuron is nourished by a separate capillary. Signaling molecules are used by neurons to communicate (ions, neurotransmitters, neuromodulators, and neuropeptides), synaptic and action potentials, and electrical signals. Unintended changes in these molecules must therefore be avoided for neurons and other brain cells to function effectively, and waste products from cerebral metabolic processes must be continuously eliminated. Furthermore, protecting the adult central nervous system (CNS) from toxins (such as xenobiotics or metabolites from various metabolic reactions) in the blood circulation is essential because the CNS lacks a significant capacity for regeneration. Because of the unique morphological and biochemical characteristics of the numerous interfaces and their functional relationships with auxiliary brain parenchymal cells, the cerebral microenvironment is therefore kept in check by the strict control of molecular traffic.[1] As a result, the brain creates special protections for the (CNS) by capillaries, known as the blood–brain barrier (BBB). For appropriate functioning, neurons need a unique microenvironment and micromilieu that are very different from peripheral organs in terms of their cellular and molecular makeup. All vertebrate species have evolved a BBB to create and maintain the physical separation of compartments of the blood from the brain. Direct control at the blood–brain interface is the greatest way to regulate the flow of chemicals from the blood to the neurons. As a result, the BBB is restricted to the brain capillary endothelial cells (BCEC), which tightly regulate the entry and exit of metabolites from the CNS. BCECs create complex and continuous interendothelial tight connections to provide these regulation tight junctions (TJs). This microvessel network serves as a mediator for the delivery of nutrients, a flexible regulator of ion balance, and a defense against toxic products. This problem also poses a serious impediment to the development of CNS medications.[2] The brain normally excludes all big molecules and more than 98% of macromolecules, such as recombinant peptides and chemicals. Although CNS vessels are continuous nonfenestrated vessels, they also have some other characteristics that allow them to precisely control the transport of chemicals, ions, and cells, blood, and the CNS. This severely limiting barrier capacity enables them to closely control CNS. Homeostasis is essential for enabling proper neuronal activity and CNS protection from infections, poisons, inflammation, damage, and illness. The BBB's stringent requirements create a barrier to the delivery of medicines to the CNS; therefore, significant works have been made to develop approaches to modify or obstruct the BBB for the administration of medications.[3]

In most mammals and other species with a fully developed CNS, the cerebral capillaries that enter the brain and spinal cord to form the BBB are lined by microvascular endothelial (MVE) cells (ECs). Given that the average adult's total surface area is estimated to be between 12 and 18 m^2 and that the average microvessel surface area/g of tissue is between 150 and 200 cm^2, it is the greatest interface for blood–brain interaction. A BBB tune plays an essential function in safeguarding the brain parenchyma from blood-borne pathogens and posing a major challenge for medicines and other foreign substances entering the brain and spinal cord. The BBB serves as the barrier. The epithelial cells of the blood–brain–stem–cell-derived from the choroid plexus The choroid plexus epithelial cells regulate CSF secretion into the ventricular brain system. Contrarily, the interstitial fluid (ISF), which is made up of the remaining extracellular fluid in the brain, is produced at least in part by secretion through the BBB's capillary endothelium. ISF freely exchanges information with CSF at several points, which is thought to contribute between 10 and 60% of CSF. The avascular epithelium of the arachnoid mater, which is regarded as the third barrier, is located underneath the dura mater. The CNS extracellular fluids are sealed off from the rest of the body by the dura mater, which covers the CNS. Its contribution to the flow of blood to the brain is minimal because of its avascular structure and comparatively small surface area compared to other barriers.[4] BBB along with the blood–CSF barrier have pretended hurdle in achieving effective drug delivery into the brain.[5] The drug or large protein molecule of molecular weight more than 400–600 Da cannot cross the BBB.[6]

2.2 HISTORICAL PERSPECTIVE ON THE BBB

German immunologist Paul Ehrlich conducted the first experiments that demonstrated the barrier's existence in 1885. He noticed that distant brain tissue was not colored by the given dye, while animal organs were stained. This finding's first interpretation was based on various binding affinities. Later pharmacological research by Lewandowsky and Bield as well as Bield and Kraus caused a barrier to exist at the level of the cerebral arteries in 1900, interestingly, when Lewandowsky investigated the minimal potassium ferrocyanate permeability through the head. Goldmann referred to this barrier as the "blood–brain barrier." Goldmann (a student of Ehrlich) also carried out staining studies on dogs and rabbits, demonstrating distinct, unique staining of the choroid plexus following injection of dyes into the peripheral circulation. Cerebrospinal fluid (CSF) and surrounding brain tissue were colorless, which confirms earlier findings made by other experts. Goldmann also discovered that aside from the choroid, the brain was dyed following subarachnoidal injection, and concluded that the plexus epithelium constituted the exact barrier blocking the dye transport to the brain. However, the Russian biologist Lina Stern discovered that after being administered intravenous (IV), some test chemicals could be identified preferentially in the brain and cerebrospinal fluid as opposed to others. She named this phenomenon "barrier he matoence phalique."[1] After a while, Spatz and colleagues proposed the idea of two distinct CNS barriers—the BBB and the liquor–blood barrier. The first scientific article was written by H. Foertig in 1929. The article was titled "Die Bluthirnschranke," which is meant in German as "the blood–brain barrier."[5] Additionally, Broman claimed that the barrier function of the BBB but not the astrocytic ECs were localized to the capillary ECs.[6] Additionally, he asserted that the BBB demonstrated flaws in brain disorders and displayed a fleeting BBB breakdown or opening following intracarotid arterial hypertonic solution administration.[7]

2.3 STRUCTURE OF BLOOD-BRAIN BARRIER

2.3.1 BLOOD-BRAIN BARRIER (BBB)

The two main cell types that make up blood vessels are ECs which form the blood vessel walls, and mural cells, which rest on the EC layer's abluminal surface. Characteristics of the BBB are mostly seen in the ECs, and they are also significantly induced and regulated by interactions with mural cells, along with immune cells, glial cells, and brain parenchyma that take place within the neurovascular unit (NVU) shown in (Figure 2.1).[8]

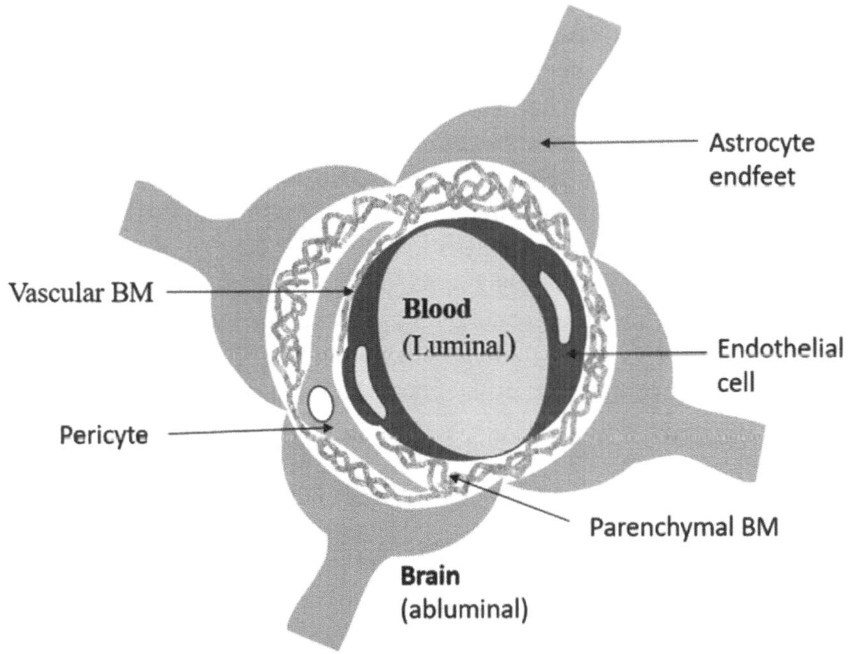

FIGURE 2.1 Neurovascular unit.

2.3.1.1 ENDOTHELIAL CELLS

The cells that make up the blood vessel walls are called ECs, which are modified simple squamous epithelial cells originating from mesoderm. The very small capillary is created by a one-time EC folding over itself thereby forming the lumen, but the diameter of big arteries and also veins might be made up of many dozens of ECs. The lumenal and parenchymal surfaces of these CNS microvascular ECs are separated by less than a quarter of a micron, making them incredibly thin cells that are 39% thinner than muscle ECs. As they can closely control the movement of ions, chemicals, and also cells between the blood and the brain, CNS ECs differentiate from ECs in other tissues. TJs, which hold CNS ECs together and significantly reduce the paracellular flux of solutes CNS ECs transcytosis at relatively low rates in comparison to peripheral ECs, which significantly restricts the transport of solutes between cells via vesicles[9] This tight paracellular barrier and transcellular barrier results in a polarized cell with different lumenal and abluminal membrane compartments, making it possible to precisely control the flow of blood to the brain by regulating cellular transport proteins. The CNS ECs express two different kinds of transporters. The initial is efflux transporters, they are oriented towards the lumenal surface and move a diverse range of lipophilic substances toward the blood in place of those that would otherwise diffuse from across the membrane of the cell. The second category consists of highly specialized nutrient transporters which enable the removal of specialized waste products from the CNS into the blood as well as the transportation of specialized nutrients across the BBB into the CNS. Compared to other ECs, CNS ECs have more mitochondria, which is considered to be essential for producing adenosine triphosphate (ATP) to power the ion gradients required for transport tasks.[10] Leukocyte adhesion molecules (LAMs) are also expressed at a very low level in CNS ECs compared to ECs in other organs, which significantly reduces the number of immune cells that can reach the CNS. Additionally, it is hypothesized that CNS ECs' altered vascular metabolism creates a barrier by changing the physical characteristics of molecules, which can affect their reactivity and transport characteristics. The ECS can closely control CNS homeostasis because of a mix of molecular barrier features (efflux transporters, specialized metabolism, and low LAMs), structural barrier properties (TJs and lower transcytosis), and specific transporters to deliver required nutrients. Whether the BBB in various parts of the brain has particular qualities necessary for the operation of the regional neuronal circuitry remains a significant open subject. For example, the growth or function of particular neuronal subtypes may depend on the localized delivery of particular nutrients. Although capillaries with BBB properties are present in the majority of the CNS's vascularized regions, The subfornical organ, region postrema, pineal gland, and central eminence are among the nuclei close to the third and fourth ventricles that contain vessels with noticeably higher passive permeability. These circumventricular organs' capillaries are continuous, and fenestrated channels with high solute permeability. Based on their high permeability, these nuclei either detect blood solute concentrations or release substances into the blood.[11]

TABLE 2.1 Cells of the BBB and their Functions.

S. No.	Type of cell	Functions	Reference
1	ECs	1. To make up the blood vessel walls 2. Control the movement of ions, chemicals, and cells in between the blood and brain 3. Sense concentration of solute in blood or secrete chemicals in the blood	
2	Mural cells	1. These cells can contract to regulate the capillary's width 2. These cells function in controlling angiogenesis, deposition at the extracellular matrix, wound healing, infiltration of cells' immune system, and blood flow modulation in response to brain activity	
3	Basement membrane	1. To give anchor to cellular components 2. Maintaining their interaction and ensuring the stability of the microvasculature	11
4	Astrocytes	1. Crucial regulators of BBB formation and function 2. Act as progenitor cells	
5)	Immune cells	1. By phagocytosing cellular waste, these cells serve as the initial line of defense for innate immunity 2. These cells can serve as antigen-presenting cells in adaptive immunity and are important in controlling neuronal development, innate immune response, and tissue repair	

2.3.1.2 MURAL CELLS

Mural cells contain pericytes (PC) and vascular smooth muscle cells that encircle the major arteries. These are cellular components implanted in the vascular BM and rest on the abluminal surface of the micro-VE tube. The lack of a distinct marker that PCs express exclusively makes it challenging to investigate PCs because these cells are frequently confused with other perivascular cells. Anpep (CD13), and desmin, these biomarkers are used to identify PCs, but none of them are sharp biomarkers of this cell type. Currently, the widely acknowledged molecular identification of CNS PCs is a positive reaction to PDGFR-b. Long cellular processes that frequently cover many

EC bodies are extended along the endothelium's abluminal surface by PC. These cells can contract to regulate the capillary's width since they contain contractile protein. Although they line up the endothelial tube, the majority of the cell body and the processes remain apart from the endothelium due to the BM they are embedded in. The mechanisms do result in peg-and-socket junctions, or cellular adhesions with the endothelium, at specific locations, and they are regulated by the integrin N-cadherin. Other PC–EC adhesions, such as adhesion plaques, gap junctions, and TJs, have also been discovered. It has been demonstrated that CNS PCs differ from PCs in other tissues in several ways. In contrast to PCs in the CNS, PCs in numerous peripheral tissues are produced from the mesodermal origin, which is formed from the neural crest.[12] The endothelial: PC ratio in the CNS microvasculature is believed to be between 1:1 and 3:1, whereas its ratio in muscle is 100:1. In addition, the CNS microvasculature does have the largest coverage of CNS PCs of any tissue. PC is believed to be multipotent CNS stem cells because of their significant functions in controlling angiogenesis, extracellular matrix deposition, healing of wounds, infiltration of immune system cells, and blood flow modulation in response to brain activity.[13] These cells have also been demonstrated to play a crucial role in maintaining the BBB's functionality during adulthood and aging as well as controlling its creation throughout development. One of the chief issues in PC biology is if there are multiple subgroups of PCs that might have different types of functions. Due to the lack of identifying markers Whether the various PC-attributed duties are carried out by all the same cells, by various subsets of PCs, or even by non-PC cells that are present close to the vasculature, is still a mystery. These queries will be addressed by the discovery of novel PC-specific biomarkers and perhaps the discovery of identifiers for subgroups of PCs.[11]

2.3.1.3 BASEMENT MEMBRANE (BM)

Two BMs, known as the outermost parenchymal BM and the vascular glia limitans, respectively, surround the perivascular and vascular tube. The outermost BM is largely released by an astrocytic process that extends near the vasculature, as opposed to the vascular BM, which is a matrix extracellular in origin released by the ECs and PCs. Numerous secreted molecules, such as type IV collagens, nidogen, heparin sulfate proteins, and other glycoproteins, make up these BMs.[14] The compositions of the vascular and parenchymal BMs differ; for example, the former contains laminins α4 and α5, whereas the second does α1 and α2. Many signaling mechanisms at the vasculature are anchored by these BMs, but they also act as a further barrier for chemicals and cells. before reaching the neural tissue, cross. In several different neurological illnesses, leukocyte infiltration and BBB malfunction are seen as a result of matrix metalloproteinase (MMP) disruption of these BMs.[14]

2.3.1.4 ASTROCYTES

Astrocytes, which extend polarized cellular processes that envelop either blood vessels or neural processes, are one of the most prevalent forms of glial cells. The vascular tube is almost entirely enshrouded by the endfeet of the basal process, which also houses a variety of proteins such as dystroglycan, dystrophin, and aquaporin 4. The re-binding, of the dystroglycan-dystrophin complex, is crucial for connecting the endfeet framework to the BM. Aquaporin 4 is coordinated into the orthogonal structure of particles by this connection, which is essential for controlling water homeostasis in the brain.[15] The cellular connection between blood arteries and neural circuitry is provided by astrocytes. Astrocytes can send signals that control blood flow by neuronal activity due to this neurovascular coupling. This includes controlling the vascular smooth muscle cells surrounding arterioles and PCs surrounding capillaries to contract or dilate. Purified astrocytes' capacity to produce barrier characteristics in grown ECs in vitro coculture paradigms as well as non-CNS blood arteries in transplantation experiments has led to the identification of astrocytes as crucial regulators of BBB formation and function. These studies have a problem in that the astrocytes are frequently cultivated using newborn rodent brains and undergo multiple cycles of cell division, indicating that the cells being studied are progenitor cells rather than mature ones.[11,16] Recent studies on the BBB in dissected mouse embryos show that the BBB forms before astrocyte production and the ensheathing of the vasculature, indicating that these cells are not involved in the first generation of the BBB. The discovery of substances produced by astrocytes that do control BBB function raises the possibility that mature astrocytes modify and maintain the barrier after it has been created.[17]

2.3.1.5 IMMUNE CELLS

Different immune cell types within the blood and the CNS interact with CNS blood arteries. Perivascular monocytes and microglial cells make up the CNS's two major cell groups. Perivascular macrophages are cells of the monocyte lineage that are located at the abluminal side of the vascular tube that is frequently found in, a tiny canal that is filled with fluid and borders the abluminal surface of the arteries and veins that enter and exit the CNS which is also known as the Virchow–Robin space. These cells come from blood-borne progenitors, and chimeric tests indicate that they can enter the BBB which can be replaced to an extent of 80% in 3 months. By phagocytosing cellular waste, these types of cells serve as the initial line of defense for innate immunity.[18] Microglial cells are parenchymal immune cells that live in the CNS and enter the brain during embryogenesis. They are produced from progenitors in the yolk sac. These cells can serve as antigen-presenting cells in adaptive immunity and are important in controlling neuronal development, innate immune response, and tissue repair. Additionally, several blood-borne immune cell types, including neutrophils, T cells, and macrophages, can interact with CNS arteries when activated and are hypothesized to modulate BBB properties in response to an infection, injury, and disease by generating reactive oxygen species (ROS), which could make the vessels more permeable. Understanding the processes by which immune cells and the BBB are "activated" to interact may be crucial to understanding how the BBB is disrupted during various neurological disorders.[19]

2.4 MOLECULES OF THE BBB

The identification of significant structural and transport elements of the BBB was made possible by the discovery of chemicals expressed by CNS ECs. Recent advances in the molecular biology of the BBB have been made possible using extensive proteomic and genome-wide experimental methods. Using microarray technology, RNA sequencing, mass spectrometry, and proteomic analysis, acutely pure microvascular fragments acutely purified ECs, and cultured ECs have allowed for extensive gene expression studies of brain ECs with neural cells and ECs from other organs. Understanding the distinctive molecular makeup of the BBB has been facilitated in part by an analysis of the molecular differences between ECs from nonneural tissues and those from the CNS.[20]

2.4.1 TIGHT JUNCTIONS

TJs, which polarize the luminal and abluminal compartments by forming a high-resistance paracellular barrier to molecules and ions, hold CNS ECs together.[21] The majority of the information on TJs comes from research on ECs, which has revealed that these types of cellular adhesions are created through homotypic and heterotypic contacts of transmembrane molecules, which are related to the cytoskeleton via interactions with cytoplasmic adaptors, on the apical portion of the lateral membrane. Work in cell culture reveals that the strength of these junctions changes significantly based on the tissue in which they are present. Among the transmembrane molecules are junctional adhesion molecules (JAMs), occludins, and claudins. The more than 25 distinct claudin family members, which are tetraspanins, are distinguished from one another by the W-GLW-C-C motif in the first external loop.[11]

2.4.2 CLAUDINS

The TJs connecting cells in epithelial cell sheets are home to claudins, which are molecules that promote cell-cell adhesion. 27 four-transmembrane domain proteins make up the claudin family in mammals. Claudins are in charge of the paracellular barrier function of TJs, and they occasionally provide the paracellular barriers of TJs with paracellular channel functions. The hypothetical "antiparallel double row model," which explains how claudins polymerize linearly and form TJ strands with paracellular barrier functions, was put forth in light of recent advances in the molecular structure of claudins. The strong and adaptable paracellular barrier, and also channel activities of the claudin-based TJs, which coordinates with many biological systems, are currently being clarified by ongoing studies at the cell and tissue levels.[22]

Claudins are necessary for the establishment of paracellular barriers, according to in vitro evidence. Claudin expression is necessary for the formation of TJ strands in fibroblasts, and disruption of claudin reduces the paracellular barrier characteristics of the canine kidney cells. The dimensions and charge selectivity of the pore inside the cellular junction are determined by residues of amino acids in the first extracellular loop, according to research with chimeric claudins. As a result, the claudin composition and the accessibility of the paracellular barriers can vary depending on the cell in question. Different members of the claudin family are expressed by different epithelial barriers in different tissues, and mouse knockout studies have shown that specific members of the family are necessary for certain barriers (such as the claudin-1 epidermal barrier, claudin-16 renal epithelia, claudin-11,and CNS myelin; so many of which have been connected to human disease.[21]

At the BBB, other claudins have also been discovered, including cldn12 and cldn3. It has been shown that CNS ECs strongly express claudin-5, and animals lacking the protein exhibit a size-specific BBB leak. Occludin, tetraspanins produced by epithelial cells and CNS ECs, may be crucial for the barrier's resistance, according to an in vitro experiment that disrupted its homotypic connections. Occludin is significantly more abundant in CNS ECs than in ECs from nonneural tissues, suggesting that it might represent a crucial part of the barrier. However, it turns out that mice lacking occludin have a sound high-resistance epithelial barrier as well as a functional BBB. These animals do have calcified CNS, which suggests that occludin may play a specific role in regulating calcium transit over the BBB.[23]

2.4.3 OCCLUDIN

At TJs, a wide variety of structural and signaling proteins have been found. Occludin is always expressed in all epithelial and endothelial TJs, whereas distinct members of the claudin family have varied expressions at TJs. Occludin is a protein with a molecular weight of 60–65 kDa with four transmembrane motifs two extracellular loops that cross the intercellular cleft, and carboxyl and amino terminals that face the cytoplasm. It is consistently found on CNS EC margins.[11] the cellular through accessory proteins, the C-terminal region of occludin is connected to the EC's cytoskeleton Increased paracellular permeability for low-molecular-weight molecules can be explained by the production of C-terminally shortened versions of occludin, which regulates that permeability.[24]

2.4.4 JUNCTIONS OF ADHESION

The presence of adhesion molecules, which are pervasive throughout the vasculature, mediates the adherence of ECs to one another. These chemicals have a significant impact on endothelial polarity remodeling, vascular development, and to some extent, the control of paracellular permeability. The major element of adhesion junctions is VE-cadherin, a Ca^{2+}-regulated protein that promotes cell–cell adhesion by homophilic interactions between the extracellular motifs of proteins generated in the surrounding cells. The stability of adhesion molecules-mediated cell–cell interaction requires the interaction of VE-cadherin to catenin and plakoglobin, which then in turn bind to the actin cytoskeleton through catenin, and actinin.[25]

2.4.5 JUNCTIONAL ADHESION MOLECULES (JAMS)

JAMs are immunoglobulin superfamily members that interact homotypically with epithelial cells and ECs at TJs. JAMs have been demonstrated to control paracellular permeability and leukocyte extravasation. For instance, mice's BBB has been found to contain JAM. The paracellular barrier must be sealed at the contact points of three cells, and it has recently been demonstrated that this requires special chemical elements. Lipolysis-stimulated receptor (LSR) is a component of these tricellular junctional complexes that are necessary for directing tricellular adhesions. It is still unknown what type of size/charge-selective pore is produced by the particular combination of tight-junction proteins expressed by CNS ECs, as well as whether or not all this pore's permeability is constant or changes dynamically in response to neuronal activity.[24]

The cytoskeleton and the transmembrane adhesion complexes are connected by many cytoplasmic adaptors, such as zonula occludens (ZO) (ZO-1, ZO-2, cingulin, and membrane-associated guanylate kinase (MAGUKs), well as MPPs It's interesting to note that several of the reported TJ proteins, such as cldn5, cldn12, ZO-1, and also ZO-2, seem to be expressed by the ECs across all tissues. Therefore, a crucial topic is why ECs in other tissues do not form this tight barrier, but only ECs in the CNS do. Several cytoplasmic adaptors, such as Jacob and MPP7, and at the BBB, tricellular TJ proteins, LSR, and marveld2 are prevalent, indicating that such molecules may be essential for the formation of this barrier, according to transcriptional research comparing CNS ECs with peripheral ECs.[26]

2.4.6 ACCESSORY PROTEINS

Supplementary proteins several auxiliary proteins are connected to the TJ complex's constituents. These primarily consist of the MAGUK-like protein homologs. Multiple protein–protein interactions are made possible by the Src homolog-3 domain, guanylate kinase-like domain, and numerous postsynaptic dense protein-95/discs-large/ZO-1-binding motifs of these proteins The formation of specific domains within the membranes of ECs and the clustering of protein complexes to the cell membrane are both mediated by MAGUK proteins. ZO-1, zona occludin-2 (ZO-2), and zona occludin-3 are the three main MAGUK proteins found at the TJ complex (ZO-3). ZO-1, an EC-expressed 220-kDa phosphoprotein, which has been linked to adhesion molecules and gap junction proteins ZO-1, connects the membrane proteins of the TJ complexes to the actin cytoskeleton of the cell, ensuring the stability and efficient operation of TJ proteins. A common side effect of ZO-1 displacement from the junctional complex is enhanced permeability. By communicating details about just the TJ complex to the inner of the EC or vice versa, ZO-1 can act as a signaling molecule.[27] Additionally, it has been demonstrated that ZO-1 localizes inside the nucleus of ECs when there is proliferation and damage. A phosphoprotein of 160 kDa called ZO-2 has a strong sequence homology to ZO-1. It can bind to signaling molecules like transcription factors and other structural elements of TJ complexes in addition to those localized into the nucleus during circumstances of stress and proliferation ZO-3, a protein with molecular weight 130-kDa homolog has been discovered in some tissues' TJs, but not in the BBB.[28]

2.5 ADDITIONAL BBB COMPONENTS

Signaling cascades that are activated in CNS ECs have been discovered using extensive genomic and proteomic methods. For example, it has been demonstrated that Wnt/catenin signaling through Lef1 and Sonic hedgehog signaling through Gli are important for controlling the formation and functioning of the BBB. Additionally, it has been suggested that by metabolizing potential poisons or changing the characteristics of molecules, vascular metabolism controls the barrier qualities of the CNS vasculature. Certain enzymes, such as g-glutamyl transpeptidase and carbonic anhydrase IV, are more abundant in CNS vasculature than in vessels from nonneural tissues. There is still research to be done to ascertain which of these BBB-enriched genes are crucial for each aspect of the BBB, if there is significant variation in these genes at different portions of the vascular tree and in various brain regions, and if the expression and action of each protein are adaptively regulated by neurotransmission. Understanding the BBB's gene expression has benefited from the huge proteomic and genomic techniques. Beyond genomics, various regulatory systems that are essential for BBB formation and function are being investigated, including proteome, microRNAs (miRNAs), noncoding RNAs, lipoproteins, metabolomics, and epigenetics.[29]

2.6 BBB REGULATION AND HOMEOSTASIS

Although the ECs exhibit crucial BBB characteristics, significant transplantation studies show that these features are controlled by interactions with the

CNS's milieu. The BBB is not one physiological phenomenon, but rather a collection of physiological characteristics that CNS ECs must either activate (through TJs, transporters, and metabolic enzymes) or block (by transcytosis, and LAMs). Recent studies have analyzed the cellular and molecular processes governing this process demonstrating that its induction and regulation are complex processes that involve interactions between CNS ECs.[30]

2.7 FUNCTIONS OF THE BLOOD–BRAIN BARRIER

2.7.1 ION REGULATION

The BBB maintains the ideal ionic composition for synaptic signaling function in addition to providing a network of specific ion channels and transporters to provide a steady environment for neuronal function. Thus, despite potential fluctuations in plasma [K+] brought on by exercise or a meal, enforced during an experiment, or brought on by pathology, the level of potassium in CSF and the ISF of the CNS is kept constant at 2.5–2.9 mM. This is even though the potassium concentration in mammalian plasma is approximately 4.5 mM. At the BBB and BCSFB, Ca^{2+}, Mg^{2+}, and pH are all actively controlled.[31]

2.7.2 NEUROTRANSMITTERS

The neuroexcitatory amino acid glutamate is present in high concentrations in the plasma, although these levels change considerably following food consumption. If glutamate is uncontrollably released into the brain ISF, Neural tissue can sustain significant and long-lasting neurotoxic/neuroexcitatory damage, as from, say, hypoxic neurons after an ischemic stroke. The BBB also aids in keeping the central and peripheral transmitter reservoirs separate, minimizing "crosstalk," as the central and peripheral nervous systems utilize several neurotransmitters that are the same.[4]

2.7.3 MACROMOLECULES

Numerous macromolecules cannot reach the brain because of the BBB. CSF has a far lower protein level than plasma, and individual protein composition varies greatly. Plasma proteins that activate cells and cause apoptosis, such as albumin, prothrombin, and plasminogen, harm brain tissue. The thrombin receptor PAR1 is abundantly expressed in the CNS, and factor Xa, which turns prothrombin into thrombin, is present in the brain. Similar to this, tissues of the CNS include a tissue plasminogen activator (tPA), which turns plasminogen into plasmin. If present in the brain ISF, thrombin, and plasmin can set off a chain of occurrences that result in glial activation, cell death, scarring, and division. Therefore, if these big molecular weight serum proteins leak into the brain through a damaged BBB, the pathogenic implications could be very serious. Cystatin-C, a protein that is synthesized locally within the CNS, is one of the few that is present in higher concentrations in CSF than in plasma. A high quantity of cystatin-C, a serine protease inhibitor, in the CSF may act as a preventative mechanism against the BBB's ongoing, spontaneous microleaks, otherwise, it would allow components of plasma to permeate the brain.[32]

2.7.4 NEUROTOXINS

The BBB serves as a barrier that protects the CNS from toxic chemicals flowing through the blood. These toxic chemicals are harmful to neurons (neurotoxins) and could be endogenous proteins or metabolites, xenobiotics consumed in food, or something else eaten from the surrounding environment. Many of these substances are actively pumped out of the brain by several ATP-binding cassette transporters (ABC energy-dependent efflux transporters). If injured and completely differentiated neurons are unable to split and replace themselves normally, the adult CNS does not have a considerable capability for regeneration. The human brain is healthy, yet there is a continual, steady pace of neuronal cell death of neurons from birth to death with very modest levels of neurogenesis. Any increase in the rate of neurotoxins entering the brain would hasten the natural rate of cell death, which would be prematurely debilitating.[33]

2.7.5 NUTRITION FOR THE BRAIN

The passive type of permeability of the BBB is very low for several nutrients which are vital and water soluble, and metabolites needed by neural tissue. Therefore, the BBB expresses specific transport networks to guarantee a sufficient supply of these compounds. Beginning with embryonic angiogenesis the endothelium begins to differentiate into a barrier layer. In adults, this differentiation is mostly maintained by intimate inductive associations with various cell types, particularly the endfeet of astrocytic glial cells This induction promotes the upregulation of TJ protein and the formation of polarity in ECs because the luminal and abluminal membrane expresses certain transporter proteins differently. In addition to being tightly linked to the endothelium, PC, microglia, and nerve terminals also contribute to barrier induction, maintenance, and function This induction promotes the overexpression of TJ proteins and the formation of polarity in ECs because of the differential expression of certain transporter proteins in the luminal and abluminal membranes. In addition to being tightly linked to the endothelium, PC, microglia, and nerve terminals also contribute to barrier induction, maintenance, and function.[4]

2.8 BBB CELLULAR INTERACTIONS

The BBB structure is described as a complex of cells, which suggests more than just a morphological collection of very few different cell types and the structures that surround them. Not only physically and biologically, but also biochemically and autonomically, the cells that make up the BBB are dependent on one another. A biochemical–anatomical network called the BBB allows for extensive cellular communication. The local concentration of released chemicals is high because ECs and astrocytes are near one another. A distinct "microdomain" in which one EC is attached to one astrocyte is suggested by three-dimensional microanatomical representations of glial–endothelial interactions. To govern cerebral blood flow, microvessels, neurons, and glia are precisely organized into NVUs. In these units, even the proper spatial (apical/basal) polarity of the EC/astrocyte mixture matters. Numerous studies demonstrate that astrocytes play a critical role in the physical, transportation, and metabolic aspects of BBB growth and operation. The results of experiments showed that astrocytes are essential for the EC- and PC-derived tube-like structures. These studies demonstrate that for the morphogenesis and growth of a vessel wall, direct EC-astrocyte interactions are essential. Both the influence of ECs on astrocytes and the participation of other BBB-located cells in barrier formation have been demonstrated. The upregulation of the expression of numerous transporter systems, such as glutamyl transpeptidase (GTP), GLUT-1, and Pgp, has also been recognized as a way for ECs to show glial influence. The reversed impact has also been observed. The number of astrocyte-derived components required for proper EC growth in the brain is constantly increasing. The evidence points to astrocyte-derived factors such as TGF being the cause of the decreased expression of the thrombomodulin (TM) and endothelium tPA genes. BBB maturation is also brought on by glial-derived neurotrophic factor (GDNF). Additionally, the endothelium-specific receptor tyrosine kinase 2 (TIE2) is affected by angiopoietin 1 (ANG1). Hydrocortisone, interleukin-6 (IL-6), and basic fibroblast growth factor (bFGF) have all been given a part. A further unanswered subject is how the brain endothelium affects astrocytes and neuron precursor cells. Several substances that promote astrocyte development come from ECs.[34,35]

2.9 FACTORS AFFECTING BLOOD–BRAIN PERMEABILITY

The NVU structurally regulates the BBB permeability. Additionally, the BBB permeability is impacted by a variety of chemical modulators in the milieu in which the NVU is present.

2.9.1 INFLAMMATORY AGENT

According to numerous research, inflammatory chemicals such as bradykinin (BK), substance P (SP), histamine, and ET-1 can make the BBB more permeable. According to studies, BK increases BBB permeability by downregulating claudin-5 and acting on B2 receptors, whereas SP, another neuropeptide, and SP antagonist have a similar effect by inhibiting the induction of cytokine-stimulated BBB permeability decrease. Histamine is one of the few neurotransmitters in the CNS that attaches to the H2 receptor to increase BBB permeability, while the H1 receptor's role in permeability reduction is connected by an increase in cAMP. Furthermore, cAMP levels are elevated in permeability. Additionally, it is hypothesized that thrombin damages the BBB acutely by activating the Src kinase phosphorylation of molecules and causing edema via its PAR receptors. The involvement of ET-1 in disrupting the BBB is also supported by in vivo and in vitro experimental models. Through ETB receptor signaling in the brain ECs, ET-1 helps to facilitate the passage of monocytes engaged in BBB inflammation, and ET-1 overexpression worsens BBB collapse in subarachnoid hemorrhage (SAH) rats. inflammatory mediators and associated inflammatory cytokines Additionally, numerous studies have demonstrated the impact of inflammatory mediators such as free radicals, MMPs, eicosanoids, tumor necrosis factor (TNF), and inflammatory cytokines on the BBB.[35] New research reveals that neuroinflammation affects the BBB's integrity as a risk factor and that the production of multiple cytokines, including IL-1, TNF-, and eicosanoids, is primarily responsible for BBB disruption. Changes in BBB integrity are mediated by cytokines, which control occludin expression. Through the stimulation of the ATP/P2X7R signaling pathway, the release of IL-1 in the BBB mode in vitro condition can cause the degradation of the proteins occluding and ZO-1. Additionally, occludin and ZO-1 protein redistribution caused by IL-1 causes BBB rupture in cultured human corneal epithelial cells via disrupting the nuclear factor kappa B (NFB) pathway. Occludin and ZO-1 protein expression is increased when IL-1 and montelukast are inhibited, which prevents BBB breakdown. Occludin degradation and BBB destruction are both facilitated by TNF via various signaling mechanisms. TNF also reduces the expression of occludin by triggering the HIF-1/VEGF/VEGFR2/ERK signaling pathway. Additionally, research has shown that NADPH promotes TNF-induced barrier dysfunction in human astrocytes, along with activation of MMP and a decrease in expression of occludin, whereas inhibiting TNF downregulates NADPH activation and promotes BBB function by enhancing the expression of occludin proteins. It has been found, however, that proinflammatory cytokines, for example, TNF, IL-1, and IL-6 can mediate the production of ABC transporters and activity at the BBB. In guinea pig brain ECs, it has been demonstrated through experimental investigations that IL-1, IL-6, and TNF reduce P-gp activity while also lowering mRNA levels. Eicosanoids, which come from arachidonic acid, are generated in response to inflammation and comprise prostaglandin (PG) and leukotrienes (LTs), which are responsible for cyclooxygenase-1 (COX-1) and COX-2 discharge. Numerous studies demonstrated how PGs and LTs affect the hyperpermeability of BBB. According to the latest research, increasing PG expression makes a model of in vitro BBB model in human BMECs more permeable, and PGs make the barrier more permeable in mice which have given LPS and TNF. Additionally, infusing LTs into the brain cells directly increases BBB permeability, but inhibitors of lipoxygenase can reduce this impact.

ROS and also reactive nitrogen species (RNS) production is frequently related to the development of neuroinflammatory responses and is crucial for both early and delayed BBB breakdown. Production of ROS is a crucial factor in opening the BBB during disease, and BBB disruption is caused by several pathways, including the following: Protein, lipid, and DNA oxidative damage; alteration of TJ proteins; rearrangement of the cytoskeleton; elevation of inflammatory mediators; and activation of MMP. Other research has demonstrated that ROS can affect cerebral blood flow by changing vascular tone, which in turn raises platelet aggregability and EC permeability. Additionally, ROS alters the ABC transporters, which disrupts the BBB's normal operation. Increased inflammatory cytokine expression, ROS, and RNS, as well as MMP secretion and pro-MMP activation, can occur during inflammation. MMPs can also activate preforms of cytokines, such as TNF- and IL-1.[36]

2.9.2 NEUROTRANSMITTERS

Additionally, some neurotransmitters, including NO and glutamate, impact the BBB's integrity. Although the particular chemical pathways are yet unknown, it is typically hypothesized that NO can help to open the BBB. Several studies have demonstrated that NO can facilitate the opening of the BBB which is mediated by MMP, induce vascular dilatation, and promote vessel remodeling to change the permeability of the BBB. This is consistent with the observation that NO plays a role in the activation of MMP, breakdown of the BBB, and the emergence of temporary cerebral edema. The TJ-related protein levels also show a verified decrease following NO generation.

Barrier function is also altered by other chemical mediators, such as the transcriptional factors the vascular endothelial growth factor (VEGF) and hypoxia-inducible factor 1 (HIF-1). HIF-1 is a complex heterodimeric unit made up of the constitutively produced protein HIF-1b and the hypoxia-inducible subunit HIF-1a. The results of this study imply that HIF-1 may contribute to BBB leakage by increasing MMP expression as a result of increased MMP activities during ischemia, which causes occludin and claudin-5 to fragment and relocalize. The fact that VEGF is one of the most well-known HIF-1 target genes provides more evidence that the HIF-1/VEGF pathway is strongly associated with TJ protein loss and increases BBB paracellular permeability. VEGF overexpression is one method by which HIF1 disrupts the BBB, and YC-1's suppression of HIF-1 lowers VEGF levels and decreases the increase in blood–brain permeability.

Some additional factors such as age, sex, microRNAs temperature, anesthetics, and exercise can also have an impact on BBB function.[4]

Age-related changes in the BBB and a reduction in the blood vessel density in the brain have an impact on brain homeostasis and raise the risk of developing a variety of neurodegenerative illnesses. A more recent study found that PC loss or degeneration, low levels of TJ proteins, and other structural factors can all contribute to BBB leakage. Occludin levels and

ZO-1 expression are consistently substantially lower in 24-month-old mice than in young adult mice. The degenerative proinflammatory features of an old, healthy BBB in the absence of injury support the idea that a chronic inflammatory state is a substantial contributing cause to increasing BBB permeability. current research has demonstrated that persistent inflammatory mediators, for example, IL-1, IFN, and TNF, rise in the CNS with aging and are accompanied by the activation of microglia.[37]

2.9.3 SEX

It is generally established that gender difference affects ischemic stroke treatment and could have an effect on its effectiveness. Aging female mice had lower estrogen levels than young adult female mice, which is accompanied by an increase in gonadotropins and higher BBB permeability. Recent research has shown that estrogen can alter BBB permeability by attaching to key TJ sites such as claudin-5 or key regulators of TJ integrity such as Annexin A1. In an in vivo investigation, estrogen therapy reduced the BBB rupture and edema development brought on by ischemia through a variety of mechanisms. Additionally, estradiol reduced MMP transcription and activity and improved the related TJ degradation following ischemia.[38]

Most of the evidence points towards the protective impacts of androgens on the BBB under physiological circumstances in males. Whereas but the 5-dihydrotestosterone has detrimental effects on the integrity of the BBB under pathological conditions, as in a stroke model, by down-regulating of claudin-5 and increasing the expression of the proinflammatory molecule chemokine CCL2. Similar to this, additional research shows that persistent gonadal testosterone deficiency causes inflammation and BBB malfunction in male rats.[35]

2.9.4 miRNAs

According to recent research, miRNAs are a novel class of BBB permeability controllers that negatively regulate the production of protein as nonprotein-coding short RNA molecules. Several miRNAs, which are present in BMECs, astrocytes, and microglia, can participate in several cellular signaling pathways and help regulate EC activities and BBB permeability. By inhibiting the NF-B signaling pathway, the anti-inflammatory miRNA

(miRNA-146a-5p) can reduce P-gp expression in the cerebral arteries in SE rats. Furthermore, VE-cadherin and ZO-1 junctional complexes formed by BMECs overexpressing miRNA-125a-5p are thicker and more continuous, which improves barrier function. On the other hand, some studies have demonstrated how miRNAs impair BMEC and BBB function. By controlling MMP-9, DNA (cytosine-5-)-methyltransferase 3β, and miRNA-29b these can harm junction proteins and membranes. resulting in hyperpermeability of the BBB and a leaky vasculature. More research is required to fully understand how miRNAs contribute to the construction and operation of the BBB.

2.9.5 TEMPERATURE

The effects of temperature on BBB permeability have been studied recently, and hyperthermia (38–42°C) and hypothermia (32–34°C) have been linked to BBB integrity. The findings that hypothermia maintains the BM integrity by reducing the activities and translational levels of MMP-2 and MMP-9 and enhancing the endogenous MMP inhibitor are consistent with the idea that brain hypothermia has a protective effect on the integrity of the BBB. Hyperthermia can result in increased brain water content and cellular abnormalities, which indicate thermal damage. However, at low temperatures (15°C), claudin-5's subcellular localization changes from the cell membrane to the cytoplasm, which may result in a lower TEER value. However, when the temperature is raised to 37°C, the value quickly returns to normal.[39]

2.10 TRANSPORT MECHANISM ACROSS THE BLOOD-BRAIN BARRIER (BBB)

There are different transport mechanisms involved in the transport of solutes and other chemical substances across the BBB. Hydrophilic substances cross the brain endothelium membrane through a paracellular pathway by the simple diffusion mechanism. Small lipophilic substances including alcohol and corticosteroid transported through the transcellular pathway to cross the BBB. Apart from that, some other mechanisms are involved in the transport of the substances across the endothelial membrane of brains such as carrier-mediated transport pathway, RMT, and efflux transporter sown in (Figure 2.2).[40]

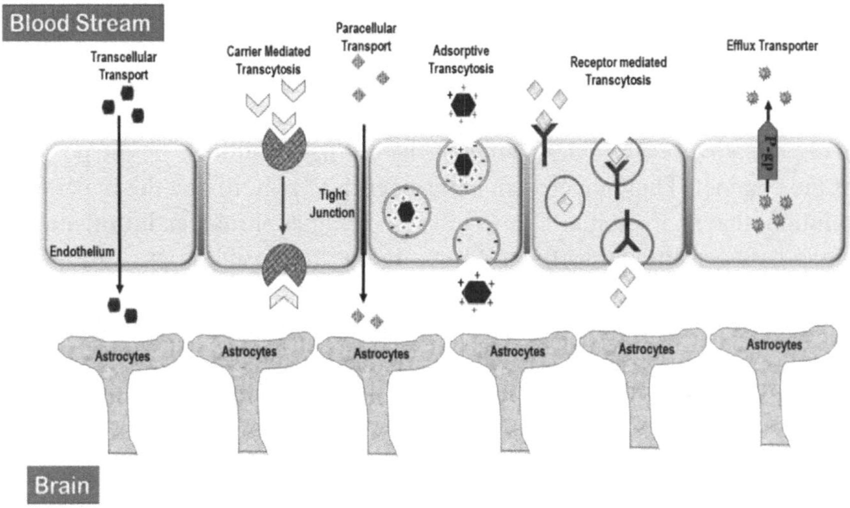

FIGURE 2.2 Transport mechanism across BBB.

2.10.1 PARACELLULAR PATHWAY

Paracellular pathway act by the passive transport process. The paracellular transport route is composed of narrow, winding channels that twisted across gaps in the intercellular junctional complex in peripheral, continuous capillaries. This pathway only allows those molecules having a width of 5–10 nm to diffuse through this channel. There are very complex intracellular junctions made up of the adherence junction (zonula adhesion), a TJ on the blood–brain EC which exhibits a higher level of continuity, due to which paracellular transportation of solute and water is restricted from the bloodstream to BBB. Furthermore, ZO, also named TJs, are domains of occluded intercellular clefts where the distance between the opposing membranes is nearly zero. The crucial rate-limiting step for the penetration of hydrophilic drugs through the paracellular route is a TJ. It is made up of three integral proteins including ZO-1, ZO-2, and ZO-3 along with the junction of adhesion molecules such as occludin, claudin, and other molecules shown in (Figure 2.3).[41]

The protein and peptide are not able to enter through biological membranes including the BBB and intestinal mucosa due to the physical characteristics of the molecule and size. The paracellular pathway is also utilized to transport the large hydrophilic molecule, that is, peptides and proteins to enter the

BBB. Due to containing TJs, its restricted the passive diffusion of molecules to transportation. Mainly researchers used several techniques for improving the entry of peptides and proteins through paracellular pathways. Researchers attempt various strategies to influence the porosity of TJs.[41] Irudayanathan et al., use a method to deliver an anticancer drug by influencing the porosity of the channel. They injected an anticancer drug by utilizing the hypertonic solution, that is, mannitol. Due to this, the cell gets shrunk and formation of a gap between the intracellular TJ due to the high osmotic pressure of the solution. As a result, the anticancer drug reaches the efficiently to brain. Also recognized that the interactivity of TJ proteins including claudin–occludin enhances the entry of hydrophilic molecules (peptide and protein) by the paracellular route.[42]

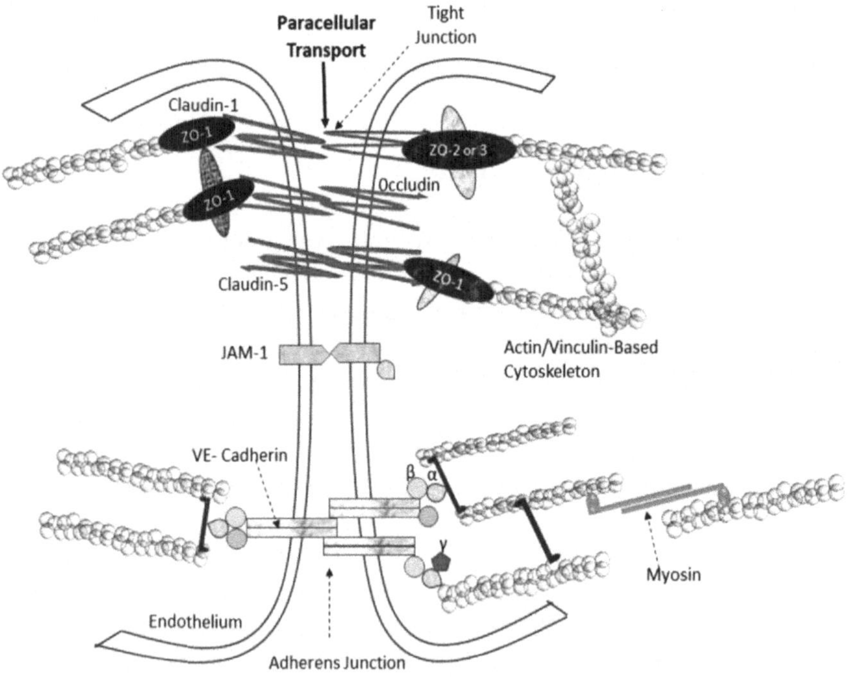

FIGURE 2.3 Paracellular pathway through TJ.

2.10.2 TRANSCELLULAR PATHWAY

Passive diffusion is crucial in the transcellular route because it efficiently delivers the therapeutic molecule across the BBB. The apical and basolateral sides are present in the biological membrane. Therapeutic molecules split across the cell membrane through the apical side into the cytoplasmic zone in the transcellular pathway and the therapeutic gets partitioned into the basolateral side of the biological membrane, where it travels to the systemic circulation or brain. Therapeutic molecules have to face off with both lipid bilayer membranes, that is, apical and basolateral membranes, which causes the restriction to delivery of the drug and acts as a rate-limiting step to deliver the therapeutic molecule to a target site.[43] Physiochemical properties of therapeutic substances, that is, hydrophilicity, size, charge, and log*P*, play a vital role in membrane partition. Lipophilic and low molecular weight molecules (<700 Da but typically <300 Da) can efficiently enter the BBB through the endothelial membrane of the brain by passive diffusion mechanisms such as benzodiazepine and barbiturate. The rate of the substance entering the BBB depends on the lipid solubility which considers the neutral and ionized species present in the solution. If the lipophilic molecule is the substrate of efflux ABC transporters, it will not accumulate in the brain. Less hydrogen bonding, that is, less than six hydrogen bonds, smaller size (less than 300 Da), lipophilicity, additionally the unavailability of free rotational bonds (less than eight rotational bonds) is desirable to transport the substance across BBB. The shape of the substances also plays a major role to cross the BBB, the spherical shape moiety is preferred over the rod shape molecule, when the molecule contains more than six hydrogen bonds present, It takes more net free energy to go from aqueous into the lipid phase which hinders transcellular diffusion. The ionization of molecules has an important role to permeate the substance through the endothelial membrane of the brain, Basic molecules are more easily penetrating than acidic and neutral molecules because the basic molecule contains a positive charge at physiological pH which can efficiently interact with anionic biological membrane enhances the penetration of the molecule. The metabolic steadiness of the molecule should be desirable, the molecule with a higher metabolic rate can easily eliminate the therapeutic molecule from the circulation without sufficient penetration of therapeutic across BBB.[44,45] Stella et al. modulate the physicochemical property of therapeutic molecules to enhance the penetration across the endothelial membrane of BBB by the transcellular route. This method involves changing the therapeutic molecule's physiochemical property to generate the prodrug through promoiety. To enhance the penetration across BBB and have the intended to impact, the property is added to prodrug. After passing through the BBB moiety is eliminated. For instance, it was found that the utilization of ester prodrugs such as S-acetylthiorphan and m-nitro phenyl nipecotic ester increases brain-focused delivery.[46]

2.10.3 CARRIER-MEDIATED TRANSPORT PATHWAY

There are several endogenous molecules situated in the body that cannot enter the BBB such as neuropeptides, glucose, vitamins, and amino acids. Certain specialized carrier transporters are located in BBB, and through these transporters, endogenous substances can be transported to the BBB which is important for the body. Certain therapeutics that must target the brain are chemically altered as a structure similar to the endogenous molecule, which allows them to be an appropriate transporter or specialized carrier-mediated transporter. One appropriate example is levodopa. Dopamine is converted into levodopa to treat Parkinson's disease. Dopamine cannot be able to cross the BBB, so levodopa is chemically modified from which it can easily enter through the endothelial membrane of the brain under the support of an amino acid transporter. Several other therapeutics such as methyldopa, and gabapentin, utilization of amino acid transporter to enter the therapeutics across the BBB.[47] Dhanawat et al. formed a prodrug form of nipecotic acid to demonstrate the permeability of the drug across the brain barrier in a mouse model and observed that nipecotic acid-L-serine ester prodrug has higher antiepileptic activity and BBB permeation across BBB than nipecotic acid.[48]

There are several solute carriers (SLCs) present on BBB including SLC2, SLC7, and SLC 16. SLC2A, that is, glucose; SLC16A1, that is, lactate pyruvate; SLC7A, that is, cationic amino acids; and SLC7A5, that is, neutral amino acids, all the members of the SLC class of facilitated transporters. SLC2A1, also known as GLUT-1, has mostly been investigated for its function in supplying glucose to the CNS. All these transporters are substantially expressed in CNS ECs compared to EC in nonneural tissues, and help make it easier for glucose to go from the blood into the brain along its concentration gradient. A high-ketone diet is used to treat the epileptic condition that results from Glut1 deficiency in humans. Recent studies were reported to develop poor penetrable drugs. One of the scientists developed niosomes that are coated with dual ligands that target brain endothelial transporters to increase the penetration of cargo, that is, serum albumin attached with Evan Blue. The SLC ligands and glutathione (abbreviated as GSH) such as alanine and glucopyranose were used to advanced niosomes. The absorption of the cargo molecule by the brain endothelial membrane was boosted by the presence of targeting ligands present on niosomes, particularly dual labeling. After treatment with targeted nanocarriers, the absorption of the cargo was increased by adding a positively charged lipid to the biological membrane of the negatively charged surface or dissolving the glycocalyx using neuraminidase. Niosome treatment enhanced plasma membrane permeability, which suggests that nanovesicles and EC membranes have fused. Targeting ligands increased the cargo's permeability across the BBB in the mouse and culture model, and niosomes decorated with two ligands performed better than those decorated with one ligand. resulting that dual labeling with ligands of several SLC transporters being extensively utilized to transport the nanoparticles (NPs) within the BBB. In a comparison with another glucose transporter, the GLUT-1 transporter is situated on both the areas of the abluminal and luminal membrane of the EC of BBB. Apart from these advantages, this method is restricted to only transporting substances that are highly homologous to the intracellular ligands since they can only be carried by intracellular carriers. Additionally, because the carriers are found on the biological membranes, even the size of the drug molecules should be comparable to those of endogenous ligands. Designing peptide nanocarriers is being tested as a means of overcoming these restrictions. A synthetic peptide carrier called K16 apolipoprotein E (ApoE) was developed. The permeability of the BBB might briefly change due to a unique feature of this carrier. Cetuximab and K16ApoE were premixed, and then seven distinct chemotherapeutic substances were administered for various medications, using K16ApoE as a carrier enhanced BBB penetration by a factor of 34–92. Substances that are closely related to D-glucose can be easily transported by insulin-independent glucose transporters. GLUT-1 plays a vital role in the absorption of glucose, and hypoglycemia causes GLUT-1 concentration to increase in the brain. Other glucose transporters, such as GLUT-4, are also present in the brain endothelial along with the GLUT-1 transporter.[47,49] Arora et al. formed a BDNF gene containing surface conjugated mannose target liposome NPs for efficient permeability to the brain for the prevention of Alzheimer's disease (AD). Mannose acts as a GLUT-1 targeted ligand for the entry of therapeutics across BBB. They have demonstrated that mannose-conjugated liposomes showed a 50% higher brain penetration than unmodified liposomes for the prevention of AD.[50]

The transport of particles with GSH functionalization has also been transported by using GSH carrier proteins. After an IV infusion of 7 mg/kg of GSH, functionalized PEG–doxorubicin (DOX) encapsulated liposomes have a 4.9 times enhanced brain-to-blood ratio as compared to PEG–DOX-loaded liposomes without altering the structure of BBB. Antiviral medications might also be transported to the brain via GSH-functionalized pegylated liposomes using the GSH transporter 1.[51] The greatest candidates for delivering substrates to the brain are the hexose and big neutral amino acid nanocarriers since they have the maximum incorporation capacity. To successfully target medications to a particular nutrition transporter, one must have a detailed understanding of both the transporter and the drug.

2.10.4 TRANSCYTOSIS

Though far less frequent in CNS ECs than in ECs in nonneural tissues, transcytosis is upregulated as a key factor in BBB disruption after damage and disorder. Trafficking of caveolin-based vesicles is the mechanism that controls transcytosis through ECs. All ECs express caveolin-1, which is upregulated at the BBB after traumatic brain injury. When compared to CNS ECs, peripheral ECs exhibit higher levels of plasmalemma vesicle-associated protein (PLVAP), which has been linked to leukocyte extravasation, fenestra development, and vesicle trafficking in these leaky vascular. In addition, this substance is elevated in CNS ECs in several disorders where the BBB is leaking. Therefore, it appears that restricting permeability requires the absence of PLVAP in normal CNS ECs. The immune system is very poorly regulated in the healthy CNS, and the parenchyma almost entirely lacks neutrophils and lymphocytes. Rolling adhesion, firm adhesion, and extravasation are all steps in the process by which leukocytes from the blood enter a tissue. Selectins (E-selectin and P-selectin) and members of the immunoglobulin family are required for firm adherence as well as a variety of other leukocyte adhesion molecules. These adhesion molecules are expressed at higher fewer levels in the central nervous EC as compared to peripheral ECs, but at higher levels during neuroinflammatory disorders such as multiple sclerosis (MS) and stroke. It is interesting to note that different inflammatory cell subsets have been shown to invade the CNS in various illnesses. For example, in MS, T cells, B cells, neutrophils, and macrophages are infiltrated in the locations of active abrasion, but in the conditions of stroke, neutrophils, and macrophage infiltrates are present, but lymphocytes are mostly absent. The ability of each cell to traverse the BBB differently and whether discrimination occurs at the degree of the active BBB or the active immunized cell are crucial questions.

2.10.5 RECEPTOR-MEDIATED TRANSCYTOSIS

Larger molecular weight substances, macromolecules such as peptides and proteins, and several particulate formulations including functionalized NPs, drug conjugates, and antibody conjugates can easily endocytose, and all can enter the endothelial membrane of the brain by the receptor-mediated endocytosis. This method developed vesicles comprising the absorbed molecules but its subsequently regulated by receptors that are present on the basolateral surface of the ECs. Only receptor-specific substances can enter the cell through this process. RMT actively targets the therapeutics across BBB. A developed formulation containing a ligand exclusively and selectively targeted to an upregulated receptor. After the interaction of the ligand-receptor, the process of ligand-receptor endocytosis occurs. The drug is then allowed onto the abluminal surface through exocytosis, followed by the migration of the complex of drug and receptor inside the cytoplasmic endothelium. During the transit of the complex of drug and receptor inside the endothelium cytoplasm, several enzymes, endosomes, and lysosomes come into touch along with this. These may or may not break down the candidate's drug. Hence, it is necessary to create a formulation that is unaffected by lysosomes and is stable in the presence of such enzymes. The diffusely distributed transferrin (Tf) receptors, which are found throughout the biological membrane, only transfer to treated vesicles after adhering to that ligand. The majority of low-density lipoprotein receptors (LDL) are situated at the external surface of the membrane, where coated vesicles can exist even in the unavailability of a ligand and the LRP1 transporter can transport substances in both directions. To get enter the BBB, ligand-carrying vesicles can either fuse with a lysosome and exocytosis or attach to another intracellular such as transportation of iron from Tf to intracellular ferritin (Table 2.2).[52]

TABLE 2.2 Types of Receptors and Substrate of RMT Across BBB.

Receptor	Abbrevlations	Substrate
Transferin	TfR	Transferin
Melanotransferrin	MTfR	Melanotransferrin
Insulin	Insulin	Insulin
Leptin	Leptin	Leptin
LDL Receptor Related Protein 1 & 2	LRP1 LRP2	Lipoproteins, amyloid-β ApoE, Melanotransferrin
Interleukin	IL	IL1α, IL1β, IL6
Immunoglobulin G	IgG	IgG
Apolioprotein E	ApoER2	Lipoprotein and ApoE-conjugated molecules
Diptheria toxin Receptor	DTR	

2.10.5.1 TRANSFERRIN RECEPTOR

Tf receptor widely used receptor to target the formulation across BBB. Brain capillaries expressed a significant level of Tf receptors to regulate the supply of iron to enter through BBB. Iron-linked protein, that is, Tf is the natural Tf ligand-receptor ligand. The transmembrane glycoprotein known as the Tf receptor has a disulfide link connecting its two 90 kDa subunits and the components have the capacity to be attached with a single Tf protein. According to various investigations, the limited quantity of Tf is transposed across the endothelial membrane of the brain and deposited there. Tf ligand is very efficient to deliver molecules to the brain.[53] Recently, Tf-conjugated lipid NP was developed for the efficient entry of curcumin into the brain. Curcumin has anti-inflammatory and antioxidant properties to treat neurodegenerative disease, but it has poor bioavailability due to it is not able to enter through the brain barrier. To enhance, the permeability of Tf is conjugated with a lipid NP that is attached to the Tf receptor. The permeability analysis was carried out with hCMEC/D3 cell monolayers in transwell devices, and a 1.5-fold greater penetration of curcumin through the BBB was reported. Both SLNs and nanostructured lipid carriers (NLCs) show promise for the transport of curcumin to the brain because they secure the comprised curcumin and target the brain by including Tf on the surface of the NPs. Cang et al. developed a difunctional erythropoietin Tf receptor fused protein for the prevention of AD. Erythropoietin has a neuroprotective effect, but it is not able to achieve a high concentration in the brain because of less penetrability. When EOP is fused with Tf receptor McAb, leading to delivers a higher concentration of EOP in the mouse brain with AD.[54] Recently, Tf-targeted, PEGylated albumin NPs have been utilized to administer the antiviral medication azidothymidine (AZT) (PEG-NP). Using Tf-targeted PEG-NP, 21.1% of the medication was retrieved from the rat brain, compared to 9.3% for nontargeted PEG-NP after 4 h.[55]

Several studies have demonstrated that anti-Tf receptor antibodies easily transport across the endothelial membrane of BBB as compared to unspecified immunoglobulin and reach the tissue of the BBB in a larger amount. However, further research revealed that the antibody transport was restricted to the endothelial membrane of the brain alone, demonstrating that RMT could not deliver the therapeutic dose of medication across the brain membranes for antibodies such as OX26. They prepared a gold NP associated with 8D3 anti-Tf receptor antibodies that undertaken RMT which is injected into mice IV. Only a few numbers of the vesicles were able to cross by the abluminal membrane because the majority were distracted by endocytosis.[56]

To address this issue, a new approach has been developed which involves manipulation of the antibody's binding affinity. These changes are intended to mirror the natural features of transferrin (Tf), increasing attachment strength and promoting antibody's absorption in the brain. This technique attempts to solve the issue given by the small amount of vesicles that pass the abluminal membrane, since the bulk are redirected by endocytosis. Clark and Davis used a similar method to create a Tf-conjugated gold NP. They introduce an acid cleavage bond between the NP core and Tf ligand. However, allowed for an outflow from endosomal disruption and enhanced conveyance to the parenchymal area.[57] Kang et al developed a DA-containing PEG conjugated liposome, which subsequently attaches with OX26, a monoclonal antibody against the Tf receptor, to the particle. They recognized that dopamine level rises to 8-fold in the BBB tissue using a rat model of Parkinson's disease.[58] Targeted delivery or increased permeability to the brain by using the magnetic NP were evaluated. Thomsen et al., develop a magnetic NP with red fluorescent that is encapsulated in liposome and attached with antibodies (OX26) target Tf receptor in the rat. Resulting, the developed magnetic immunoliposome shows higher transportation through rat ECs of the BBB as compared to a nonconjugated and naked NP and shows the targeted delivery to the Tf receptor.

2.10.5.2 INSULIN RECEPTOR

Insulin is transported across the BBB through the insulin receptor which belongs to the tyrosine kinase-linked receptor family. Amyloid-β peptides interfere with the insulin capacity to connect to insulin receptors during AD, which impairs the brain's ability to use glucose.[59] Amphiphilic diblock copolymer poly(dimethylsiloxane)-block-poly(2-methyl-2-oxazoline) self-assembling polymersomes were utilized to conjugate the anti-insulin Ab receptor. The in vitro research employing the hCMEC/D3 cell line showed that the polymersomes were taken up specifically, resulting in effective targeting.[60] Additionally, the liposome-encapsulated formulation has been delivered across the BBB by using the Human insulin receptor mAbs. It has been demonstrated that pegylated liposomes containing 2000-Da PEG chains are attached with HIR mAbs at the end, leading to tyrosine hydrolase-specific siRNA over the BBB. It has also been investigated how the mannose 6-phosphate (M6P) receptor, popularly called the insulin-like growth factor II (IGF-II) receptor, moves through the BBB of newborn mice. The M6P receptor works by interacting with the M6P component of lysosomal enzymes, which causes internalization and lysosomal sorting. It had been demonstrated in the past that the 312 kDa enzyme β-glucuronidase (GUS) was only available to the brain during the initial 2 weeks of birth. The lysosomal storage disease mucopolysaccharidosis type VII is due to a shortage of this enzyme. P-GUS penetrated the brain when radiolabeled and phosphorylated-GUS (131I-P-GUS) and nonphosphorylated GUS were injected into newborn mice, however nonphosphorylated GUS absorption was noticeably lower. Transport of 131I-P-GUS stopped being substantial around 7 weeks of age. These findings demonstrated that RMT via the M6P/IGF-II receptor occurs in P-GUS early in postnatal development but not in adulthood.[61]

2.10.5.3 LIPOPROTEIN RECEPTOR-RELATED PROTEIN

A multifunctional protein called lipoprotein receptor-related protein (LRP) may be linked with a wide range of receptors to regulate their endocytosis, including Apoprotein E, lactoferrin, plasminogen activator, β-amyloid initiator protein, and others. Many tissues, including the CNS and malignancies, express LRP. Lipoprotein receptor-related associated protein is present in the cerebellum, neuronal cells, and astrocytes. Abnormal astrocytomas particularly glioblastomas have higher levels of LRP expression. Recently, ApoE-modified liposomes were created (AD) to increase BBB uptake and deliver rosmarinic acid (RA) and quercetin (QU) to prevent β-amyloid[1–42] and (A1-42)-caused AD. The dual-activity of apoprotein E-quercetin-rosmarinic acid-PA-liposomes' improved capacity to penetrate the brain and maintain high endothelial feasibility as compared to Tween 80-quercetin-*Rosmarinus*-PA-liposomes was confirmed by utilizing an in vitro BBB model. According to immunochemical staining images, Apoprotein E-quercetin-rosmarinic acid-PA-liposomes were able to cross the BBB due to strong interactions between ApoE and brain vascular ECs low-density lipoprotein receptors (LDLP), They also prevented the death of A1-42-insulted SK-N-MC cells by inhibiting apoptosis. ApoE-QU-RA-PA-liposomes reduced acetylcholinesterase efficiency, and lipid peroxidation concentration, as well as Aβ plaque development in an in vivo AD model. A possible method for delivering QU and RA to the brain and crossing the BBB to treat A1-42-induced neurotoxicity is surface-modified liposomes utilizing PA and ApoE.[62]

Melanotransferrin (MTf) enters the brain with the help of the LRP1 receptor. in comparison to TfR, LRP1 has a larger capable receptor that can be used to carry drugs to cross the BBB. Kalkan et al. affected the model of a mouse by intracranial tumor, LPR1 receptor was decided to the administration of DOX attached with MTf, which enhanced the survival of the mouse. Since lactoferrin is generally present at extremely less physiological concentrations, it is another intriguing vector for targeting LRP1. In a rotenone-induced model of rats in the case of Parkinson's disease, this was demonstrated by attaching lactoferrin through a PEG spacer to PAMAM dendrimers that could multipart a neurotrophic inheritable factor and provide neuroprotective effects.[63] However, ligand-derived peptides are being used in clinical research (finished phase II trials) to create a formulation for the prevention of both primary and advanced brain cancers. According to the aprotinin structural model, Angiochem has created BBB-permeable peptides known as angiopep nanoparticles. A sequence of 19-amino-acid peptides, known as angiopep nanonparticles, is transcytosis rapidly by the LRP-1 and LRP-2 receptors and is generated from the aprotinin Kunitz domain. In clinical studies with cancer patients, paclitaxel attached to the LRP receptor ligand angiopep-2, which is shown to go through receptor-mediated endocytosis, had positive results. The medicament was found secure and easily tolerable.[64,65]

2.10.5.4 FOLATE RECEPTOR

Another strategy, if executed effectively, involves reaching the brain by folate receptor-mediated endocytosis with the benefit of avoiding endosomal destruction. Based on the clinical brain tumor investigation, the utilization of micelle-type NPs for the transport of Cyt-C and the formation of redox-sensitive linkage between folic acid and NPs leads to efficient brain targeting.[66] In a different approach, for the specified administration of the antineoplastic drug, they prepare a nanocrystal embellished with folic acid for enhanced effect and targeted delivery. Cellular uptake experiments in human and glioblastoma cells of rat brains demonstrated the system undertaking RMT.[67]

2.10.5.5 GLUTAMATE RECEPTOR

Metabotropic glutamate receptors type 1 is a type of heptahelical receptor that is linked with various illnesses including anxiety, Pain, epilepsy, and drug addiction. A bi-specific Abs was created that targets BBB transmigration, and the immunoglobulin-G Abs appose to the type-1 glutamate receptor. The secondary Ab was produced from the camelid nanobodies. These antibodies effectively inhibited heat algesia and showed excellent penetration. Recently observed that metabotropic glutamate receptors type-1 inhibitor is used to treat SAH by reducing the glutamate level. By utilizing the rat SAH model, they discovered that SAH enhances the cerebrospinal fluid glutamate levels and BBB permeability in the initial phases of brain injury, that intracerebroventricular infusion of exogenous glutamate worsened BBB damage and cerebral edema, and that intraperitoneal administration of JNJ16259685, a metabotropic glutamate receptor 1 (mGluR1) inhibitor remarkably reduced SAH-induced BBB damage and cerebral human brain microvascular endothelial cells (HBMVEC) exhibited enhanced monolayer permeability in an in vitro BBB model when exposed to glutamate, but JNJ16259685 protected the integrity of the BBB after glutamate injury to HBMVEC.[68]

2.10.5.6 INTERLEUKIN- 13 RECEPTOR α2

Interleukin-13 receptor α2 is the important receptor that comes under the family of IL-13 cytokine receptors without signaling activity. IL-13Rα2 specified isoform that regulation gets increased in glioblastoma different form and goes through internalization and stimulate by ligand. Pep-1 (CGEMGWVRC) peptide is recognized to transport the medicament to enter through BBB. The same study is promoted by the development of copolymer NPs linked with pep-1 for delivery of paclitaxel. In a glioma-causing mice model with C6 glioma cells, an in vitro study was evaluated to observe the increased transportation of paclitaxel across the BBB for the prevention of glioma.[69] Further dual targeting approach utilizes the two ligands for the targeting of two receptors to transport the drug. A polymeric NP is prepared that is conjugated with IL-13 which acts as a ligand for IL-13Rα2, and arginylglycylaspartic acid (RGD) acts as a ligand for αvβ3 integrin receptors such as vitronectin, osteopontin, fibrinogen on cerebrovasculature. Dual targeting not only incorporates NPs to a higher extent but also leads to claritin-mediated endocytosis in the position of micropinocytosis of the IL-13 peptide ligand.

A further advanced approach was also developed, the utilization of one type of ligand for the targeting of two different receptors. Octa-arginine is a cell-invading enzyme that is linked with dGR and develops a tandem peptide that acts as a ligand for neuropilin-1 and αvβ3 receptors. Liposome containing paclitaxel prepared with tandem peptide. The result shows the enhanced effect of suppressing a malignant cancerous cell. Recently, Kurihara et al.

utilized a hybrid peptide to target the Interleukin-13 Receptor α2 for effective glioblastoma therapy. In this study, the IL-13R2-lytic hybrid peptide was created by joining this peptide with a lytic peptide that contained a linker sequence. In vitro testing of the IL-13R2-lytic hybrid peptide against glioblastoma cell lines revealed cytotoxic action. Additionally, the IL-13R2-lytic hybrid peptide impacted the activation of Akt and Erk1/2 after interleukin-13 administration and produced quick ATP dynamics in glioblastoma cells. After intratumoral administration, antitumor efficacy of the IL-13R2-lytic hybrid peptide was seen in a mice xenograft model of glioblastoma cells of humans. It was reported that an effective treatment alternative for glioblastoma patients may be an IL-13R2-lytic hybrid peptide.[70]

2.10.5.7 LEPTIN RECEPTOR

Leptin receptors are present on the choroid plexus and ECs of brain capillaries, leptins are bound to leptin receptors induced by the peripheral adipocytes and occupied by the parenchyma of BBB. As an endogenous protein leptin shows a larger intake in rats, Barrette et al. prepared a DNA complexed leptin conjugated pegylated poly-lysine dendrimers showing the highest gene exhibited on BBB.[71]

2.10.5.8 DIPHTHERIA TOXIN RECEPTOR/HEPARIN BINDING EPIDERMAL GROWTH FACTOR-LIKE GROWTH FACTOR

In getting to transport drugs through the endothelial membrane of the brain, Gaillard et al., used a CRM197, a harmless variant of diphtheria toxin. This mutant has a history of successful usage in human therapies, having served as a transport protein for human immunizations since the mid of 1980s and more recently exhibiting some level of anticancer action in humans Gaillard et al. investigated the ability of CRM197 for entry to the brain. CRM197 was reported to endocytose after engaging the epidermal membrane binding forerunner of heparin-attached epidermal growth factor-like growth factor (HB-EGF), also identified as the diphtheria toxin receptor. An in vitro BBB model employing rat astrocytes and bovine brain capillaries was utilized to report the transporting ability of CRM197 when it was coupled to the protein indicator, that is, horseradish peroxidase (HRP). These tests showed transcytosis, during the beginning time delay and went slowly for several hours. Furthermore, the CRM197-HRP conjugate was IV administered into the brains of guinea pigs, and the HRP resulting mixture was mostly found trapped in blood vessels of the brain, supporting the in vitro findings that suggested a stagnant frequency of transcytosis. However, some HRPs are evaluated which show complete transcytosis into the parenchyma of the brain. The utilization of neutralizing Ab apposed to CRM197 from prior vaccinations is mentioned by the authors as an issue for the CRM197, but they also mention anticancer clinical trials that recognized that the level of neutralizing Abs dropped dramatically after continuous treatment.[72]

2.10.5.9 NICOTINIC ACETYLCHOLINE RECEPTOR

Nicotinic acetylcholine receptor is evaluated by the mechanism of transportation of 29 amino acid peptide complex entered by the brain endothelial membrane which is acquired from rabies glycoprotein (RGV29). These amino acid complexes are developed by a D-arginine-9-mer along with siRNA that is attached with a short triglycine spacer. Transportation of these complexes is restricted by bungarotoxin, that is, they act like a substrate, indicating the entry of RVG29 in the brain with the help of a receptor given by the nicotinic Ach receptor substrate, that is, bungarotoxin. Cationic liposomal siRNA attached with RVG29 leads to cellular protein gene knockdown. Wilkin et al. prepared an RVG29-tagged PAMAM dendrimer gene complex. Bungarotoxin acts as a substrate for the GABA-B receptor. The transportation of these prepared gene complexes is not restricted by the GABA-B, nicotinic antagonist, and agonist receptor uptake involvement cannot be prohibited. In recent studies, RVG29 peptide was functionalized on solid lipid nanoparticles (SLNs) and nanolipid carriers containing QU to increase the uptake of the drug into the brain through the nicotinic acetylcholine receptor.[73]

2.10.6 ADSORPTIVE-MEDIATED TRANSCYTOSIS

Adsorptive-mediated transcytosis is based on the direct association of a therapeutic substance with an anionic surface of BBB and transports the drug from one side, that is, luminal side to the other side, that is, the basolateral side by the formation of a vesicle. The transportation of antibodies and albumin can be potentiated by cationic alteration. Absorptive-mediated transcytosis is regulated by the electrostatic interaction (van der Waals interaction) between the cationic charged peptide such as albumin and an anionic charged surface of BBB. Electrostatic interaction is further facilitated through the sialic acid and heparin surface group expressed on both sides of the endothelial membrane. Large molecular weight compounds and β-endorphin are not able to enter through the endothelial membrane. The permeability of these molecules gets enhanced when it is conjugated with cationic albumin. Absorptive-mediated endocytosis has a lesser binding potential as compared to RMT. Cationic molecule provides a higher binding capacity to AMT. Cationic albumin acts as a ligand, In recent studies, the author prepared cationic albumin conjugated with a chelating agent of iron, that is, deferasirox to prevent AD. Iron is involved in protein destruction and oxidative stress resulting in neuronal harm. To demonstrate the efficient delivery of formulation through AMT, in vitro and in vivo studies were reported. Results evaluated the system can protect from neuronal damage and decreases the amyloid β aggregate causing learning impairment. Cationic bovine serum c bovine serum albumin also enhances the permeability of therapeutic across BBB through AMT. In addition, polyethylene glycol-poly chic acid conjugated with cationic bovine serum albumin shows a higher transcytosis to transport the drug across BBB. In further studies, DOX encapsulated SLN were prepared that are conjugated with cationic bovine serum albumin.[74] The result showed that higher absorptive mediated transcytosis occurs in the HNGC-1 cell line and enhanced pharmacokinetic properties are also seen in in vivo studies. GM-1 is the form of glycosphingolipid, a transcytosis receptor expressed on the endothelial membrane of the brain for the permeability of cholera toxin B. GM1 targeted ganglioside polymersomes go through transcytosis across BBB. Apart from that, Numerous in vitro studies revealed that amphiphilic cell-penetrating peptides (CPPs) were more effective in crossing the BBB; however, in vivo studies suggested that cationic CPPs were superior to amphiphilic CPPs in terms of permeability into the brain parenchyma. Due to electrostatic interactions, cationic CPP was thought to be rather susceptible to being trapped by cellular organelles. A neutral cyclic heptapeptide was developed by Yamaguchi et al. as a BBB permeable peptide that could transfer conjugated macromolecules via the BBB. In contrast to the negatively charged linear CPP, it was expected that the cyclic configuration and charge neutrality show reduced electrostatic interactions and greater stability against proteases. Zhang et al. examined the therapeutic properties of CB5005 CPP and demonstrated its antitumor synergistic impact with DOX to draw attention to the issue. Their research indicates that CB5005 has considerable antitumor properties in addition to being able to enter cell nuclei and target and suppress NF-B activity in gliomas. These characteristics enable the CB5005 to work as a dual CPP. In a subsequent investigation, the CB5005 was also employed to improve the properties of the DOX-loaded liposomes to draw out both its anticancer efficacy and influence on aiding liposome transportation.[75]

There is another type of cell-permeating protein known as TAT protein. It is derived from immune deficiency virus 1. TAT peptide increases the transcription of viral genes and was originally produced from nondistracted HIV-1 infected cells. That is visible in HIV-1 infected serum and supernatant of ex vivo culture. TAT can enter infected and uninfected endothelial brain cells, but the accurate transportation mechanism of TAT is still not clear. The permeability of ciprofloxacin was improved by the joining of cholesteryl chloroformate with TAT peptide (YGRKKRRQRRR, an amino acid sequence of TAT peptide.) go through absorptive mediated transcytosis. TAT peptide contains an arginine amino acid having a higher uptake as compared to other amino acid residues such as histidine, lysine, and ornithine. In addition, pAnt TAT peptide with the sequence of RQIKIWFQNRRMKWKK and SynB5 with peptide sequence of RGGRLAYLRRRWAVLGR having a higher arginine residue shows the penetration through the endothelial membrane of the brain through AMT. Chan et al. recognized a dual strategy, absorptive mediated transcytosis along with RMT. They prepared a procationic liposome containing liposomes that are modified with lactoferrin for brain cancer. Further preparation was also developed with mannose-modified albumin along with cationic albumin that is conjugated with DOX NPs for glioma. Both the system approaches show the decreased size of a tumor in the glioma model of rats. Herve et al., cationic the antibodies to enhance the brain permeation to penetrate the BBB. The current therapy of tetanus is upgraded by employing a cationization of antitetanus Fab-2 fragment binding by forming a van der Waals interaction with the anionic charge on the surface of the EC of BBB. Liposomes containing drugs and other NPs are attached to cationic targets and can easily arrive at brain parenchyma through an absorptive mediated transcytosis.[76]

2.10.7 EFFLUX TRANSPORTER

ECs of BBB show different types of efflux transporter driven by ATP including P-glycoprotein and multi -resistant protein (MRP) (MRP1, MRP3, MRP4, and MRP6), SLC transporter (SLC12 and SLC13) having a wider role to throw out the drugs from the brain. These transporters are the subtypes of adenosine triphosphate binding cassette (ABC) transporter. This transporter restricted the brain targeting of medicament. Multidrug resistance (MDR) transporter permeates the amphiphilic, cationic, and natural substances through the BBB to blood. Numerous of these transporters carry a variety of substrates into the blood compartment and are concentrated on the lumenal surface. These transporters can block many tiny lipophilic compounds which would otherwise passively diffuse through the EC membrane thanks to the large variety of substrates they can bind to. Mdr1, also known as P-glycoprotein P-glycoprotein is mostly studied as an efflux transporter that regulates efflux transporter expressed on an EC of the brain, succeed by breast cancer resistance-associated protein and MDR protein. Larger concentrations of drugs are maintained by the inhibition of P-glycoprotein (P-gp) transporter by the use of P-glycoprotein (P-gp) inhibitors for the prevention of various types of CNS disorders and also enhance brain targeting. P-glycoprotein prevents the transportation of a wide range of substances such as antineoplastic drugs including DOX, methotrexate, and vinblastine. Recently, it was demonstrated that the ABCB1 knocked out mouse model shows the inhibitory activity on P-glycoprotein accretion and dispositioning of therapeutic in the parts of the brain. The activity of P-glycoprotein can be changed in the condition of meningitis. In the case of *Streptococcus agalactiae*, it acts as a meningitis pathogen and causes the prevention of P-glycoprotein expression and activity. In further studies, breast cancer resistance protein (Bcrp) was demonstrated, it is expressed on a cell line of breast cancer that is resistant to chemotherapeutics but it has no activity in breast malignant cells. P-glycoprotein (P-gp) and breast cancer resistance protein (Bcrp) transporter are widely overlapped with each other. Both the transporter exhibits the preventive activity from a harmful molecule. Two phosphatidylinositol 3-kinase PI3k targets of rapamycin inhibitors, GNE-317 and GDC-0980, also block efflux pumps in various ways. GNE317 has 3-fold higher permeability than GDC-0980 in an animal model of C57B6/J mice with intracranial, making them crucial for the prevention of glioblastoma.[76]

Fingolimod (FTY720) is an approved prodrug for the prevention of MS. This prodrug is transformed into phosphorylate compound that acts as an agonist on the sphingosine phosphate receptor. Fingolimod and sphingosine phosphate are observed, and both prevent the P-gp receptor. The absorption of radiolabeled verapamil, paclitaxel, and loperamide concentration increased in the brain when sphingosine phosphate and fingolimod (FTY720) were coadministered. This suggests that concomitant use of the medications with fingolimod or sphingosine 1-phosphate may increase the penetration of the therapeutics to the brain EC.[77] Further studies were also evaluated, and the activity of riluzole utilized for amyotrophic lateral sclerosis (ALS) management, is decreased because of p-glycoprotein efflux transporter causes the abnormal quantity in the brain. One of the researchers formulated a codelivery system based on liposomes which a prepared by a lipid film hydration method. Riluzole coadministered with verapamil acts as a P-glycoprotein inhibitor. Results demonstrate that the concentration of riluzole is increased by the prevention of the P-glycoprotein transporter. In recent studies, the prevention of P-gp transporter was also identified by using one more strategy. Cediranib is an inhibitor of a vascular endothelial (VE) growth factor receptor that is reported for the suppression of glioblastoma multiforme. Cediranib is a P-gp substrate, and it has limited penetration across BBB. P-gp inhibitor and P-gp/Bcrp inhibitor are coadministered with cediranib showing a higher concentration of the drug in the mice brain.[78] Similarly, simultaneous administration of elacridar (P-gp/Bcrp) with sorafenib, that is, multitargeted inhibitor of tyrosine kinase leads to higher penetration across BBB. Pluronic block copolymer, that is, Pluronic P85 is a P-gp inhibitor, and it can increase the transportation of antineoplastic drugs such as digoxin, valproic acid, and loperamide. Similarly, Pluronic P85 also prevents MDR-associated proteins such as MRP1 and MRP2. The permeability of the drug rhodamine 123 is enhanced when the concentration of Pluronic 68 is lesser than the critical micelle concentration (CMC) but if the concentration gets higher, it will not show activity. In addition, pluronic P85 was demonstrated to be a chemosensitive multiresistance tumor and enhance the activity and potency of DOX by enhancing the apoptotic signaling in the malignant cell. Chemotherapeutics are unable to reach therapeutically important quantities inside cancer cells due to efflux transporter-mediated MDR. In this work, the effects of two LAT1-using variants of probenecid (PRB), which may inhibit organic anion transporters (OATs) and MRPs, on the induction of apoptosis in cancer cells, both alone and in conjunction with vinblastine (VBL) were examined. After in vivo rat brain infusion and intraperitoneal delivery to mice, the rate and extent of vinblastine uptake in the brain along with the most promising LAT1-using efflux inhibitor were examined. Therefore, these focused inhibitors considerably enhanced the apoptosis-inducing effects of VBL and did so in a higher efficient way as compared to PRB alone. Additionally, they were harmless to live cells and hemocompatible, making them suitable for various biomedical applications.[79]

KEYWORDS

- **blood-brain barrier**
- **transport mechanisms**
- **brain endothelial cells**
- **CNS**
- **tight junction**
- **receptor-mediated transcytosis**
- **signaling molecules**

REFERENCES

1. Pandit, R.; Chen, L.; Götz, J. The Blood-brain Barrier: Physiology and Strategies for Drug Delivery. *Adv. Drug Deliv. Rev.* **2020,** *165–166,* 1–14. https://doi.org/10.1016/j.addr.2019.11.009
2. Choudhari, M.; Hejmady, S.; Narayan Saha, R.; Damle, S.; Singhvi, G.; Alexander, A.; Kesharwani, P.; Kumar Dubey, S. Evolving New-age Strategies to Transport Therapeutics Across the Blood-brain Barrier. *Int. J. Pharm.* **2021,** *599,* 120351. https://doi.org/10.1016/j.ijpharm.2021.120351
3. Benz, F.; Liebner, S. Structure and Function of the Blood-Brain Barrier (BBB). In *Handbook of Experimental Pharmacology*; 2022; Vol. 273, pp 3–31. https://doi.org/10.1007/164_2020_404
4. Abbott, N. J.; Patabendige, A. A.; Dolman, D. E.; Yusof, S. R.; Begley, D. J. Structure and Function of the Blood-brain Barrier. *Neurobiol. Dis.* **2010,** *37* (1), 13–25. https://doi.org/10.1016/j.nbd.2009.07.030
5. Pandey, P. K.; Sharma, A. K.; Rani, S.; Mishra, G.; Kandasamy, G.; Patra, A. K.; ... Gupta, U. MCM-41 Nanoparticles for Brain Delivery: Better Choline-esterase and Amyloid Formation Inhibition with Improved Kinetics. *ACS Biomater. Sci. Eng.* **2018,** *4* (8), 2860–2869. https://doi.org/10.1021/acsbiomaterials.8b00335
6. Singh, A. K.; Gothwal, A.; Rani, S.; Rana, M.; Sharma, A. K.; Yadav, A. K.; Gupta, U. Dendrimer Donepezil Conjugates for Improved Brain Delivery and Better In Vivo Pharmacokinetics. *ACS Omega* **2019,** *4* (3), 4519–4529. https://doi.org/10.1021/acsomega.8b03445
7. Terstappen, G. C.; Meyer, A. H.; Bell, R. D.; Zhang, W. Strategies for Delivering Therapeutics Across the Blood-brain Barrier. *Nat. Reviews. Drug Discov.* **2021,** *20* (5), 362–383. https://doi.org/10.1038/s41573-021-00139-y
8. Daneman, R.; Prat, A. The Blood-brain Barrier. *Cold Spring Harb. Perspect. Biol.* **2015,** *7* (1), a020412. https://doi.org/10.1101/cshperspect.a020412
9. Bernacki, J.; Dobrowolska, A.; Nierwińska, K.; Małecki, A. Physiology and Pharmacological Role of the Blood-brain Barrier. *Pharmacol. Rep.* **2008,** *60* (5), 600–622.

10. Kaplan, L.; Chow, B. W.; Gu, C. Neuronal Regulation of the Blood-brain Barrier and Neurovascular Coupling. *Nat. Rev. Neurosci.* **2020,** *21* (8), 416–432. https://doi.org/10.1038/s41583-020-0322-2
11. Pollak, T. A.; Drndarski, S.; Stone, J. M.; David, A. S.; McGuire, P.; Abbott, N. J. The Blood-brain Barrier in Psychosis. *Lancet Psychiatry* **2018,** *5* (1), 79–92. https://doi.org/10.1016/S2215-0366(17)30293-6
12. Bonney, S. K.; Sullivan, L. T.; Cherry, T. J.; Daneman, R.; Shih, A. Y. Distinct Features of Brain Perivascular Fibroblasts and Mural Cells Revealed by *in vivo* Two-photon Imaging. *J. Cereb. Blood Flow Metab.* **2022,** *42* (6), 966–978. https://doi.org/10.1177/0271678X211068528
13. Hartmann, D. A.; Coelho-Santos, V.; Shih, A. Y. Pericyte Control of Blood Flow Across Microvascular Zones in the Central Nervous System. *Annu. Rev. Physiol.* **2022,** *84,* 331–354. https://doi.org/10.1146/annurev-physiol-061121-040127
14. Xu, L.; Nirwane, A.; Yao, Y. Basement Membrane and Blood-brain Barrier. *Stroke Vasc. Neurol.* **2018,** *4* (2), 78–82. https://doi.org/10.1136/svn-2018-000198
15. Liebner, S.; Dijkhuizen, R. M.; Reiss, Y.; Plate, K. H.; Agalliu, D.; Constantin, G. Functional Morphology of the Blood-brain Barrier in Health And Disease. *Acta Neuropathol.* **2018,** *135* (3), 311–336. https://doi.org/10.1007/s00401-018-1815-1
16. Galea I. The Blood-brain Barrier in Systemic Infection and Inflammation. *Cell. Mol. Immunol.* **2021,** *18* (11), 2489–2501. https://doi.org/10.1038/s41423-021-00757-x
17. Furtado, D.; Björnmalm, M.; Ayton, S.; Bush, A. I.; Kempe, K.; Caruso, F. Overcoming the Blood-Brain Barrier: The Role of Nanomaterials in Treating Neurological Diseases. *Adv. Mater.* **2018,** *30* (46), e1801362. https://doi.org/10.1002/adma.201801362
18. Huang, X.; Hussain, B.; Chang, J. Peripheral Inflammation and Blood-brain Barrier Disruption: Effects and Mechanisms. *CNS Neurosci. Therapeut.* **2021,** *27* (1), 36–47. https://doi.org/10.1111/cns.13569
19. Alexander J. J. Blood-brain Barrier (BBB) and the Complement Landscape. *Mol. Immunol.* **2018,** *102*, 26–31. https://doi.org/10.1016/j.molimm.2018.06.267
20. Yang, C.; Hawkins, K. E.; Doré, S.; Candelario-Jalil, E. Neuroinflammatory Mechanisms of Blood-brain Barrier Damage in Ischemic Stroke. *Am. J. Physiol. Cell Physiol.* **2019,** *316* (2), C135–C153. https://doi.org/10.1152/ajpcell.00136.2018
21. Otani, T.; Furuse, M. Tight Junction Structure and Function Revisited. *Trends Cell Biol.* **2020,** *30* (10), 805–817. https://doi.org/10.1016/j.tcb.2020.08.004
22. Tsukita, S.; Tanaka, H.; Tamura, A. The Claudins: From Tight Junctions to Biological Systems. *Trends Biochem. Sci.* **2019,** *44* (2), 141–152. https://doi.org/10.1016/j.tibs.2018.09.008
23. Kadry, H.; Noorani, B.; Cucullo, L. A Blood-brain Barrier Overview on Structure, Function, Impairment, and Biomarkers of Integrity. *Fluids Barriers CNS* **2020,** *17* (1), 69. https://doi.org/10.1186/s12987-020-00230-3
24. Sharif, Y.; Jumah, F.; Coplan, L.; Krosser, A.; Sharif, K.; Tubbs, R. S. Blood-brain Barrier: A Review of Its Anatomy and Physiology in Health and Disease. *Clin. Anat.* **2018,** *31* (6), 812–823. https://doi.org/10.1002/ca.23083
25. Castro Dias, M.; Mapunda, J. A.; Vladymyrov, M.; Engelhardt, B. Structure and Junctional Complexes of Endothelial, Epithelial, and Glial Brain Barriers. *Int. J. Mol. Sci.* **2019,** *20* (21), 5372. https://doi.org/10.3390/ijms20215372
26. Hartmann, C.; Schwietzer, Y. A.; Otani, T.; Furuse, M.; Ebnet, K. Physiological Functions of Junctional Adhesion Molecules (JAMs) in Tight Junctions. *Biochim. Biophys. Acta Biomembr.* **2020,** *1862* (9), 183299. https://doi.org/10.1016/j.bbamem.2020.183299

27. Li, J.; Zheng, M.; Shimoni, O.; Banks, W. A.; Bush, A. I.; Gamble, J. R.; Shi, B. Development of Novel Therapeutics Targeting the Blood-Brain Barrier: From Barrier to Carrier. *Adv. Sci. (Weinh.)* **2021,** *8* (16), e2101090. https://doi.org/10.1002/advs.202101090
28. Profaci, C. P.; Munji, R. N.; Pulido, R. S.; Daneman, R. The Blood-brain Barrier in Health and Disease: Important Unanswered Questions. *J. Exp. Med.* **2020,** *217* (4), e20190062. https://doi.org/10.1084/jem.20190062
29. Palomer, E.; Buechler, J.; Salinas, P. C. Wnt Signaling Deregulation in the Aging and Alzheimer's Brain. *Front. Cell. Neurosci.* **2019,** *13,* 227. https://doi.org/10.3389/fncel.2019.00227
30. Benz, F.; Liebner, S. Structure and Function of the Blood-Brain Barrier (BBB). In *Handbook of Experimental Pharmacology*; 2022; Vol. 273, pp 3–31. https://doi.org/10.1007/164_2020_404
31. Rhea, E. M.; Banks, W. A. Role of the Blood-Brain Barrier in Central Nervous System Insulin Resistance. *Front. Neurosci.* **2019,** *13,* 521. https://doi.org/10.3389/fnins.2019.00521
32. Preston, J. E.; Joan Abbott, N.; Begley, D. J. Transcytosis of Macromolecules at the Blood-brain Barrier. *Adv. Pharmacol.* **2014,** *71,* 147–163. https://doi.org/10.1016/bs.apha.2014.06.001
33. Shackleton, B.; Ringland, C.; Abdullah, L.; Mullan, M.; Crawford, F.; Bachmeier, C. Influence of Matrix Metallopeptidase 9 on Beta-Amyloid Elimination Across the Blood-Brain Barrier. *Mol. Neurobiol.* **2019,** *56* (12), 8296–8305. https://doi.org/10.1007/s12035-019-01672-z
34. Bernacki, J.; Dobrowolska, A.; Nierwińska, K.; Małecki, A. Physiology and Pharmacological Role of the Blood-brain Barrier. *Pharmacol. Rep.* **2008,** *60* (5), 600–622.
35. Zhao, Y.; Gan, L.; Ren, L.; Lin, Y.; Ma, C.; Lin, X. Factors Influencing the Blood-brain Barrier Permeability. *Brain Res.* **2022,** *1788,* 147937. https://doi.org/10.1016/j.brainres.2022.147937
36. Lasek-Bal, A.; Jedrzejowska-Szypulka, H.; Student, S.; Warsz-Wianecka, A.; Zareba, K.; Puz, P.; Bal, W.; Pawletko, K.; Lewin-Kowalik, J. The Importance of Selected Markers of Inflammation and Blood-Brain Barrier Damage for Short Term Ischemic Stroke Prognosis. *J. Physiol. Pharmacol.* **2019,** *70* (2), https://doi.org/10.26402/jpp.2019.2.04
37. Bowman, G. L.; Dayon, L.; Kirkland, R.; Wojcik, J.; Peyratout, G.; Severin, I. C.; Henry, H.; Oikonomidi, A.; Migliavacca, E.; Bacher, M.; Popp, J. Blood-brain Barrier Breakdown, Neuroinflammation, and Cognitive Decline in Older Adults. *Alzheimer's Dement'.* **2018,** *14* (12), 1640–1650. https://doi.org/10.1016/j.jalz.2018.06.2857
38. Solarz, A.; Majcher-Maślanka, I.; Chocyk, A. Effects of Early-life Stress and Sex on Blood-Brain Barrier Permeability and Integrity in Juvenile and Adult Rats. *Dev. Neurobiol.* **2021,** *81* (7), 861–876. https://doi.org/10.1002/dneu.22846
39. Małkiewicz, M. A.; Szarmach, A.; Sabisz, A.; Cubała, W. J.; Szurowska, E.; Winklewski, P. J. Blood-brain Barrier Permeability and Physical Exercise. *J. Neuroinflam.* **2019,** *16* (1), 15. https://doi.org/10.1186/s12974-019-1403-x
40. Harilal, S.; Jose, J.; Parambi, D.; Kumar, R.; Unnikrishnan, M. K.; Uddin, M. S.; Mathew, G. E.; Pratap, R.; Marathakam, A.; Mathew, B. Revisiting the Blood-brain barrier: A Hard Nut to Crack in the Transportation of Drug Molecules. *Brain Res. Bull.* **2020,** *160,* 121–140. https://doi.org/10.1016/j.brainresbull.2020.03.018
41. Choudhari, M.; Hejmady, S.; Narayan Saha, R.; Damle, S.; Singhvi, G.; Alexander, A.; Kesharwani, P.; Kumar Dubey, S. Evolving New-age Strategies to Transport

Therapeutics Across the Blood-brain Barrier. *Int. J. Pharm.* **2021,** *59 9*, 120351. https://doi.org/10.1016/j.ijpharm.2021.120351
42. Irudayanathan, F. J.; Wang, N.; Wang, X.; Nangia, S. The Architecture of the Paracellular Channels Formed by Claudins of the Blood-brain Barrier Tight Junctions. *Ann. N. Y. Acad. Sci.* **2017,** *1405* (1), 131–146. https://doi.org/10.1111/nyas.13378
43. Azarmi, M.; Maleki, H.; Nikkam, N.; Malekinejad, H. Transcellular Brain Drug Delivery: A Review on Recent Advancements. *Int. J. Pharm.* **2020,** *586*, 119582. https://doi.org/10.1016/j.ijpharm.2020.119582
44. De Bock, M.; Van Haver, V.; Vandenbroucke, R. E.; Decrock, E.; Wang, N.; Leybaert, L. Into Rather Unexplored Terrain-transcellular Transport Across the blood-brain Barrier. *Glia* **2016,** *64* (7), 1097–1123. https://doi.org/10.1002/glia.22960
45. Lalatsa, A.; Butt, A. M. Physiology of the Blood-brain Barrier and Mechanisms of Transport Across the BBB. In *Nanotechnology-Based Targeted Drug Delivery Systems for Brain Tumors*; Academic Press, 2018; pp 49–74.
46. Stella, V. J.; Nti-Addae, K. W. Prodrug Strategies to Overcome Poor Water Solubility. *Adv. Drug Deliv. Rev.* **2007,** *59* (7), 677–694. https://doi.org/10.1016/j.addr.2007.05.013
47. Tsuji, A.; Tamai, I. I.; Carrier-mediated or Specialized Transport of Drugs Across the Blood-brain Barrier. *Adv. Drug Deliv. Rev.* **1999,** *36* (2 and 3), 277–290. https://doi.org/10.1016/s0169-409x(98)00084-2
48. Dhanawat, M.; Gupta, S.; Mehta, D. K.; Das, R. Design, Synthesis and Enhanced BBB Penetration Studies of L-serine-Tethered Nipecotic Acid-Prodrug. *Drug research* **2021,** *71* (2), 94–103. https://doi.org/10.1055/a-1290-0119
49. Liu, X. SLC Family Transporters. *Adv. Exp. Med. Biol.* **2019,** *1141*, 101–202. https://doi.org/10.1007/978-981-13-7647-4_3
50. Arora, S.; Sharma, D.; Singh, J. GLUT-1: An Effective Target to Deliver Brain-Derived Neurotrophic Factor Gene Across the Blood Brain Barrier. *ACS Chem. Neurosci.* **2020,** *11* (11), 1620–1633. https://doi.org/10.1021/acschemneuro.0c00076
51. Birngruber, T.; Raml, R.; Gladdines, W.; Gatschelhofer, C.; Gander, E.; Ghosh, A.; Kroath, T.; Gaillard, P. J.; Pieber, T. R.; Sinner, F. Enhanced Doxorubicin Delivery to the Brain Administered through Glutathione PEGylated Liposomal Doxorubicin (2B3-101) as Compared with Generic Caelyx, (®)/Doxil(®)—A Cerebral Open Flow Microperfusion Pilot Study. *J. Pharm. Sci.* **2014,** *103* (7), 1945–1948. https://doi.org/10.1002/jps.23994
52. Kadry, H.; Noorani, B.; Cucullo, L. A Blood-brain Barrier Overview on Structure, Function, Impairment, and Biomarkers of Integrity. *Fluids Barriers CNS* **2020,** *17* (1), 69. https://doi.org/10.1186/s12987-020-00230-3
53. Jones, A. R.; Shusta, E. V. Blood-brain Barrier Transport of Therapeutics via Receptor-mediation. *Pharm. Res.* **2007,** *24* (9), 1759–1771. https://doi.org/10.1007/s11095-007-9379-0
54. Chang, R.; Al Maghribi, A.; Vanderpoel, V.; Vasilevko, V.; Cribbs, D. H.; Boado, R.; Pardridge, W. M.; Sumbria, R. K. Brain Penetrating Bifunctional Erythropoietin-Transferrin Receptor Antibody Fusion Protein for Alzheimer's Disease. *Mol. Pharm.* **2018,** *15* (11), 4963–4973. https://doi.org/10.1021/acs.molpharmaceut.8b00594
55. Mishra, V.; Mahor, S.; Rawat, A.; Gupta, P. N.; Dubey, P.; Khatri, K.; Vyas, S. P. Targeted Brain Delivery of AZT via Transferrin Anchored Pegylated Albumin Nanoparticles. *J. Drug Target.* **2006,** *14* (1), 45–53. https://doi.org/10.1080/10611860600612953
56. Cabezón, I.; Manich, G.; Martín-Venegas, R.; Camins, A.; Pelegrí, C.; Vilaplana, J. Trafficking of Gold Nanoparticles Coated with the 8D3 Anti-Transferrin Receptor

Antibody at the Mouse Blood-Brain Barrier. *Mol. Pharm.* **2015,** *12* (11), 4137–4145. https://doi.org/10.1021/acs.molpharmaceut.5b00597

57. Clark, A. J.; Davis, M. E. Increased Brain Uptake of Targeted Nanoparticles by Adding an Acid-cleavable Linkage between Transferrin and the Nanoparticle Core. *Proc. Natl Acad. Sci. USA.* **2015,** *112* (40), 12486–12491. https://doi.org/10.1073/pnas.1517048112
58. Kang, Y. S.; Jung, H. J.; Oh, J. S.; Song, D. Y. Use of PEGylated Immunoliposomes to Deliver Dopamine Across the Blood-Brain Barrier in a Rat Model of Parkinson's Disease. *CNS Neurosci. Ther.* **2016,** *22* (10), 817–823. https://doi.org/10.1111/cns.12580
59. Rhea, E. M.; Rask-Madsen, C.; Banks, W. A. Insulin Transport Across the Blood-brain Barrier can Occur Independently of the Insulin Receptor. *J. Physiol.* **2018,** *596* (19), 4753–4765. https://doi.org/10.1113/JP276149
60. Dieu, L. H.; Wu, D.; Palivan, C. G.; Balasubramanian, V.; Huwyler, J. Polymersomes Conjugated to 83-14 Monoclonal Antibodies: In Vitro Targeting of Brain Capillary Endothelial Cells. *Eur. J. Pharm. Biopharm.* **2014,** *88* (2), 316–324. https://doi.org/10.1016/j.ejpb.2014.05.021
61. Pardridge W. M. shRNA and siRNA Delivery to the Brain. *Adv. Drug Deliv. Rev.* **2007,** *59* (2 and 3), 141–152. https://doi.org/10.1016/j.addr.2007.03.008
62. Storck, S. E.; Kurtyka, M.; Pietrzik, C. U. Brain Endothelial LRP1 Maintains Blood-brain Barrier Integrity. *Fluids Barriers CNS*, **2021,** *18* (1), 27. https://doi.org/10.1186/s12987-021-00260-5
63. Karkan, D.; Pfeifer, C.; Vitalis, T. Z.; Arthur, G.; Ujiie, M.; Chen, Q.; Tsai, S.; Koliatis, G.; Gabathuler, R.; Jefferies, W. A. A Unique Carrier for the Delivery of Therapeutic Compounds beyond the Blood-brain Barrier. *PLoS One* **2008,** *3* (6), e2469. https://doi.org/10.1371/journal.pone.0002469
64. Kuo, Y. C.; Chen, I. Y.; Rajesh, R. Use of Functionalized Liposomes Loaded with Antioxidants to Permeate the Blood-brain Barrier and Inhibit β-amyloid-induced Neurodegeneration in the Brain. *J. Taiwan Inst. Chem. Eng.* **2018,** *87,* 1–14.
65. Song, X.; Li, R.; Deng, H.; Li, Y.; Cui, Y.; Zhang, H.; Dai, W.; He, B.; Zheng, Y.; Wang, X.; Zhang, Q. Receptor-mediated Transcytosis in Biological Barrier: The Influence of Receptor Character and their Ligand Density on the Transmembrane Pathway of Active-targeting Nanocarriers. *Biomaterials* **2018,** *180,* 78–90. https://doi.org/10.1016/j.biomaterials.2018.07.006
66. Morales-Cruz, M.; Cruz-Montañez, A.; Figueroa, C. M.; González-Robles, T.; Davila, J.; Inyushin, M.; Loza-Rosas, S. A.; Molina, A. M.; Muñoz-Perez, L.; Kucheryavykh, L. Y.; Tinoco, A. D.; Griebenow, K. Combining Stimulus-Triggered Release and Active Targeting Strategies Improves Cytotoxicity of Cytochrome c Nanoparticles in Tumor Cells. *Mol. Pharm.* **2016,** *13* (8), 2844–2854. https://doi.org/10.1021/acs.molpharmaceut.6b00461
67. Dong, S.; Cho, H. J.; Lee, Y. W.; Roman, M. Synthesis and Cellular Uptake of Folic Acid-conjugated Cellulose Nanocrystals for Cancer Targeting. *Biomacromolecules* **2014,** *15* (5), 1560–1567. https://doi.org/10.1021/bm401593n
68. Zhang, C.; Jiang, M.; Wang, W. Q.; Zhao, S. J.; Yin, Y. X.; Mi, Q. J.; Yang, M. F.; Song, Y. Q.; Sun, B. L.; Zhang, Z. Y. Selective mGluR1 Negative Allosteric Modulator Reduces Blood-Brain Barrier Permeability and Cerebral Edema After Experimental Subarachnoid Hemorrhage. *Transl. Stroke Res.* **2020,** *11* (4), 799–811. https://doi.org/10.1007/s12975-019-00758-z
69. Wang, B.; Lv, L.; Wang, Z.; Jiang, Y.; Lv, W.; Liu, X.; Wang, Z.; Zhao, Y.; Xin, H.; Xu, Q. Improved Anti-glioblastoma Efficacy by IL-13Rα2 Mediated Copolymer Nanoparticles Loaded with Paclitaxel. *Sci. Rep.* **2015,** *5,* 16589. https://doi.org/10.1038/srep16589

70. Liu, Y.; Mei, L.; Xu, C.; Yu, Q.; Shi, K.; Zhang, L.; Wang, Y.; Zhang, Q.; Gao, H.; Zhang, Z.; He, Q. Dual Receptor Recognizing Cell Penetrating Peptide for Selective Targeting, Efficient Intratumoral Diffusion, and Synthesized Anti-Glioma Therapy. *Theranostics* **2016,** *6* (2), 177–191. https://doi.org/10.7150/thno.13532
71. Kuo, Y. C.; Wang, I. H.; Rajesh, R. Use of Leptin-conjugated Phosphatidic Acid Liposomes with Resveratrol and Epigallocatechin Gallate to Protect Dopaminergic Neurons Against Apoptosis for Parkinson's Disease Therapy. *Acta Biomater.* **2021,** *119*, 360–374. https://doi.org/10.1016/j.actbio.2020.11.015
72. Buzzi, S.; Rubboli, D.; Buzzi, G.; Buzzi, A. M.; Morisi, C.; Pironi, F. CRM197 (nontoxic diphtheria toxin): Effects on Advanced Cancer Patients. *Cancer Immunol. Immunother.* **2004,** *53* (11), 1041–1048. https://doi.org/10.1007/s00262-004-0546-4
73. Pinheiro, R.; Granja, A.; Loureiro, J. A.; Pereira, M. C.; Pinheiro, M.; Neves, A. R.; Reis, S. RVG29-Functionalized Lipid Nanoparticles for Quercetin Brain Delivery and Alzheimer's Disease. *Pharm. Res.* **2020,** *37* (7), 139. https://doi.org/10.1007/s11095-020-02865-1
74. Lu, W.; Wan, J.; She, Z.; Jiang, X. Brain Delivery Property and Accelerated Blood Clearance of Cationic Albumin Conjugated Pegylated Nanoparticle. *J. Controll. Release* **2007,** *118* (1), 38–53. https://doi.org/10.1016/j.jconrel.2006.11.015
75. Patel, M. M.; Goyal, B. R.; Bhadada, S. V.; Bhatt, J. S.; Amin, A. F. Getting into the Brain: Approaches to Enhance Brain Drug Delivery. *CNS Drug.* **2009,** *23* (1), 35–58. https://doi.org/10.2165/0023210-200923010-00003
76. Patel, M. M.; Patel, B. M. Crossing the Blood-Brain Barrier: Recent Advances in Drug Delivery to the Brain. *CNS Drugs* **2017,** *31* (2), 109–133. https://doi.org/10.1007/s40263-016-0405-9
77. Roy, R.; Alotaibi, A. A.; Freedman, M. S. Sphingosine 1-Phosphate Receptor Modulators for Multiple Sclerosis. *CNS Drugs* **2021,** *35* (4), 385–402. https://doi.org/10.1007/s40263-021-00798-w
78. Wang, T.; Agarwal, S.; Elmquist, W. F. Brain Distribution of Cediranib is Limited by Active Efflux at the Blood-brain Barrier. *J. Pharmacol. Exp. Ther.* **2012,** *341* (2), 386–395. https://doi.org/10.1124/jpet.111.190488
79. Montaser, A.; Markowicz-Piasecka, M.; Sikora, J.; Jalkanen, A.; Huttunen, K. M. L-type Amino Acid Transporter 1 (LAT1)-Utilizing Efflux Transporter Inhibitors can Improve the Brain Uptake and Apoptosis-inducing Effects of Vinblastine in Cancer Cells. *Int. J. Pharm.* **2020,** *586*, 119585. https://doi.org/10.1016/j.ijpharm.2020.11958

CHAPTER 3

Nanodiamonds as Emerging Nanotherapeutics for Brain-Targeted Drug Delivery in the Management and Diagnosis of Neurodegenerative Disorders

BHAGAWATI SAXENA[1], FAGUN PATHAK[1], BHAVNA BOHRA[1], and VIRAL SHAH[2]

[1]*Department of Pharmacology, Institute of Pharmacy, Nirma University, Ahmedabad, Gujarat, India*

[2]*Department of Pharmaceutics, Sal Institute of Pharmacy, Sola, Ahmedabad, Gujarat, India*

ABSTRACT

Neurodegenerative diseases are a range of illnesses that can produce different levels of cognitive and motor impairments. Neurodegenerative disorders tend to be one of the most complex diseases, with major challenges in diagnosis, management, and therapy. Conventional drugs are not able to target neurodegenerative diseases effectively, especially because of the blood–brain barrier (BBB) and efflux-transporters (p-glycoprotein). Nanodiamonds, having the size range of millionth of a meter, are considered to be an emerging and effective tool to deliver the medicine into the targeted region of the brain. Nanodiamonds have qualities like biocompatibility, intrinsic fluorescence without photobleaching, tunable surface, and nonreactivity, making them well tolerated and suitable for both diagnostic and therapeutic purposes. Recent studies have also suggested that the neurotransmitter uptake can

Nanomedicine for Neurodegenerative Disorders: Selective Treatment Strategies. Rishabha Malviya, Kamla Pathak, & Swati Verma (Eds.)

be changed by nanodiamonds, thus exerting neuroprotective action to the degenerating neuron. Compatibility of nanodiamonds with other biological molecules also makes it much more suitable as a carrier for transporting the medicines across BBB, for example albumin-coated nanodiamonds. Currently, scientists have been able to demonstrate the intraneuronal axonal transport within the degrading neurons with the help of fluorescent nanodiamonds which is found to be the crucial tool to understand the genetic factors behind the pathogenesis of neurodegenerative disorders. This chapter emphasizes and discusses the vast potential of nanodiamonds in the detection and treatment of neurodegenerative disorders that represent a significant threat to human health.

3.1 INTRODUCTION

Neurodegenerative diseases are a comprehensive term, which is used to indicate a group of conditions that can cause varying degrees of motor and cognitive impairment. Neurodegenerative diseases are broadly classified by their clinical presentation which includes Parkinson's disease (PD), Alzheimer's disease (AD), Frontotemporal dementia, Amyotrophic lateral sclerosis (ALS), multiple sclerosis, Huntington's disease (HD), Batten disease, Creutzfeldt–Jakob disease (CJD), and Spinocerebellar ataxias.[1] Among all the neurodegenerative disorders, AD, PD, and ALS are the most common. The health of people is seriously threatened by neurodegenerative illnesses. According to WHO, neurodegenerative disorders are the second leading cause of mortality. These are age-dependent illnesses, becoming more and more frequent in the last few years partially because of the rise in the population of elderly individuals over past decades due to better healthcare systems.[2] Around 36.5 million people worldwide were diagnosed with dementia in 2010. Dementia cases are predicted to almost quadruple every 20 years and are expected to reach around sixty-six million in 2030 and around one hundred sixteen million in 2050.[3] These forms of dementia are overwhelmingly caused by AD, which contributes for 60–80% of all cases of dementia.[4] In the elderly population, it is projected that five to seven million AD's new cases are identified each year.[5] The onset of AD before the age of 50 is uncommon, with the exception of familial AD. The prevalence rate of AD is around 30% among people aged 85 and above. The incidence rate for AD also climbs steeply from 0.5% per year for the age range 65–75 to directly 6–8% per year for the age group 85 and above.[6] Just like AD, incidences of PD are rarer before the age of 50. Beyond this age limit incidence and prevalence rates, both sharply rise through the late 80s age. Annual incidence rates of PD are around 10–15 per 100,000 have been noted in many surveys. The possibility of a 2% prevalence in individuals aged 65 years and above has been observed.[8]

In the majority of brain-related illnesses, neurodegeneration has been defined as the gradual functional and structural loss of neurons that results in crucial pathophysiological alterations and worsening of the brain's functional architecture.[9,10] The underlying pathological process causing the neuronal loss is still unidentified, but it is considered that environmental, genetic, and endogenous features related to aging conditions play a major role in neuronal loss[11] Neurodegeneration is allied with the deposition of physiochemically altered protein, dysfunction of synapses, and neuronal network.[12–15] Neurodegenerative disorders are noted to be more difficult to detect at an early stage when compared to other illnesses. Thus, neurodegenerative diseases may be serious and life-threatening.

Many medical treatments and surgical method are available that cure the disease symptomatically, reduce the pain if present, and restore cognition, balance, and mobility. Despite the ongoing efforts of contemporary science to develop novel medicinal and surgical procedures, in the case of the neurodegenerative disease, the outcomes are found to be unfavorable. The clinical acceptance of highly evasive techniques and surgeries is limited because their tendency to harm the brain barrier raises questions regarding their long-term advantages. Another challenge is that most of these medications fail to cross the barriers of the brain. Thus, for halting or reversing neurodegeneration and managing these neurodegenerative diseases, a new therapeutic approach is needed.[16] Utilization of nanotherapeutic methods is gaining attention when compared to conventional dosage forms because of their several benefits including the potential to cross the blood–brain barrier (BBB).[17,18] Even after great progress, it is necessary to refine nanotherapeutics to ensure maximum outcomes.[19] Nanodiamonds have become potentially designed nanotherapeutics for a variety of biomedical applications because of their distinctive chemical, structural, and biological characteristics.[20] Nanodiamonds come under the subset group of diamondoids, which is a larger group consisting of structurally similar nanocarbon compounds also known as condensed adamantanes. According to the recent advancements this group is being considered one of the most promising building blocks in nanomedicine.[21] In this review, challenges in delivering the drug to brain targets including the BBB are discussed. This book chapter also highlightened properties of nanodiamonds, synthesis strategies for formulating and characterization of nanodiamonds, the application of nanodiamonds in neurodegenerative disorders, and enormous potential nanodiamonds have in the detection and treatment of neurodegenerative disorders that represent a significant threat to human health.

3.2 CHALLENGES ASSOCIATED WITH BRAIN TARGETED DRUG DELIVERY

3.2.1 BLOOD–BRAIN BARRIER

Current development in the treatment, management as well as diagnosis of neurodegenerative illnesses have made it possible to impede the progression of condition and improved the life span of the patients suffering with neurodegenerative disorders. However, most of these medications fail to cross the barriers of the central nervous system (CNS). These barriers are basically against the introduction of foreign substances into the CNS. However, these barriers cause extreme difficulty to deliver medications to the CNS and especially the brain. Thus, the effective therapy of neurodegenerative illnesses is restricted by the failure to transport the necessary concentrations of medicines to the brain's desired target because of these barriers of CNS. Three important barriers include the ependymal barrier, blood–cerebrospinal fluid barrier, and most importantly the BBB, which partitioned the circulation of peripheral system from the brain.[22] Machineries of the BBB consist of several components which include mural cells, endothelial cells, basement membrane (BM), immune cells, and astrocytes. The detailed structure of BBB is shown in Figure 3.1.

3.2.1.1 ENDOTHELIAL CELLS

The blood vessel walls are made of endothelial cells, which are originating from the mesoderm. Modified simple squamous epithelial cells are endothelial cells. A single endothelial cell folds over on itself to produce the vessel's lumen, forming the perimeter of the microvascular capillary and partitioning the parenchymal from the luminal surface.[23,24] The endothelial cells within the CNS are very thin cells, measuring less than a quarter of a micron.[25] Endothelial cells within CNS in contrast to the endothelial cells present in other tissue systems have distinctive features. Firstly, the tight junctions, which are responsible for holding endothelial cells within the CNS together, significantly reduce the paracellular flow of solutes.[26] Secondly, compared

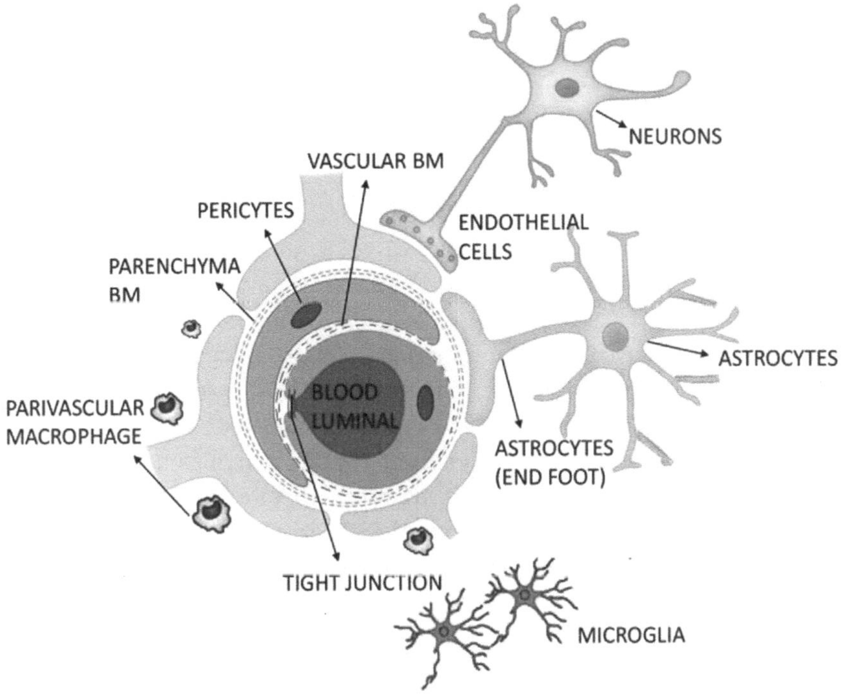

FIGURE 3.1 Structure and components of blood–brain barrier.

to peripheral endothelial cells, endothelial cells within CNS transcytosis at incredibly low rates, which severely limits the transfer of solutes between cells via vesicles.[25] Thirdly, endothelial cells within CNS have more mitochondria.[27] It is believed that mitochondria are necessary for ATP synthesis in order to maintain the ion gradients necessary for transport operations. It is very well known that endothelial cells within CNS consist of two main categories of transporter, i.e., efflux transporter[28,29] and particularly specialized nutrient transporter that aids in the elimination of particular waste items from the CNS into the circulation as well as the passage of particular nutrients entering the CNS via the BBB.[30] Fourth, leukocyte adhesion molecules (LAMs) are also particularly poorly expressed by endothelial cells within CNS compared to endothelial cells in other organs, severely restricting how many immune cells may enter the CNS.[23,31–32] Fifth, it is believed that endothelial cells within CNS have differential vascular metabolism that alters the physical properties of molecules, which may have an impact on their solubility, reactivity, and transport capabilities, to produce a molecular barrier. Thus, the endothelial cells are able to closely control CNS homeostasis because of an amalgamation of qualities of physical barrier (tight junctions, low transcytosis), efflux transporters, specific transporters to distribute needed nutrients, and molecular barrier (low LAMs, particular metabolism).

3.2.1.2 MURAL CELLS

Mural cells comprise pericytes and vascular smooth muscles. Pericytes are originated from the neural crest.[33] and are found to be immersed into the vascular BM. These cells are located on the microvascular endothelial tube's abluminal surface and only partially encase the endothelial walls of the microvasculature.[34] Pericytes include contractile proteins; hence they can constrict in a bid to regulate the capillary diameter.[35] Pericytes line the endothelial tube, but they are not in direct contact with the endothelium and are segregated from each other by the basement membrane, in which they are embedded. However, cellular adhesion is observed between pericytes and endothelium at discrete points. These pericyte-endothelial cellular adhesions include peg-and-socket junctions enriched with the N-cadherin adhesion molecule,[36] gap junctions, tight junctions, and adhesion plaques.[37–39] In addition to controlling extracellular matrix deposition, angiogenesis, infiltration of immune cells, wound healing, and blood flow modulation in accordance with the brain conditioning, investigations indicate that pericytes may also be multipotent CNS stem cells[40] and show a chief role in controlling BBB formation throughout development stage as well as maintaining its function over the course of the body's lifespan.[41–42]

3.2.1.3 BASEMENT MEMBRANE

The two BMs that surround the vascular tube include the outer parenchymal BM and the inner vascular BM.[43,44] Parenchymal BM, also termed as the vascular glia limitans perivascular, is principally formed by the secretions from the astrocytic end feet while the vascular BM is an extracellular matrix formed by the secretion from the pericytes and endothelial cells. Both the BMs consisted of various secreted molecules including heparin sulfate, proteoglycans, collagens type IV, nidogen, laminin, and various other glycoproteins. The compositions of parenchymal and vascular BMs are substantially distinctive, for example, parenchymal BM contains α1 and α2 laminins while vascular BM contains α4 and α5 laminins.[44] On the top of acting as a barrier for cells and molecules trying to enter the brain tissue, these BMs act as an attachment point for a number of signal transduction pathways inside the vasculature. In many different neurological illnesses, leukocyte infiltration and BBB failure are seen as a result of disruption of these BMS by matrix metalloproteinases.[45]

3.2.1.4 ASTROCYTES

Astrocyte is one of the glial cell types. Vasculature and neurons are both covered by the endfeet of the astrocyte's basal process. They consist of numerous proteins (aquaporin 4, dystroglycan, and dystrophin). The dystroglycan–dystrophin complex with binding agrin is crucial for connecting the cytoskeleton of the endfeet of astrocyte to the BM.[46,47] Earlier research work shows that astrocytes are responsible for playing a significant part in mediating BBB development and function.[48,49] Recent findings show that the early development of the BBB is not significantly influenced by astrocytes.[41] The discovery of substances released by astrocytes that do control BBB functions leads to the conclusion that mature astrocytes modify and sustain the integrity of barrier after it has been created.

3.2.1.5 IMMUNE CELLS

Various immune cell populations in the blood and the CNS interact with the blood arteries of the CNS. The two major immune cell types in the CNS include microglial cells and perivascular macrophages. A crucial component of both the innate and adaptive immune response is played by microglial cells. In adaptive immunity, microglial cells serve as antigen-presenting cells. They also play a chief role in controlling neuronal growth and wound healing.[50] Perivascular macrophages consist of monocyte lineage cells that are placed over the abluminal part of the vasculature.[51] These immune cells can cross the BBB because they are generated from blood-borne progenitors.[52,53] These cells by phagocytosing cellular waste act as the initial line of defence for innate immunity. Additionally, when these immune cells (macrophages, neutrophils, and T cells) are activated, they interact with CNS vessels. In response to injury, infection, and illness, these immune cells are hypothesized to enhance vascular permeability and altered the BBB integrity.[54]

With the presence of various types of above-mentioned specialized cells and their specific arrangement, the architecture of BBB prevents harmful toxins or effective treatments from entering the brain parenchyma. BBB is also essential for maintaining homeostasis and providing an unchanged environment for optimum neuronal growth and protection even in new-borns at their early developmental stage.[55] Consequently, the BBB is not only accountable for maintaining the brain's homeostasis but also prevents drugs from reaching the brain's active regions as well. Restriction in the entry of dissolved polar solutes across BBB is also attributed to the presences of continuous tight junctions and a lack of aqueous pathways.[56] This restriction in the entry is also enforced by basal lamina, endothelial cells, pericytes, and astrocytes.[57] However, the brain is not totally inaccessible for certain compounds to entre via certain mechanisms and transporter systems. Studies of BBB at cellular, metabolic, kinetic, and molecular levels have revealed several transporter systems which are present across the BBB to strategically facilitate the brain drug delivery. These systems of transporters include transferrin receptor, insulin transporter, glucose transporter 1, etc.[58] The integrity of BBB is also disrupted in some neurological diseases, which facilitates the permeation of certain molecules and toxins into the brain.[59–63] Manipulation of physicochemical properties of drugs which can include molecular weight, size, surface activity, surface charge, and lipid solubility also helps to achieve optimum transportation of drugs across the BBB.[58,64] In this sense, one of the most crucial instruments for the transmission of drugs cargos across highly specific biological barriers may be nanoparticles.

3.2.2 PHARMACOKINETIC PRINCIPLES AFFECTING BRAIN-TARGETED DRUG DELIVERY

Pharmacokinetic properties of therapeutic agent have a crucial influence on affecting the efficiency of medications that are taken systematically.[65] The route taken by therapeutics to reach the target from the site of administration is typically arduous and unfavorable. The target site of all the medications for the neurological disease is some or other regions of the brain. The presence of numerous embedded plasma proteins is the first thing which is needed to be addressed. Numerous medications used to treat neurodegenerative diseases are strongly bound to these proteins, lowering their availability in circulation and, ultimately, lowering the quantity of free medication accessible for the delivery to the brain.[66] Additionally, only a minimal quantity of drugs is left in circulation after some of them are eliminated by the main clearance organs at a substantial pace. Moreover, the extent of drug absorption is restricted by the interaction of the drug and target cells. More precisely, pharmacological compounds can have an impact on cells that prevent channels from opening, modify the membrane potential, or even change the conformation of the cell. This transient impact may restrict the reaction of the cell toward the medication molecule being supplied and its absorption.[67]

3.2.3 EFFLUX TRANSPORTERS

In addition to the BBB, the existence of several efflux transporters causes decreased drug penetration into the brain. These transporters are essential for the transit of a variety of medicines, endogenous substrates, and xenobiotics into the blood from the CNS. They are also accountable for restraining the effective transportation of drugs into the CNS from the blood and thereby reducing the quantity of drug inside the brain.[68] Among several regulatory mechanisms which make difficultly in the brain-targeted delivery of drugs, one of them is P-glycoprotein (P-gp). It is a crucial active efflux transporter present at the BBB[68] and an ATP-dependent drug efflux transporter protein which is mainly found in the blood luminal membrane of the endothelial cells of the brain capillary which makes up the BBB. These efflux pumps are essential in hindering the passage of medications into the brain. It also prevents the entry of toxins inside the brain. This transporter protein is accountable for the active transport of a variety of hydrophobic drugs out of the cell into the blood, thus resulting in the poor concentration of these drugs inside the CNS. Thus, this efflux mechanism imparts significant challenges in transporting the drug across BBB.[69,70]

P-gp efflux transporters are also crucial for the clearance of toxic compounds from the brain. The findings of a study confirm the linking of p-gp to amyloid-β clearance throughout the BBB and have important implications in the prognosis of AD.[71] A study using [^{11}C]-verapamil positron emission tomography (PET) brain imaging technique published in 2008 showed correlation between decreased functionality of P-gp efflux transport at BBB and progression of neurodegenerative diseases like PD, multisystem atrophy, and progressive supranuclear palsy.[72] These studies suggested that diminished functionality of P-gp efflux transporter affects the prognosis and severity of these neurodegenerative diseases.[72] A pilot study performed in 2005 found impaired functioning of midbrain BBB P-gp in five PD patients which was measured using [^{11}C]-verapamil PET. However, the findings of the above study do not confirm the pathophysiology of PD as a primary defective BBB's P-gp export system, but they do show diminished P-gp activity at later illness stages.[73] The previous literature also shows the coexistence of β-amyloid with α-synuclein in patients with PD with dementia.[74] The coexistence of deposited proteins may also be caused by decreased P-gp activity to eject proteins in the advanced stage of PD. Hence, these studies suggested the essentiality of P-gp in reducing the accumulation of toxic moieties within the brain. Attenuation in the expression and functioning of P-gp in BBB is also one of the factors that affect the commencement, severity, and advancement of other neurodegenerative diseases including AD[75] and CJD.[76]

3.2.4 PHYSICOCHEMICAL PROPERTIES OF DRUGS

Physical and chemical characteristics such as particle size, polarity, and plasma protein–drug conjugation present another difficult aspect. The BBB averts the transportation of large molecules inside the brain. The tight connections between endothelial cells allow smaller molecules to pass through the BBB with ease. Higher polarity and water-soluble compounds are unable to get across the BBB, while small lipophilic pharmacological molecules are often appropriate for brain delivery.[77] The diffusion process allows the shuttling of nonpolar moieties across the BBB. The BBB averts the passage of drugs that have been conjugated to plasma proteins and created drug–protein complexes. Drugs that are lipophilic can easily traverse the BBB. As a result, a medicine should be lipophilic for efficient and convenient CNS drug delivery.[78]

3.3 INTRODUCTION ON NANODIAMONDS

Nanodiamonds are condensed octahedral structures, which consist of carbon-based nano-particle with 14 faces, 36 edges, and 24 corners. Observation of nanodiamonds structure was done by using the X-ray diffraction (XRD) technique and by means of a high-resolution transmission electron microscopy (HRTEM).[79,80] Nanodiamonds were suggested to be more flake-like in structure. Structure of nanodiamonds results from hybridized amorphous carbon (sp^2) with diamond core lattice (sp^3) bonds on surface.[81] These bonds are exchangeable which means that they can be switched around and provide flexibility in geometric orientation, especially on round curved surfaces. Based on their sizes, nanodiamonds can be differentiated as nanocrystalline particles (>10–150 nm or higher), ultra-nanocrystalline particles (2–10 nm), and diamondoids (1–2 nm). Owing to their distinct intrinsic properties nanodiamonds with a size of 10 nm have been widely used in bio-medicine. A dense hydration layer is formed on the surface of nanodiamond, due to its unique characteristic of a large area-to-volume ratio; which improves the stability and ability of the molecule to incorporate through cell membranes; exclusively via BBB. Rough edges were estimated to initiate deformation of the nanodiamond membrane, leading to higher absorption. Endocytosis and pinocytosis are other important mechanisms of transportation of nanodiamonds across cell membranes including the BBB.

3.4 PROPERTIES OF NANODIAMONDS

Diamond is a magnificent material, of which nanodiamonds inherit many of the best properties of parent diamond and deliver them significantly on nanoscale.[82] The nanodiamond has outstanding properties which include: chemical stability, high thermal conductivity, hardness, resistance to harsh environment, electrical resistivity, hardness, optical and fluorescence properties, and bioavailability. On the basis of these useful properties nanodiamonds cover a variety of applications. The biocompatibility studies were done using fluorescent nanodiamond powder size ranging from 100 nm and the results show that low cytotoxicity in kidney cells. Later, nanodiamond with a size range of 2–10 nm was not found to be toxic by analyzing mitochondrial function and luminescent assays of ATP production.[83] Cell morphology does not change during culture. In addition, it has excellent optical properties for utilization as a bio-label or bio-marker. In this section, we learned about how nano-diamond can be used because of their properties, like fluorescence and biocompatibility.

3.4.1 FLUORESCENT PROPERTY

Optical property is an outstanding property of the diamond. For the last few decades, it has attracted attention because of its optical initialization. Due to optical property, they can be easily analyzed by microwave or laser radiation.[84,85] Diamond has a number of color centers, which have been reported to hold unique advantages. These advantages include various kinds of atom vacancies such as nitrogen-vacancy (NV),[86–88] silicon-vacancy,[89–92] germanium vacancy,[93–96] and tin vacancy centers.[97–100] Among these, the nitrogen center, which has been studied only in basic science and applied science, is a representative example. The NV center is a place in the ambient environment where the spin coherence time is long and the spin ground state is easily manipulated. This makes it interesting for quantum information processing,[101] optical sensors,[102] and bioimaging.[103] When a laser is used to pump an NV center at room temperature, a zero-photon line can be observed. So far, scientists have studied the optical properties of nanodiamonds and have found many interesting results which can be explored further.

3.4.2 BIOCOMPATIBILITY

An agent is considered to be biocompatible when it does not cause genotoxic, cytotoxic, carcinogenic, or other adverse reactions in cells or organisms. Nanodiamonds prepared via various techniques might potentially be harmful to cells or organisms due to their nanostructures. Therefore, assessing the safety as well as toxicity associated with nanodiamonds is crucial in drug discovery. Schrand and his team studied biocompatibility of nanodiamonds and compared them with various other nanomaterials, which were also carbon-based, in terms of their effects on morphology and structure at subcellular level. It was observed that nanodiamonds in comparison to other carbon-based nanomaterials show most biocompatibility with neuroblastoma cells. Though the nanodiamonds concentration reaches 100 mol/L, it does not affect the survival of the neuroblastoma cells.[104] Additionally, the biocompatibility of nanodiamonds in neurons produced originated from embryonic cancer stem cells was also the subject of another investigation. The findings demonstrated that, throughout the process of neural differentiation, the nanodiamonds neither affect the size, shape, protein expression, development of neurons nor result in cytotoxicity or neuronal death.[105] Functionalization of nanodiamonds is very necessary for improved drug delivery. However, literature and data of biocompatibility of nanodiamonds are limited, but results of previous studies did not indicate a harmful effect of nanodiamonds. It is vital at first to execute biocompatibility and toxicity testing to authorize that the functional nanodiamonds are safe for the application in the biomedical field. For instance, carboxylated nanodiamond with a modified surface has been used for the conjugation of biological molecules like protein and DNA. -COOH group-coated nanodiamonds altered neither the profile of protein expression in lung cell nor viability of lung cells.[106]

3.4.3 SURFACE MODIFICATION

Especially small nanodiamonds of 3–5 nm in size, which are synthesized by detonation technique, have large surface specific area and plenty of functionally active groups on the surface. A surface functionalization may be obtained by targeting modification on surfaces.[107–111] Since nanodiamonds have low dispersibility in aqueous solution, it tends to agglomerate, limiting their use in biomedical applications. Nanodiamonds might be effortlessly disseminated by using mechanical polishing and ultrasonic scattering technique.[112] The researchers typically modify functional targeting groups as required and after that these modified targeting groups are covalently attached to the optimal biological macromolecule and/or other nanoparticles to form nano-composites for various domains. Nanodiamonds are first treated with an oxidizing agent, which adds oxygen atoms to the surface, followed by carboxylating agent, which adds carboxyl group to the surface. Finally, a surface modification is applied on nanodiamonds to obtain salinized nanodiamonds (NDs-NH2).[113–115] Due to a large variety of functional groups, nanodiamonds can be easily modified. Nanodiamonds with modified surfaces have excellent dispersion ability and they can be also combined with multiple different drugs, luminance materials, antibodies, and genetic materials to respond to the needs of various situations.

3.4.4 *SURFACE AREA-TO-VOLUME RATIO*

Nanodiamonds may bound to a range of molecules effectively, due to their enormous surface area.[116,117] Nanodiamond's surface can be altered by noncovalent and covalent bonds, preventing attachment of drugs or other chemical reagents. In particular, when a targeted drug, especially water insoluble drug, is modified or immobilized on the nanodiamonds surface, the water-insoluble drug can easily enter the cells and release the drug into the target cell more precisely.[118] Hence, nanodiamonds may use a variety of biotherapeutic molecules, enabling multimodal therapy.[119]

3.5 SYNTHESIS STRATEGIES FOR FORMULATING NANODIAMOND

Several techniques are used for synthesizing nanodiamonds of varied sizes and morphologies. Most commonly used strategies for the synthesis of nanodiamonds include: (1) detonation techniques, (2) high pressure-high temperature (HPHT) technique, (3) ball milling technique, (4) ablation using laser beam, and (5) chemical vapor deposition. Different synthesis methods produce different types of nanodiamonds. Various synthesis strategies for formulating the nanodiamonds are summarized in Figure 3.2.

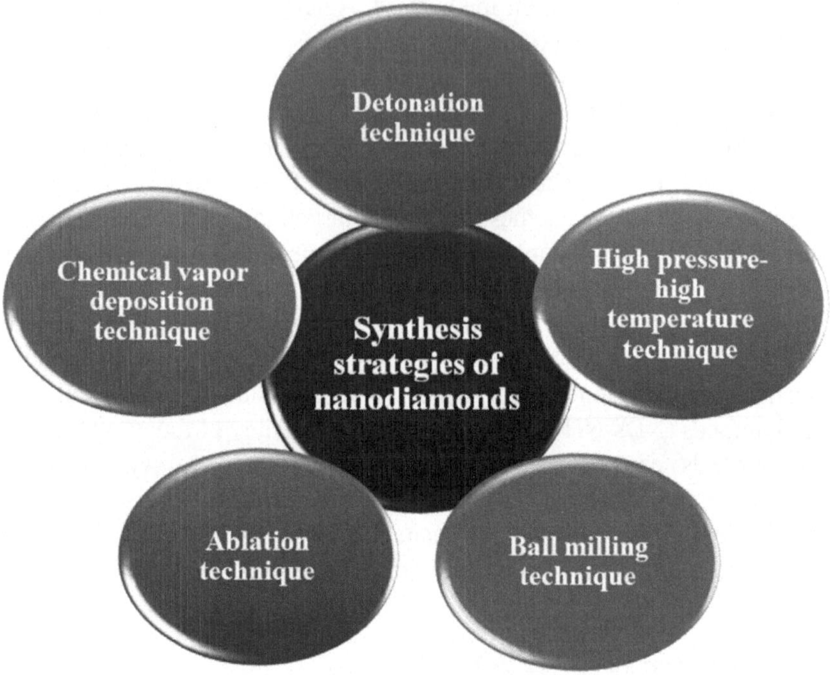

FIGURE 3.2 Synthesis strategies for formulating nanodiamond.

3.5.1 DETONATION TECHNIQUE

Explosive synthesis technology based on explosive impact method was traditionally used for synthesis of nanodiamonds. In this traditional approach due to explosion, high temperature and shock wave pressure are generated that transforms the phase of graphite precursors into nanodiamonds. The limitation of the above-mentioned traditional approach is relatively low synthesis yield and recovery rate.[120] Detonation is a newer approach that utilizes explosive technology as the precursor for synthesis of nanodiamonds through an explosive having oxygen atom deficiency. Due to benefits of detonation technique like fast reaction speed, ease in operation procedure, low cost, and relatively simple equipment have become a popular and most widely used technique for synthesizing nanodiamonds.[20,109,120] Moreover, detonated nanodiamonds (DNDs) exhibit good chemical stability, biocompatibility, high wear resistance, relatively high hardness, and large specific surface area. Limitation of detonation technique is because of the presence of oxygen containing as well as other functional groups on the nanodiamond's surface. Because of different treatment methods the surface potential of nanodiamonds is altered which may eventually lead to agglomeration of nanodiamonds. Detonated products are usually in aggregated form having mean crystalline size of 4–5 nm, strategies for deagglomeration are additionally needed in DNDs to obtain monodisperse-isolated particles. Furthermore, DNDs may contain impurities of trace metal, amorphous carbon; thus, purification is also an additional step required in the detonation process.[109] Two types of deagglomeration strategies namely mechanical and chemical are used for obtaining monodispersed and isolated nanodiamond particles. Ball grinding, ultrasonic crushing, or combination of these techniques are mechanical techniques used for de-aggregating nanodiamonds, whereas liquid phase reaction and gas phase treatment are chemical techniques used for deagglomeration.

3.5.2 HIGH PRESSURE HIGH TEMPERATURE (HPHT) SYNTHESIS TECHNIQUE

Naturally, diamonds are obtained deep under-earth in high-temperature and high-pressure conditions. Thus, it was presumed that pristine carbon sources can be converted into diamonds by mimicking the identical conditions. Conventionally, 5–6 GPa pressure and 1300–1500°C temperature conditions along with metal catalysts were used to synthesize nanodiamonds from graphite.[121] Nanodiamonds obtained through the HPHT technique are of high quality, nano-sized, thermally stable, wear resistant, free from metallic impurities and highly biocompatible.[20,121] Nitrogen, boron, and silicon-doped nanodiamonds can be successfully prepared utilizing the HPHT method. Additionally, hydrocarbons, fluorocarbons, and organosilicon-based growth systems along with high hydrostatic pressure are a novel approach to formulate micro- and nano-sized particles using the HPHT technique.[121] As nanodiamonds are synthesized from organic compounds, they are devoid of metallic impurities and because of this reason they are also highly biocompatible thus making them suitable for medical applications.[122]

3.5.3 BALL MILLING

Ball mill works on the principal of impact and attrition. In this technique due to rotation and vibration, the balls would crush the filled raw material to nano size (within 100 nm) by grinding the filled material due to impact and agitation. Nanodiamonds obtained through detonation and HPHT techniques can be nanosized using the ball milling technique. The nanosized diamonds obtained after the ball milling technique would have high fluorescence properties which increase their application in bioimaging and drug delivery.[121]

3.5.4 LASER ABLATION

Ablating the diamonds from micron to nanosize using laser beam is known as laser ablation. Nanodiamonds obtained through detonation and HPHT techniques can be nanosized using the laser ablation technique.[123] Laser ablation can also be used as an independent technique to formulate nanodiamonds. In this technique graphite micro-powder used as a precursor is dispersed in liquid medium (ethanol, ketone, water, benzene) and laser beam is focused on the suspended graphite powder which in turn brings alterations in the carbon structure leading to nanodiamond formation.[123] A cavitation bubble is created by laser beam with solid boundary which in turn initiates nucleation, its growth, and solidification under rapid quenching conditions to form nanodiamonds. Benefit of laser ablation technique is low level of impurities and limitations are low production levels and high consumption energy.[20,109,121,123]

3.5.5 CHEMICAL VAPOR DEPOSITION

This technique is based on a chemical reaction between gas phase compounds and target product elements on the surface of the substrate to formulate a product. This technique is useful in preparing large-scale, high-purity diamonds. Nanodiamonds can be synthesized using the microwave plasma chemical vapor deposition method, wherein plasma environment generated by microwave is utilized and gas phase oxygen molecules can be dissociated into ions which in turn would create an environment favorable for the hydrocarbons substances to convert into diamonds. The advantages of the chemical vapor deposition technique are no additional steps of purification are required and the limitations of the technique are its slow deposition rate, flammable resources used which sometimes are toxic and explosive and relatively high cost.[124]

3.6 CHARACTERIZATION TECHNIQUES FOR NANODIAMONDS

Efficacy of nanodiamonds as a drug delivery formulation is characterized through varied physical as well as chemical evaluation parameters. The characterization techniques used for nanodiamonds are summarized in Figure 3.3.

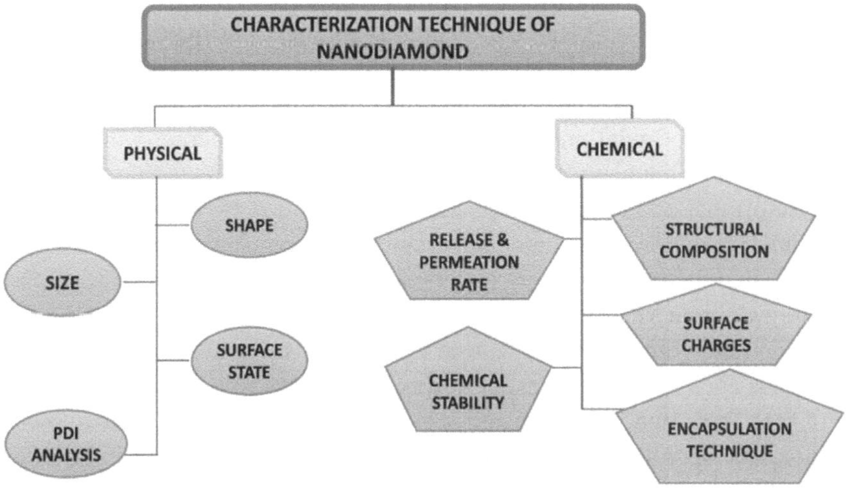

FIGURE 3.3 Characterization techniques for nanodiamonds.

3.6.1 PHYSICAL CHARACTERIZATION

Structure, surface state, and size are the important physical attributes of nanodiamonds that would significantly affect the efficacy and quality of nanodiamonds formulations. Optical analysis techniques like HRTEM and scanning electron microscopy are utilized to evaluate the properties of surface as well as to identify agglomeration in nanodiamond formulations. Particle size and poly dispersity index (PDI) of nanodiamonds can be analyzed using size analyzer based on dynamic light scattering (DLS) approach. DLS is size measurement of particles based on their Brownian motion in the dispersed medium through light which is scattered at varied angles due to motion of particles. PDI is the parameter that would reflect the uniformity in the size of formulated nanodiamonds.[125–129]

3.6.2 CHEMICAL CHARACTERIZATION

Several chemical parameters like structural composition, surface charges, encapsulation efficiency, release rate of entrapped drug substance, permeation rate across BBB, and physico-chemical stability would also impact the efficacy of formulated nanodiamonds. Structural composition and presence of impurities in nanodiamond formulations can be determined using techniques like energy diffraction spectroscopy, Fourier transform infrared spectroscopy (FTIR), XRD, differential scanning calorimeter, and Raman spectroscopy (Raman). Presence of surface charges due to the synthesis technique employed can be evaluated by measuring the zeta potential of the nanodiamond formulations. Zeta potential and surface charges would reveal the potential of the nanodiamonds for aggregation. Encapsulation efficiency of the formulated nanodiamonds can be determined by extracting out the entrapped drug from nanodiamonds in suitable solvent and then analyzing the solvent quantitatively by using a suitable spectroscopic or chromatographic technique. Drug release rate from nanodiamonds and permeation rate of nanodiamonds through BBB can be determined by using USP dissolution apparatus and Franz diffusion cell respectively. Both release and permeation parameters are important indicators to detect the efficacy of nanodiamond as drug delivery formulations in neurodegenerative disorders. In addition to the listed methods, mechanical strength and environmental stability of nanodiamonds are some other characterization parameters evaluated to determine the efficacy of nanodiamonds.[125–131]

3.7 NANODIAMONDS AS A PROMISING TOOL FOR BRAIN TARGETING

A summary of nanodiamond formulations is given in Table 3.1. As discussed earlier, transporting the drug in its active form across the BBB poses significant challenges. Although recent in-silico, in-vitro, and in-vivo models have uncovered the substantial potential of nanodiamonds under nanotheranostics in diagnosing and managing neurodegenerative disorders, nanodiamonds is one of the nanotherapeutics which have the potential to facilitate the shuttling of drugs into the CNS by penetrating BBB.

The BBB consists of an intracellular space with a thickness of 20 nm. The BBB has the boundary connecting the CNS and the peripheral circulations.[132] However, the BBB is one of the major hurdles for drug deliveries and for

TABLE 3.1 A Summary of Nanodiamond Formulations as Given in the Following Table.

No.	Formulation	Class/type of drug	Biological mechanism	Methods used to assess the activity of formulation	Application	Reference
1.	PEG-HSA (Polyethylene glycol-HSA complex) coated onto the nanodiamonds	–	Passive diffusion and transcytosis of the formulation through the endothelial layer of BBB	Transwell BBB model consisting of bEnd.3 cells	Formulation can be used to transport a variety of drugs across the BBB without peripheral loss	138
2.	EFV-coated nanodiamonds	EFV: Non-nucleoside reverse transcriptase inhibitor	Formulation crosses the BBB and binds with noncatalytic site of HIV reverse transcriptase thus inhibiting its activity	– XRD – Raman Spectroscopy – MTS assay to assess cell viability	HAND	125,147
3.	Adamantine- based nanodiamonds	Structurally and functionally similar with the drug memantine	–Inhibits toxicity caused by over activity of NMDA receptor –Increases level of BDNF	In-vivo study performed on albino Wistar rats by administrating formulation through *i.p* route	-AD	140
4.	Anti TGF-β1 coated nanodiamonds	Transforming growth factor β1: cytokine responsible for immunosuppressive and neuroprotective effect	Causes modulation of TGF-β1 (up regulation) pathway thereby decreasing the production and accumulation of amyloid plaques	– Stability of the formulation was measured via: – Transmission electron microscopy (TEM) – UV-visible spectroscopy – ELISA	AD	119,148, 149

TABLE 3.1 *(Continued)*

No.	Formulation	Class/type of drug	Biological mechanism	Methods used to assess the activity of formulation	Application	Reference
5.	Amlodipine loaded nanodiamonds	Amlodipine: Calcium channel blocker of dihydropyridine class	Inhibits influx of calcium which leads to decreased generation of ROS as well as pro-apoptotic factors	– Loading of the drug on the surface of nanodiamonds were examined by – High Performance Liquid Chromatography (HPLC) – FTIR – TEM	AD	150–152
6.	Nanodiamonds bound with -O functional group and coated with TCPS	–	In-vitro study demonstrated adhesion of the formulation to hNSCs and promoted neuronal growth	– Roughness was measured by Atomic force microscopy – X-ray photoelectron Spectroscopy – Cell adhesion was determined by labeling the hNSCs using Hoechst dye and Alexa Fluro® 488 Phallodin	– AD – Potential application in PD and HD – HAND	142
7.	DNDs	–	Reduces toxicity associated with over active excitatory system	Formulation was tested through isolated rat brain nerve terminals	AD, HD	[144,145

managing the various neurological diseases. Researchers have found ways to improve the chances of a compound getting through the BBB, but so far these efforts have not been very successful in clinical trials.[133,134] Researchers have shown that very small particles (smaller than 200 nm) can easily travel through the BBB.[135] Hence, recently, the focus of the researchers is on synthesizing and developing nanoparticles, because of their smaller particle size, they can effortlessly cross BBB and penetrate into the brain.[135] To overcome the limitation of other brain imaging technologies, nanodiamonds render outstanding circumstances for in-vivo brain imaging and a tractable vehicle for drug delivery, combining diagnostic and therapeutic modalities.

As discussed earlier, nanodiamonds are characterized by unusual magnetic and optical properties, electric resistivity, less toxicity and higher biocompatibility, chemical stability, high thermal conductivity, less diameter in size molecule, an elevated surface area-to-volume ratio, and nondegradability even in a harsh biological environment.[136] However, because of the hydrophobic nature of nanodiamonds, they also exhibit nonspecific biomolecular absorption, which creates hindrance in the cellular uptake of the nanodiamonds. To overcome these limitations and to achieve brain-targeted delivery across the BBB, mainly two types of modifications can be done, i.e., change in average particle size and modification of surface structure. Between these two types of modifications surface structure modification has been employed predominantly to achieve brain-targeted drug delivery in various types of *in-silico*, *in-vitro*, *ex-vivo*, and *in-vivo* models. Functionalization of nanodiamonds surface is done by a bioactive molecule of choice, e.g., coating with biocompatible polymers, silica, protein, and lipid.[137] Promising bioactive molecules which were tested by different means include: (1) Human serum albumin (HSA) coating on nanodiamonds results in nanodiamonds having cationic properties, with which these can easily penetrate the BBB. Furthermore, studies have also shown covalent attachment of poly ethylene glycol (PEG) with HAS termed as PEGlytion of HAS-coated fluorescent nanodiamonds (FNDs) by PEG 2000 increases the colloidal stability while decreasing the plasma protein binding which results in a higher concentration of the formulation inside the CNS.[138] (2) Studies have also shown that denatured and cationized albumin bound with nanodiamonds cross the BBB efficiently by the transcytosis process. (3) *Ex-vivo* studies have demonstrated the penetration ability of transferrin-coated nanodiamonds by endothelial cells present in the blood capillaries of BBB.[139] (4) *In-vivo* studies in neurological disease induced mice model injected with the intravenous formulation of HAS-NDs showed promising results by crossing the BBB efficiently. Flurochemistry studies showed that this transportation across the BBB takes place via transcytosis and active endocytosis.[138]

Human immunodeficiency virus associated neurodegenerative disorders (HAND) are a major problem associated with later stages of HIV infection. Efavirenz (EFV), an antiretroviral medication, is used to manage HAND, but it has 99.5% of plasma protein binding. Because of this high plasma protein binding EFV has very poor bioavailability in CNS and high toxicity. A study done by using surface-modified nanodiamonds which are loaded with EFV showed promising results in terms of low neuronal toxicity, maintained % cell viability, and improved loading capacity of drug. EFV-coated nanodiamonds (EFV-NDs) have also shown effective results in controlling HIV replication on primary human macrophage infected by HIV. It indicates the potential utilization of nanodiamonds as a promising carrier for brain-targeted delivery of drugs.[125]

Nanodiamonds also have a unique property. It has an admantane nucleus which makes it stand apart among other nano formulations. Admante is typically described as a fusion of three cyclohexane rings having specific bioactivity. This admantane nucleus imitates the organization of drug memantine, a medication used to manage progression of AD. Histopathological examinations performed in cognitively impaired rats treated with nanodiamonds showed neuroprotection by reducing the excitation of N-Methyl-D-Aspartate (NMDA) glutamate receptors. They exhibit the ability to limit the secretion of inflammatory cytokines including tumor necrosis factor and IL-6 and enhance release of brain-derived neurotrophic factor (BDNF). Nanodiamonds were also able to affect the clearance rate of phosphorylated Tau protein and amyloid β plaques which are the main causing factor of cognitive as well as behavioral problems associated with AD.[140] Another study in accordance with the involvement of escalated level of transforming growth factor β1 (TGF-β1) in the pathogenesis of AD was done where nanodiamonds were conjugated with anti-TGF-β1 antibody and were tested in Dulbecco's modified eagle medium (DMEM). Activity of anti-TGF-β1 antibody liberated in DMEM (+) serum was established using an enzyme-linked immunosorbent assay (ELISA). This study showed high degree of adsorption and functioning of antibody when conjugated with nanodiamonds.[119]

Amlodipine, a potent dihydropyridine calcium channel blocker, treats numerous neurologic illnesses by reversing calcium-induced excitotoxicity and also by preventing the release of reactive oxygen species (ROS) due to mitochondrial dysfunction. This property of amlodipine can be of great importance in the management of symptoms associated with AD as well as brain stroke. However, conventional amlodipine formulation is not able to cross the BBB effectively. Studies have revealed that putting amlodipine onto the nanodiamonds is a successful method of overcoming this specific issue. This loading was done by first oxidizing nanodiamonds by using acid mixture of HNO_3 and H_2SO_4 and thereafter loading of amlodipine on the surface of nanodiamonds by using 2 mM concentration of NaOH. This particular method showed 41% drug binding on the nanodiamonds surface. The results of this study raise the possibility of using nanodiamonds as a drug delivery system to deliver amlodipine inside CNS and pave the way for other medications with a similar mechanism of action.[141]

One more study was done in the case of AD, where nanodiamonds were made functionalized by means of hydrogen and oxygen functional group (H-ND & O-ND) and then they were laminated by protein tissue culture polystyrene (TCPS), an amalgamation of laminin (LN) and poly-L-lysine. It has shown to exert positive generation of human neuronal stem cells (hNSC). The results of this study indicate that TCPS-coated O-NDs showed improved cellular adhesion to the target cells when compared with TCPS-coated H-NDs. This phenomenon took place because TCPS-coated nanodiamonds had a rough surface area which resulted in a more available surface area. Thus, there is higher cell adhesion, which in turn results in better proliferation of hNSC indicated by high neuronal density, increase in the length, and higher amount of branching. O-NDs also promoted expression of specific biomarker namely glia fibrillary acidic protein, neurospecific endolase, neurofilament protein 200, and a neuro epithelial stem protein named Nestin which confirmed the possible role of O-NDs in the application of managing disorders like AD and HAND.[142,143]

A different type of class of nanodiamonds called detonated DNDs have shown to exert modulatory effects on the level of neurotransmitters like Gamma amino butyric acid (inhibitory) and glutamate (excitatory). DNDs decrease the cellular transporter-mediated uptake of these neurotransmitters, thus increasing their extracellular concentration at the synapse. This increased neurotransmitter concentration at synapses inhibits the release of more neurotransmitter particularly of glutamate. This decreased release of glutamate can help to modulate glutamate-mediated excitotoxicity, one of the pathological features in the prognosis of AD.[144] This glutamate-induced excitotoxicity is also one of the major causative factors in the pathogenesis of HD. These types of DNDs can also be employed in the patient with early diagnosis of the disease to prevent further neuronal degeneration.[145]

3.8 NANODIAMONDS AS A PROMISING TOOL FOR NEXT-GENERATION BIOMARKER FOR NEURODEGENERATIVE DISORDERS

Various examinations have shown the potential use of nanodiamonds as a versatile biomarker. One study demonstrated the ability of PEGylated denatured HSA (dcHSA-PEG)-coated nanodiamonds to penetrate the intact BBB in both in-vitro and in-vivo conditions. dcHSA-PEG nanodiamonds unlike other newer brain targeting nanoplatforms for diagnostic purposes exhibit the following ideal features simultaneously, namely, (1) biocompatibility, (2) colloidal stability, (3) stable fluorescence, (4) temperature sensing, (5) capability of attaching multiple functional groups on the surface, and most importantly (6) possibility of nuclear spin hyperpolarization for magnetic resonance imaging (MRI). These properties allow the transportation of dcHSA-NDs through the BBB when given by the intravenous route and it opened the new horizons for treatment tracking via MRI and sensing the temperature changes in the brain.[138] Furthermore, the capacity to change the nanodiamond's lattice structure has enabled the creation of several variants with different applications. For instance, replacement of a carbon atom with a nitrogen atom creates a so-called "flawed diamond" which can be easily diagnosed by imaging studies like MRI, once it crosses the BBB and enters the brain, providing a diagnostic tool for many neurological diseases. Another study showed the capacity of cell-penetrating peptides to aid the transport of FNDs over the BBB which helps them to initiate the release of amino acids like leucine, phenylalanine, aspartic acid etc, which detect the fibrillar amyloid beta plaques, a biomarker of AD.[146]

3.9 CONCLUSION

Neurodegenerative disorders are a set of disorders which affect almost 30% of the population aged 85 years and above. Neurodegenerative diseases still remain one of the most complex conditions in terms of pathophysiology as well as treatment options and it also worsens with age. AD, PD, and ALS are the most commonly occurring neurodegenerative diseases. Conventional medications are unable to efficiently target neurodegenerative disorders because of extremely selective biological barriers. The BBB is one of them. Presence of various types of specialized cells like astrocytes, pericytes, various types of transporter proteins in the BBB imparts difficulties in the transportation of biologically active molecules. Other challenges of effective drug delivery at the target site of CNS include efflux transporter, pharmacokinetic factors, as well as physiochemical property of therapeutic agents. As an encouraging remedy to these challenges, nanodiamonds, having a size range of a millionth of a meter, are considered to be an emerging and effective tool to deliver medicine into the targeted region of the brain. Nanodiamonds are carbon-based nanoparticles with truncated octahedral geometry and with a diameter ranging from 2 to 8 nm and having qualities like biocompatibility, intrinsic fluorescence without photobleaching, tuneable surface and nonreactivity, colloidal stability, and also temperature-sensing properties which make them well tolerated and suitable for both diagnostic and therapeutic purposes. Multiple synthesis methods available for the production of nanodiamonds make them economically viable as well. Moreover, the compatibility of nanodiamonds with other biologically occurring molecules also makes it much more suitable as a carrier for transporting the medicines across BBB for example, amlodipine coated on nanodiamonds. Currently, scientists have been able to demonstrate the intraneuronal axonal transport within the degrading neurons with the help of FNDs which are found to be the crucial tool to understand the genetic factors behind the pathogenesis of neurodegenerative disorders. dcHSA-PEG nanodiamonds have been also proven to be versatile for loading of multiple drugs onto the surface of nanodiamonds while opening new strategies for treatment tracking through imaging studies. Apart from the use of nanodiamonds as imaging probes, scientists have also found various techniques to incorporate pharmaceutical ingredients with nanodiamonds like drugs, antibodies etc. Nanodiamonds also provide numerous superior advantages over the conventional drug delivery system; one such important and unique advantage is that nanodiamonds can be used in their original form, i.e., it does not need to go through oxidative modification and acidic treatment like in the case of loading of amlodipine onto the nanodiamonds where they undergo modification by means of combination of acidic mixture. Thus, they can be used as such as a remedy; this property is attributed because nanodiamonds have structural similarities with the drug memantine. Multiple unique properties like this make nanodiamonds an interesting and promising topic to study and explore for the delivery of therapeutic agents in the management and hopefully treatment of neurodegenerative disorders in near future.

KEYWORDS

- **neurodegenerative diseases**
- **nanodiamonds**
- **blood–brain barrier**
- **P-glycoprotein**
- **targeted drug delivery**
- **Alzheimer's disease**
- **Parkinson's disease**
- **Huntington's disease**

REFERENCES

1. Gitler, A. D.; Dhillon, P.; Shorter, J. Neurodegenerative Disease: Models, Mechanisms, and a New Hope. *Dis. Model Mech.* **2017,** *10,* 499–502.
2. Heemels, M.-T. Neurodegenerative Diseases. *Nature* **2016,** *539,* 179.
3. Chauhan, H.; Gupta, P.; Saxena, B. MicroRNAs as Future Treatment Tools and Diagnostic Biomarkers in Alzheimer's Disease. *Alzheimers Dis.* **2022**. https://doi.org/10.5772/intechopen.103173.
4. Sosa-Ortiz, A. L.; Acosta-Castillo, I.; Prince, M. J. Epidemiology of Dementias and Alzheimer's Disease. *Arch. Med. Res.* **2012,** *43,* 600–608.
5. Robinson, M.; Lee, B. Y.; Hane, F. T. Recent Progress in Alzheimer's Disease Research, Part 2 : Genetics and Epidemiology. *J. Alzheimer's Dis. 57,* 317–330.
6. Ferri, C. P.; Prince, M.; Brayne, C.; et al Global Prevalence of Dementia: A Delphi Consensus Study. *Lancet* **2005,** *366,* 2112–2117.
7. Elbaz, A.; Bower, J. H.; Maraganore, D. M.; Mcdonnell, S. K.; Peterson, B. J.; Ahlskog, J. E.; Schaid, D. J.; Rocca, W. A. Risk Tables for Parkinsonism and Parkinson's Disease. *J. Clin. Epidemiol.* **2002,** *55,* 25–31.
8. Logroscino, G. Incidence of Amyotrophic Lateral Sclerosis in Southern Italy: A Population Based Study. *J. Neurol. Neurosurg. Psychiatry* **2005,** *76,* 1094–1098.
9. Jellinger, K. A. Basic Mechanisms of Neurodegeneration: A Critical Update. *J. Cell. Mol. Med.* **2010,** *14,* 457–487.
10. Przedborski, S.; Vila, M.; Jackson-Lewis, V. Series Introduction: Neurodegeneration: What is it and where are we? *J. Clin. Invest.* **2003,** *111,* 3–10.
11. Jellinger, K. A. Recent Advances in Our Understanding of Neurodegeneration. *J. Neural. Transm. (Vienna)* **2009,** *116,* 1111–1162.
12. Hoover, B. R.; Reed, M. N.; Su, J.; et al Tau Mislocalization to Dendritic Spines Mediates Synaptic Dysfunction Independently of Neurodegeneration. *Neuron* **2010,** *68,* 1067–1081.

13. Milnerwood, A. J.; Raymond, L. A. Early Synaptic Pathophysiology in Neurodegeneration: Insights from Huntington's Disease. *Trends Neurosci.* **2010,** *33,* 513–523.
14. Scott, D. A.; Tabarean, I.; Tang, Y.; Cartier, A.; Masliah, E.; Roy, S. A Pathologic Cascade Leading to Synaptic Dysfunction in Alpha-Synuclein-Induced Neurodegeneration. *J. Neurosci.* **2010,** *30,* 8083–8095.
15. Kovacs, G. G. Molecular Pathology of Neurodegenerative Diseases: Principles and Practice. *J. Clin. Pathol.* **2019,** *72,* 725–735.
16. Saraf, J.; Kalia, K.; Bhattacharya, P.; Tekade, R. K. Growing Synergy of Nanodiamonds in Neurodegenerative Interventions. *Drug Discov. Today* **2019,** *24,* 584–594.
17. Harilal, S.; Jose, J.; Parambi, D. G. T.; Kumar, R.; Mathew, G. E.; Uddin, M. S.; Kim, H.; Mathew, B. Advancements in Nanotherapeutics for Alzheimer's Disease: Current Perspectives. *J. Pharm. Pharmacol.* **2019,** *71,* 1370–1383.
18. Hinge, N. S.; Kathuria, H.; Pandey, M. M. Engineering of Structural and Functional Properties of Nanotherapeutics and Nanodiagnostics for Intranasal Brain Targeting in Alzheimer's. *Appl. Mater. Today* **2022,** *26,* 101303.
19. Montazersaheb, S.; Ahmadian, E.; Dizaj, S. M.; Jahanbani, Y.; Davaran, S.; Huseynova, I.; Zhdanov, R. I.; Keskin, C.; Khalilov, R.; Eftekhari, A. (2021) *Emerging Nanotherapeutic Strategies in Alzheimer's Disease*; pp 173–203.
20. Kaur, R.; Badea, I. Nanodiamonds as Novel Nanomaterials for Biomedical Applications: Drug Delivery and Imaging Systems. *Int. J. Nanomed.* **2013,** *8,* 203–20.
21. Ali Mansoori, G. *Adv. Chemi. Phys.* **2011,** https://doi.org/10.1002/9781118135242.
22. Bhavsar, N.; Saxena, B.; Shah, J. Blood-Brain Barrier and Central Nervous System Drug Delivery: Challenges and Opportunities. In: *Nanocarriers for Drug-Targeting Brain Tumors*; Elsevier, 2022; pp 31–48.
23. Aird, W. C. Phenotypic Heterogeneity of the Endothelium. *Circ. Res.* **2007,** *100,* 174–190.
24. Aird, W. C. Phenotypic Heterogeneity of the Endothelium. *Circ. Res.* **2007,** *100,* 158–173.
25. Coomber, B. L.; Stewart, P. A. Morphometric Analysis of CNS Microvascular Endothelium. *Microvasc. Res.* **1985,** *30,* 99–115.
26. Westergaard, E.; Brightman, M. W. Transport of Proteins across Normal Cerebral Arterioles. *J. Comp. Neurol.* **1973,** *152,* 17–44.
27. Oldendorf, W. H.; Cornford, M. E.; Brown, W. J. The Large Apparent Work Capability of the Blood-Brain Barrier: A Study of the Mitochondrial Content of Capillary Endothelial Cells in Brain and other Tissues of the Rat. *Ann. Neurol.* **1977,** *1,* 409–417.
28. Cordon-Cardo, C.; O'Brien, J. P.; Casals, D.; Rittman-Grauer, L.; Biedler, J. L.; Melamed, M. R.; Bertino, J. R. Multidrug-Resistance Gene (P-Glycoprotein) is Expressed by Endothelial Cells at Blood-Brain Barrier Sites. *Proc. Natl Acad. Sci.* **1989,** *86,* 695–698.
29. Löscher, W.; Potschka, H. Blood-Brain Barrier Active Efflux Transporters: ATP-Binding Cassette Gene Family. *Neurorx* **2005,** *2,* 86–98.
30. Mittapalli, R. K.; Manda, V. K.; Adkins, C. E.; Geldenhuys, W. J.; Lockman, P. R. Exploiting Nutrient Transporters at the Blood–Brain Barrier to Improve Brain Distribution of Small Molecules. *Ther. Deliv.* **2010,** *1,* 775–784.
31. Daneman, R.; Zhou, L.; Agalliu, D.; Cahoy, J. D.; Kaushal, A.; Barres, B. A. The Mouse Blood-Brain Barrier Transcriptome: A New Resource for Understanding the Development and Function of Brain Endothelial Cells. *PLoS One* **2010,** *5,* E13741.
32. Henninger, D. D.; Panés, J.; Eppihimer, M.; Russell, J.; Gerritsen, M.; Anderson, D. C.; Granger, D. N. Cytokine-Induced VCAM-1 and ICAM-1 Expression in Different Organs of the Mouse. *J. Immunol.* **1997,** *158,* 1825–1832.

33. Majesky, M. W. Developmental Basis of Vascular Smooth Muscle Diversity. *Arterioscler. Thromb. Vasc. Biol.* **2007,** *27,* 1248–1258.
34. Sims, D. E. The Pericyte—A Review. Tissue Cell **1986,** *18,* 153–174.
35. Peppiatt, C. M.; Howarth, C.; Mobbs, P.; Attwell, D. Bidirectional Control of CNS Capillary Diameter by Pericytes. *Nature* **2006,** *443,* 700–704.
36. Gerhardt, H.; Wolburg, H.; Redies, C. N-Cadherin Mediates Pericytic-Endothelial Interaction during Brain Angiogenesis in the Chicken. *Dev. Dyn.* **2000,** *218,* 472–479.
37. Courtoy, P. J.; Boyles, J. Fibronectin in the Microvasculature: Localization in the Pericyte-Endothelial Interstitium. *J. Ultrastruct. Res.* **1983,** *83,* 258–273.
38. Cuevas, P.; Gutierrez-Diaz, J. A.; Reimers, D.; Dujovny, M.; Diaz, F. G.; Ausman, J. I. Pericyte Endothelial Gap Junctions in Human Cerebral Capillaries. *Anat. Embryol. (Berl.)* **1984,** *170,* 155–159.
39. Larson, D. M.; Carson, M. P.; Haudenschild, C. C. Junctional Transfer of Small Molecules in Cultured Bovine Brain Microvascular Endothelial Cells and Pericytes. *Microvasc. Res.* **1987,** *34,* 184–199.
40. Armulik, A.; Genové, G.; Betsholtz, C. Pericytes: Developmental, Physiological, and Pathological Perspectives, Problems, and Promises. *Dev. Cell* **2011,** *21,* 193–215.
41. Daneman, R.; Zhou, L.; Kebede, A. A.; Barres, B. A. Pericytes are Required for Blood–Brain Barrier Integrity During Embryogenesis. *Nature* **2010,** *468,* 562–566.
42. Armulik, A.; Genové, G.; Mäe, M.; et al Pericytes Regulate the Blood–Brain Barrier. *Nature* **2010,** *468,* 557–561.
43. Del Zoppo, G. J.; Milner, R.; Mabuchi, T.; Hung, S.; Wang, X.; Koziol, J. A. Vascular Matrix Adhesion and the Blood–Brain Barrier. *Biochem. Soc. Trans.* **2006,** *34,* 1261–1266.
44. Sorokin, L. The Impact of the Extracellular Matrix on Inflammation. *Nat. Rev. Immunol.* **2010,** *10,* 712–723.
45. Daneman, R.; Prat, A. The Blood–Brain Barrier. *Cold Spring Harb. Perspect. Biol.* **2015,** *7,* A020412.
46. Noell, S.; Wolburg-Buchholz, K.; Mack, A. F.; Beedle, A. M.; Satz, J. S.; Campbell, K. P.; Wolburg, H.; Fallier-Becker, P. Evidence for a Role of Dystroglycan Regulating the Membrane Architecture of Astroglial Endfeet. *Eur. J. Neurosci.* **2011,** *33,* 2179–2186.
47. Wolburg, H.; Wolburg-Buchholz, K.; Fallier-Becker, P.; Noell, S.; Mack, A. F. Structure and Functions of Aquaporin-4-Based Orthogonal Arrays of Particles. *Int. Rev. Cell Mol. Biol.* **2011,** *287,* 1–41.
48. Janzer, R. C.; Raff, M. C. Astrocytes Induce Blood–Brain Barrier Properties in Endothelial Cells. *Nature* **1987,** *325,* 253–257.
49. Abbott, N. J.; Rönnbäck, L.; Hansson, E. Astrocyte–Endothelial Interactions at the Blood–Brain Barrier. *Nat. Rev. Neurosci.* **2006,** *7,* 41–53.
50. Streit, W. J.; Conde, J. R.; Fendrick, S. E.; Flanary, B. E.; Mariani, C. L. Role of Microglia in the Central Nervous System's Immune Response. *Neurol. Res.* **2005,** *27,* 685–691.
51. Hickey, W. F.; Kimura, H. Perivascular Microglial Cells of the CNS are Bone Marrow-Derived and Present Antigen In Vivo. *Science* **1988,** *239,* 290–292.
52. Vass, K.; Hickey, W. F.; Schmidt, R. E.; Lassmann, H. Bone Marrow-Derived Elements in the Peripheral Nervous System. An Immunohistochemical and Ultrastructural Investigation in Chimeric Rats. *Lab. Invest.* **1993,** *69,* 275–282.
53. Williams, K.; Alvarez, X.; Lackner, A. A. Central Nervous System Perivascular Cells are Immunoregulatory Cells that Connect the CNS with the Peripheral Immune System. *Glia* **2001,** *36,* 156–164.

54. Persidsky, Y.; Ghorpade, A.; Rasmussen, J.; et al. Microglial and Astrocyte Chemokines Regulate Monocyte Migration through the Blood-Brain Barrier in Human Immunodeficiency Virus-1 Encephalitis. *Am. J. Pathol.* **1999,** *155,* 1599–1611.
55. Interlandi, J. Breaking the Brain Barrier. *Sci. Am.* **2013,** *308,* 52–57.
56. Begley, D. J. The Blood-Brain Barrier: Principles for Targeting Peptides and Drugs to the Central Nervous System. *J. Pharm. Pharmacol.* **2011,** *48,* 136–146.
57. Serlin, Y.; Shelef, I.; Knyazer, B.; Friedman, A. Anatomy and Physiology of the Blood–Brain Barrier. *Semin. Cell Dev. Biol.* **2015,** *38,* 2–6.
58. Lockman, P. R.; Mumper, R. J.; Khan, M. A.; Allen, D. D. Nanoparticle Technology for Drug Delivery across the Blood-Brain Barrier. *Drug Dev. Ind. Pharm.* **2002,** *28,* 1–13.
59. Argaw, A. T.; Asp, L.; Zhang, J.; et al Astrocyte-Derived VEGF-A Drives Blood-Brain Barrier Disruption in CNS Inflammatory Disease. *J. Clin. Invest.* **2012,** *122,* 2454–2468.
60. Arora, S.; Sharma, D.; Singh, J. GLUT-1: An Effective Target to Deliver Brain-Derived Neurotrophic Factor Gene across the Blood Brain Barrier. *ACS Chem. Neurosci.* **2020,** *11,* 1620–1633.
61. Kook, S.-Y.; Seok Hong, H.; Moon, M.; Mook-Jung, I. Disruption of Blood-Brain Barrier in Alzheimer Disease Pathogenesis. *Tissue Barriers* **2013,** *1,* E23993.
62. Lee, H. Disruption of the Blood-Brain Barrier in Parkinson's Disease: Curse or Route to a Cure? *Front. Biosci.* **2014,** *19,* 272.
63. Sengillo, J. D.; Winkler, E. A.; Walker, C. T.; Sullivan, J. S.; Johnson, M.; Zlokovic, B. V. Deficiency in Mural Vascular Cells Coincides with Blood-Brain Barrier Disruption in Alzheimer's Disease. *Brain Pathol.* **2013,** *23,* 303–310.
64. van de Waterbeemd, H.; Camenisch, G.; Folkers, G.; Chretien, J. R.; Raevsky, O. A. Estimation of Blood-Brain Barrier Crossing of Drugs Using Molecular Size and Shape, and H-Bonding Descriptors. *J. Drug Target.* **1998,** *6,* 151–165.
65. Dong, X. Current Strategies for Brain Drug Delivery. *Theranostics* **2018,** *8,* 1481–1493.
66. Ghuman, J.; Zunszain, P. A.; Petitpas, I.; Bhattacharya, A. A.; Otagiri, M.; Curry, S. Structural Basis of the Drug-Binding Specificity of Human Serum Albumin. *J. Mol. Biol.* **2005,** *353,* 38–52.
67. Krol, S. Challenges in Drug Delivery to the Brain: Nature is against us. *J. Control. Release* **2012,** *164,* 145–55.
68. Patel, M. M.; Goyal, B. R.; Bhadada, S. V.; Bhatt, J. S.; Amin, A. F. Getting into the Brain. *CNS Drugs* **2009,** *23,* 35–58.
69. Schinkel, A. H. P-Glycoprotein, a Gatekeeper in the Blood-Brain Barrier. *Adv. Drug Deliv. Rev.* **1999,** *36,* 179–194.
70. Correale, J.; Villa, A. Cellular Elements of the Blood-Brain Barrier. *Neurochem. Res.* **2009,** *34,* 2067–2077.
71. Wang, W.; Bodles-Brakhop, A. M.; Barger, S. W. A Role for P-Glycoprotein in Clearance of Alzheimer Amyloid B-Peptide from the Brain. *Curr. Alzheimer Res.* **2016,** *13,* 615–620.
72. Bartels, A. L.; Willemsen, A. T. M.; Kortekaas, R.; de Jong, B. M.; de Vries, R.; de Klerk, O.; van Oostrom, J. C. H.; Portman, A.; Leenders, K. L. Decreased Blood-Brain Barrier P-Glycoprotein Function in the Progression of Parkinson's Disease, PSP and MSA. *J. Neural. Transm. (Vienna)* **2008,** *115,* 1001–9.
73. Kortekaas, R.; Leenders, K. L.; Van Oostrom, J. C. H.; Vaalburg, W.; Bart, J.; Willemsen, A. T. M.; Hendrikse, N. H. Blood-Brain Barrier Dysfunction in Parkinsonian Midbrain In Vivo. *Ann. Neurol.* **2005,** *57,* 176–179.

74. Irwin, D. J.; Lee, V. M.-Y.; Trojanowski, J. Q. Parkinson's Disease Dementia: Convergence of α-Synuclein, Tau and Amyloid-β Pathologies. *Nat. Rev. Neurosci.* **2013,** *14,* 626–36.
75. Vogelgesang, S.; Cascorbi, I.; Schroeder, E.; Pahnke, J.; Kroemer, H. K.; Siegmund, W.; Kunert-Keil, C.; Walker, L. C.; Warzok, R. W. Deposition of Alzheimer's??-Amyloid is Inversely Correlated with P-Glycoprotein Expression in the Brains of Elderly Non-demented Humans. *Pharmacogenetics* **2002,** *12,* 535–541.
76. Vogelgesang, S.; Glatzel, M.; Walker, L. C.; Kroemer, H. K.; Aguzzi, A.; Warzok, R. W. Cerebrovascular P-Glycoprotein Expression is Decreased in Creutzfeldt–Jakob Disease. *Acta Neuropathol.* **2006,** *111,* 436–443.
77. Lawther, B. K.; Kumar, S.; Krovvidi, H. Blood-Brain Barrier. Continuing Education in Anaesthesia, *Crit. Care Pain* **2011,** *11,* 128–132.
78. Abbott, N. J.; Patabendige, A. A. K.; Dolman, D. E. M.; Yusof, S. R.; Begley, D. J. Structure and Function of the Blood–Brain Barrier. *Neurobiol. Dis.* **2010,** *37,* 13–25.
79. Barnard, A. S.; Ōsawa, E. The Impact of Structural Polydispersivity on the Surface Electrostatic Potential of Nanodiamond. *Nanoscale* **2014,** *6,* 1188–1194.
80. Gunawan, M. A.; Poinsot, D.; Domenichini, B.; Dirand, C.; Chevalier, S.; Fokin, A. A.; Schreiner, P. R.; Hierso, J.-C. The Functionalization of Nanodiamonds (*Diamondoids*) as a Key Parameter of their Easily Controlled Self-Assembly in Micro- and Nanocrystals from the Vapor Phase. *Nanoscale* **2015,** *7,* 1956–1962.
81. Ashek-I-Ahmed, G. L.; Mandal, S.; Song, C.-Y.; Williams, O. A.; Sarmiento, M. N.; Cheng, C.-L. Facile Amine Termination of Nanodiamond Particles and their Surface Reaction Dynamics. *ACS Omega* **2019,** *4,* 16715–16723.
82. Bhosale, R. R. Nanodiamonds: A New-Fangled Drug Delivery System. 2013.
83. El-Say, K. M. Nanodiamond as a Drug Delivery System: Applications and Prospective. *J. Appl. Pharm. Sci.* **2011,** *1,* 29–39.
84. Hu, W.; Li, Z.; Yang, J. Surface and Size Effects on the Charge State of NV Center in Nanodiamonds. *Comput. Theor. Chem.* **2013,** *1021,* 49–53.
85. Shenderova, O. A.; Shames, A. I.; Nunn, N. A.; Torelli, M. D.; Vlasov, I.; Zaitsev, A. Review Article: Synthesis, Properties, and Applications of Fluorescent Diamond Particles. *J. Vac. Sci. Technol. B* **2019,** *37,* 030802.
86. Schirhagl, R.; Chang, K.; Loretz, M.; Degen, C. L. Nitrogen-Vacancy Centers in Diamond: Nanoscale Sensors for Physics and Biology. *Annu. Rev. Phys. Chem.* **2014,** *65,* 83–105.
87. Manson, N. B.; Harrison, J. P.; Sellars, M. J. Nitrogen-Vacancy Center in Diamond: Model of the Electronic Structure and Associated Dynamics. *Phys. Rev. B* **2006,** *74,* 104303.
88. Mittiga, T.; Hsieh, S.; Zu, C.; et al Imaging the Local Charge Environment of Nitrogen-Vacancy Centers in Diamond. *Phys. Rev. Lett.* **2018,** *121,* 246402.
89. Sipahigil, A.; Jahnke, K. D.; Rogers, L. J.; Teraji, T.; Isoya, J.; Zibrov, A. S.; Jelezko, F.; Lukin, M. D. Indistinguishable Photons from Separated Silicon-Vacancy Centers in Diamond. *Phys. Rev. Lett.* **2014,** *113,* 113602.
90. Dhomkar, S.; Zangara, P. R.; Henshaw, J.; Meriles, C. A. On-demand Generation of Neutral and Negatively Charged Silicon-Vacancy Centers in Diamond. *Phys. Rev. Lett.* **2018,** *120,* 117401.
91. Becker, J. N.; Becher, C. Coherence Properties and Quantum Control of Silicon Vacancy Color Centers in Diamond. *Phys. Status Solidi A* **2017,** *214,* 1700586.
92. Fehler, K. G.; Antoniuk, L.; Lettner, N.; Ovvyan, A. P.; Waltrich, R.; Gruhler, N.; Davydov, V. A.; Agafonov, V. N.; Pernice, W. H. P.; Kubanek, A. Hybrid Quantum

Photonics Based on Artificial Atoms Placed Inside One Hole of a Photonic Crystal Cavity. *ACS Photon.* **2021,** *8,* 2635–2641.
93. Chen, D.; Mu, Z.; Zhou, Y.; Fröch, J. E.; Rasmit, A.; Diederichs, C.; Zheludev, N.; Aharonovich, I.; Gao, W. Optical Gating of Resonance Fluorescence from a Single Germanium Vacancy Color Center in Diamond. *Phys. Rev. Lett.* **2019,** *123,* 033602.
94. Iwasaki, T.; Ishibashi, F.; Miyamoto, Y.; et al Germanium-Vacancy Single Color Centers in Diamond. *Sci. Rep.* **2015,** *5,* 12882.
95. Siampour, H.; Wang, O.; Zenin, V. A.; et al Ultrabright Single-Photon Emission from Germanium-Vacancy Zero-Phonon Lines: Deterministic Emitter-Waveguide Interfacing at Plasmonic Hot Spots. *Nanophotonics* **2020,** *9,* 953–962.
96. Siyushev, P.; Metsch, M. H.; Ijaz, A.; et al Optical and Microwave Control of Germanium-Vacancy Center Spins in Diamond. *Phys. Rev. B* **2017,** *96,* 081201.
97. Iwasaki, T.; Miyamoto, Y.; Taniguchi, T.; Siyushev, P.; Metsch, M. H.; Jelezko, F.; Hatano, M. Tin-Vacancy Quantum Emitters in Diamond. *Phys. Rev. Lett.* **2017,** *119,* 253601.
98. Liu, G.-Q.; Pan, X.-Y. Quantum Information Processing with Nitrogen–Vacancy Centers in Diamond. *Chin. Phys. B* **2018,** *27,* 020304.
99. Rugar, A. E.; Dory, C.; Sun, S.; Vučković, J. Characterization of Optical and Spin Properties of Single Tin-Vacancy Centers in Diamond Nanopillars. *Phys. Rev. B* **2019,** *99,* 205417.
100. Trusheim, M. E.; Pingault, B.; Wan, N. H.; et al Transform-Limited Photons from a Coherent Tin-Vacancy Spin in Diamond. *Phys. Rev. Lett.* **2020,** *124,* 023602.
101. Maletinsky, P.; Hong, S.; Grinolds, M. S.; Hausmann, B.; Lukin, M. D.; Walsworth, R. L.; Loncar, M.; Yacoby, A. A Robust Scanning Diamond Sensor for Nanoscale Imaging with Single Nitrogen-Vacancy Centres. *Nat. Nanotechnol.* **2012,** *7,* 320–324.
102. Balasubramanian, G.; Lazariev, A.; Arumugam, S. R.; Duan, D. Nitrogen-Vacancy Color Center in Diamond—Emerging Nanoscale Applications in Bioimaging and Biosensing. *Curr. Opin. Chem. Biol.* **2014,** *20,* 69–77.
103. Bradac, C.; Gaebel, T.; Chrisi, P.; Say, J. M.; Zvyagin, A V, Rabeau, J. R. Effect of the Nanodiamond Host on a Nitrogen-Vacancy Color-Centre Emission State. *Small* **2013,** *9,* 132–139.
104. Schrand, A. M.; Huang, H.; Carlson, C.; Schlager, J. J.; Ōsawa, E.; Hussain, S. M.; Dai, L. Are Diamond Nanoparticles Cytotoxic? *J. Phys. Chem. B* **2007,** *111,* 2–7.
105. Hsu, T.-C.; Liu, K.-K.; Chang, H.-C.; Hwang, E.; Chao, J.-I. Labeling of Neuronal Differentiation and Neuron Cells with Biocompatible Fluorescent Nanodiamonds. *Sci. Rep.* **2015,** *4,* 5004.
106. Liu, K.-K.; Cheng, C.-L.; Chang, C.-C.; Chao, J.-I. Biocompatible and Detectable Carboxylated Nanodiamond on Human Cell. *Nanotechnology* **2007,** *18,* 325102.
107. Reina, G.; Zhao, L.; Bianco, A.; Komatsu, N. Chemical Functionalization of Nanodiamonds: Opportunities and Challenges Ahead. *Angew. Chem. Int. Ed.* **2019,** *58,* 17918–17929.
108. Qin, J.-X.; Yang, X.-G.; Lv, C.-F.; Li, Y.-Z.; Liu, K.-K.; Zang, J.-H.; Yang, X.; Dong, L.; Shan, C.-X. Nanodiamonds: Synthesis, Properties, and Applications in Nanomedicine. *Mater. Des.* **2021,** *210,* 110091.
109. Tinwala, H.; Wairkar, S. Production, Surface Modification and Biomedical Applications of Nanodiamonds: A Sparkling Tool for Theranostics. *Mater. Sci. Eng. C* **2019,** *97,* 913–931.
110. Vervald, A. M.; Laptinskiy, K. A.; Burikov, S. A.; Laptinskaya, T V.; Shenderova, O. A.; Vlasov, I. I.; Dolenko, T. A. Nanodiamonds and Surfactants in Water: Hydrophilic and Hydrophobic Interactions. *J. Colloid Interface Sci.* **2019,** *547,* 206–216.

111. Wahab, Z.; Foley, E. A.; Pellechia, P. J.; Anneaux, B. L.; Ploehn, H. J. Surface Functionalization of Nanodiamond with Phenylphosphonate. *J. Colloid Interface Sci.* **2015,** *450,* 301–309.
112. Shenderova, O.; Panich, A. M.; Moseenkov, S.; Hens, S. C.; Kuznetsov, V.; Vieth, H.-M. Hydroxylated Detonation Nanodiamond: FTIR, XPS, and NMR Studies. *J. Phys. Chem. C* **2011,** *115,* 19005–19011.
113. Arnault, J. C.; Girard, H. A. Hydrogenated Nanodiamonds: Synthesis and Surface Properties. *Curr. Opin. Solid State Mater. Sci.* **2017,** *21,* 10–16.
114. Lisichkin, G. V.; Korol'kov, V. V.; Tarasevich, B. N.; Kulakova, I. I.; Karpukhin, A. V.. Photochemical Chlorination of Nanodiamond and Interaction of its Modified Surface with C-Nucleophiles. *Russ. Chem. Bull.* **2006,** *55,* 2212–2219.
115. Reina, G.; Gismondi, A.; Carcione, R.; Nanni, V.; Peruzzi, C.; Angjellari, M.; Chau, N. D. Q.; Canini, A.; Terranova, M. L.; Tamburri, E. Oxidized and Amino-Functionalized Nanodiamonds as Shuttle for Delivery of Plant Secondary Metabolites: Interplay Between Chemical Affinity and Bioactivity. *Appl. Surf. Sci.* **2019,** *470,* 744–754.
116. Khalid, A.; Mitropoulos, A. N.; Marelli, B.; Tomljenovic-Hanic, S.; Omenetto, F. G. Doxorubicin Loaded Nanodiamond-Silk Spheres for Fluorescence Tracking and Controlled Drug Release. *Biomed. Opt. Express* **2016,** *7,* 132.
117. Krüger, A.; Kataoka, F.; Ozawa, M.; Fujino, T.; Suzuki, Y.; Aleksenskii, A. E.; Aya, V. '.; Ōsawa, E. Unusually Tight Aggregation in Detonation Nanodiamond: Identification and Disintegration. *Carbon N Y* **2005,** *43,* 1722–1730.
118. Chen, M.; Pierstorff, E. D.; Lam, R.; Li, S.-Y.; Huang, H.; Osawa, E.; Ho, D. Nanodiamond-Mediated Delivery of Water-Insoluble Therapeutics. *ACS Nano* **2009,** *3,* 2016–2022.
119. Smith, A. H.; Robinson, E. M.; Zhang, X.-Q.; Chow, E. K.; Lin, Y.; Osawa, E.; Xi, J.; Ho, D. Triggered Release of Therapeutic Antibodies from Nanodiamond Complexes. *Nanoscale* **2011,** *3,* 2844.
120. Whitlow, J.; Pacelli, S.; Paul, A. Multifunctional Nanodiamonds in Regenerative Medicine: Recent Advances and Future Directions. *J. Control. Release* **2017,** *261,* 62–86.
121. Jariwala, D. H.; Patel, D.; Wairkar, S. Surface Functionalization of Nanodiamonds for Biomedical Applications. *Mater. Sci. Eng. C* **2020,** *113,* 110996.
122. Stehlik, S.; Varga, M.; Ledinsky, M.; et al Size and Purity Control of HPHT Nanodiamonds Down to 1 nm. *J. Phys. Chem. C* **2015,** *119,* 27708–27720.
123. Mitev, D. P.; Alsharabasy, A. M.; Morrison, L.; Wittig, S.; Diener, C.; Pandit, A. Plasma & Microwaves as Greener Options for Nanodiamond Purification: Insight into Cytocompatibility. *Front. Bioeng. Biotechnol.* **2021.** https://doi.org/10.3389/fbioe.2021.637587.
124. Giussani, A.; Janssens, S. D.; Vázquez-Cortés, D.; Fried, E. Evolution of Nanodiamond Seeds during the Chemical Vapor Deposition of Diamond on Silicon Substrates in Oxygen-Rich Plasmas. *Appl. Surf. Sci.* **2022,** *581,* 152103.
125. Roy, U.; Drozd, V.; Durygin, A.; Rodriguez, J.; Barber, P.; Atluri, V.; Liu, X.; Voss, T. G.; Saxena, S.; Nair, M. Characterization of Nanodiamond-Based anti-HIV Drug Delivery to the Brain. *Sci. Rep.* **2018,** *8,* 1603.
126. Wang, H.; Lee, D.-K.; Chen, K.-Y.; Chen, J.-Y.; Zhang, K.; Silva, A.; Ho, C.-M.; Ho, D. Mechanism-Independent Optimization of Combinatorial Nanodiamond and Unmodified Drug Delivery Using a Phenotypically Driven Platform Technology. *ACS Nano* **2015,** *9,* 3332–3344.

127. Aleksenskiy, A.; Baidakova, M.; Osipov, V.; Vul', A. The Fundamental Properties and Characteristics of Nanodiamonds. In *Nanodiamonds*; Springer US: Boston, MA, 2010; pp 55–77.
128. Li, J.; Ge, X.; Cui, C.; Zhang, Y.; Wang, Y.; Wang, X.; Sun, Q. Preparation and Characterization of Functionalized Graphene Oxide Carrier for Sirna Delivery. *Int. J. Mol. Sci.* **2018,** *19,* 3202.
129. Mochalin, V. N.; Shenderova, O.; Ho, D.; Gogotsi, Y. The Properties and Applications of Nanodiamonds. *Nat. Nanotechnol.* **2011,** *7,* 11–23.
130. Schrand, A. M., Hens, S. A. C.; Shenderova, O. A. Nanodiamond Particles: Properties and Perspectives for Bioapplications. *Critical Rev. Solid State Mat. Sci.* **2009,** *34*(1-2), 18–74.
131. Shah, V.; Jobanputra, A.; Saxena, B.; Nivsarkar, M. Development and Characterization of Saturated Fatty Acid-Engineered, Silica-Coated Lipid Vesicular System for Effective Oral Delivery of Alfa-Choriogonadotropin. *AAPS Pharmscitech.* **2021,** *22,* 118.
132. Ding, S.; Khan, A. I.; Cai, X.; Song, Y.; Lyu, Z.; Du, D.; Dutta, P.; Lin, Y. Overcoming Blood–Brain Barrier Transport: Advances in Nanoparticle-Based Drug Delivery Strategies. *Mater. Today* **2020,** *37,* 112–125.
133. Banks, W. A. From Blood–Brain Barrier to Blood–Brain Interface: New Opportunities for CNS Drug Delivery. *Nat. Rev. Drug Discov.* **2016,** *15,* 275–292.
134. Liu, C.-C.; Kanekiyo, T.; Xu, H.; Bu, G. Apolipoprotein E and Alzheimer Disease: Risk, Mechanisms and Therapy. *Nat. Rev. Neurol.* **2013,** *9,* 106–118.
135. Henna, T. K.; Raphey, V. R.; Sankar, R.; Ameena Shirin, V. K.; Gangadharappa, H. V.; Pramod, K. Carbon Nanostructures: The Drug and the Delivery System for Brain Disorders. *Int. J. Pharm.* **2020,** *587,* 119701.
136. Zhu, Y.; Li, J.; Li, W.; Zhang, Y.; Yang, X.; Chen, N.; Sun, Y.; Zhao, Y.; Fan, C.; Huang, Q. The Biocompatibility of Nanodiamonds and Their Application in Drug Delivery Systems. *Theranostics* **2012,** *2,* 302–312.
137. Terada, D.; Genjo, T.; Segawa, T. F.; Igarashi, R.; Shirakawa, M. Nanodiamonds for Bioapplications–Specific Targeting Strategies. *Biochim. Biophys. Acta* **2020,** *1864,* 129354.
138. Moscariello, P.; Raabe, M.; Liu, W.; Bernhardt, S.; Qi, H.; Kaiser, U.; Wu, Y.; Weil, T.; Luhmann, H. J.; Hedrich, J. Unraveling In Vivo Brain Transport of Protein-Coated Fluorescent Nanodiamonds. *Small* **2019,** *15,* 1902992.
139. Šimková, V.; Freislebenová, H.; Neuhöferová, E.; Petráková, V.; Amini, A.; Benson, V. Coated Nanodiamonds Interact with Tubulin beta-III Negative Cells of Adult Brain Tissue. *Biointerphases* **2020,** *15,* 061009.
140. Alawdi, S. H.; El-Denshary, E. S.; Safar, M. M.; Eidi, H.; David, M.-O.; Abdel-Wahhab, M. A. Neuroprotective Effect of Nanodiamond in Alzheimer's Disease Rat Model: A Pivotal Role for Modulating NF-Kb and STAT3 Signaling. *Mol. Neurobiol.* **2017,** *54,* 1906–1918.
141. Alawdi, S. H.; Eidi, H.; Safar, M. M.; Abdel-Wahhab, M. A. Loading Amlodipine on Diamond Nanoparticles: A Novel Drug Delivery System. *Nanotechnol. Sci. Appl.* **2020,** *12,* 47–53.
142. Taylor, A. C.; González, C. H.; Miller, B. S.; Edgington, R. J.; Ferretti, P.; Jackman, R. B. Surface Functionalisation of Nanodiamonds for Human Neural Stem Cell Adhesion and Proliferation. *Sci. Rep.* **2017,** *7,* 7307.

143. Taylor, A. C.; González, C. H.; Ferretti, P.; Jackman, R. B. Spontaneous Differentiation of Human Neural Stem Cells on Nanodiamonds. *Adv. Biosyst.* **2019,** *3,* 1800299.
144. Pozdnyakova, N.; Pastukhov, A.; Dudarenko, M.; Galkin, M.; Borysov, A.; Borisova, T. Neuroactivity of Detonation Nanodiamonds: Dose-Dependent Changes in Transporter-Mediated Uptake and Ambient Level of Excitatory/Inhibitory Neurotransmitters in Brain Nerve Terminals. *J. Nanobiotechnol.* **2016,** *14,* 25.
145. Kim, A.; Lalonde, K.; Truesdell, A.; Welter, P. G.; Brocardo, P. S.; Rosenstock, T. R.; Gil-Mohapel, J. New Avenues for the Treatment of Huntington's Disease. *Int. J. Mol. Sci.* **2021,** *22,* 1–50.
146. Morales-Zavala, F.; Casanova-Morales, N.; Gonzalez, R. B.; et al Functionalization of Stable Fluorescent Nanodiamonds Towards Reliable Detection of Biomarkers for Alzheimer's Disease. *J. Nanobiotechnol.* **2018,** *16,* 60.
147. McDonagh, E. M.; Lau, J. L.; Alvarellos, M. L.; Altman, R. B.; Klein, T. E. PharmGKB Summary: Efavirenz Pathway, Pharmacokinetics. *Pharmacogenet. Genomics* **2015,** *25,* 363–376.
148. Caraci, F.; Battaglia, G.; Bruno, V.; Bosco, P.; Carbonaro, V.; Giuffrida, M. L.; Drago, F.; Sortino, M. A.; Nicoletti, F.; Copani, A. TGF-β1 Pathway as a New Target for Neuroprotection in Alzheimer's Disease. *CNS Neurosci. Ther.* **2011,** *17,* 237–249.
149. Chen, J.-H.; Ke, K.-F.; Lu, J.-H.; Qiu, Y.-H.; Peng, Y.-P. Protection of TGF-β1 Against Neuroinflammation and Neurodegeneration in Aβ1-42-Induced Alzheimer's Disease Model Rats. *PLoS One* **2015,** *10,* E0116549.
150. Chomova, M.; Racay, P. Mitochondrial Complex I in the Network of Known and Unknown Facts. *Gen. Physiol. Biophys.* **2010,** *29,* 3–11.
151. Decuypere, J.-P.; Monaco, G.; Bultynck, G.; Missiaen, L.; De Smedt, H.; Parys, J. B. The IP3 Receptor–Mitochondria Connection in Apoptosis and Autophagy. *Biochim. Biophys. Acta* **2011,** *1813,* 1003–1013.
152. Rizzuto, R.; Marchi, S.; Bonora, M.; et al Ca2+ Transfer from the ER to Mitochondria: When, How and Why. *Biochim. Biophys. Acta* **2009,** *1787,* 1342–1351.

CHAPTER 4

The Real Issue in Targeting Neurodegenerative Disease

SMRITI OJHA[1], ANUBHAV ANANAD[2], HINA CHADHA[3], and SUDHANSHU MISHRA[1]

[1]Department of Pharmaceutical Science & Technology, Madan Mohan Malviya University of Technology, Gorakhpur, Uttar Pradesh, India

[2]Department of Pharmaceutics, Hygia Institute of Pharmaceutical Education and Research, Lucknow Uttar Pradesh, India

[3]Department of Pharmacy, Vishveshwarya Group of Institutions, Greater Noida, Uttar Pradesh, India

ABSTRACT

"Neurodegenerative disease" (ND) refers to numerous disorders that predominantly damage the neurons in the brain. Nanocarriers are engineered materials or devices with vast potential to integrate with biological tissues at cellular, molecular, and genetic levels. These are appropriate resources for the diagnosis and cure of neurodegenerative diseases. The multifunction property of drug-loaded nanocarriers and their flexibility toward surface and charge modification have put an effort into developing nanocarriers that can pass the blood–brain barrier (BBB) in a crucial chance to treat or manage various neurological disorders. Traditional medication delivery techniques frequently fail to cross the BBB, making treatment ineffective. Although research ensures the progression of nano-theranostic techniques from animal to human modeling, aspects of translational applicability and feasibility must be considered by understanding these body tissues' molecular interaction

Nanomedicine for Neurodegenerative Disorders: Selective Treatment Strategies. Rishabha Malviya, Kamla Pathak, & Swati Verma (Eds.)

with nanocarriers. Decoding and understanding complex and multifactorial neural networks, receptor-mediated and adsorptive-mediated transcytosis mechanisms, and their correlation with physicochemical properties of potential nanocarrier will be able to target various stages mechanisms and could effectively reduce the progress of the disease.

4.1 INTRODUCTION

A vast network of interconnected, specialized regions makes up the central nervous system (CNS). The entire system depends on a delicate equilibrium, which is occasionally threatened by various disturbing inputs. The developing degradation of the structural and functional units of the central nervous system or peripheral nervous system characterizes the diverse group of disorders known as neurodegenerative diseases.[1] Neurodegenerative illnesses impact millions of individuals globally. Alzheimer's disease may affect up to 6.2 million Americans by 2022, according to a report from the Alzheimer's Disease Association.[2] According to the Parkinson's Foundation, about a million Americans are affected by Parkinson's disease.[3] Even though certain treatments can alleviate certain neurodegenerative disease symptoms, there is no cure and just a slowdown of the disease's progression.[4] Regardless of the relatively high blood flow, the central nervous system poses a significant barrier to drug delivery. The central nervous system is covered by the blood–brain barrier (BBB), blood–cerebrospinal fluid (CSF) barrier, blood–spinal cord barrier, and blood–retinal barrier (CNS). The two physiological barriers dividing the brain from its blood supply are the blood–brain barrier and the blood–cerebrospinal fluid barrier (BCSFB).[5]

4.2 BLOOD–BRAIN BARRIER

Humans and other complex organisms rely on the ability to maintain a stable internal environment, or homeostasis. The brain is the one place where this dependence is most pronounced. Hormone, amino acid, and ion concentrations, such as potassium, fluctuate slightly throughout the body, especially after meals and exercise. Because certain biological chemical substances play a role in neurotransmitters and some electrolytes like potassium ions affect the threshold of nerve cell electrical potential when exposed to such fluctuation, the brain may experience the uncontrolled nervous activity as a result. Therefore, the brain needs to stay out of the way of any changes in blood composition.[6]

The BBB offers selectively permeation only that allows specific biomolecules to pass through while restricting water-soluble substances. As a result, it restricts the use of active medicaments and diagnostic agents in the management of various ND disorders. At their margins, the continuous cerebral endothelial intercellular barrier builds up tight junctions and closes the hydrophilic water-based diffusional pathway regulating only selective movement of important solutes between the cells and tissue fluid.[7] Pericytes relatively encircle the endothelial tissues and are dispersed irregularly alongside cerebral capillaries. The structure of the local basement membrane BL1, in which both the cerebral endothelial cells and pericytes come up with the surrounding, is distinct from that of the extracellular matrix of the glial end foot (BL2). The activities from these cells build integrated connections encircling the fine capillaries, thus forming intimate cell fusion or amalgamation which is necessary to sustain the qualities of junction or barrier.[8]

The cells that construct the blood vessel walls are called endothelial cells (ECs), which are modified simple squamous epithelial cells produced from the mesoderm.[9] In contrast to ECs in other tissues, CNS ECs possess special features that enable them to carefully maintain the passage of ions, chemicals, or cellular structures between the blood and brain fluid.[10,11] Tight junctions (TJs) significantly hinder the paracellular flow of solutes through CNS ECs. The CNS ECs express two different kinds of transporters. The first is efflux transporters, which help to move many lipophilic molecules away from the cell membrane where they might otherwise diffuse. The second category consists of highly specialized nutrient transporters that enable the shifting of specialized unwanted materials from the CNS toward systemic circulation as well as the transportation of specialized beneficial and essential substances through the BBB into the CNS.[12]

4.2.1 BASEMENT MEMBRANE (BM)

Two BMs surround the vascular tube: the inner vascular BM and the touter parenchymal BM.[13] These BMs serve as an anchor for numerous signaling events and as an additional barrier for chemicals to traverse before reaching the CNS tissues. Matrix metalloproteinases play a significant role in the malfunctioning of the blood–brain barrier (BBB) and leukocyte infiltration found in numerous neurological diseases.[14]

4.2.2 ASTROCYTES

Astrocytes are a predominant type of glial cell that stretch polarized tissue processes that sheath neuronal network functioning or blood vessels.[15] Astrocytes serve as a connection between neural circuitry and blood vessels. In reaction to nerve cell action, this neuronal activity and vascularity of the endothelial area together empower and allow astrocytes to transmit electrical signals that coordinate blood flow regulation. These cells are better known as crucial mediators of BBB formation and function due to their potential to produce barrier characteristics in non-CNS blood arteries in vitro coculture settings with cultured ECs and transplantation research.[16]

Li et al. constructed a model for BBB permeability and found that the BM and the astrocyte work and orient around the endothelium giving a good barrier to aqueous substances and other hydrophilic solutes transport over the BBB. These present an important part of preserving the BBB's potential for offering high-grade selective permeation.[17]

4.2.3 TIGHT JUNCTIONS

The key to the BBB is "tight junctions" which are extremely characterized by offering very low permeability (*zonulae occludentes*), and can considerably limit the penetration of polar solutes from blood plasma to brain extracellular fluid via paracellular diffusional routes.[18] Between endothelial cells, a few junctional complexes such as adherents (AJs) and tight junctions (TJ) are available. AJs contain cadherin proteins, providing structural orientation and barrier to the junction. To give the tissue its structural support, the adherens junctions uphold the tissues adequately.[19] Barrier disruption can occur when AJs are disrupted, reflecting AJs as an essential and integrated component of BBB's tight junctions. Occludin and claudin proteins, as well as JAMs, make up the tight junctions.[20,21] Claudin has around 20 different isoforms that have been identified so far (claudins 1–20).[22]

To prevent macromolecules from entering the endothelial cells via the paracellular diffusional pathway, these tight junctions' primary work is to provide an efficient restriction of this pathway. The junctions exhibit a size-based permeability proving selective entry to up to 4-mm size range, but a limited entry for bigger molecules, according to cell culture research. Because of ion movement being impeded, the BBB has an in vivo electrical resistance of about 1800 Ω cm^2.[23] Because the potential paracellular channel has high electrical resistance, the closure of this track by the tight junction through the effective reduction of ion transport is highlighted.[24,25]

4.2.4 TRANSPORTERS

Previously, it was believed that medication availability from the bloodstream to the brain fluid was through passive transport depending on the drug's physical as well as chemical nature and qualities. These qualities of medicine affect its bioavailability and access to target tissues, the focused expression of transporter proteins in tissues such as the brain has a big impact on the overall drug distribution process.[26] Two major types of transporters expressed by central nervous system-derived endothelial cells (CNS ECs) are efflux transporters and nutrient transporters. Nutrient transporters allow certain nutrients to go along their particular concentration gradients. CNS ECs present a large array of these carriers to carry or transport only important or permitted substances or ions across this junction and reach into the CNS parenchyma. There are two main categories of transporters with well-defined involvement in medication effectiveness: solute carrier (SLC) transporters superfamily (slc2a1 (glucose), slc16a1 (lactate, pyruvate), slc7a1 (cationic amino acids), and slc7a5 (cationic amino acids) (neutral amino acids, L-DOPA) and adenosine triphosphate (ATP)-binding cassette (ABC) transporters superfamily. The ABC transporter superfamily contains medically significant members such as the breast cancer resistance protein (BCRP), multidrug resistance-associated protein 2 (MRP2), and MDR1 (also known as PGP), which are localized at the apical membrane whereas multidrug resistance-associated protein 1 (MRP1) is present at the basolateral plasma membrane. MDR1, BCRP, and MRP efflux transporters use ATP hydrolysis to move substrates up concentration gradients. This extensive variety of substrates enables these transporters to act as a barrier for several minute lipophilic substances which may permeate via EC membrane following the passive diffusion process. Additionally, increased MDR1 expression has been linked with multidrug-resistant epilepsy and cancers.

In addition, CNS ECs express a multitude of receptor-mediated transport systems, including low-density receptor-related lipoprotein (LRP)1/LRP8, the transferrin receptor (transferrin/iron), and Ager (amyloid). Most of the transport ways are generally utilized as Trojan horses to expedite medicine availability to the central nervous system. Even though the bulk of these transporters (slc2a1, slc16a1, slc7a5, Tfr) transfer biomolecules from the systemic fluid to the brain fluid, a few of them seem to be crucial for eliminating unwanted material in the brain.

4.2.5 TRANSCYTOSIS

Transcytosis is the movement of chemicals or agents transcellular via the vesicular system. On one side of the cell, macromolecular structures are first engulfed or absorbed by vesicles, then stored with congestion in vesicles, and finally exocytosed or discharged. Transcytosis could be classified into two different classes: receptor-mediated transcytosis, which, as in the cases of insulin and transferrin, attachment to receptors induces endocytosis and transcytosis (nonselective), which is facilitated by charged contacts between the molecule and plasma membrane, as with albumin.[27] The rate of transcytosis in CNS ECs is far less although it is upregulated as a key factor in BBB failure during tissue damage due to any disorder or wound, it is lower than in ECs from non-neural tissues. In ECs, caveolin-dependent vesicle trafficking regulates transcytosis. In these "leaky" vascular beds, plasmalemma vesicle-associated protein (PLVAP) expression is higher in peripheral ECs and has been linked to vesicle trafficking, and fenestra development. Therefore, it appears that the absence of PLVAP in normal CNS ECs is crucial for limiting permeability.

4.3 BLOOD–CEREBROSPINAL FLUID BARRIER (BCSFB)

Internally and externally, the brain and spinal cord are enclosed having specific CSF around them, which is secreted by the epithelial cells of the choroid plexus (CP) in each cerebral ventricle. CP is present outside the lateral, third, and fourth ventricles of the brain. In addition to forming a confluence between CSF and surrounding blood, CP can account for more than fifty percent of all CSF. The basic purpose of the CP is productivity. The blood–CSF barrier is composed of mainly impermeable junctions that permit tissues at the junction to govern and manage the movement of ions or chemicals between the blood and CSF.[30] The CP of the blood–CSF barrier (BCSFB) has distinct features compared to the BBB.[31]

There are three potential routes for a cerebrospinal fluid (CSF)-injected drug to reach the brain parenchyma: First Pathway: is hematogenic or blood-borne, in which medication in CSF goes through and migrates away from blood and then traverses the BBB to recur again into the brain. Second

Pathway: diffusion, wherein the medicines present in the fluid, permeate through diffusion into the brain over the ependymal cellular membrane or lining of the CSF flow corridors. The third Pathway: is convection, wherein medication in CSF reaches the brain via heavy fluid flow along perivascular gaps emanating from the CSF surface of the brain.[32]

Due to the continual absorption of CSF into the peripheral venous system, the injection of a medication into CSF is analogous to a slow intravenous infusion. Every four to five hours, or five times a day, the CSF is absorbed into the bloodstream. Some high molecular weight inert molecules (360 to 5000 Dalton) for example sucrose and inulin are not able to cross the BBB, and they enter CSF with a rate of diffusion inversely proportional to their molecular weight when they pass through the choroid plexus.

In the case when the CSF compartment was steady with no change within the environment and lacking flow, albumin protein diffusion will be only approximately up to 2.4 millimeters in twenty-four hours. CSF is a fluid compartment whose volume is completely regenerated every 5 h in the human brain. The quick and fast CSF emigration from the brain to the circulation via mass flow and the slower rate of drug diffusion into the brain leads to a decrement in drug concentration in a logarithmic manner within the brain for every millimeter removed from the CSF surface.

The choroid plexus operates as a good barrier for various physical agents, immune agents, and biological enzymes that facilitate drug transportation, biotransformation, and signaling activity, and prevent further transfer into the CSF.[33] The CP strongly monitors the amount of substances concentration in the fluid, along with diverse movements or shifting via activating secretion channels in the CP epithelial tissues preparing them satisfactory for controlling the ionic content of brain fluid as well as in CSF, along with the arachnoid membrane, which serves as a strong barrier between the blood and CSF.

The medication injected into the CSF does not reach the deeper brain parenchyma, but rather the bloodstream. Due to the fast transit of the drug from the CSF to the circulation following CSF injection, pharmacologic effects may show in peripheral organs.

The 5-kDa peptide insulin-like growth factor (IGF)-1 was administered intravenously (IV) or intravenously (LV) to rats. Similar IGF1 plasma patterns were observed 20 minutes after intravenous or intrathecal administration. Diffusion from the CSF into the brain parenchyma is the major route from which CSF-borne drugs reach the brain parenchyma. Autoradiography can also demonstrate the minimum distribution of medication into the brain following CSF injection.

Following ventriculocisternal perfusion, the distribution of CSF in the primate brain was investigated. Examined were both tiny substances with good tissue permeability, like thiotepa, and substances with less tissue penetration, such as hydroxyurea or methotrexate. At a distance of 1 to 2 mm away from the CSF lining, the number of active ingredients in the brain decreased 10-fold. Because this medicine is consumed by tissues with good rate than methotrexate or hydroxyurea, its levels decreased more rapidly.

4.4 BLOOD–SPINAL CORD BARRIER (BSCB)

The spinal cord (SC) is separated from other body tissues by a barrier termed BSCB, which regulates and protects the molecule or ion exchange between the SC parenchyma and circulation. Similar to the BBB, spinal cord capillary barrier function is supported by a particular arrangement of non-fenestrated endothelial cells and their supporting tissues, such as the basement membrane, pericytes, and astrocytic end foot processes.[34]

Thus, an environment containing biological chemicals and immunological substances in the subcutaneous tissue is efficient enough to reduce susceptibility to pathogenic insult and minimize the relative damaging action.[9] From a therapeutic aspect, this im-permeability of barrier hinders or obstructs the passage of various important medications that must enter the SC. In addition, degrading enzymes may remove substances carried within the cytosol of endothelial cells,[11] so further restricting SC passage into the surrounding environment. 100 percent of large molecules (> 500 Da) and 98 percent of tiny molecules (500 Da) are rejected, according to scientific evidence.[35,36]

Approximately all high molecular weight medications and approx 98 percent of small-drug molecules are not capable of passing the blood–brain barrier (BBB) today, and therapeutic candidates have demonstrated poor biopharmaceutical and pharmacokinetic qualities.[7] As a result, effective drug delivery systems that do not harm healthy organs and tissues are an absolute necessity. Even though the chemical stability of nanoparticles administered systemically is superior, there are drawbacks associated with their preparation. Further research is needed into the safety of nanoparticles when injected, as well as their effect on CNS function after they penetrate the BBB.[7–15,16] Advanced therapy options for ND disorders include implant therapy and the use of anticancer moieties loaded within compatible and biodegradable polymers, such as hydrogels.[17,18]

TABLE 4.1 Various Strategies for Drug Delivery to the Brain.

Approach	Advantages	Disadvantages
BBB interference	Clinical utility Improved stability with non-immunological reactions	Nonselective; neurotoxic
Biotechnological delivery	Effective in diseases like brain cancer and neurodegenerations	Long-lasting effects are difficult to be seen
Chemistry based delivery	Prodrugs could be utilized	Adverse pharmacokinetic parameters enhanced molecular weight of prodrug
Intracerebral delivery	Sustained release, good drug concentration in brain fluid	The slow movement of active medicament
Intrathecal delivery	Low therapy cost, more effective with the minimum adverse effects	Highly invasive, poor patient compliance
Intranasal delivery	good absorption; enhanced bioavailability	Drug degradation via mucosal enzymes
Non-invasive delivery	Good permeability while crossing BBTB	Extensive drug distribution

For example, senile plaques, neurofibrillary tangles, neuronal loss, and cholinergic insufficiency are characteristics of Alzheimer's disease. The identification of disease-specific cellular markers and the characterization of cell loss patterns have assisted in nosologic classification. Figure 4.1 reflects some diseases born due to neurological degeneration.

The development of new drugs to cure various brain diseases, and brain proteins are interesting targets. The great majority of current drug targets are proteins because they are frequently the last executors of cellular operations and are typically stable. Moreover, neurodegenerative illnesses frequently exhibit aberrant protein accumulation, conformations, and interactions.[37] The difficulty that brain mRNA levels are typically not well connected with available protein abundance[38] can be avoided by studying brain proteins directly rather than transcripts. This is probably because there are many layers of post-transcriptional, and posttranslational control. Last, but not the least, proteins that share a biological pathway frequently interact physically, which can be used to deduce similar pathophysiology.[39]

Galectins are lectins, which have conserved galactoside-binding sites inside their distinctive 130 amino acid carbohydrate recognition domains (CRDs). The expression of some of these lectins is constitutive, while that of others is stimulated. Physiological and pathologic circumstances alter glycosylation patterns, which affects how galectins operate.

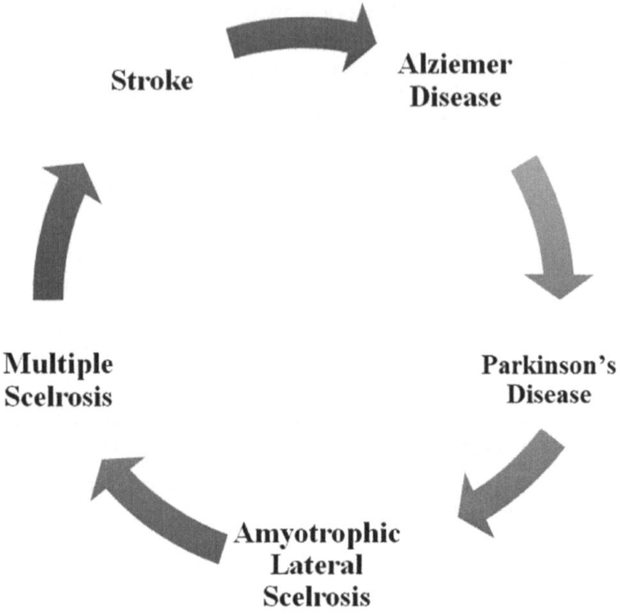

FIGURE 4.1 Some diseases associated with neurodegeneration.

APP is a type I transmembrane protein essential for neurological development and homeostasis. It is mostly recognized for its function in the etiology of Alzheimer's disease (AD). In humans, alternative splicing generates three major isoforms of APP. Figure 4.2 explains various possible mechanisms which lead to neurodegeneration.

All proteins and organelles within a cell are subject to quality control. When repair is impossible and repurposing of changed cell level parts. The autophagic breakdown of proteins and organelles in the lysosomal system is an evolutionarily conserved cellular process.[40] Various neurological disorders have been linked to dysfunctional autophagy. Autophagy is an efficient neuroprotective process that aggressively removes pathogenic polypeptides, but in a few cases, it acts as the target of the harmful impact of available polypeptides.

The method of cargo transport to the lysosomes has been linked to three distinct types of autophagy in mammals. In macroautophagy, double-membrane vesicles (autophagosomes) first engulf cytosolic cargo before merging with lysosomes to completely degrade the cargo. The subset of genes and proteins that assist in this process are known as genes and proteins associated with autophagy. In chaperone-mediated autophagy, a cytosolic

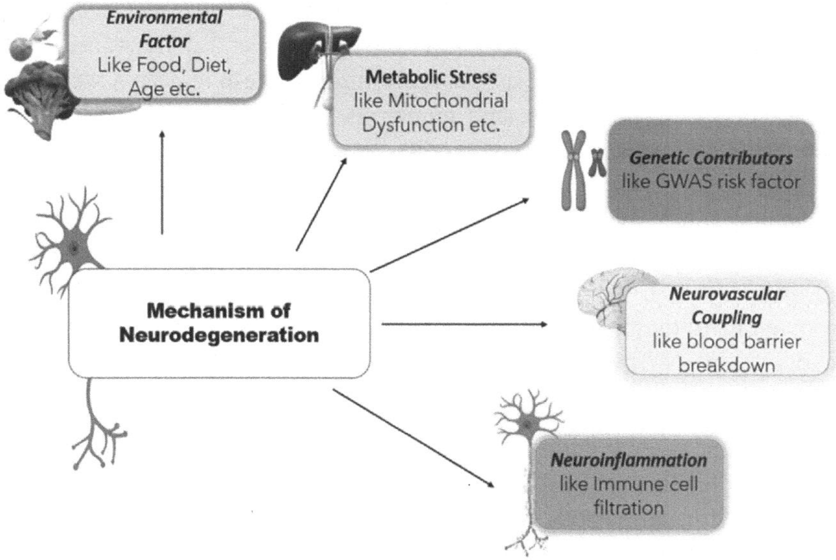

FIGURE 4.2 The mechanism responsible for neurodegeneration.

chaperone identifies and moves certain proteins to the lysosomal surface for translocation across this membrane. Cargo is ultimately absorbed during microautophagy and endosomal microautophagy by invaginations in the lysosomal and endosomal membranes.[41]

When the therapeutic target is a unicellular prokaryotic organism, such as a bacterium, virus, or another agent, the target could be achieved by taking the advantage of various metabolic pathways and their differences between the diseased and infectious agents. This is explained by the strategy where the pharmacological agent is having enough systemic availability but only shows its activity at the target tissues or cells. The method has gained considerable achievements with antibiotics and its area, which often interact with a metabolic pathway important to the organism's growth but minor for the host. Due to the brief reproduction cycles of microorganisms, mutations that prevent or circumvent the effects of the medication can emerge, leading to the development of drug resistance. A second issue involves the place of infection. For instance, if the organism gains entry to the CNS, medication therapy will be challenging because of the low permeation of these therapeutics through the BBB, even in the presence of meningitis.

It is tempting to use tiny substances like liposomal vesicles,[42,43] micro- and nanotherapeutics,[44–46] or macromolecules such as naturally occurring

DNA and synthetic polymers[47] including cellular components[48] to protect and conceal therapeutic moiety in the bloodstream and deliver this drug-containing package to the desired target. Initially, these concepts were met with tremendous enthusiasm, and numerous studies were done to demonstrate their potential. Numerous studies demonstrated increased transport of liposome-encapsulated medicines to cultured cells. Liposomes were prominent, and numerous studies demonstrated their efficacy.[49–51] Early in vivo studies were also promising in that the usage of entrapped medications and drugs coupled with polymer carriers such as DNA could increase the survival rate of tumor-bearing animals. However, the carrier-vehicle strategy has drawbacks, such as

- methods of preparation,
- carrier stability during storage, and in-vivo activity
- drug loading
- need for intravenous administration
- restricted capacity to pass capillary endothelium
- ability to be eliminated by RES
- immunogenicity
- recognition ability
- degradability

The failure of the carrier-vehicle paradigm to considerably increase drug selectivity *in vivo* has resulted in the incorporation of additional components to enhance targetability.

4.5 BIOPHYSICAL APPROACH

The biophysical technique is based on biological macromolecular recognition. The fundamental idea underlying the utilization of high molecular weight polymers is carriers identify the target site, bind to it, and permit the drug to exert its activity. Since most carriers lack this property, numerous studies have been conducted on the use of biogenic substances as pharmaceutical drug delivery vectors which can guide direction toward it tissue deposition showing maximum concentration which could be achieved by adding or attaching suitable surface ligands. The said strategy seems promising in theory, but its present degree of success has been unsatisfactory and some drawbacks are the same as the carrier vehicle approach. Other components emerge from the features of the recognizable substances, most notably the fact that these molecules must be frequently generated on an individual basis and that any chemical alteration must be performed with care to avoid loss of recognition ability. In addition, they are frequently rapidly inactivated in vivo and, as alien macromolecules, may induce immune reactions.

4.6 NANOTECHNOLOGY FOR NEURODEGENERATIVE DISEASE

Nanotechnology involves manipulating a material's size and shape at the nanoscale for applications of designing, characterization, formulation, and application (1 to 100 nm). Micro- to nanometer-sized nanosystems are created utilizing top-down lithographic and nonlithographic fabrication techniques. Due to their large surface-to-volume ratio, nanoparticles exhibit a variety of optical, magnetic, and physiological features inside the human body. Organic (like Liposomes) and inorganic nanoparticles are two different types of nanoparticles (e.g., gold nanoparticles). Polymeric nanoparticles can conceal a medicine from degradation because they are constructed of biocompatible and biodegradable polymers. Nanotechnology in neurodegenerative disorders focuses mostly on targeting the brain and providing local medication release after crossing the BBB. The following are some findings of various types of nanoformulations for neurodegenerative disease:

- Rivastigmine Liposomes were formulated by Ismail et al. using a combination of heating and hydration of lipids. With nearly suppressing amyloid plaque development in the histological examination of rat brains, rivastigmine liposomes (RLs) over rivastigmine solution (RS) demonstrated considerable therapeutic efficacy, which come to the conclusion that RLs might be a useful and effective delivery system for treating Alzheimer's disease.[52]
- In the study by M.R. et al., albumin was added to the surface of the nanosystems to enhance the interaction with specific endothelial cell membrane receptors, facilitating nanoparticles to cross through the BBB and reach to the site of action. As a whole, the use of dopamine-loaded albumin/PLGA nanoformulation increases the possibility of a unique and effective delivery of drugs for the symptomatic management of Parkinson's disease.[53]
- Ajit et al. prepared a dendrimer for the treatment of fibril toxicity which acts as carrier matric for piperin. Through the carbodiimide coupling procedure, tocopheryl polyethylene glycol succinate-1000-

multifunctional polyamidoamine (TPGS-PAMAM) was developed, and Piperin was then embedded in dendrimer using the solvent injection method to create PIP-TPGS-PAMAM. PIP-TPGS-PAMAM demonstrated a reduction of A1-42-induced toxicity in neuronal cells, providing a high potential for neuroprotection and treatment of Alzheimer's disease.[54]

4.7 CHALLENGE AND CONCLUSION

Our understanding of neurodegenerative illnesses has evolved over the last few decades as a result of extensive study on numerous fronts. Genetics and neural pathogenesis have made significant contributions, generated a wealth of information, and served as the foundation for advanced technology and a variety of treatment targets for various neurodegenerative disorders. From a clinical standpoint, it is obvious that more accurate and targeted disease biomarkers are required. These would enable the early detection of neurodegenerative disorders when they are most treatable and the monitoring of disease development, which is crucial when evaluating the effectiveness of new treatments. Genetic profile is a significant consideration when choosing a medication. In recent years, it has been evident that a person's genetic profile will affect how they react to medication therapies. This was particularly evident in recent studies on Alzheimer's disease when people with the apoE4 allele did not benefit from the treatment intervention. Genetic background and environmental effects must now be taken into consideration when planning new clinical trials because personalized treatment is a long-term objective of the health sector.

Diverse chronic conditions linked to the progressive motor, sensory, and perceptual dysfunctions that result in cognitive and behavioral deficiencies are referred to as neurodegenerative diseases. The pharmaceutical industry is attempting to develop medicines for neurodegenerative diseases, which is undoubtedly its most difficult challenge. The future of the development of neurodegenerative therapies rests on successful disease-modifying approaches focusing on intensively explored targets. The necessary advancements will be made through pharmaceutical research projects that look for a much better understanding of disease pathophysiology and explain how adaptive or compensatory mechanisms might be used to slow the onset or course of the disease.

KEYWORDS

- **nanotechnology**
- **neurodegenerative disease**
- **blood-brain barrier**
- **molecular level**

REFERENCES

1. Zang, X.; Chen, S.; Zhu, J. Y.; Ma, J. et al. The Emerging Role of Central and Peripheral Immune Systems in Neurodegenerative Diseases. *Front. Aging Neurosci.* **2022,** *14*, 366.
2. *2022 Alzheimer's Disease Facts and Figures*; John Wiley & Sons Ltd, 2022.
3. DeMaagd, G.; Philip, A.; Parkinson's Disease and Its Management: Part 1: Disease Entity, Risk Factors, Pathophysiology, Clinical Presentation, and Diagnosis. *Pharm. Therap.* **2015,** *40*, 504.
4. Mortada, I.; Farah, R.; Nabha, S.; Ojcius, D. M. et al. Immunotherapies for Neurodegenerative Diseases. *Front. Neurol.* **2021,** *12*, 873.
5. Redzic, Z. Molecular Biology of the Blood-Brain and the Blood-Cerebrospinal Fluid Barriers: Similarities and Differences. *Fluids Barriers CNS* **2011,** *8*, 1–25.
6. Goldstein, G. W.; Betz, A. L. The Blood-Brain Barrier. *Sci. Am.* **1986,** *255*, 74–83.
7. Bellettato, C. M.; Scarpa, M. Possible Strategies to Cross the Blood–Brain Barrier. *Ital. J. Pediatr.* **2018,** *44*, 1.
8. Macvicar, B. A.; Newman, E. A. Astrocyte Regulation of Blood Flow in the Brain. *Cold Spring Harb. Perspect. Biol.* **2015,** *7*, 1–15.
9. Daneman, R.; Prat, A. The Blood–Brain Barrier. *Cold Spring Harb. Perspect. Biol.* **2015,** *7*.
10. Archie, S. R.; Al Shoyaib, A.; Cucullo, L. Blood-Brain Barrier Dysfunction in CNS Disorders and Putative Therapeutic Targets: An Overview. *Pharmaceutics* **2021,** *13*, 1779.
11. Kadry, H.; Noorani, B.; Cucullo, L. A Blood–Brain Barrier Overview on Structure, Function, Impairment, and Biomarkers of Integrity. *Fluids Barriers CNS* **2020,** *17*, 1–24.
12. Gawdi, R.; Shumway, K. R.; Emmady, P. D. *Physiology, Blood Brain Barrier*; StatPearls Publishing: Treasure Island, 2022.
13. Thomsen, M. S.; Routhe, L. J.; Moos, T. The Vascular Basement Membrane in the Healthy and Pathological Brain. *J. Cereb. Blood Flow Metabol.* **2017,** *37*, 3300.
14. Lakhan, S. E.; Kirchgessner, A.; Tepper, D.; Leonard, A. Corrigendum: Matrix Metalloproteinases and Blood-Brain Barrier Disruption in Acute Ischemic Stroke. *Front. Neurol.* **2018,** *9*, 32.
15. Sofroniew, M. V.; Vinters, H. V. Astrocytes: Biology and Pathology. *Acta Neuropathol.* **2010,** *119*, 7.
16. Attwell, D.; Buchan, A. M.; Charpak, S.; Lauritzen, M. et al. Glial and Neuronal Control of Brain Blood Flow. *Nature* **2010,** *468*, 232.
17. Li, G.; Yuan, W.; Fu, B. M. A Model for the Blood–Brain Barrier Permeability to Water and Small Solutes. *J. Biomech.* **2010,** *43*, 2133–2140.

18. Abbott, N. J.; Patabendige, A. A. K.; Dolman, D. E. M.; Yusof, S. R. et al. Structure and Function of the Blood-Brain Barrier. *Neurobiol. Dis.* **2010,** *37*, 13–25.
19. Hartsock, A.; Nelson, W. J. Adherens and Tight Junctions: Structure, Function and Connections to the Actin Cytoskeleton. *Biochim. Biophys. Acta* **2008,** *1778*, 660.
20. Wolburg, H.; Lippoldt, A. Tight Junctions of the Blood–Brain Barrier: Development, Composition and Regulation. *Vascul. Pharmacol.* **2002,** *38*, 323–337.
21. Wolburg, H.; Noell, S.; Mack, A.; Wolburg-Buchholz, K. et al. Brain Endothelial Cells and the Glio-Vascular Complex. *Cell Tissue Res.* **2009,** *335*, 75–96.
22. Abbott, N. J.; Patabendige, A. A. K.; Dolman, D. E. M.; Yusof, S. R. et al. Structure and Function of the Blood-Brain Barrier. *Neurobiol. Dis.* **2010,** *37*, 13–25.
23. Greene, C. *The Blood-Brain Barrier in Neuropsychiatric Disorders*; Trinity College, 2018.
24. Paolinelli, R.; Corada, M.; Orsenigo, F.; Dejana, E. The Molecular Basis of the Blood Brain Barrier Differentiation and Maintenance: Is It Still a Mystery? *Pharmacol. Res.* **2011,** *63*, 165–171.
25. Liu, W. Y.; Wang, Z. bin, Zhang, L. C.; Wei, X. et al. Tight Junction in Blood-Brain Barrier: An Overview of Structure, Regulation, and Regulator Substances. *CNS Neurosci. Ther.* **2012,** *18*, 609–615.
26. Girardin, F. Membrane Transporter Proteins: A Challenge for CNS Drug Development. *Dialogues Clin. Neurosci.* **2006,** *8*, 311–321.
27. Ayloo, S.; Gu, C. Transcytosis at the Blood-Brain Barrier. *Curr. Opin. Neurobiol.* **2019,** *57*, 38.
28. Hartmann, D. A.; Coelho-Santos, V.; Shih, A. Y. Pericyte Control of Blood Flow Across Microvascular Zones in the Central Nervous System. *Annu. Rev. Physiol.* **2022,** *84*, 331–354.
29. Armulik, A.; Genové, G.; Mäe, M.; Nisancioglu, M. H. et al. Pericytes Regulate the Blood–Brain Barrier. *Nature* **2010,** *468*, 557–561.
30. Johansson, P. A.; Dziegielewska, K. M.; Liddelow, S. A.; Saunders, N. R. The Blood–CSF Barrier Explained: When Development Is Not Immaturity. *BioEssays* **2008,** *30*, 237–248.
31. Johanson, C. E.; Stopa, E. G.; McMillan, P. N. The Blood-Cerebrospinal Fluid Barrier: Structure and Functional Significance. In: *The Blood-Brain and Other Neural Barriers. Methods in Molecular Biology*; Nag, S., Ed.; Humana Press: Clifton, 2011; pp 101–131.
32. Hladky, S. B.; Barrand, M. A. Elimination of Substances from the Brain Parenchyma: Efflux via Perivascular Pathways and via the Blood–Brain Barrier. *Fluids Barriers CNS* **2018,** *15*, 1–73.
33. Demeestere, D.; Libert, C.; Vandenbroucke, R. E. Therapeutic Implications of the Choroid Plexus–Cerebrospinal Fluid Interface in Neuropsychiatric Disorders. *Brain Behav. Immun.* **2015,** *50*, 1–13.
34. Bartanusz, V.; Jezova, D.; Alajajian, B.; Digicaylioglu, M. The Blood–Spinal Cord Barrier: Morphology and Clinical Implications. *Ann. Neurol.* **2011,** *70*, 194–206.
35. Rossi, F.; Perale, G.; Papa, S.; Forloni, G. et al. Current Options for Drug Delivery to the Spinal Cord. *Expert Opin. Drug Deliv.* **2013,** *10*, 385–396.
36. Popovich, P. G.; Horner, P. J.; Mullin, B. B.; Stokes, B. T. A Quantitative Spatial Analysis of the Blood–Spinal Cord Barrier: I. Permeability Changes after Experimental Spinal Contusion Injury. *Exp Neurol* **1996,** *142*, 258–275.
37. Gameiro, M.; Silva, R.; Rocha-Pereira, C.; Carmo, H. et al. Cellular Models and In Vitro Assays for the Screening of Modulators of P-gp, MRP1 and BCRP. *Molecules* **2017,** *22*, 600.

38. Liu, Y.; Beyer, A.; Aebersold, R. On the Dependency of Cellular Protein Levels on mRNA Abundance. *Cell* **2016,** *165*, 535–550.
39. Wingo, T. S.; Liu, Y.; Gerasimov, E. S.; Vattathil, S. M. et al. Shared Mechanisms Across the Major Psychiatric and Neurodegenerative Diseases. *Nat. Commun.* **2022,** *13*, 1–19.
40. Parzych, K. R.; Klionsky, D. J. An Overview of Autophagy: Morphology, Mechanism, and Regulation. *Antioxid. Redox. Signal* **2014,** *20*, 460.
41. Yang, Z.; Klionsky, D. J. An Overview of the Molecular Mechanism of Autophagy. *Curr. Top. Microbiol. Immunol.* **2009,** *335*, 32.
42. Nsairat, H.; Khater, D.; Sayed, U.; Odeh, F. et al. Liposomes: Structure, Composition, Types, And Clinical Applications. *Heliyon* **2022,** *8*, e09394.
43. Bozzuto, G.; Molinari, A. Liposomes as Nanomedical Devices. *Int. J. Nanomed.* **2015,** *10*, 999.
44. Wong, H.; Wu, X. Y.; Bendayan, R. Nanotechnological Advances for the Delivery of CNS Therapeutics. *Adv. Drug Deliv. Rev.* **2012.**
45. Tosi, G.; Forni, F.; Vandelli, M. A.; Costantino, L. et al. Polymeric Nanoparticles for the Drug Delivery to the Central Nervous System. *Expert Opin. Drug Deliv.* **2008,** *5*, 155–174.
46. Reynolds, J. L.; Mahato, R. I. Nanomedicines for the Treatment of CNS Diseases. *J. Neuroimmune Pharmacol.* **2017,** *12*, 1–5.
47. Chirila, T. V.; Rakoczy, P. E.; Garrett, K. L.; Lou, X. et al. The Use of Synthetic Polymers for Delivery of Therapeutic Antisense Oligodeoxynucleotides. *Biomaterials* **2002,** *23*, 342.
48. Xia, Q.; Zhang, Y.; Li, Z.; Hou, X. et al. Red Blood Cell Membrane-Camouflaged Nanoparticles: A Novel Drug Delivery System for Antitumor Application. *Acta Pharm. Sin. B* **2019,** *9*, 675–689.
49. Eliaz, R.; Szoka, F. C. Liposome-Encapsulated Doxorubicin Targeted to CD44: A Strategy to Kill CD44-Overexpressing Tumor Cells. *Cancer Res.* **2001.**
50. Zhan, W.; Wang, C.-H. Convection Enhanced Delivery of Liposome Encapsulated Doxorubicin for Brain Tumour Therapy. *J Control Release* **2018.**
51. Pinzõn-Daza, M. L.; Garzõn, R.; Couraud, P. O.; Romero, I. et al. The Association of Statins Plus LDL Receptor-Targeted Liposome-Encapsulated Doxorubicin Increases In Vitro Drug Delivery Across Blood–Brain Barrier Cells. *Br. J. Pharmacol.* **2012,** *167*, 1431–1447.
52. Ismail, M. F.; ElMeshad, A. N.; Salem, N. A. H. Potential Therapeutic Effect of Nanobased Formulation of Rivastigmine on Rat Model of Alzheimer's Disease. *Int. J. Nanomed.* **2013,** *8*, 393.
53. Monge-Fuentes, V.; Biolchi Mayer, A.; Lima, M. R. et al. Dopamine-Loaded Nanoparticle Systems Circumvent the Blood–Brain Barrier Restoring Motor Function in Mouse Model for Parkinson's Disease. *Sci. Rep.* **2021,** *11*, 15185.
54. Singh, A.; Ujjwal, R. R.; Naqvi, S.; Verma, R. K.; Tiwari, S.; Kesharwani, P.; Shukla, R. Formulation Development of Tocopherol Polyethylene Glycol Nanoengineered Polyamidoamine Dendrimer for Neuroprotection and Treatment of Alzheimer Disease. *J. Drug Target.* **2022,** 1–15.

CHAPTER 5

Strategies to Cross the Blood-Brain Barrier

SHRADDHA DWIVEDI

Government Degree College, Department of Zoology, Haripur, Nihastha, Raibareliy Uttar Pradesh, India

ABSTRACT

The restrictiveness of blood–brain barrier (BBB) is vital to maintain the homeostatic microenvironment of the brain. BBB consists of endothelial cell, pericytes, basal lamina, and astrocytic foot processes of astrocyte. The paracellular, transcellular, carrier-mediated transport (CMT), and transcytosis are the transport systems that allow nutrients or essential solute to cross BBB depending upon their size and chemical nature. Through the above-mentioned pathways some harmful or unwanted substances also reach the brain that quickly sends back by the second level regulators called efflux transporters viz., Pgp, MRPs, and BCRP. These tight regulations also restrict therapeutic penetrations, which encourage researchers to develop strategies that overcome the restrictiveness of BBB and enhance therapeutic uptake into the brain parenchyma. In this sequence several innovative strategies have been explored as a possible gateway; some of them are transient disruption of tight junction, inhibition of efflux transporter, utilization of transport/carrier systems that modulate BBB or other alternative ways like intranasal, intra-cerbroventricular (ICV), intrathecal infusion intracerebral/intra-parenchymal and intra-tympanic are discussed in detail.

5.1 GENERAL BACKGROUND

The selective permeable blood–brain interface called blood–brain barrier (BBB) tightly regulates molecular trafficking to maintain the homeostatic

Nanomedicine for Neurodegenerative Disorders: Selective Treatment Strategies. Rishabha Malviya, Kamla Pathak, & Swati Verma (Eds.)

state of brain's microenvironment. Its anatomical architecture comprises monolayer endothelial lining of brain capillaries and neighboring perivascular cells, astrocyte a glial cell that communicate with the associated neurons by their end feet's and pericytes that encircles the abluminal surface of capillary which provide physical support and stability to BBB.[5,9] Structurally, neuro-vascular network of BBB are continuous non-fenestrated type that offers limited permeability for solutes.[3,4] Further, two adjacent endothelial cells are cemented with the junctional complexes (Tight, Adherens, and Gap junctions) that provide high trans-endothelial resistance by blocking paracellular permeability.[36].This paracellular blockage or limited inter-endothelial spaces for solute is primarily a distinctive feature of tight junctions with the associated transmembrane proteins like claudin, ocludins, and junctional adhesion molecules.[29]

5.2 BLOOD–BRAIN BARRIER TRANSPORT FUNCTION

The normal physiological function of BBB allows influx of certain molecules into the brain tissue either by gaps between endothelial cells or by transcytosis. The hydrophilic molecules cross BBB paracellularly (Figure 5.1A), that is, through the cleft present between endothelial cells and the hydrophilic molecule such as O_2 and CO_2 diffuse freely transcellularly (Figure 5.1B) following their concentration gradient.[37] In addition, transport of small polar molecules like carbohydrates (GLUT1) and large or neutral amino acids (LAT1) occurs through carrier-mediated transport (CMT) (Figure 5.1C) and larger solutes like albumins are transported through BBB by adsorptive-mediated transcytosis (AMT) and insulin (IR), leptin, lipoproteins, and transferrin (TfR) are transported through receptor-mediated transcytosis (RMT) (Figure 5.1D).[1,7,31]

Thus, these influx transporters allow only essential nutrients into the brain and block 90% smaller and almost all large-sized unwanted solutes or therapeutics entry in the brain.[31] The new drugs or solutes that are designed to cross BBB further transported back into the systemic circulation by the activity of efflux transporters, thus providing an additional barrier. The efflux transporters (Figure 5.1E) are majorly an active ATP-driven adenosine triphosphate binding cassette (ABC), localized in the luminal and abluminal surface of the blood–brain interface.[26] The primary and most studied efflux transporters are P-glycoprotein (Pgp), glutathione-dependent multidrug resistance transporters (MRPs), breast cancer resistance protein (BCRP), and organic anion transporting polypeptide.[24,32] The down transcriptional regulation or decreased functional integrity of these transporters has been a prime cause behind several neurological disorders, whereas an increased expression has been associated with the therapeutic resistances.[25,45] Consequently, the active efflux transporters restrict the success and effectiveness of brain therapeutics either by preventing its entry into the brain or by removing it from brain into systemic circulation.[16] Thus, it results in the failure of most of the therapeutic treatments given to neurological disorders.[28,39]

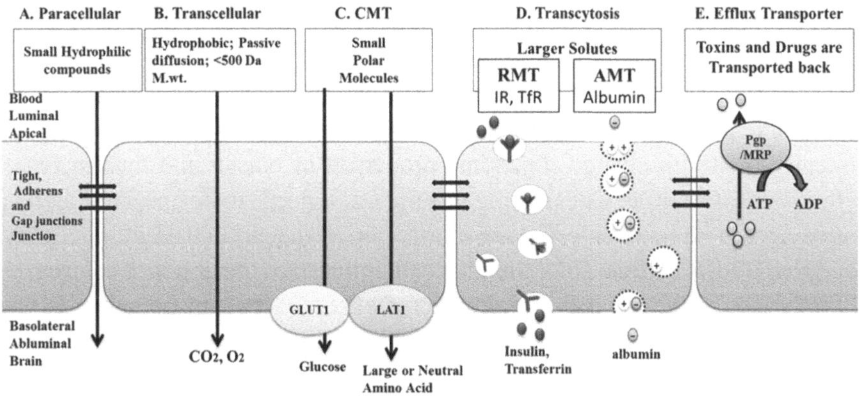

FIGURE 5.1 Diagrammatic representation of transport mechanism at the blood brain interface. (A) Paracellular pathway for small hydrophilic molecules; (B) transcellular transport of gases; (C) carrier-mediated transport (CMT) of small polar molecule; (D) receptor-mediated (RMT) and adsorptive-mediated (AMT) transcytosis of large solutes; and (E) efflux pump that removes unwanted molecules and drugs into systemic circulation.

5.3 POTENTIAL STRATEGIES FOR SUCCESSFUL DRUG DELIVERY INTO THE BRAIN

With all the gathered structural and functional knowledge and considering the negative impact of tight regulation of the blood-brain barrier in association with the treatment of neurological disorders, it changes the direction of research. Now therapeutic delivery is considered equally crucial for successful treatment of neurological diseases along with the development of drug. In this accordance several approaches have been explored like enhancing brain penetration, ranging from disruption of tight junctional complex to inhibiting efflux transporters by modifying the solutes and their carriers or by exploring other advanced alternate pathways like development of nanoparticles and drug conjugates that will bypass secondary regulatory pathway of BBB. Overall there are two gateways that either utilize and modulate existing pathways through which the desired drugs can reach to the targeted brain site or directly administer drugs into the brain parenchyma by various bypass routes. Thus, these potential gateways are either crossing the BBB or bypassing it; here possible mechanisms through which these gateways can be utilized to overcome BBB are discussed in detail.

5.4 STRATEGIES TO CROSSING THE BBB

As we know that the restrictive permeability of BBB is the major hurdle in the efficient drug delivery, one obvious approach is to disturb its structural integrity that will change functional properties of barrier and thus increase effectiveness of drug. Considering this option, it needs to be ensured that this opening will be reversible and for shorter period that ensures high specificity and thus allows entrance of systemically administered therapeutics in targeted brain tissue without causing any adverse effects. This can be achieved by disrupting junctional complex primarily tight junction and by modulating efflux pumps.

5.4.1 TRANSIENT DISRUPTION OF JUNCTIONAL COMPLEX

On intra-arterial injection of 25% hyperosmotic solution such as mannitol or arabinose causes two fold alteration in endothelial cell; firstly cells shrink due to the osmotic loss of water and secondly endothelial membrane stretches by vasodilation of blood vessel.[30,42] These alterations create tractive forces on tight junction and disintegrate it; this process relaxes BBB more than 20-folds and increases brain penetration that allows high concentrations of systemically administered therapeutics to reach the brain.[20] The other biological and chemical alternative stimuli that can breach the BBB are zonula occludens toxin, histamine, bradykinin,[13] cereport (synthetic analog of bradykinin), and alkylglycerol.[17] However, major limitation of this is that this opening is not specific for therapeutics only and allows other unwanted molecules or neurotoxins too into the brain that will lead to further neurological disorders. Recent research focuses on more specific approaches that use radiation and ultrasound for the modulation of BBB.[2,11]

5.4.2 INHIBITING EFFLUX TRANSPORTER

Active efflux transporter as discussed earlier selectively eliminates unwanted molecules or therapeutic drugs out from the brain to blood. Therefore, inhabiting regulatory pathways of these transporters could check their function or occurrence at the luminal and abluminal surface of enthothelial cells that reduces possible elimination of drug from brain.[34] This increases effectiveness of drug by its longer stay into the brain. Direct inhibition[8] or inhibiting the transcriptional activation[15] is the mechanisms through which the activities of these transporters are modulated. Several inhibitors (Table 5.1) *viz.*, verapamil, cyclosporin A, benzbromarone, probenecid, and quinidine have been found successfully taking up the therapeutics into brain through both competitive and noncompetitive inhibition.[18] Jekerle et al.[23] also mentioned new inhibitor, WK-X-34, which targets both Pgp and BCRP efflux transporters in tested models.

Inhibition of signaling pathway (Table 5.2) that upregulates Pgp expression provides a feasible route to overcome Pgp-mediated resistance of therapeutics.[15] In epileptic brains, signaling pathway of glutamate through N-methyl-D-aspartate receptor (NMDA) activates cascade of signals that induce expression of Pgp and BCRP efflux transporters at the BBB. However this signaling pathway can be inhibited by cyclooxygenase 2 (CoX-2) inhibitor or by prostaglandin E_2 receptor antagonist.[41,44] For example, antagonist MK-801 of NMDA receptor, CoX-2 inhibitors indomethacin and celecoxib and Prostaglandin E_2 receptor antagonist SC-51089 can effectively down regulate the expression of glutamate-induced Pgp expression and enhance the delivery of antiepileptic drugs.[6]

5.4.3 BY UTILIZING TRANSPORT/CARRIER SYSTEMS

The transport/carrier systems provide a route to transfer polar molecules from blood to brain that would otherwise be restricted by BBB. Based on the information of the stereochemical necessities for transport by these carriers, potential drugs are designed that mimic endogenous substrates for these carriers and provide easy access to the brain.[38] The modified drugs should be more lipophilic; or in the form of prodrugs that are therapeutically inactive and after crossing BBB modified into a biologically active form.[22] Moreover, sometimes ligand conjugated drug or antibody conjugated drugs trigger endogenous RMT pathway and easily transport drug across the endothelial cell. The RMT monoclonal antibodies act as Trojan horses, crossing the BBB and internalizing the receptor-attached drug through endocytosis into the endothelial cell.[34] The drug diffuses into the brain parenchyma and receptors are sent back to the endothelial membrane. In this technique to cross BBB chimeric peptides are formed by covalently conjugating non-transportable therapeutic with the BBB transportable peptide vector that makes therapeutics accessible to the brain tissues. The most commonly used transporters are GLUT1 transport glucose, LAT1 that transport large neutral amino-acids, and CAT1 that transports cation.[27]

TABLE 5.1 Different Modes That Inhibit Efflux Transporters.

Direct inhibitor	
Verapamil	
Cyclosporine A	
Quinidine	
Second-generation inhibitor	
Valspodar (PSC-833)	Pgp inhibitors
Third-generation inhibitor	
Tariquidar	Pgp inhibitors
Laniquidar	Pgp inhibitors
Zosuquidar	Pgp inhibitors
Elacridar	Pgp inhibitors
Noval inhibitor	
WK-X-34	Pgp/ BCRP

TABLE 5.2 Inhibiting Efflux Transporter by Targeting Regulatory Pathway.

Target receptor	
Pregnane X receptor (PXR)	Pgp expression upregulation
Steroid and xenobiotic receptor (SXR)	Pgp expression upregulation
Target receptor in epileptic	
Glutamate-NMDA receptor	MK-801
Glutamate-COX-2 (selective)	Celecoxib
Glutamate-COX (nonselective)	Indomethacin

5.5 POSSIBLE PATHWAYS TO BYPASS THE BBB

5.5.1 INTRANASAL OLFACTORY MUCOSA FOR DRUG DELIVERY

Drug administration through intranasal olfactory mucosa is a simple, noninvasive way to bypass BBB efficiently and targets brain injury sites better than the intravenous route. Here drug is sprayed into the nasal cavity till it reaches the cribriform plate; now drug is absorbed by the olfactory and respiratory mucosa. From the olfactory mucosa, the drug reaches the brain through three possible pathways: extracellular diffusion, directing the drug to the subarachanoid spaces and then the CSF of the brain; through axonal transport, the drug reaches the brain stem and then the brain via the trigeminal nerve and olfactory sensory neuron.[14] This bypass route has been utilized to deliver a number of therapeutics to the brain such as Melanocortin, Neurotrophins, Glutathione, Insulin, Perillyl Alcohol, Cytokines, Angiotensin II, and Sumatriptan.[21] However, efficacy of delivery will be further dependent on the administration factors (patient's head position) and chemical feature of the drug.[40]

5.5.2 INTRA-CERBROVENTRICULAR (ICV) AND INTRATHECAL INFUSION

Intrathecal infusion and intra-cerbroventricular (ICV) involves the direct delivery of drug into the lumbar sub-arachnoid space or alternatively into the brain ventricles respectively, thereby avoiding the restrictiveness of BBB. The ICV administration involves invasive or surgical procedure to deliver drugs through implant or directly infuse drug into the brain parenchyma through injections.[10] The implant used may be polymeric-controlled release or convection-enhanced delivery that infuses drug into the brain tissues in a slow continued manner for longer period.[35] Among them convection-enhanced delivery is a least invasive implant procedure that involves placement of small diameter catheters into the parenchymal interstitial space.[10] However, there are certain drawbacks associated with this approach like implant will damage the nearby and implanted area of the brain. The other issue with this is that the entire CSF pool is replaced every 4–5 h and the penetration of infused drug into brain parenchyma is slow; therefore, most often drug exits the CSF before it can diffuse into the brain tissue.[33]

In intrathecal administration drug was directly injected into the CSF by lumber puncture and usually delivers drug in a significant amount.[43] However, the drug administrated through intrathecal route fails to accumulate in deeper brain tissues that were not in direct contact with CSF. Thus, this made it one of the best options for the treatment of disseminated meningeal or spinal disease.[19]

5.5.3 INTRACEREBRAL/INTRA-PARENCHYMAL

This approach involves direct delivery of drug through injection or implant into the brain parenchyma similar as ICV. In this method, drug moves to the nearby tissue only through passive diffusion. This is a slow process and allows only limited penetration into the surrounding tissues. Also some displacement of tissue over time has been recorded at the implanted area.

5.5.4 INTRA-TYMPANIC

Intra-cochlear administration emerges as one of the potential and promising alternatives to the central nervous system (CNS) drug delivery. The inner ear fluid perilymph communicates with the similar ionic composition CSF of the subarachnoid space, through the duct called cochlear aqueduct or perilymphatic duct. It was suggested that this communication transfers a limited amount of fluid in CSF. This transfer of fluid becomes a possibility, through which CNS drug can deliver. For this drug was injected into the middle ear cavity which then crosses round window membrane through pinocytosis and reaches perilymph. From perilymph the drug is transferred to the CSF of subarachnoid space by bypassing BBB. Chen et al.[12] have reported successful brain targeted drug delivery through intra-tympanic route.

5.6 SUMMARY

The strict regulation of BBB is the prime reason for the failure of CNS therapeutics used for neurological disorders. However, stressed life style and increasing cases of neurological diseases establish the need of improved CNS drug delivery. Current advances target transient modulation in BBB either by relaxing tight junctions or by inhibiting or downregulating the expression of efflux transports. However, these regulations are not specific and allow the entry of other unwanted solutes that may induce other neurological toxicity. To minimize the risk of associated toxicity other bypass methods are involved such as intranasal, intra-cerbroventricular (ICV), intrathecal infusion, intra-cerebral/intra-parenchymal, and intra-tympanic drug delivery system was explored that directly delivers drug to the target tissue. Although these bypass methods have their own drawbacks like in intranasal degradation of drugs is seen by mucosal enzymes and others are highly invasive and expensive methods with poor distribution of drug. Therefore, more research is needed for clinical translation to find an easier, safer delivery method.

KEYWORDS

- **blood-brain barrier**
- **paracellular**
- **efflux transporters**
- **tight junction and intrathecal**

REFERENCES

1. Abbott, N. J.; Patabendige, A. A. K.; Dolman, D. E. M. et al. Structure and Function of the Blood-Brain Barrier. *Neurobiol. Dis.* **2010,** *37*, 13–25. DOI: 10.1016/j.nbd.2009.07.030
2. Abrahao, A.; Meng, Y.; Llinas, M. et al. First-in-Human Trial of Blood–Brain Barrier Opening in Amyotrophic Lateral Sclerosis Using MR-Guided Focused Ultrasound. *Nat. Commun.* **2019,** *10*, 1–9. DOI: 10.1038/s41467-019-12426-9
3. Aird, W. C. Phenotypic Heterogeneity of the Endothelium: II. Representative Vascular Beds. *Circ. Res.* 2007a, *100*, 174–190. DOI: 10.1161/01.RES.0000255690.03436.ae
4. Aird, W. C. Phenotypic Heterogeneity of the Endothelium: I. Structure, Function, and Mechanisms. *Circ. Res. 100*, 158–173. DOI: 10.1161/01.RES.0000255691.76142.4a
5. Anny-Claude, L.; Artus, C.; Glacial, F. et al. Tight Junctions at the Blood-Brain Barrier: Physiological Architecture and Disease-Associated Dysregulation. *Fluids Barriers CNS* **2012,** *9*, 23.
6. Bankstahl, J. P.; Hoffmann, K.; Bethmann, K.; Löscher, W. Glutamate Is Critically Involved in Seizure-Induced Overexpression of P-glycoprotein in the Brain. *Neuropharmacology* **2008,** *54*, 1006–1016. DOI: 10.1016/j.neuropharm.2008.02.008
7. Barar, J.; Rafi, M. A.; Pourseif, M. M.; Omidi Y Blood-Brain Barrier Transport Machineries and Targeted Therapy of Brain Diseases. *BioImpacts* **2016,** *6*, 225–248. DOI: 10.15171/bi.2016.30
8. Bauer, B.; Hartz, A. M. S.; Fricker, G.; Miller, D. S. Modulation of p-glycoprotein Transport Function at the Blood-Brain Barrier. *Exp. Biol. Med.* **2005,** *230*, 118–127. DOI: 10.1177/153537020523000206

9. Begley, D. J. Delivery of Therapeutic Agents to the Central Nervous System: The Problems and the Possibilities. *Pharmacol. Ther.* **2004,** *104*, 29–45. DOI: 10.1016/j.pharmthera.2004.08.001
10. Bennewitz, M. F.; Saltzman, W. M. Nanotechnology for Delivery of Drugs to the Brain for Epilepsy. *Neurotherapeutics* **2009,** *6*, 323–336. DOI: 10.1016/j.nurt.2009.01.018
11. Brown, W. R.; Thore, C. R.; Moody, D. M. et al. Vascular Damage After Fractionated Whole-Brain Irradiation in Rats. *Radiat. Res.* **2005,** *164*, 662–668. DOI: 10.1667/RR3453.1
12. Chen, G.; Hou, S.; Hu, P. et al. Preliminary Study on Brain-Targeted Drug Delivery via Inner Ear. *Yao Xue Xue Bao* **2007,** *42*, 1102–1106.
13. Côté, J.; Bovenzi, V.; Savard, M. et al. Induction of Selective Blood-Tumor Barrier Permeability and Macromolecular Transport by a Biostable Kinin B1 Receptor Agonist in a Glioma Rat Model. *PLoS One* **2012,** *7*, 1–17. DOI: 10.1371/journal.pone.0037485
14. Crowe, T. P.; Greenlee, M. H. W.; Kanthasamy, A. G.; Hsu, W. H. Mechanism of Intranasal Drug Delivery Directly to the Brain. *Life Sci.* **2018,** *195*, 44–52. DOI: 10.1016/j.lfs.2017.12.025
15. Ekins, S.; Ecker, G. F.; Chiba, P.; Swaan, P. W. Future Directions for Drug Transporter Modelling. *Xenobiotica* **2007,** *37*, 1152–1170. DOI: 10.1080/00498250701646341
16. Engelhardt, B.; Vajkoczy, P.; Weller, R. O. The Movers and Shapers in Immune Privilege of the CNS. *Nat. Immunol.* **2017,** *18*, 123–131. DOI: 10.1038/ni.3666
17. Erdlenbruch, B.; Schinkhof, C.; Kugler, W. et al. Intracarotid Administration of Short-Chain Alkylglycerols for Increased Delivery of Methotrexate to the Rat Brain. *Br. J. Pharmacol.* **2003,** *139*, 685–694. DOI: 10.1038/sj.bjp.0705302
18. Fox, E.; Bates, S. E. Tariquidar (XR9576): A P-glycoprotein Drug Efflux Pump Inhibitor. *Expert Rev. Anticancer Ther.* **2007,** *7*, 447–459. DOI: 10.1586/14737140.7.4.447
19. Groothuis, D. R.; Benalcazar, H.; Allen, C. V. et al Comparison of Cytosine Arabinoside Delivery to Rat Brain by Intravenous, Intrathecal, Intraventricular and Intraparenchymal Routes of Administration. *Brain Res.* **2000,** *856*, 281–290. DOI: 10.1016/S0006-8993(99)02089-2
20. Haluska, M.; Anthony, M. L. Osmotic Blood-Brain Barrier Modification for the Treatment of Malignant Brain Tumors. *Clin. J. Oncol. Nurs.* **2004,** *8*, 263–267. DOI: 10.1188/04.cjon.263-267
21. Hanson, L. R.; Frey, W. H. Intranasal Delivery Bypasses the Blood-Brain Barrier to Target Therapeutic Agents to the Central Nervous System and Treat Neurodegenerative Disease. *BMC Neurosci.* **2008,** *9*, 1–4. DOI: 10.1186/1471-2202-9-s3-s5
22. Hersh, D. S.; Wadajkar, A. S.; Roberts, N. et al. Evolving Drug Delivery Strategies to Overcome the Blood Brain Barrier. *Curr. Pharm. Des.* **2016,** *22*, 1177–1193. DOI: 10.2174/1381612822666151221150733
23. Jekerle, V.; Klinkhammer, W.; Scollard, D. A. et al. In Vitro and In Vivo Evaluation of WK-X-34, a Novel Inhibitor of P-glycoprotein and BCRP, Using Radio Imaging Techniques. *Int. J. Cancer* **2006,** *119*, 414–422. DOI: 10.1002/ijc.21827
24. Kadry, H.; Noorani, B.; Cucullo, L. A Blood–Brain Barrier Overview on Structure, Function, Impairment, and Biomarkers of Integrity. *Fluids Barriers CNS* **2020,** *17*, 1–24. DOI: 10.1186/s12987-020-00230-3
25. Löscher, W.; Potschka, H. Blood-Brain Barrier Active Efflux Transporters: ATP-Binding Cassette Gene Family. *NeuroRx* **2005,** *2*, 86–98. DOI: 10.1602/neurorx.2.1.86

26. Mahringer, A.; Fricker, G. ABC Transporters at the Blood-Brain Barrier. *Expert Opin. Drug Metab. Toxicol.* **2016,** *12*, 499–508. DOI: 10.1517/17425255.2016.1168804
27. Mikitsh, J. L.; Chacko, A. M. Pathways for Small Molecule Delivery to the Central Nervous System Across the Blood-Brain Barrier. *Perspect. Med. Chem.* **2014,** 11–24. DOI: 10.4137/PMc.s13384
28. Nies, A. T. The Role of Membrane Transporters in Drug Delivery to Brain Tumors. *Cancer Lett.* **2007,** *254*, 11–29. DOI: 10.1016/j.canlet.2006.12.023
29. O'Keeffe, E.; Campbell, M. Modulating the Paracellular Pathway at the Blood–Brain Barrier: Current and Future Approaches for Drug Delivery to the CNS. *Drug Discov. Today Technol.* **2016,** *20*, 35–39. DOI: 10.1016/j.ddtec.2016.07.008
30. Pandit, R.; Chen, L.; Götz, J. The Blood-Brain Barrier: Physiology and Strategies for Drug Delivery. *Adv. Drug Deliv. Rev.* **2020,** *165–166*, 1–14. DOI: 10.1016/j.addr.2019.11.009
31. Pardridge, W. M. Drug Transport Across the Blood-Brain Barrier. *J. Cereb. Blood Flow Metab.* **2012,** *32*, 1959–1972. DOI: 10.1038/jcbfm.2012.126
32. Pardridge, W. M. Blood-Brain Barrier Delivery. *Drug Discov. Today* **2007,** *12*, 54–61. DOI: 10.1016/j.drudis.2006.10.013
33. Pardridge, W. M. Drug Transport in Brain via the Cerebrospinal Fluid. *Fluids Barriers CNS* **2011,** *8*, 2–5. DOI: 10.1186/2045-8118-8-7
34. Sanchez-Covarrubias, L.; Slosky, L.; Thompson, B. et al. Transporters at CNS Barrier Sites: Obstacles or Opportunities for Drug Delivery? *Curr. Pharm. Des.* **2014,** *20*, 1422–1449. DOI: 10.2174/13816128113199990463
35. Sawyer, A. J.; Piepmeier, J. M.; Saltzman, W. M. New Methods for Direct Delivery of Chemotherapy for Treating Brain Tumors. *Yale J. Biol. Med.* **2006,** *79*, 141–152
36. Stamatovic, S. M.; Johnson, A. M.; Keep, R. F.; Andjelkovic, A. V. Junctional Proteins of the Blood-Brain Barrier: New Insights into Function and Dysfunction. *Tissue Barriers* **2016,** *4*, 1 12. DOI: 10.1080/21688370.2016.1154641
37. Sweeney, M. D.; Zhao, Z.; Montagne, A. et al. Blood-Brain Barrier: From Physiology to Disease and Back. *Physiol. Rev.* **2019,** *99*, 21–78. DOI: 10.1152/physrev.00050.2017
38. Tamai, I.; Tsuji, A Transporter-Mediated Permeation of Drugs Across the Blood-Brain Barrier. *J. Pharm. Sci.* **2000,** *89*, 1371–1388. DOI: 10.1002/1520-6017(200011)89:11<1371:AID-JPS1>3.0.CO;2-D
39. Thuerauf, N.; Fromm, M. F. The Role of the Transporter P-glycoprotein for Disposition and Effects of Centrally Acting Drugs and for the Pathogenesis of CNS Diseases. *Eur. Arch. Psychiatry Clin. Neurosci.* **2006,** *256*, 281–286. DOI: 10.1007/s00406-006-0662-6
40. Ugwoke, M. I.; Verbeke, N.; Kinget, R. The Biopharmaceutical Aspects of Nasal Mucoadhesive Drug Delivery. *J. Pharm. Pharmacol.* **2010,** *53*, 3–21. DOI: 10.1211/0022357011775145
41. van Vliet, E. A.; Zibell, G.; Pekcec, A. et al. COX-2 Inhibition Controls P-glycoprotein Expression and Promotes Brain Delivery of Phenytoin in Chronic Epileptic Rats. *Neuropharmacology* **2010,** *58*, 404–412. DOI: 10.1016/j.neuropharm.2009.09.012
42. Witherspoon, B.; Ashby, N. E. The Use of Mannitol and Hypertonic Saline Therapies in Patients with Elevated Intracranial Pressure: A Review of the Evidence. *Nurs. Clin. North Am.* **2017,** *52*, 249–260. DOI: 10.1016/j.cnur.2017.01.002
43. Yi, X.; Manickam, D. S.; Brynskikh, A.; Kabanov, A. V. Agile Delivery of Protein Therapeutics to CNS. *J. Control Release* **2014,** *190*, 637–663. DOI: 10.1016/j.jconrel.2014.06.017

44. Zibell, G.; Unkrüer, B.; Pekcec, A. et al. Prevention of Seizure-Induced Up-Regulation of Endothelial P-glycoprotein by COX-2 Inhibition. *Neuropharmacology* **2009,** *56*, 849–855. DOI: 10.1016/j.neuropharm.2009.01.009
45. Zlokovic, B. V. Neurovascular Pathways to Neurodegeneration in Alzheimer's Disease and Other Disorders. *Nat. Rev. Neurosci.* **2011,** *12*, 723–738. DOI: 10.1038/nrn3114

CHAPTER 6

Nanotechnology-Based Drug Delivery Systems for the Treatment of Neurodegenerative Disorders

HIMANSHU PALIWAL[1], BHUPENDRA G. PRAJAPATI[2,3], and TEERAPOL SRICHANA[1]

[1]*Marwadi University Research Center Department of Pharmaceutics, Faculty of Pharmacy, Marwadi University, Rajkot, Gujarat, India*

[2]*Department of Pharmaceutics and Pharmaceutical Technology, Shree S.K. Patel College of Pharmaceutical Education and Research, Ganpat University, Kherva, India*

[3]*Faculty of Pharmacy, Silpakorn University, Nakhon Pathom, Thailand*

ABSTRACT

The disorders associated with the central nervous system (CNS) are challenging for healthcare professionals, mainly due to complicated anatomical features of physiological barriers and unknown causative factors responsible for such diseases. Serious neurodegenerative disorders (NDs) may be caused due to genetic defects that lead to the localization of antigens at specific sites, followed by systemic inflammation or immunoassociated diseases provoking the number of neurodegenerative processes. These neurodegenerative pathways are progressive and impart incurable damage to the neuronal cells. Since degenerated neurons are delicate and lack self-repair capacity, the exploration of advanced therapeutic approaches for CNS disorders is of utmost importance. The efficient delivery of drugs for the treatment of CNS disorders, such as brain tumors, epilepsy, stroke, multiple sclerosis, Alzheimer's disease, Huntington's disease, Parkinson's

Nanomedicine for Neurodegenerative Disorders: Selective Treatment Strategies. Rishabha Malviya, Kamla Pathak, & Swati Verma (Eds.)

disease, etc., is hampered mainly due to the blood-brain barrier (BBB) and blood-cerebrospinal fluid barrier. The therapeutic strategies proposed in the past few decades are still lacking concerning the substantial mitigation of NDs. The therapeutic products used in the present time are mostly dedicated to the management of disease symptoms and preventing subsequent neuronal degeneration. There is a need for a clear understanding of disease pathophysiology, the involvement of the BBB, and the precise molecular and submolecular features of the regions affected by the disease. This will provide substantial support for more patient-specific therapy. The emergence of nanotechnology-based delivery systems has been showing a lot of promise for the efficient treatment of neurological diseases by evading the challenges faced by conventional therapeutic products. One of the approaches is nanoengineering the molecules for conveying several functions, like targeting a particular cell, tissue, or signaling pathway, enhancing crossing through the BBB, responding to endogenous stimuli, carrier for the delivery of genes, assisting the regeneration of nerves, and ensuring the survival of the cell. Furthermore, there are several nanotechnology-based materials and devices that may offer an efficient platform for the identification, bioimaging, diagnosis, medication, and regeneration of various NDs. In recent times, several nanocarriers have been investigated for the delivery of drugs to the CNS, such as solid lipid nanoparticles/nanostructured lipid carriers (SLNs/NLCs), dendrimers, liposomes, nanoemulsions, microemulsions, polymeric nanoparticles, etc. This chapter aims at discussing pertinent characteristics of delivery to the CNS for NDs and emphasizing that nanoparticle-based delivery systems are appropriate and flexible for improving the therapeutic benefits of the drugs and biologicals in the treatment of neurodegenerative conditions.

6.1 INTRODUCTION

Recently, numerous advancements have been put forth in comprehending the biochemical, molecular, and genetic mechanisms of neurodegenerative disorders (NDs).[131,140] These disorders involve intricate processes characterized by the intracellular and extracellular accumulation of misfolded proteins, leading to progressive neuronal dysfunction, degradation, or even death.[28,88,139] The series of events after protein misfolding includes, firstly, malfunction of the ubiquitin-proteasome system (UPS), followed by the failure of autophagy. These events contribute to oxidative strain, lack of mitochondrial energy, impairment of neutrophins, along with the predominant generation of free radicals.[42,132,133] Amongst the group of disorders, Alzheimer's disease (AD), Parkinson's disease (PD), and Huntington's disease (HD) are known to be more widely occurring NDs. These diseases have some similar clinical presentations at the subcellular and molecular level, like synaptic anomalies, glial cell activation, accumulation of misfolded proteins, and diminution of neuronal linkages of synaptic circuits. Mostly, these diseases emerge in adulthood and progressively get critical, primarily accompanying impairments of mental, cognitive, and motor functions.[2,56]

6.2 COMMON NEURODEGENERATIVE DISORDERS

6.2.1 ALZHEIMER'S DISEASE

AD is a commonly diagnosed neurodegenerative disease throughout the world and the primary cause of dementia among old-age people. Globally, it is one of the foremost causes of death in developed countries.[34,104] The major manifestation of the disease seen in patients with AD is neurodegeneration, which further induces protein deposition or synaptic damage, leading to the loss of neurons, which causes cognitive impairment, loss of memory, and an alteration in the behavioral performance of the patients.[76,104] The suitable mechanisms for the precise description of the occurrence of AD are still unclear.[20] A popular mechanism for explaining the disorder is the overactivity of a signaling protein known as cyclin-dependent kinase-5 (CDK5). This protein is vital for the development of neurons and gets activated by the production of p35 or p39, which eventually leads to the formation of a particular complex, which is highly imperative for the neuroplasticity induced during disease pathogenesis.[120,143]

6.2.2 PARKINSON'S DISEASE

PD is considered the second most common neurodegenerative disease after AD, which affects the central nervous system (CNS), thereby resulting in the impairment of motor functions in individuals.[1] The disease involves functional loss of neurons in the substantia nigra region and may even worsen with the death of the neurons. The production of dopamine is reduced, leading to the death of neurons and defects in movement and body functions. Limb stiffness, tremor in hands and joints, slow movement, lack of balance and coordination, etc. are some of the major symptoms of PD.[40,58,78] The disease mechanism is still not clearly understood, but there are several molecular mechanisms put forward to elucidate the emergence of the disease.[87] One of the popularly reported mechanisms is the association of the occurrence of PD with the aggregation of α-synuclein (filamentous protein structure in the brain), which may in turn produce toxic materials. Apart from this, the aggregation of proteins into Lewy bodies, eventually producing α-synucleinopathies, is another mechanism for PD.[21,50]

6.2.3 HUNTINGTON'S DISEASE

HD is an autosomal dominant type of neurodegenerative disease that is inheritable and arises due to a monogenic mutation in the huntingtin (*Htt*) gene on chromosome 4. This mutation results in the generation of unusually elongated polyglutamine-repeated tracts adjacent to the N-terminus of the *Htt* gene.[47] The primary feature of the mutated Htt protein is its tendency to localize and aggregate to produce neuronal inclusions, leading to neuronal impairment and death via numerous mechanisms.[30,138] Further, these involve ramifications such as fragmentation of Htt, prone to abnormal aggregates, along with unpredictable impacts on axonal transport, transcription, translation, cellular proteostasis, etc.[68]

6.2.4 AMYOTROPHIC LATERAL SCLEROSIS

Amyotrophic lateral sclerosis (ALS) is a motor neuron disease marked by progressive paralysis of muscles leading to the degeneration of motor neurons. The disease presentation is extremely variable and dependent upon progression rate, the contribution of upper and lower motor neurons, onset body part, and cognitive dysfunction.[109,134] Generally, the disease remains unidentified because its early signs, such as muscle cramps, twitches, stiffness, involuntary jerking movements, a lack of capacity to regulate the bowel or bladder, etc., may seem mild. ALS is diagnosed clinically, and one of the pivotal tests for facilitating the diagnosis is electromyography.[41,65,127]

6.3 CHALLENGES OF DRUG DELIVERY TO THE BRAIN FOR NDS

Several therapeutic agents have been discovered for dealing with NDs; however, their therapeutic potential has been unsatisfactory owing to undesirable in vivo features, like poor blood-brain barrier (BBB) permeability, poor stability in the biological fluid, enzymatic degradation, clearance by the immune system, unsuitable release profiles, etc.[128,142] The challenges to the brain delivery of drugs are discussed in different sections below.

6.3.1 BLOOD-BRAIN BARRIER (BBB)

BBB is highly selective in allowing the passage of substances across the endothelial membrane while restricting the entry of pathogens or toxic substances.[107] Along with that, this restricted entry also impedes the delivery of therapeutic drugs for the treatment of NDs. It is known to obstruct close to 90% of small-molecule drugs and almost all biologicals.[96] Furthermore, the barrier also regulates the excretion of the drug and endogenous compounds from the brain to the blood with the help of efflux transporters, such as P-glycoprotein (P-gp). The efflux activity of P-gp is the main reason for the failure to maintain the required concentration of therapeutics at the site of action.[64,77] Apart from this, there are a variety of phase I and phase II enzymes that are present in capillary endothelial cell membranes associated with transporter proteins and control the movement of therapeutic agents through the BBB.[145]

6.3.2 BIOAVAILABILITY AND STABILITY

The inadequate bioavailability and stability of the therapeutics are other issues that restrict the potential of therapy because about half of the newly synthesized drugs exhibit extremely poor water solubility.[53] Olesoxime, a neuroprotective agent, is one such example that has low water solubility because of its structural similarity with cholesterol.[136] Most of the drugs utilized for neurological diseases are small-sized lipid-based molecules that utilize active transmembrane diffusion for crossing the BBB. Although the absorption of the drug by capillary endothelial cells of the brain requires delivery through the interstitial fluid of the brain tissues, in such cases, a highly lipophilic drug may get sequestrated by accumulating at the capillary bed and eventually be unable to cross the BBB. Hence, it is critical to transform drugs with adequate lipid solubility to ensure their satisfactory localization in the brain.[38,60]

6.3.3 DISTRIBUTION AND CLEARANCE

The brain-targeted delivery of the drugs may also be hindered due to the systemic distribution of many lipophilic drugs. Although lipophilic drugs can passively diffuse to enter the CNS, these drugs, upon intravenous administration, are also liable to be quickly absorbed by cells in other tissues. Therefore, the dose required to produce the necessary therapeutic action may have to be increased.[13] The nonspecific distribution of the therapeutics may also be responsible for systemic toxicity, producing serious life-threatening consequences.[98] In addition, the rapid rate of clearance for several drugs may also reduce the ability of the drug to attain therapeutic concentration in the brain. The main issue is that hydrophilic drugs are quickly cleared off owing to poor reabsorption, while lipophilic moieties are mostly converted to hydrophilic metabolites in the liver.[3,113]

6.4 BENEFITS OF USING NANOCARRIER-BASED DRUG DELIVERY FOR NDS

Nanotechnology is an evolving field in which nanomaterials can be fabricated to attain desired clinical outcomes for managing NDs. Drug delivery through nanoparticles (NPs) allows multifunctional delivery of the therapeutic agents to regions that are difficult to access, like the brain, along with providing neuroprotection and targeted delivery to the degenerated areas of the brain.[16,141] Some nanocarriers have provided dynamic approaches in the form of polymeric nanoparticles, solid lipid nanoparticles, dendrimers, nanoemulsions, microemulsions, liposomes, nanomicelles, etc. for precise delivery of the drugs to the particular molecular targets in a specific region of the brain.[91] These nanocarriers may be useful in controlling the release of the drug, allowing the safe release of the drug, and minimizing the required dose. The modified NPs found their utility in the pharmaceutical and biomedical fields for diagnosis or treatment due to their versatility.[27,37,95] Even though there are several published research studies and well-known discoveries, the available treatment strategies are mostly unreliable, and additional studies are essential to explicate the mechanisms associated with NDs.[76] In contrast, the rising number of aging populations facing the wrath of neurological diseases throughout the world needs better diagnostic and therapeutic approaches for NDs.[25,86] Figure 6.1 is a pictorial representation of nanotechnology-based drug delivery systems for the management of NDs. Several major advantages of using nanocarriers as drug delivery systems are as follows:

a) Improvement in BBB permeation of the active drug leads to higher localization in the brain.[11,112]
b) Facilitating the higher uptake of NPs to increase the release of drugs in neuronal cells.[63]
c) Bioavailability enhancement of drugs and/or biologicals by increasing their water solubility and permeation.[52,123]
d) Imparting sustained release characteristics for prolonging the drug, reducing the dosing frequency, and reducing the chances of toxicity.[4]
e) Attainment of desired physicochemical features, such as particle size, encapsulation efficiency, stability, etc.[103,130]
f) Intranasal administration of the nanoparticulate carriers is known to improve brain-specific delivery.[6,108]
g) Amelioration of the neuroprotective potential of therapeutic agents and diminishing the neurotoxic effects.[70,119]
h) Enabling the long-term circulation of the nanocarriers for increasing the chance of brain uptake of the drug.[70]
i) Higher brain-targeted delivery of the drug particles from the nano-carrier systems and surface-modified carrier systems.[8]

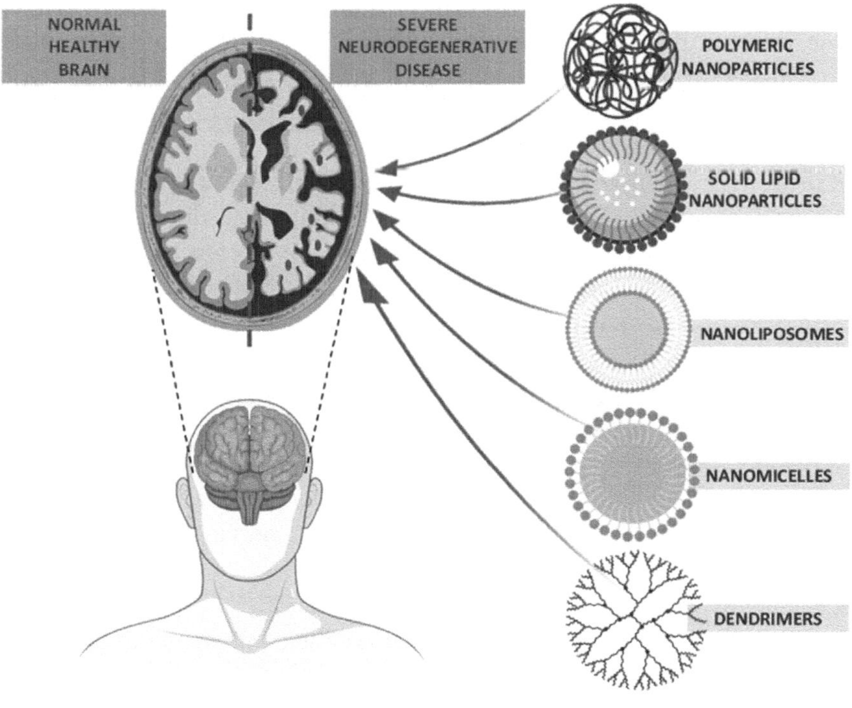

FIGURE 6.1 Nanotechnology-based drug delivery systems for the management of NDs.

6.5 APPLICATION OF NPS FOR THE TREATMENT OF NDS

6.5.1 NPS FOR ALZHEIMER'S DISEASE

AD is one of the most common NDs, which has impaired the cognitive abilities of millions of people all over the world.[118,125] It has been the cause of a huge healthcare burden, especially due to the great difficulty in early diagnosis and intervention of the disease. Although the disease was discovered a century ago, there is still a lack of a concrete therapeutic strategy to combat AD.[39,55] The major reason behind the lack of efficient drugs is the heterogeneity of the disease and its intricate pathological manifestations.[35,135] The delivery of the drug is also hampered because of the BBB around the CNS, which confines the bioavailability of drugs.[97] The nanocarriers could be useful in improving penetrability and sustaining the release of the drug for prolonged action.[12,66]

Sathya et al.[115] evaluated the neuroprotective action of α-bisabolol-loaded solid lipid nanoparticles against the toxicity of Aβ25–35-induced toxicity in Neuro-2a cell lines. The NPs were successful in inhibiting the generation of free radicals, which resulted in protection against damage to macromolecules and mitochondrial membrane potential. Apart from this, the neuroprotective action was also indicated by the considerable reduction in the actions of β-secretase, caspase-3, and cholinesterase.[115,116] Some researchers have found a novel therapeutic strategy of employing the small molecule MC111, which is known to induce the activity of the two transporters, P-glycoprotein (P-gp) and breast cancer resistance protein (BCRP). The induction of the expression of these transporters in the endothelial cells can eliminate Aβ peptides from the brain. However, this approach had some restrictions due to the toxicity of MC111 and the pathological expression of transporters in various parts of the body. To resolve these limitations, NLCs functionalized with transferrin were used as a nanocarrier for the targeted delivery of MC111 in the brain. The novel NLCs were able to avoid the side effects by inducing the targeted expression of P-gp and BRCP in brain endothelial cells.[5] Figure 6.2 illustrates the selective delivery of transferrin-functionalized NLCs and activation of the transporters.

Sadegh et al.[111] developed NLCs and SLNs containing curcumin for enhancing its localization in the brain and improving the therapeutic potential for AD. The brain accumulation of curcumin-containing NLCs was considerably higher in comparison with curcumin-SLNs and free curcumin. The study involved the utilization of an optimum combination of lipids and surfactants to produce biocompatible and sustainable NLCs and SLNs of curcumin with high penetrability to reach the brain.[111] Further, the NLCs were evaluated for brain uptake and biodistribution of curcumin, as well as progression of the disease, memory performance, and microscopic plaque generation in a rat model. The study depicted that the accumulation of curcumin was considerably higher in the serum and brain of the rat. The results showed an evident reduction in oxidative stress factors in the hippocampus and an enhancement of spatial memory. The sequence of events depicted the neuroprotective ability of curcumin-loaded NLCs to decrease the amyloid β peptide in the animal model.[112] Yasir et al.[144] reported the fabrication of SLNs of donepezil for targeting the brain through the nasal route. The NPs were found to possess physicochemical characteristics within an acceptable range and optimum stability. The intranasal administration of SLNs leads to the localization of a high concentration of donepezil in the brains of Wistar albino rats. The selective delivery of drugs to the brain was also confirmed by the biodistribution studies.[144]

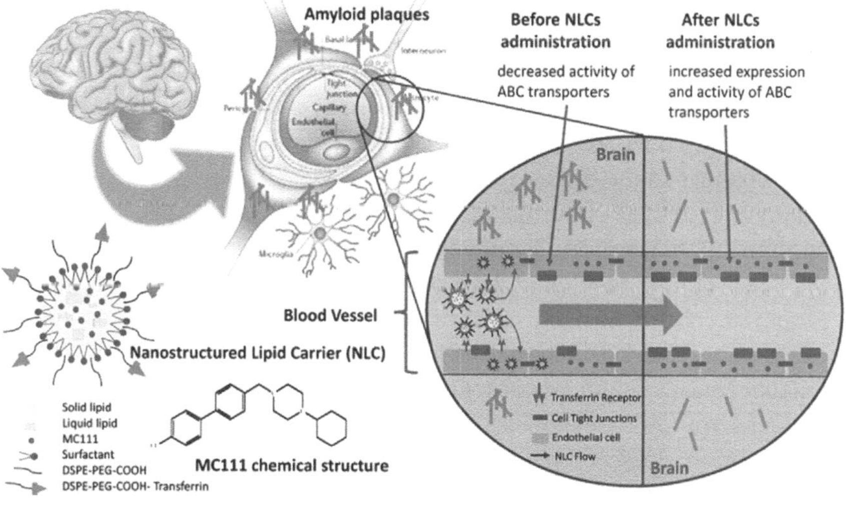

FIGURE 6.2 Pictorial representation of utilization of transferrin-functionalized NLCs for inducing the selective expression and activity of P-gp and BCRP transporters in the endothelial cells of the brain.

Source: Reprinted from Ref. [5] with permission from Elsevier.

A group of scientists studied the effect of polyethylene glycol (PEG)-ceramide nanomicelles on inducing autophagy to remove the tau protein from N2a neuroblastoma cells. PEG-ceramide nanomicelles triggered a rise in the ratio of light chain 3 proteins (LC3-II/LC3-I), whereas p62 protein levels were reduced. There was a considerable upsurge in the number of dots, which indicated the activation of autophagosomes and autolysosomes. PEG-ceramide nanomicelles displayed good potential to trigger autophagy and the elimination of tau proteins, slowing down the progression of AD. Neurodegeneration in AD involves the formation of β-amyloid (Aβ) fibrils in amyloid plaques, which hampers neural synaptic transmission.[22,48] Mirzaie et al.[84] developed polymeric nanomicelles containing curcumin for impeding amyloidogenesis by selectively targeting Aβ fibrils via the glycation method of bovine serum albumin. Polymeric nanomicelles of curcumin were able to significantly reduce the thioflavin T (ThT) fluorescence, which in turn reduced the formation of Aβ-sheets and advanced glycation end (AGE) products. Although there is no clearly defined mechanism for the action of nanomicelles, it could possibly be due to the ability of micelles to keep the protein fibers in α-helical conformation.[84] Muthukumaran et al.[89] investigated the neuroprotective potential of nanomicelle of coenzyme Q10 (CoQ10), called Ubisol-Q10. It was observed in the study that fortifying drinking water with Ubisol-Q10 decreased the circulating Aβ peptide, which further led to improvements in long-term memory and protection of working memory. The author suggested that supplementing AD patients with Ubisol-Q10 has the capacity to slow down the progression of degenerative changes in the brain.[89]

Intranasal delivery of drugs incorporated in nanoemulsions is one of the propitious approaches to circumventing the BBB for the management of AD.[93] Kaur et al.[63] developed a nanoemulsion of memantine and evaluated it for physicochemical characteristics, antioxidant potential, in vivo pharmacokinetics, and biodistribution. The nanoemulsion formulation with suitable physicochemical characteristics (Table 6.1) indicated 98% cell viability and long-term antioxidative activity. The results of pharmacokinetic and biodistribution studies showed high brain uptake of memantine from the nanoemulsion after intranasal administration.[63] Naringenin, a bioflavonoid that has been accounted to display neuroprotective effects in AD,[54,94] was incorporated into the nanoemulsion formulation to improve its delivery to the brain. The formulation displayed a neuroprotective effect by preserving the SH-SY5Y neuroblastoma cell line against beta-amyloid (Aβ) peptide. The neuroprotective effect was mainly related to the suppression of amyloid precursor protein (APP) and β-secretase (BACE), thereby decreasing amyloidogenesis. Apart from this, the naringenin-loaded nanoemulsion also reduced the phosphorylated tau in SH-SY5Y cells, which are prone to Aβ peptide.[82]

In recent times, several studies have been published focusing on using nanosized vesicular carriers for brain delivery.[60,110] A coumarin compound known as Osthole (Ost) is believed to consolidate the neurons around the hippocampus and neuron stem cells, thereby providing neuroprotection against Aβ oligomer-induced neurotoxicity.[29,75] To enhance its brain targeting and bioavailability, transferrin-modified liposomes of Ost were developed by the thin film hydration method. The intracellular uptake of the drug by the brain microvascular endothelial (hCMEC/D3) cell line and APP-SH-SY5Y cells was considerably increased, along with providing additional neuroprotection to the APP-SH-SY5Y cells. The accumulation and cycle time of Ost in the brain was high, and there was improvement in the therapeutic potential of Ost in AD.[70] Arora et al.[8] developed liposomes comprising an apolipoprotein E (ApoE)-encoding plasmid functionalized with glucose transporter-1 (glut-1) for targeting ligand mannose (MAN) and a cell-penetrating peptide (CPP) to improve penetration of ApoE in the brain and cellular internalization. Cell-penetrating enhancers, such as rabies virus glycoprotein peptide (RVG) or penetratin (Pen), were used during the fabrication of liposomes. The functionalized liposomes exhibited two times higher expression of protein as compared to the control formulations. The efficacy was also higher, as deduced from in vivo studies, due to the better transfection of ApoE-encoding plasmids with no indications of toxicity.[8]

Cubosomal dispersion of donepezil HCl containing mucoadhesive *in situ* gel was developed by Patil et al.[101] to augment the brain delivery of the drug. The diffusion study showed the biphasic release pattern of the drug from in situ gel, that is, rapid initial release followed by sustained release over time. The in vivo biodistribution study demonstrated that intranasal delivery of cubosomal in situ gel was successful in better transnasal penetration and localization of drugs in the brain.[101] Sintov[123] reported the use of amylolipid nanovesicles incorporated with curcumin and delivered to the brain through the intranasal route. The nanovesicles showed improved bioavailability of curcumin through intranasal administration in comparison with the intravenous route. The vesicle-type nanoformulation showed a lot of promise due to its high drug loading capacity, simple preparation, ease of scaling up, etc. However, the exploration of the complete pharmacokinetic profile of the formulation will validate its potency. Ansari and Eslami[4] developed niosomal nanocarriers containing *Artemisia absinthium* for reducing amyloid aggregation for the management of AD. The study displayed controlled drug release characteristics of niosomes, and the inhibitory effect was confirmed by using ThT fluorescence and atomic force microscopy methods.[4] Intranasal delivery of niosomes containing pentamidine has also been attempted to achieve the delivery of the drug to the brain. Niosome vesicles were stable in artificial cerebrospinal fluid, and there was no bursting or shrinkage of vesicles during the study. The changes in size and zeta potential shown by vesicles when in contact with mucin were suitable for the penetrating ability of the niosomal nanocarrier. Estabragh et al.[103] prepared niosomes of rivastigmine for enhancing brain functions in AD. The formulation showed high drug efficacy and targetability to deliver rivastigmine into the brain.[103] Table 6.1 summarizes the significant outcomes of research investigations involving NPs-based delivery systems for AD.

6.5.2 NPS FOR PARKINSON'S DISEASE

The drugs used for PD are mostly concentrated on enhancing and protecting the life quality of patients and easing the symptoms of the disease. However, these medications are not able to cure the disease, nor they can modify its progression.[18,73] The traditional delivery systems used for NDs are limited to the presence of a restrictive BBB.[49,61] There is a need for advanced delivery systems for brain-targeted delivery, neuroprotection, and reducing the severity of existing drugs for Parkinson's disease.[51] The nanocarriers have furnished numerous advantages, such as high solubility, better penetrability, maintenance of the stability of drugs, and selective delivery to the brain.[92,122] With the aid of nanotechnology, there are chances of improving the regeneration and function of degenerated neurons, restricting the state of the disease, and providing neuroprotection by achieving the delivery of drugs for PD and escaping the impermeable BBB.[91]

The NP formation may be induced by the self-assembly of polymers into spherical micelles, followed by crystallization under appropriate conditions.[46,146] Levodopa containing emulsion-based crystallized NPs known as "crystalosomes" was prepared for the management of PD. The NP formulation showed a slow release of levodopa to reduce its side effects. The therapeutic efficacy of levodopa increased, as depicted by the reduction in pathological changes and improvement in behavioral performances. The crystalosomes should be further examined for toxicity and pharmacokinetic profile to confirm their viability in the treatment of PD patients.[74] The therapeutic potential of levodopa is limited due to issues, such as low bioavailability and undesirable side effects, which can be resolved by designing biocompatible nanocarriers for levodopa.[121] Poly(lactic-co-glycolide) acid (PLGA) NPs of levodopa were developed using a double

TABLE 6.1 List of Research Investigations Comprising the NP-Based Delivery Systems for AD.

Nanocarrier	Bioactive agent	Composition	Physicochemical characterization	Applications	References
SLNs	α-bisabolol	Soy lecithin, Tween 80, and cholesterol	d_{mean}: 139.5 nm, PDI: 0.244, ZP: −31.7 mV, %EE: 98.44%, %DL: 60.41%	Neuroprotective activity against different neurotoxic mechanisms associated with AD	[116, 117]
NLCs	MC111	Cetyl palmitate, oleic acid, DSPE-PEG (2000)-COOH, Pluronic F68, and transferrin	d_{mean}: 119.6 nm, PDI: 0.177, ZP: −31.7 mV, %EE: 50.1%.	Brain targeting of MC111, allows selective induction of P-gp and BRCP in endothelial cells of the brain to remove amyloid β peptide	[5]
SLNs and NLCs	Curcumin	Cetyl palmitate, Tween 80, oleic acid, and cholesterol	For SLNs; PS: 204.76 nm, PDI: 0.194, %EE: 82%, %DL: 4.60% For NLCs; PS: 117.36 nm, PDI: 0.188, %EE: 94%, %DL: 4.50%	Higher brain uptake of bioactive agent to improve the therapeutic potential in the treatment of AD	[112]
NLCs	Curcumin	Cetyl palmitate, Tween 80, oleic acid, and cholesterol	For NLCs; PS: 117.36 nm, PDI: 0.188, %EE: 94%, %DL: 4.50%	High accumulation rate of curcumin in serum and brain of the animal model. Marked reduction in amyloid β peptide	[113]
SLNs	Donepezil	Glyceryl monostearate, Tween 80, and Poloxamer 188	PS: 121.0 nm, PDI: 0.194, ZP: −24.1 mV, %EE: 67.95%, %DL: 12.15%	Superior brain localization capacity upon intranasal administration of SLNs	[145]
Nanomicelles	Ceramide	PEG-ceramide: N-palmitoyl-sphingosine-1-succinyl [methoxy (polyethylene glycol)-2000]	PS: 17.69 nm, ZP: 0.75 mV	Induction of autophagy to eliminate tau proteins	[47]

TABLE 6.1 *(Continued)*

Nanocarrier	Bioactive agent	Composition	Physicochemical characterization	Applications	References
Polymeric nanomicelles	Curcumin	Phosphatidylethanolamine-distearoyl methoxypolyethylene glycol conjugates	PS: 21.0 nm, ZP: −16.64 mV	Reduction of Aβ protein fibrillation and glycation, thereby decreasing the formation of amyloid plaques	[85]
Polymeric nanomicelles	CoQ10	PEG-derivatized α-tocopherol	–	Inhibition of Aβ plaque formation results in enhanced long-term memory and preservation of working memory	[90]
Nanoemulsion	Memantine	Labrasol, Tween 20, and propylene glycol	PS: 11.0 nm, PDI: 0.080, ZP: −19.6 mV, %DTE: 207.23%	High brain uptake with 98**%** cell viability on neuroblastoma cells	[64]
Nanoemulsion	Naringenin	Capryol 90, Tween 20, and ethanol	PS: 113.83 nm, PDI: 0.312, ZP: 12.4 mV, %DTE: 207.23%	Alleviation of neuro-toxic activity of Aβ peptide on SH-SY5Y cells by suppressing the amyloidogenesis and tau phosphorylation	[83]
Liposomes	Osthole	Transferrin, egg yolk phosphatidylcholine, cholesterol, polyethylene glycol-distearoyl phosphatidylethanolamine, and 1.2-distearoyl-sn-glycero-3-phosphoethanolamine-N [carboxy (polyethylene glycol)-2000]	PS: 104.28 nm, PDI: 0.194, ZP: −6.95 mV, %EE: 92.79%, %DL: 3.71%	Long-term circulation, targeted release of OST, and neuroprotection in AD	[71]

TABLE 6.1 *(Continued)*

Nanocarrier	Bioactive agent	Composition	Physicochemical characterization	Applications	References
Liposomes	ApoE-encoding plasmid	Dioleoyl-3-trimethylammonium-propane chloride, dioleoyl-sn-glycero-3- phosphoethanolamine, CPP-conjugated PEGylated 1,2-distearoyl-sn-glycero-3-phosphorylethanolamine (DSPE), MAN-conjugated PEGylated DSPE, and cholesterol	RVG-liposomes; PS: 172.0 nm, PDI: 0.191, ZP: 19.0 mV, %EE: 86.30% PEN-liposomes; PS: 167.8 nm, PDI: 0.132, ZP: 19.8 mV, %EE: 84.50%	Brain targeted delivery of plasmid, protection of the encapsulated gene from endonuclease digestion, and enhanced levels of ApoE expression	[8]
Cubosomal	Donepezil HCl	Glycerol mono-oleate, Poloxamer 407, gellan gum, and konjac glucomannan	PS: 143.6 nm, PDI: 0.38, ZP: −40 mV, %EE: 48.48%	Biphasic release pattern and brain accumulation of the drug	[102]
Amylolipid nanovesicles	Curcumin	Polyoxyl 40 hydrogenated castor oil, cocoa butter, tetraglycol and glyceryl oleate, and corn starch	PS: 147.8 nm, PDI: 0.18	Improved bioavailability of curcumin in brain	[124]
Niosomes	*Artemisia absinthium*	Phosphatidylcholine, span 60, cholesterol, and DSPE-PEG2000	PS: 174 nm, PDI: 0.373, ZP: 26.5 mV, %EE: 66%	Sustained drug release and inhibition of amyloid aggregation	[4]
Niosomes	Pentamidine	Tween 20, cholesterol, dicetyl phosphate, and chitosan glutamate	d_{mean}: 180.2 nm, PS: 182.0 nm, PDI: 0.248, ZP: −29.5, %EE: 10.96%	Brain delivery of drug through nasal route	[109]
Niosomes	Rivastigmine	Sorbitan esters, their water-soluble derivatives, and cholesterol	-	Uniform size distribution, high encapsulation efficiency (more than 70**%**), and good stability of vesicles	[104]

PS, Particle size; d_{mean}, Mean hydrodynamic diameter; ZP, Zeta potential; %EE, % encapsulation efficiency; %DL, % drug loading; %DTE, % drug targeting efficiency.

emulsion and solvent evaporation method for intranasal delivery of levodopa. The surface of the formulation was modified with the wheat germ agglutinin (WGA) graft to improve nasal absorption of the nanocarriers. The strategy was successful in showing high tissue targeting along with a low level of dopamine in the blood. The formulation was tolerated by animals with little signs of cytotoxicity as compared to plain levodopa.[6]

Tan et al. conjugated apomorphine to phenylboronic acid and functionalized it with polycarbonate to avoid oxidation and improve its efficiency in PD. The encapsulation of the drug protects it from oxidative degradation. The release of the drug was rapid in acidic conditions due to endolysosomes, while the release was very low at pH 7.4. The NPs were able to pass through the BBB to get localized in the brain tissue, and the accumulation of drugs was found to increase with time.[129] Although ropinirole hydrochloride is effective in PD, its activity is restricted due to substantial first-pass metabolism after oral administration.[36,148] To resolve these issues and improve brain uptake, the chitosan NPs of ropinirole hydrochloride were prepared by using the emulsification-crosslinking method. The formulation showed a biphasic release pattern, that is, a rapid initial release followed by a slow release for 10 h. The biodistribution studies revealed a considerably higher localization of drug in the brain as compared to the kidney, liver, and spleen. The surface coating of the NPs was useful in achieving an increase in brain accumulation of active ingredients.[106] Wang et al.[137] developed biodegradable poly(ethylene glycol)-b-poly(trimethylene carbonate) (PEG-PTMC) NPs containing ginkgolide B for enhancing its oral bioavailability and accumulation in the blood and brain. The polymer-based NPs were able to sustain the release of ginkgolide B for 48 h and avoid occurrences of 1-methyl-4-phenylpyridine (MPP+)-induced neuronal cytotoxicity. The pharmacokinetic studies indicated that accumulation was considerably higher in the blood and the brain in comparison with a plain drug.[137]

The microneedle patch-based SLNs of *Bacopa monnieri* were prepared by Joy et al.[59] for the effective management of PD. The microneedle arrays were believed to be a bloodless and painless strategy for delivering drugs through the transdermal route. The nonirritant microneedle was observed to possess good mechanical stability without displaying any concerning signs of bradykinesia. The approach was able to impart high motor coordination and balancing ability at a relatively low effective dose. It showed good neuroprotective activity in the rotenone-induced PD rat model.[59] Khotimah et al.[67] encapsulated *Centella asiatica* into SLNs and then formulated the NPs into orally disintegrating tablets, particularly suitable for older PD patients. The physicochemical features of the SLNs and tablets were found to be within an acceptable range. The formulation is expected to show better BBB penetrability and good performance in PD and dysphagia.[67]

A group of scientists has tried out developing a vitamin E-containing naringenin nanoemulsion for intranasal administration for the management of PD. Behavioral studies, such as the narrow beam test, grip strength test, akinesia, etc., conducted in a rat model, showed a reversion of symptoms in PD-induced rats. To potentiate the effect of therapy, levodopa was also administered intranasally along with a nanoemulsion formulation. The biochemical estimation showed that although the levels of glutathione and superoxide dismutase were higher, the malonaldehyde in the brain tissue was considerably lower.[44] Gupta et al.[52] fabricated a nanoemulsion of coenzyme Q_{10} (CoQ_{10}) to enhance its solubility and thereby enhance oral bioavailability. CoQ_{10} nanoemulsions were examined for their effect on the behavioral performance of the haloperidol-challenged rats. The nanoformulation considerably improved behavioral activities as compared to plain CoQ_{10} suspension by decreasing nigrostriatal dopamine exhaustion, which is useful in controlling the effects of PD. The bioavailability of the CoQ_{10} released from the nanoemulsion formulation was 1.81 folds higher than the CoQ_{10} suspension. The outcomes of biochemical studies showed a marked increase in glutathione and a relative reduction of thiobarbituric acid-reactive substances.[52] Mandal et al.[79] loaded ibuprofen into sodium hyaluronate mucoadhesive nanoemulsion for nose-to-brain delivery for controlling dopaminergic neurodegeneration in PD. The nasal administration of the formulation was found to reduce 1-methyl-4-phenyl-1,2,3,6-tetrahydropyridine (MPTP)-mediated dopamine diminution, which in turn resulted in a reduction in MPTP intoxication. Apart from this, the motor and behavioral performance of the treated mice was significantly improved after administration of the nanoemulsion formulation of ibuprofen.[79]

The liposomal complex comprising 1,2-distearoyl-sn-glycero-3-phosphocholine, dihexadecyl phosphate (DHDP), cholesterol, and 1-palmitoyl-2-oleoyl-sn-glycero-3-phosphate (PA) was employed for the delivery of resveratrol and epigallocatechin gallate (ECG). The surface of liposomes was linked with leptin to enable penetration through the BBB and impart neuroprotection. The liposomes with the modified surface showed substantially higher penetration through the BBB and cellular uptake as compared to the nonmodified liposomes. Additionally, cell viability and target efficiency were also observed to be higher in the study. The results of immunofluorescence and western blot analysis indicated that a modified liposome complex may serve as a reasonable neural protection approach by decreasing the Bcl-2-associated X protein and α-synuclein.[71] Kahana et al.[62] prepared liposomes comprising amyloid precursor protein linked to the diacylglycerol moiety, which can bind to a particular receptor in the BBB for the efficient delivery of dopamine. The intraperitoneal administration of dopamine through liposomes presented a dose-dependent improvement in behavioral activities in mice, and the optimal dose was significantly less than the dose used for levodopa. The targetability of the formulation was indicated because no increase in the concentration of dopamine was observed in the heart or liver.[62] Liposomal nanocarriers can also be used for the delivery of natural-derived organic antioxidants, like polyphenols, which are known to counter the abrupt rise in reactive oxygen species (ROS) and oxidative stress-induced necrosis in PD.[9] A study reported the utilization of nanoliposomes functionalized with antitransferrin receptor antibodies for the delivery and efficient BBB crossing of polyphenol-rich extracts from grape seeds and pomace. The liposomes were observed to complete the restoration of the ROS levels and avoid the aggregation of α-synuclein fibrils. Apart from this, the in vitro studies performed using the rot-induced PD model showed maintenance of cell viability and suppression of β3-tubulin diminution.[80]

Monge-Fuentes et al.[85] designed the albumin and PLGA-based NPs for brain delivery and to enhance the neurotherapeutic potential of dopamine. It was evident from the physicochemical features that NPs allow permeation through BBB, thereby allowing delivery of the drug. The highest dose used in the study showed considerable improvements in the symptoms of PD. Moreover, the dopamine-loaded NPs were successful in reinstating motor coordination and sensorimotor activities in the treated animals.[85] Chen et al.[26] developed NPs containing puerarin for prolonging the in vivo half-life and enhancing its bioavailability. The NPs helped puerarin attain better cellular internalization, penetration, and neuroprotection; along with that, the accumulation of the drug in plasma and the brain was considerably higher as compared to free drug. The outcomes of the study have indicated that the formulation improved PD-associated behavioral deficits and the depletion of dopamine.[26] Poly(ethylene glycol)-co-poly(ϵ-caprolactone)-based NPs were designed for poorly bioavailable ginkgolide B to sustain its release and increase its accumulation in the brain. The study showed that these NPs were internalized through multiple nonspecific mechanisms, followed by localization in the endoplasmic reticulum and lysosomes. The nanocarriers exhibited the neuroprotective ability and requisite pharmacokinetic profile, which were significantly better than free drug.[146] Table 6.2 provides an outlook on research investigations comprising NP-based delivery systems for PD.

TABLE 6.2 List of Research Investigations Comprising the NP-Based Delivery Systems for the PD.

Nanocarrier	Bioactive agent	Composition	Physicochemical characterization	Applications	References
Crystalosomes (Emulsion-based crystallized NPs)	Levodopa	Poly (L-lactic acid), p-xylene, and cetyltrimethyl ammonium bromide	PS: 254.1 nm, ZP: 6.87 mV, %EE: 56%	Reduction in behavioral impairments and pathological changes	[74]
Polymeric nanoparticles	Levodopa	PLGA, polyvinyl alcohol (PVA), and WGA	PS: 329.0 nm, PDI: 0.384, ZP: −4.47 mV, %EE: 72.95%	Enhanced nasal absorption, high tissue targeting, and low cytotoxicity	[6]
Polymeric nanoparticles	Apomorphine	Phenylboronic acid-functionalized polycarbonate	PS: 92.0 nm, PDI: 0.18, %DL: 24.1%	pH-specific drug release, protection of the drug from oxidation, and enhanced brain accumulation	[129]
Polymeric nanoparticles	Ropinirole hydrochloride	Chitosan, span 80, liquid paraffin, and glutaraldehyde	PS: 233.0 nm, PDI: 0.276, ZP: −4.48 mV, %EE: 38.75%	Biphasic release pattern, high brain accumulation, and low accumulation in other organs	[106]
Polymeric nanoparticles	Ginkgolide B	Poly(ethylene glycol)-poly(trimethylene carbonate) and D-tocopheryl polyethylene glycol succinate	PS: 77.58 nm, PDI: 0.124, ZP: −10.37 mV, %DL: 19.43%, %EE: 92.08%	Negligible toxicity, rapidly cross BBB, and high brain uptake	[137]
Solid lipid nanoparticles	*Bacopa monnieri*	Glyceryl monostearate and Tween 80	PS: 77.58 nm, PDI: 0.124, ZP: −10.37 mV, %DL: 19.43%, %EE: 92.08%	Better neuroprotective activity with no irritation and sensitivity	[59]
Solid lipid nanoparticles	*Centella asiatica*	Stearic acid, Tween 80, and PVP K-30	PS: 37.91 nm, PDI: 0.14, ZP: −10.27 mV, %DL: 3.99%, %EE: 95.07%	Management of PD and dysphagia in elder patients	[67]

TABLE 6.2 *(Continued)*

Nanocarrier	Bioactive agent	Composition	Physicochemical characterization	Applications	References
Nanoemulsion	Naringenin	Capryol 90: Vitamin E (1:1), Tween 80, and Transcutol-HP	PS: 38.70 nm, PDI: 0.14, ZP: −27.4 mV, %DTE: 822.71%	High targeting efficiency, reversion of PD effects, and high brain bioavailability	[44]
Nanoemulsion	Coenzyme Q_{10}	Labrafac lipophile WL 1349, Solutol HS 15, and Transcutol P	PS: 60.00 nm, PDI: 0.121, ZP: −24.40 mV	Bioavailability enhancement, better permeation, and improved behavioral activities	[52]
Nanoemulsion	Ibuprofen	Labrafil M 1944 CS, Accenon CC, Transcutol P, and sodium hyaluronate	PS: 46.3 nm, PDI: 0.286, ZP: −28.5 mV	High brain uptake and improvement in motor and behavioral activities	[79]
Liposomes	Resveratrol and epigallocatechin gallate (ECGC)	1,2-distearoyl-sn-glycero-3-phosphocholine, dihexadecyl phosphate (DHDP), cholesterol, 1-palmitoyl-2-oleoyl-sn-glycero-3-phosphate (PA), 1-(3-dimethylaminopropyl)-3-ethylcarbodiimide hydrochloride, and N-hydroxysuccinimide	PS: ~150.0 nm, ZP: −18 to −30 mV, %EE: 54.18% (Resveratrol) and 39.52% (ECGC)	BBB penetration, rescuing degenerated dopaminergic neurons, improved cell viability, and target efficiency	[71]
Liposomes	Dopamine	Cholesterol, 1,2-dioleyl-sn-glycero-3-phosphocholine, and L-α-phosphatidic acid	PS: ~100.0 nm, ZP: −33.7 mV	Brain targeted delivery, improvement in behavioral performance at a low optimal dose, and sustained release of dopamine	[62]

TABLE 6.2 *(Continued)*

Nanocarrier	Bioactive agent	Composition	Physicochemical characterization	Applications	References
Liposomes	Polyphenol-rich extracts from grape seeds and pomace	Brain lipids, biotin-PEG-DSPE, and antitransferrin receptor antibody	d_{mean}: 139.2 nm, ZP: −31.1 mV	Rescue the ROS levels, avoidance of aggregation of α-synuclein fibrils, and restoration of cell viability	[80]
Polymeric nanoparticles	Dopamine	Lipoid S100, PLGA, aluminum chloride phthalocyanine, soybean oil, and Pluranix-68	d_{mean}: 497 nm, PDI: 0.6, ZP: −29 mV	Effective BBB crossing, dopamine replenishment at the nigrostriatal pathway, improvement in motor symptoms, restoration of motor coordination, and sensorimotor performance	[85]
Polymeric nanoparticles	Puerarin	6-s-PLGA and TPGS	PS: 88.36 nm, PDI: 0.047, ZP: −18.85 mV, %DL: 42.97%, %EE: 89.52%	Sustained-release characteristics, superior neuroprotective activity, high brain uptake, reduction in behavioral deficits, and dopamine depletion	[26]
Polymeric nanoparticles	Ginkgolide B	Poly(ethylene glycol)-co-poly(ϵ-caprolactone) and Poloxamer 188	PS: 91.26 nm, PDI: 0.17, ZP: −12.09, %DL: 26.93%, %EE: 87.52%	Enhance cellular uptake (MDCK cells), multiple nonspecific internalization mechanisms, transport across BBB, enhanced brain uptakes, reduction in behavioral deficits, and dopamine depletion	[146]

**PS, Particle size; d_{mean}, Mean hydrodynamic diameter; ZP, Zeta potential; %EE, % encapsulation efficiency; %DL, % drug loading; %DTE, % drug targeting efficiency.*

6.5.3 NPS FOR HUNTINGTON'S DISEASE

HD is marked by the progressive degeneration of medium-spiny neurons (GABAergic inhibitory cells in the human striatum); subsequently, the neurodegeneration advances throughout the brain.[83] The clinical manifestations of the disease involve cognitive disablement, involuntary movements, and other psychiatric indications.[10,81] Presently, there is no established therapeutic approach to control the onset or progression of HD.[69] The available active drug molecules are limited due to their failure to cross the BBB and their lack of brain targeting capacity, like other NDs. NP-based drug carriers may be suitable for allowing the delivery of drugs or biologicals to the brain. The site-specific delivery may prove useful in reducing the side effects of therapy.[72]

One of the most common approaches for the treatment of HD is selective inhibition of huntingtin (HTT) protein aggregation.[32] However, the therapies based on the approach produced an insufficient effect, owing to the reduction in selenium levels in the brains of HD patients.[124] The selenium NPs were developed to control the neurodegeneration associated with HD and cognitive impairment. The selenium NPs were observed to produce lesser toxicity with sufficient selenium bioavailability. The optimized dose of selenium from the NPs was successful in the reduction of neuronal necrosis, adequate behavioral performance, and protection from impairment due to stress conditions. The study displayed a diminution of oxidative stress, suppression of the aggregation of HTT proteins, and downregulation of the expression of histone deacetylase family members. Figure 6.3 portrays the neuroprotective activity of selenium NPs in *Caenorhabditis elegans* HD model.[31]

Sava et al.[117] fabricated nanocarriers containing siRNA against the human *HTT* gene and examined their effects in the HD mouse model (YAC128 transgenic mouse). It was evident from the measurements in brain tissue that formulations efficiently lowered the expression of HTT mRNA. The nanocarriers were dispersed using chitosan as a matrix because of its polymerizing tendency to generate compact NPs stabilized by electrostatic interactions and cross-linking agents (Mangafodipir). However, the chitosan NPs do not bind very tightly to the siRNA, which permits the release of siRNA to induce gene silencing.[117] Birolini et al.[17] evaluated the PLGA NPs modified with a heptapeptide for their disposition, release, kinetics, and safety. The study tried to indicate that cholesterol-containing NPs were able to accumulate in various cells of the brain and deliver cholesterol to regulate neuronal functions. It was observed that systemic and repeated injections of the modified polymeric NPs augmented the biosynthesis of endogenous cholesterol, resulting in averting cognitive impairment and enhancing motor activities in the HD animal model.[17] Belletti et al. fabricated hybrid NPs using a fixed combination of g7-PLGA, PLGA, and cholesterol as the components to observe the design and reorganization of cholesterol in the nanoparticulate system. The results showed the extensive absorption of NPs by neurons with the ability to circumvent lysosomes and release cholesterol in the cells. There was an apparent modification in the expression of synaptic receptors and N-methyl-D-aspartate (NMDA) receptors, which could be useful in HD.[14]

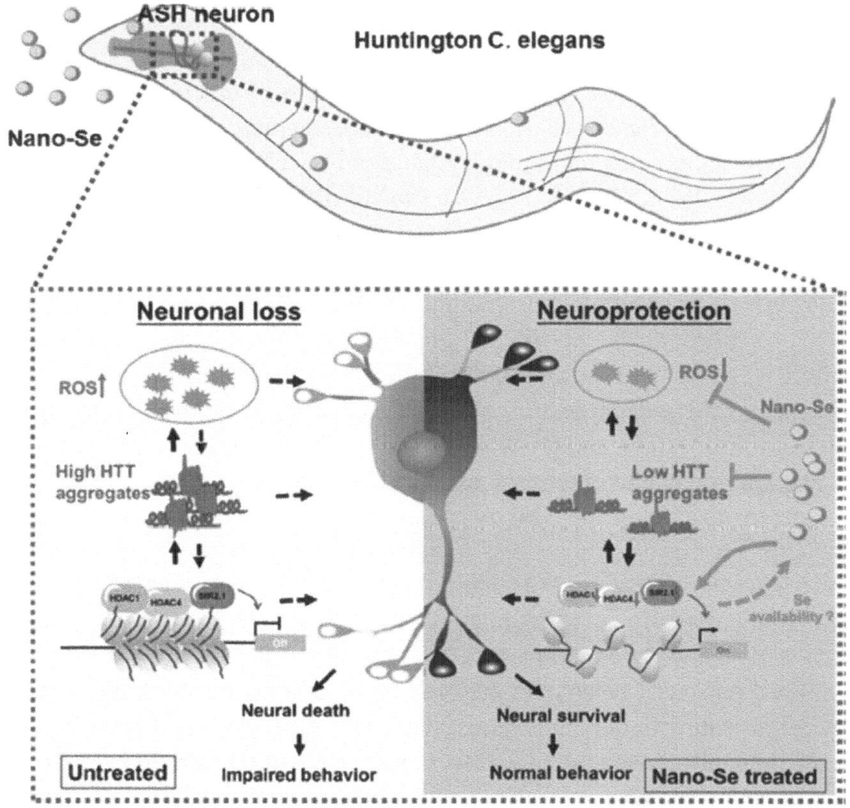

FIGURE 6.3 Illustration of neuroprotective activity of selenium NPs in NDs model for HD in *Caenorhabditis elegans*.

Source: Reprinted with permission from Ref. [31], Copyright © 2019 American Chemical Society.

The therapeutic effects of nanocapsules of epigallocatechin-3-gallate were investigated for their efficiency in decreasing motor defects in the mouse model. The authors reported enhanced movement agility, body posture, gait, etc., which were comparable to the control group. Additionally, the formulation was able to reduce neuroinflammation, which was estimated by examining astrocyte activation and enhanced glial fibrillary acidic protein (GFAP) expression.[23] Debnath et al. developed NPs containing poly (trehalose) for impeding the aggregation of amyloid or polyglutamine and reducing cytotoxicity due to aggregation. The outcomes of the study showed that trehalose NPs possessing zwitterionic charge on the surface and multivalency are critical for the effective targeting of the brain, neuronal cell uptake, and inhibition of HTT aggregation. The nanoparticulate form of trehalose in micromolar concentrations had more potent antiamyloidogenic activity than molar concentrations of molecular trehalose.[33] Pepe et al. reported the production of biodegradable polymers of curcumin to augment bioavailability in the brain. The strategy was to employ hyaluronic materials along with fatty acids and biodegradable polysaccharides to self-assemble into stable NPs. The study showed site-specific release of the drug with reasonable cell uptake and a reduction in the probability of apoptosis in the HD model.[102]

Thymoquinone SLNs were designed by Ramachandran and Thangarajan et al. to alleviate the behavioral impairments in locomotor and rotarod activities, along with the neuroprotective activity. The SLNs were also able to suppress the overexpression of proinflammatory cytokines, p-p65 NFκB nuclear translocation, and GFAP in animal models. In addition, the treatment showed improvement in tyrosine hydroxylase (TH) immunoreactive neurons and desensitization of the NMDA-NR2B-subtype receptor. These resulted in the deterrence of oxidation stress, evading damage to dopaminergic neurons and Ca^{2+} overload in cells.[105] The brain-targeting efficiency of rosmarinic acid can be improved by encapsulating it in SLNs for intranasal delivery. The in vivo study showed that intranasal administration of SLNs of rosmarinic acid exhibited enhanced behavioral performance and inhibited oxidative damage in comparison with the intravenous route. The optimum distribution of drug in the brain also favors intranasal over intravenous administration.[15]

Tetrabenazine decreases the symptoms of cholera linked with HD after the reduction of monoamine in presynaptic vesicles.[114] The intranasal nanoemulsion of tetrabenazine is for the efficient management of hyperkinesia in HD patients. The permeation and brain uptake of the tetrabenazine were higher in the nanoemulsion formulation in comparison with the tetrabenazine suspension. The pharmacokinetic study showed considerably higher values of AUC and C_{max} in the brain for intranasal tetrabenazine nanoemulsion as compared to intravenously administered tetrabenazine solution.[7] Srinageshwar et al. developed novel poly-amidoamine dendrimers with slight surface modifications to allow better BBB permeation and efficient delivery of drugs to the brain. The intracranial administration of the formulation allowed the crossing through the BBB and accumulation within neurons and glial cells by migrating through the corpus callosum. The outcomes suggested these modified dendrimers are suitable to deliver drugs or biologicals with minimum invasiveness for HD or other neurological disorders.[126] Table 6.3 covers the results of some of the recent publications on NP-based delivery systems for HD.

6.5.4 AMYOTROPHIC LATERAL SCLEROSIS

Currently, there are two USFDA-approved drugs available for the treatment of ALS, namely riluzole and edaravone.[57] On the one hand, riluzole works by inhibiting the release of glutamate to further decrease excitotoxicity potential and overaccumulation of glutamate in the brain,[19] while on the other hand, edaravone is an efficient free radical scavenging agent that can reduce the extreme oxidative stress in the brain.[24] Even though both drugs can retard the disease symptoms in patients, their impact on the treatment of ALS is insufficient. Additionally, the presence of biological barriers and restrictions, due to the nature of drugs, poses a lot of difficulties in their effective delivery to the brain, slowing down the clinical progression of ALS[43].

To improve the brain targeting of riluzole, NLCs were developed and functionalized with lactoferrin to enhance movement across the BBB. The physicochemical characteristics of NLCs were suitable for delivery to the brain with the requisite stability. The success of the conjugation of riluzole with lactoferrin was substantiated by employing FTIR and protein quantification studies. It was deduced from the MTT assay that NLC showed no observable signs of cytotoxicity up to 10 μM of drug concentration.[130] Parikh et al. developed a nanoemulsion of riluzole using phase titration to improve its direct brain delivery. A highly stable formulation showed no considerable indications of nasal ciliotoxicity. Further, the intranasal administration of the formulation exhibited high brain uptake in comparison with its oral administration.[99] Riluzole-based mesoporous silica NPs were developed using Santa Barbara Amorphous type material (SBA-15) for enhancing dissolution and bioavailability. The approach was suitable for developing a stable amorphous riluzole with a significantly enhanced rate of dissolution in comparison with a pure crystal of the drug. However, there is still a need to examine the in vivo performance of the NPs to verify improvements in bioavailability and brain uptake.[100] Nabi et al. reported the fabrication of

TABLE 6.3 List of Research Investigations Comprising the NP-Based Delivery Systems for the HD.

Nanocarrier	Bioactive agent	Composition	Physicochemical characterization	Applications	References
Selenium NPs	Sodium selenite	Glutathione and bovine serum albumin	PS: 48.0 nm, ZP: −22.3 mV	Reduction in neuronal death, alleviating behavioral dysfunction, and protection of *C. elegans* under stress	[31]
Polymeric nanoparticles	anti-HTT siRNA	Chitosan, chitosan lactate, and mangafodipir trisodium	PS: 143.0 nm, ZP: 48.7 mV	Lowering HTT mRNA expression	[117]
Polymeric nanoparticles	Cholesterol	PLGA, cholesterol, Pluronic-F68, and trehalose	PS: 303.0 nm, PDI: 0.25, ZP: −25.0 mV	Uptake of NPs by different brain cell types, accumulation in the brain over time, and no signs of inflammatory reactions	[17]
Polymeric nanoparticles	Cholesterol	PLGA, g7-PLGA, and Pluronic F-68	PS: 235.0 nm, PDI: 0.26, ZP: −25.0 mV	Escaping lysosomes, efficient neuronal uptake, and increase cholesterol release in the cells	[14]
Polymeric nanoparticles	Epigallocatechin-3-gallate	PLGA, PEG, ascorbic acid, and Tween 80	PS: 124.8 nm, PDI: 0.054, ZP: −15.7 mV	Restored locomotor performance and neurological activity, reduction of depression-like behavior, neuroinflammation, and neurodegeneration	[23]
Polymeric nanoparticles	Trehalose	3-sulfopropyl methacrylate (sulfo-acrylate), N-(3-aminopropyl) methacrylamide hydrochloride (amino-acrylate), poly(ethylene glycol) methacrylate (PEG-acrylate), and N,N-methylenebis (acrylamide)	d_{mean}: 20 to 30 nm, ZP: −3 to −15 mV	Inhibition of amyloid/ polyglutamine and HTT protein aggregation and effective in low concentration.	[33]

TABLE 6.3 *(Continued)*

Nanocarrier	Bioactive agent	Composition	Physicochemical characterization	Applications	References
Polymeric nanoparticles	Curcumin	Hyaluronic acid (HA)-fatty acid conjugates of oleic acid, linoleic acid, and palmitic acid	PS: 186.7 nm, PDI: 0.236, ZP: −30.6 mV	Self-assembling feature, high neuronal uptake, and decreased susceptibility to apoptosis	[102]
Solid lipid nanoparticles	Thymoquinone	Stearic acid, lecithin, and taurocholate	–	Inhibition of microglial activation, NMDA receptor sensitization, and neuroinflammation	[105]
Solid lipid nanoparticles	Rosmarinic acid	Glycerol monostearate, Tween 80, soya lecithin, and soya phosphatidyl choline	PS: 149.2 nm, PDI: 0.290, ZP: −38.27 mV, %EE: 61.9%	Improved behavioral activities and inhibition of oxidative stress	[15]
Nanoemulsion	Tetrabenazine	Capmul MCM, Tween 80, and Transcutol P	PS: 106.8 nm, PDI: 0.198, ZP: −9.63 mV	High permeability, enhanced bioavailability, and optimum pharmacokinetic features	[7]
Dendrimers	–	Ethanolamine, ethylenediamine, and diaminobutane	PS: ~1 to 4 nm	Permeation through BBB and accumulation within neuronal and glial cells	[126]

**PS, Particle size; d_{mean}, Mean hydrodynamic diameter; ZP, Zeta potential; %EE, % encapsulation efficiency; %DL, % drug loading; %DTE, % drug targeting efficiency.*

chitosan NPs loaded with riluzole along with transferrin as a ligand to achieve better brain targeting. The NPs improved the brain uptake and effectiveness of riluzole. Though the riluzole NPs showed good neuroprotective potential, the incorporation of transferrin further augmented the benefit by improving the targeting efficiency.[90]

To enhance the neuroprotective effect, polymeric micelles of edaravone were designed by employing polymethoxy ethylene glycol-polylactic-co-glycolic acid (mPEG-b-PLGA). The study reported a considerable reduction in lactate dehydrogenase, intracellular ROS, nitric oxide activity, and rate of apoptosis after administration of edaravone-containing micelles. Additionally, the preparation displayed a reduction in the expression of the proapoptotic gene and an increase in the expression of antiapoptotic genes. The results confirmed the neuroprotective potential of the polymeric micelles of edaravone.[119] Bao et al. prepared ceria NPs loaded with edaravone and surface modified by Angiopep-2 and poly(ethylene glycol). The modified NPs featured highly efficient crossing through the BBB to attain therapeutic concentrations in brain tissues and synergistic removal of ROS. Moreover, the edaravone-loaded ceria NPs showed low toxicity and exceptional hemo- and histocompatibility.[11] Table 6.4 outlines the outcomes of some of the latest research investigations on NP-based delivery systems for ALS.

6.6 CONCLUSION AND FUTURE PERSPECTIVE

The rise in incidences of incapacitating, life-threatening, and untreatable NDs is suspected to have disturbing effects on the lives of people. The need of the hour is efficient strategies for early diagnosis, along with therapeutic products, to decrease the occurrence and progression of these diseases. Common NDs are known to emerge in the adult stage of the individual with some symptoms and perniciously progress into severe form with age. To suppress the disease progression or even ease out their symptoms, several therapeutic mechanisms have been discovered, but they are evinced to be mostly inefficient owing to poor permeability through the BBB, low bioavailability, a lack of brain targeting and neuronal uptake, etc. The diagnosis and treatment of neuronal dysfunctions with the aid of nanotechnology tools have come forth as an exciting prospect. A nanotechnology-based carrier shows a promising resolution to overcome the hindrances related to brain delivery and furnishes an innovative approach for the management of NDs. The nanocarriers can evade the limitations associated with conventional therapeutic strategies; therefore, a lot of researchers have lately been investigating the utilization of

TABLE 6.4 List of Research Investigations Comprising the NP-Based Delivery Systems for ALS.

Nanocarrier	Bioactive agent	Composition	Physicochemical characterization	Applications	References
Nanostructured lipid carriers	Riluzole	Precirol® ATO5, Mygliol® 812, Polysorbate 80, Poloxamer 188, and stearic acid	PS: 221.9 nm, PDI: 0.219, ZP: −16.41 mV, %EE: 94.21%	Physicochemical properties compatible with brain application, high stability, and no cytotoxicity	[130]
Nanoemulsion	Riluzole	Sefsol 218, Tween 80, and Carbitol	PS: 23.92 nm	Stable formulation, free from nasal ciliotoxicity, and high brain uptake	[99]
Mesoporous silica NPs	Riluzole	SBA-15 mesoporous NPs, Pluronic P123, Poly(ethylene glycol)-block-poly(propylene glycol)-block-poly(ethylene glycol), and tetraethyl-orthosilicate	–	Enhancement of dissolution of the drug, degradable, and safely excreted	[100]
Polymeric nanoparticles	Riluzole	Chitosan, sodium tripolyphosphate, and holotransferrin	PS: 207.0 nm, PDI: 0.406	Improve brain uptake and potent neuroprotective agent	[90]
Polymeric micelles	Edaravone	mPEG-b-PLGA	PS: 155.0 nm, PDI: 0.11, ZP: −15, %DL: 13%, %EE: 65%	Significantly high rate of neuroprotective effects	
Ceria NPs	Edaravone	$Ce(NO_3)_3.6H_2O$, oleylamine, 1-octadecene, Angiopep-2, and aminepoly-(ethylene glycol)	PS: 20 to 25 nm, ZP: ~ 5 mV	Effective crossing through the BBB, synergistic removal of ROS, low toxicity, and exceptional hemo- and histocompatibility	[11]

**PS, Particle size; ZP, Zeta potential; %EE, % encapsulation efficiency; %DL, % drug loading.*

nanoformulations for the brain delivery of drugs. Moreover, the nanocarriers can be adequately designed and even modified to deliver multiple agents with particular functions. In recent times, the intranasal administration of the drug has found interest in many researchers as a potential means of improving the delivery of the drug to the brain.

KEYWORDS

- **nanotechnology**
- **central nervous system**
- **neurodegenerative disorders**
- **Alzheimer's disease**
- **Parkinson's disease**
- **blood-brain barrier**
- **nanoparticles**

REFERENCES

1. Aarsland, D.; Batzu, L.; Halliday, G. M.; Geurtsen, G. J.; Ballard, C.; Ray Chaudhuri, K.; Weintraub, D. Parkinson Disease-Associated Cognitive Impairment. *Nat. Rev. Dis. Primers* **2021,** *7* (1), 47. DOI: 10.1038/s41572-021-00280-3
2. Ahmad, K.; Baig, M. H.; Mushtaq, G.; Kamal, M. A.; Greig, N. H.; Choi, I. Commonalities in Biological Pathways, Genetics, and Cellular Mechanism between Alzheimer Disease and Other Neurodegenerative Diseases: An In Silico-Updated Overview. *Curr Alzheimer Res.* **2017,** *14* (11), 1190–1197. DOI: 10.2174/1567205014666170203141151
3. Ahmed, T. A. *Pharmacokinetics of Drugs Following IV Bolus, IV Infusion, and Oral Administration*, 2015.
4. Ansari, M.; Eslami, H. J. N. J. Preparation and Study of the Inhibitory Effect of Nano-Niosomes Containing Essential Oil from Artemisia Absinthium on Amyloid Fibril Formation. **2020,** *7* (3), 243–250.
5. Arduino, I.; Iacobazzi, R. M.; Riganti, C.; Lopedota, A. A.; Perrone, M. G.; Lopalco, A. et al. Induced Expression of P-gp and BCRP Transporters on Brain Endothelial Cells Using Transferrin Functionalized Nanostructured Lipid Carriers: A First Step of a Potential Strategy for the Treatment of Alzheimer's Disease. *Int. J. Pharm.* **2020,** *591*, 120011. DOI: 10.1016/j.ijpharm.2020.120011
6. Arisoy, S.; Sayiner, O.; Comoglu, T.; Onal, D.; Atalay, O.; Pehlivanoglu, B. In Vitro and In Vivo Evaluation of Levodopa-Loaded Nanoparticles for Nose to Brain Delivery. *Pharm. Dev. Technol.* **2020,** *25* (6), 735–747. DOI: 10.1080/10837450.2020.1740257

7. Arora, A.; Kumar, S.; Ali, J.; Baboota, S. Intranasal Delivery of Tetrabenazine Nanoemulsion via Olfactory Region for Better Treatment of Hyperkinetic Movement Associated with Huntington's Disease: Pharmacokinetic and Brain Delivery Study. *Chem. Phys. Lipids* **2020,** *230,* 104917. DOI: https://doi.org/10.1016/j.chemphyslip. 2020. 104917.
8. Arora, S.; Layek, B.; Singh, J. Design and Validation of Liposomal ApoE2 Gene Delivery System to Evade Blood–Brain Barrier for Effective Treatment of Alzheimer's Disease. *Mol. Pharm.* **2021,** *18* (2), 714–725. DOI: 10.1021/acs.molpharmaceut.0c00461.
9. Ataie, A.; Shadifar, M.; Ataee, R. Polyphenolic Antioxidants and Neuronal Regeneration. *Basic Clin. Neurosci.* **2016,** *7* (2), 81–90. DOI: 10.15412/j.Bcn.03070201.
10. Bachoud-Lévi, A.-C.; Ferreira, J.; Massart, R.; Youssov, K.; Rosser, A.; Busse, M. et al. International Guidelines for the Treatment of Huntington's Disease. **2019,** *10.* DOI: 10.3389/fneur.2019.00710
11. Bao, Q.; Hu, P.; Xu, Y.; Cheng, T.; Wei, C.; Pan, L.; Shi, J. Simultaneous Blood–Brain Barrier Crossing and Protection for Stroke Treatment Based on Edaravone-Loaded Ceria Nanoparticles. *ACS Nano* **2018,** *12* (7), 6794–6805. DOI: 10.1021/acsnano. 8b01994
12. Beaman, E. E.; Bonde, A. N.; Ulv Larsen, S. M.; Ozenne, B.; Lohela, T. J.; Nedergaard, M. et al. Blood–Brain Barrier Permeable β-Blockers Linked to Lower Risk of Alzheimer's Disease in Hypertension. *Brain* **2022.** DOI: 10.1093/brain/awac076
13. Bellettato, C. M.; Scarpa, M. Possible Strategies to Cross the Blood–Brain Barrier. *Ital. J. Pediatr.* **2018,** *44* (2), 131. DOI: 10.1186/s13052-018-0563-0
14. Belletti, D.; Grabrucker, A. M.; Pederzoli, F.; Menrath, I.; Vandelli, M. A.; Tosi, G. et al. Hybrid Nanoparticles as a New Technological Approach to Enhance the Delivery of Cholesterol into the Brain. *Int. J. Pharm.* **2018,** *543* (1), 300–310. DOI: https://doi.org/10.1016/j.ijpharm.2018.03.061
15. Bhatt, R.; Singh, D.; Prakash, A.; Mishra, N. Development, Characterization and Nasal Delivery of Rosmarinic Acid-Loaded Solid Lipid Nanoparticles for the Effective Management of Huntington's Disease. *Drug Deliv.* **2015,** *22* (7), 931–939. DOI: 10.3109/10717544.2014.880860
16. Bhattacharya, T.; Soares, G.; Chopra, H.; Rahman, M. M.; Hasan, Z.; Swain, S. S.; Cavalu, S. Applications of Phyto-Nanotechnology for the Treatment of Neurodegenerative Disorders. *Materials* **2022,** *15* (3). DOI: 10.3390/ma15030804
17. Birolini, G.; Valenza, M.; Ottonelli, I.; Passoni, A.; Favagrossa, M.; Duskey, J. T. et al. Insights into Kinetics, Release, and Behavioral Effects of Brain-Targeted Hybrid Nanoparticles for Cholesterol Delivery in Huntington's Disease. *J. Controll. Release* **2021,** *330,* 587–598. DOI: https://doi.org/10.1016/j.jconrel.2020.12.051
18. Bloem, B. R.; Okun, M. S.; Klein, C. Parkinson's Disease. *Lancet* **2021,** *397* (10291), 2284–2303. DOI: https://doi.org/10.1016/S0140-6736 (21)00218-X
19. Blyufer, A.; Lhamo, S.; Tam, C.; Tariq, I.; Thavornwatanayong, T.; Mahajan, S. S. Riluzole: A Neuroprotective Drug with Potential as a Novel Anti-Cancer Agent (Review). *Int. J. Oncol.* **2021,** *59* (5). DOI: 10.3892/ijo.2021.5275
20. Bogdanovic, B.; Eftimov, T.; Simjanoska, M. In-Depth Insights into Alzheimer's Disease by Using Explainable Machine Learning Approach. *Sci. Rep.* **2022,** *12* (1), 6508. DOI: 10.1038/s41598-022-10202-2
21. Bridi, J. C.; Hirth, F. Mechanisms of α-Synuclein Induced Synaptopathy in Parkinson's Disease. *Front. Neurosci.* **2018,** *12,* 80. DOI: 10.3389/fnins.2018.00080

22. Brown, M. R.; Radford, S. E.; Hewitt, E. W. Modulation of β-Amyloid Fibril Formation in Alzheimer's Disease by Microglia and Infection. **2020,** *13*. DOI: 10.3389/fnmol.2020.609073
23. Cano, A.; Ettcheto, M.; Espina, M.; Auladell, C.; Folch, J.; Kühne, B. A. et al. Epigallocatechin-3-gallate PEGylated Poly (Lactic-co-glycolic) Acid Nanoparticles Mitigate Striatal Pathology and Motor Deficits in 3-Nitropropionic Acid Intoxicated Mice. *16* (1), 19–35. DOI: 10.2217/nnm-2020-0239
24. Cha, S. J.; Kim, K. Effects of the Edaravone, a Drug Approved for the Treatment of Amyotrophic Lateral Sclerosis, on Mitochondrial Function and Neuroprotection. **2022,** *11* (2), 195.
25. Chen-Plotkin, Alice S. Unbiased Approaches to Biomarker Discovery in Neurodegenerative Diseases. *Neuron* **2014,** *84* (3), 594–607. DOI: https://doi.org/10.1016/j.neuron.2014.10.031
26. Chen, T.; Liu, W.; Xiong, S.; Li, D.; Fang, S.; Wu, Z. et al. Nanoparticles Mediating the Sustained Puerarin Release Facilitate Improved Brain Delivery to Treat Parkinson's Disease. *ACS Appl. Mater. Interfaces* **2019,** *11* (48), 45276–45289. DOI: 10.1021/acsami.9b16047
27. Chenthamara, D.; Subramaniam, S.; Ramakrishnan, S. G.; Krishnaswamy, S.; Essa, M. M.; Lin, F.-H.; Qoronfleh, M. W. Therapeutic Efficacy of Nanoparticles and Routes of Administration. *Biomater. Res.* **2019,** *23* (1), 20. DOI: 10.1186/s40824-019-0166-x
28. Chi, H.; Chang, H.-Y.; Sang, T.-K. Neuronal Cell Death Mechanisms in Major Neurodegenerative Diseases. **2018,** *19* (10), 3082.
29. Chu, Q.; Zhu, Y.; Cao, T.; Zhang, Y.; Chang, Z.; Liu, Y. et al. Studies on the Neuroprotection of Osthole on Glutamate-Induced Apoptotic Cells and an Alzheimer's Disease Mouse Model via Modulation Oxidative Stress. *Appl. Biochem. Biotechnol.* **2020,** *190* (2), 634–644. DOI: 10.1007/s12010-019-03101-2
30. Chung, C. G.; Lee, H.; Lee, S. B. Mechanisms of Protein Toxicity in Neurodegenerative Diseases. *Cell. Mol. Life Sci.* **2018,** *75* (17), 3159–3180. DOI: 10.1007/s00018-018-2854-4
31. Cong, W.; Bai, R.; Li, Y.-F.; Wang, L.; Chen, C. Selenium Nanoparticles as an Efficient Nanomedicine for the Therapy of Huntington's Disease. *ACS Applied Materials & Interfaces, 11* (38), 34725–34735. DOI: 10.1021/acsami.9b12319
32. Dash, D.; Mestre, T. A. Therapeutic Update on Huntington's Disease: Symptomatic Treatments and Emerging Disease-Modifying Therapies. *Neurotherapeutics* **2020,** *17* (4), 1645–1659. DOI: 10.1007/s13311-020-00891-w
33. Debnath, K.; Pradhan, N.; Singh, B. K.; Jana, N. R.; Jana, N. R. Poly (trehalose) Nanoparticles Prevent Amyloid Aggregation and Suppress Polyglutamine Aggregation in a Huntington's Disease Model Mouse. *ACS Appl. Mater. Interfaces* **2017,** *9* (28), 24126–24139. DOI: 10.1021/acsami.7b06510
34. DeTure, M. A.; Dickson, D. W. The Neuropathological Diagnosis of Alzheimer's Disease. *Mol. Neurodegen.* **2019,** *14* (1), 32. DOI: 10.1186/s13024-019-0333-5
35. Devi, G.; Scheltens, P. Heterogeneity of Alzheimer's Disease: Consequence for Drug Trials? *Alzheimer's Res. Therapy* **2018,** *10* (1), 122. DOI: 10.1186/s13195-018-0455-y
36. Di Prima, G.; Campisi, G.; De Caro, V. Amorphous Ropinirole-Loaded Mucoadhesive Buccal Film: A Potential Patient-Friendly Tool to Improve Drug Pharmacokinetic Profile and Effectiveness. **2020,** *10* (4), 242.
37. Din, F. U.; Aman, W.; Ullah, I.; Qureshi, O. S.; Mustapha, O.; Shafique, S.; Zeb, A. Effective Use of Nanocarriers as Drug Delivery Systems for the Treatment of Selected Tumors. *Int. J. Nanomed.* **2017,** *12*, 7291–7309. DOI: 10.2147/ijn.S146315

38. Dong, X. Current Strategies for Brain Drug Delivery. *Theranostics* **2018,** *8* (6), 1481–1493. DOI: 10.7150/thno.21254
39. dos Santos Picanco, C. L.; Ozela, F. P.; de Fatima de Brito Brito, M.; Pinheiro, A. A.; Padilha, C. E.; Braga, S. F. et al. Alzheimer's Disease: A Review from the Pathophysiology to Diagnosis, New Perspectives for Pharmacological Treatment. *Curr. Med. Chem.* **2018,** *25* (26), 3141–3159. DOI: http://dx.doi.org/10.2174/0929867323666161213101126
40. Emamzadeh, F. N.; Surguchov, A. Parkinson's Disease: Biomarkers, Treatment, and Risk Factors. *Front. Neurosci.* **2018,** *12*, 612. DOI: 10.3389/fnins.2018.00612
41. Farooqui, A. A. Chapter 5—Contribution of Gut Microbiota in the Pathogenesis of Amyotrophic Lateral Sclerosis and Huntington's Disease. In: Farooqui, T., Farooqui, A. A., Eds.; *Gut Microbiota in Neurologic and Visceral Diseases*; Academic Press, 2021; pp 87–100.
42. Fu, H.; Hardy, J.; Duff, K. E. Selective Vulnerability in Neurodegenerative Diseases. *Nat. Neurosci.* **2018,** *21* (10), 1350–1358. DOI: 10.1038/s41593-018-0221-2
43. Furtado, D.; Björnmalm, M.; Ayton, S.; Bush, A. I.; Kempe, K.; Caruso, F. Overcoming the Blood-Brain Barrier: The Role of Nanomaterials in Treating Neurological Diseases. *Adv. Mater.* **2018,** *30* (46), e1801362. DOI: 10.1002/adma.201801362
44. Gaba, B.; Khan, T.; Haider, M. F.; Alam, T.; Baboota, S.; Parvez, S.; Ali, J. Vitamin E Loaded Naringenin Nanoemulsion via Intranasal Delivery for the Management of Oxidative Stress in a 6-OHDA Parkinson's Disease Model. *BioMed. Res. Int.* **2019,** 2382563. DOI: 10.1155/2019/2382563
45. Gao, J.; Chen, X.; Ma, T.; He, B.; Li, P.; Zhao, Y. et al. PEG-Ceramide Nanomicelles Induce Autophagy and Degrade Tau Proteins in N2a Cells. *Int. J. Nanomed.* **2020,** *15*, 6779–6789. DOI: 10.2147/ijn.S258311
46. Gao, M.; Yang, Y.; Bergfel, A.; Huang, L.; Zheng, L.; Bowden, T. M. Self-Assembly of Cholesterol End-Capped Polymer Micelles for Controlled Drug Delivery. *J. Nanobiotechnol.* **2020,** *18* (1), 13. DOI: 10.1186/s12951-020-0575-y
47. Gatto, E. M.; Rojas, N. G.; Persi, G.; Etcheverry, J. L.; Cesarini, M. E.; Perandones, C. Huntington Disease: Advances in the Understanding of Its Mechanisms. *Clin. Parkin sonism Relat. Disorders* **2020,** *3*, 100056. DOI: https://doi.org/10.1016/j.prdoa.2020.100056
48. Ghosh, U.; Thurber, K. R.; Yau, W.-M.; Tycko, R. Molecular Structure of a Prevalent Amyloid-β Fibril Polymorph from Alzheimer's Disease Brain Tissue. **2021,** *118* (4), e2023089118. DOI: DOI: 10.1073/pnas.2023089118
49. Gosselet, F.; Loiola, R. A.; Roig, A.; Rosell, A.; Culot, M. Central Nervous System Delivery of Molecules Across the Blood-Brain Barrier. *Neurochem. Int.* **2021,** *144*, 104952. DOI: https://doi.org/10.1016/j.neuint.2020.104952
50. Gracia, P.; Camino, J. D.; Volpicelli-Daley, L.; Cremades, N. Multiplicity of α-Synuclein Aggregated Species and Their Possible Roles in Disease. *Int. J. Mol. Sci.* **2020,** *21* (21). DOI: 10.3390/ijms21218043
51. Gunay, M. S.; Ozer, A. Y.; Chalon, S. Drug Delivery Systems for Imaging and Therapy of Parkinson's Disease. *Curr. Neuropharmacol.* **2016,** *14* (4), 376–391. DOI: 10.2174/1570159x14666151230124904
52. Gupta, B. K.; Kumar, S.; Kaur, H.; Ali, J.; Baboota, S. Attenuation of Oxidative Damage by Coenzyme Q (10) Loaded Nanoemulsion Through Oral Route for the Management of Parkinson's Disease. *Rejuvenation Res.* **2018,** *21* (3), 232–248. DOI: 10.1089/rej.2017.1959

53. Haider, M. S.; Ahmad, T.; Groll, J.; Scherf-Clavel, O.; Kroiss, M.; Luxenhofer, R. The Challenging Pharmacokinetics of Mitotane: An Old Drug in Need of New Packaging. *Eu. J. Drug Metabol. Pharmacokinetics* **2021,** *46* (5), 575–593. DOI: 10.1007/s13318- 021-00700-5
54. Haider, S.; Liaquat, L.; Ahmad, S.; Batool, Z.; Siddiqui, R. A.; Tabassum, S. et al. Naringenin Protects AlCl3/D-Galactose Induced Neurotoxicity in Rat Model of AD via Attenuation of Acetylcholinesterase Levels and Inhibition of Oxidative Stress. *PLoS One* **2020,** *15* (1), e0227631. DOI: 10.1371/journal.pone.0227631
55. Hippius, H.; Neundörfer, G. The discovery of Alzheimer's disease. *Dialogues Clin Neurosci, 5* (1), 101–108. DOI: 10.31887/DCNS.2003.5.1/hhippius
56. Hussain, R.; Zubair, H.; Pursell, S.; Shahab, M. Neurodegenerative Diseases: Regenerative Mechanisms and Novel Therapeutic Approaches. *Brain Sci.* **2018,** *8* (9). DOI: 10.3390/brainsci8090177
57. Jaiswal, M. K. Riluzole and Edaravone: A Tale of Two Amyotrophic Lateral Sclerosis Drugs. *Med. Res. Rev.* **2019,** *39* (2), 733–748. DOI: 10.1002/med.21528
58. Jankovic, J.; Tan, E. K. Parkinson's Disease: Etiopathogenesis and Treatment. *J. Neurol. Neurosurg. Psychiatry* **2020,** *91* (8), 795. DOI: 10.1136/jnnp-2019-322338
59. Joy, D.; Jose, J.; Bibi, S.; Bandiwadekar, A.; Gopan, G.; Mariana Gonçalves Lima, C. et al. Development of Microneedle Patch Loaded with *Bacopa monnieri* Solid Lipid Nanoparticles for the Effective Management of Parkinson's Disease. *Bioinorgan. Chem. App.* **2022, 2022,** 9150205. DOI: 10.1155/2022/9150205
60. Juhairiyah, F.; de Lange, E. C. M. Understanding Drug Delivery to the Brain Using Liposome-Based Strategies: Studies that Provide Mechanistic Insights Are Essential. *AAPS J.* **2021,** *23* (6), 114. DOI: 10.1208/s12248-021-00648-z
61. Kadry, H.; Noorani, B.; Cucullo, L. A Blood–Brain Barrier Overview on Structure, Function, Impairment, and Biomarkers of Integrity. *Fluids Barriers CNS* **2020,** *17* (1), 69. DOI: 10.1186/s12987-020-00230-3
62. Kahana, M.; Weizman, A.; Gabay, M.; Loboda, Y.; Segal-Gavish, H.; Gavish, A. et al. Liposome-Based Targeting of Dopamine to the Brain: A Novel Approach for the Treatment of Parkinson's Disease. *Mol. Psychiatry* **2021,** *26* (6), 2626–2632. DOI: 10.1038/s41380-020-0742-4
63. Kaur, A.; Nigam, K.; Srivastava, S.; Tyagi, A.; Dang, S. Memantine Nanoemulsion: A New Approach to Treat Alzheimer's Disease. *J. Microencapsulation* **2020,** *37* (5), 355–365. DOI: 10.1080/02652048.2020.1756971
64. Keogh, J.; Hagenbuch, B.; Rynn, C.; Stieger, B.; Nicholls, G. Chapter 1 Membrane Transporters: Fundamentals, Function and Their Role in ADME. In: *Drug Transporters: Volume 1: Role and Importance in ADME and Drug Development*, Vol. 1; The Royal Society of Chemistry, 2016;, pp. 1–56.
65. Keon, M.; Musrie, B.; Dinger, M.; Brennan, S. E.; Santos, J.; Saksena, N. K. Destination Amyotrophic Lateral Sclerosis. *Front. Neurol.* **2021,** *12*, 596006. DOI: 10.3389/fneur.2021.596006
66. Khan, N. H.; Mir, M.; Ngowi, E. E.; Zafar, U.; Khakwani, M.; Khattak, S. et al. Nanomedicine: A Promising Way to Manage Alzheimer's Disease. *Front. Bioeng. Biotechnol.* **2021,** *9*, 630055. DOI: 10.3389/fbioe.2021.630055
67. Khotimah, H.; Aulanni'am, A.; Nandar Kurniawan, S.; Eka Puspita, O.; Rahayu Adianingsih, O.; Mardhiyah, M.; Setiawan, A. Development and Optimization of Orally Disintegrating Tablets Containing *Centella asiatica* Solid Lipid Nanoparticles for

Supportive Therapies of Parkinson's Disease [Version 1; Peer Review: Awaiting Peer Review]. **2022,** *11* (517). DOI: 10.12688/f1000research.118951.1
68. Kim, C.; Yousefian-Jazi, A.; Choi, S. H.; Chang, I.; Lee, J.; Ryu, H. Non-Cell Autonomous and Epigenetic Mechanisms of Huntington's Disease. *Int J Mol Sci, 22* (22). DOI: 10.3390/ijms222212499
69. Komatsu, H. Innovative Therapeutic Approaches for Huntington's Disease: From Nucleic Acids to GPCR-Targeting Small Molecules. *Front. Cell. Neurosci.* **2021,** *15*, 785703. DOI: 10.3389/fncel.2021.785703
70. Kong, L.; Li, X. T.; Ni, Y. N.; Xiao, H. H.; Yao, Y. J.; Wang, Y. Y. et al. Transferrin-Modified Osthole PEGylated Liposomes Travel the Blood-Brain Barrier and Mitigate Alzheimer's Disease-Related Pathology in APP/PS-1 Mice. *Int. J. Nanomed.* **2020,** *15*, 2841–2858. DOI: 10.2147/ijn.S239608
71. Kuo, Y.-C.; Wang, I. H.; Rajesh, R. Use of Leptin-Conjugated Phosphatidic Acid Liposomes with Resveratrol and Epigallocatechin Gallate to Protect Dopaminergic Neurons Against Apoptosis for Parkinson's Disease Therapy. *Acta Biomater.* **2021,** *119*, 360–374. DOI: https://doi.org/10.1016/j.actbio.2020.11.015
72. Lamptey, R. N. L.; Chaulagain, B.; Trivedi, R.; Gothwal, A.; Layek, B.; Singh, J. A Review of the Common Neurodegenerative Disorders: Current Therapeutic Approaches and the Potential Role of Nanotherapeutics. *Int. J. Mol. Sci.* **2022,** *23* (3). DOI: 10.3390/ijms23031851
73. Lee, T. K.; Yankee, E. L. A Review on Parkinson's Disease Treatment. *Neuroimmunol. Neuroinflamm.* **2021,** *8*, 222. DOI: 10.20517/2347-8659.2020.58
74. Li, X.; Liu, Q.; Zhu, D.; Che, Y.; Feng, X. Preparation of Levodopa-Loaded Crystalsomes Through Thermally Induced Crystallization Reverses Functional Deficits in Parkinsonian Mice. *Biomater. Sci.* **2019,** *7* (4), 1623–1631. DOI: 10.1039/C8BM01098F
75. Lin, Y.; Liang, X.; Yao, Y.; Xiao, H.; Shi, Y.; Yang, J. Retracted: Osthole Attenuates APP-Induced Alzheimer's Disease Through Up-Regulating miRNA-101a-3p. *Life Sci.* **2019,** *225*, 117–131. DOI: https://doi.org/10.1016/j.lfs.2019.04.004
76. Long, J. M.; Holtzman, D. M. Alzheimer Disease: An Update on Pathobiology and Treatment Strategies. *Cell* **2019,** *179* (2), 312–339. DOI: https://doi.org/10.1016/j.cell.2019.09.001
77. Löscher, W.; Gericke, B. Novel Intrinsic Mechanisms of Active Drug Extrusion at the Blood-Brain Barrier: Potential Targets for Enhancing Drug Delivery to the Brain? *Pharmaceutics* **2020,** *12* (10). DOI: 10.3390/pharmaceutics12100966
78. Maiti, P.; Manna, J.; Dunbar, G. L. Current Understanding of the Molecular Mechanisms in Parkinson's disease: Targets for Potential Treatments. *Transl. Neurodegen.* **2017,** *6* (1), 28. DOI: 10.1186/s40035-017-0099-z
79. Mandal, S.; Das Mandal, S.; Chuttani, K.; Sawant, K. K.; Subudhi, B. B. Neuroprotective Effect of Ibuprofen by Intranasal Application of Mucoadhesive Nanoemulsion in MPTP Induced Parkinson Model. *J. Pharm. Investig.* **2016,** *46* (1), 41–53. DOI: 10.1007/s40005-015-0212-1
80. Marino, A.; Battaglini, M.; Desii, A.; Lavarello, C.; Genchi, G.; Petretto, A.; Ciofani, G. Liposomes Loaded with Polyphenol-Rich Grape Pomace Extracts Protect from Neurodegeneration in a Rotenone-Based In Vitro Model of Parkinson's Disease. *Biomater. Sci.* **2021,** *9* (24), 8171–8188. DOI: 10.1039/D1BM01202A
81. McAllister, B.; Gusella, J. F.; Landwehrmeyer, G. B.; Lee, J.-M.; MacDonald, M. E.; Orth, M. et al. The Timing and Impact of Psychiatric, Cognitive and Motor

Abnormalities in Huntington's Disease. *bioRxiv* **2020,** 2020.2005.2026.116798. DOI: 10.1101/2020.05.26.116798
82. Md, S.; Gan, S. Y.; Haw, Y. H.; Ho, C. L.; Wong, S.; Choudhury, H. In Vitro Neuroprotective Effects of Naringenin Nanoemulsion Against β-Amyloid Toxicity Through the Regulation of Amyloidogenesis and Tau Phosphorylation. *Int. J. Biol. Macromol.* **2018,** *118*, 1211–1219. DOI: https://doi.org/10.1016/j.ijbiomac.2018.06.190
83. Miguez, A.; Fernández-García, S.; Monguió-Tortajada, M.; Bombau, G.; Galofré, M.; García-Bravo, M. et al. In Vivo Progressive Degeneration of Huntington's Disease Patient-Derived Neurons Reveals Human-Specific Pathological Phenotypes. *bioRxiv* **2020,** 2020.2010.2021.347062. DOI: 10.1101/2020.10.21.347062
84. Mirzaie, Z.; Ansari, M.; Kordestani, S. S.; Rezaei, M. H.; Mozafari, M. Preparation and Characterization of Curcumin-Loaded Polymeric Nanomicelles to Interference with Amyloidogenesis Through Glycation Method. **2019,** *66* (4), 537–544. DOI: https://doi.org/10.1002/bab.1751
85. Monge-Fuentes, V.; Biolchi Mayer, A.; Lima, M. R.; Geraldes, L. R.; Zanotto, L. N.; Moreira, K. G. et al. Dopamine-Loaded Nanoparticle Systems Circumvent the Blood–Brain Barrier Restoring Motor Function in Mouse Model for Parkinson's Disease. *Sci. Rep.* **2021,** *11* (1), 15185. DOI: 10.1038/s41598-021-94175-8
86. Mortada, I.; Farah, R.; Nabha, S.; Ojcius, D. M.; Fares, Y.; Almawi, W. Y.; Sadier, N. S. Immunotherapies for Neurodegenerative Diseases. *Front. Neurol.* **2021,** *12*, 654739. DOI: 10.3389/fneur.2021.654739
87. Mou, L.; Ding, W.; Fernandez-Funez, P. Open Questions on the Nature of Parkinson's Disease: From Triggers to Spreading Pathology. *J. Med. Genet.* **2020,** *57* (2), 73. DOI: 10.1136/jmedgenet-2019-106210
88. Moujalled, D.; Strasser, A.; Liddell, J. R. Molecular Mechanisms of Cell Death in Neurological Diseases. *Cell Death Different.* **2021,** *28* (7), 2029–2044. DOI: 10.1038/s41418-021-00814-y
89. Muthukumaran, K.; Kanwar, A.; Vegh, C.; Marginean, A.; Elliott, A.; Guilbeault, N. et al. Ubisol-Q 10 (a Nanomicellar Water-Soluble Formulation of CoQ 10) Treatment Inhibits Alzheimer-Type Behavioral and Pathological Symptoms in a Double Transgenic Mouse (TgAPEswe, PSEN1dE9) Model of Alzheimer's Disease. *J. Alzheimer's Dis.* **2018,** *61*, 221–236. DOI: 10.3233/JAD-170275
90. Nabi, B.; Rehman, S.; Fazil, M.; Khan, S.; Baboota, S.; Ali, J. Riluzole-Loaded Nanoparticles to Alleviate the Symptoms of Neurological Disorders by Attenuating Oxidative Stress. *Drug Dev. Ind. Pharm.* **2020,** *46* (3), 471–483. DOI: 10.1080/03639045.2020.1730396
91. Naqvi, S.; Panghal, A.; Flora, S. J. S. Nanotechnology: A Promising Approach for Delivery of Neuroprotective Drugs. *Front. Neurosci.* **2020,** *14*, 494. DOI: 10.3389/fnins.2020.00494
92. Ndemazie, N. B.; Inkoom, A.; Morfaw, E. F.; Smith, T.; Aghimien, M.; Ebesoh, D.; Agyare, E. Multi-disciplinary Approach for Drug and Gene Delivery Systems to the Brain. *AAPS PharmSciTech* **2021,** *23* (1), 11. DOI: 10.1208/s12249-021-02144-1
93. Nirale, P.; Paul, A.; Yadav, K. S. Nanoemulsions for Targeting the Neurodegenerative Diseases: Alzheimer's, Parkinson's and Prion's. *Life Sci.* **2020,** *245*, 117394. DOI: 10.1016/j.lfs.2020.117394
94. Nouri, Z.; Fakhri, S.; El-Senduny, F. F.; Sanadgol, N.; Abd-ElGhani, G. E.; Farzaei, M. H.; Chen, J. T. On the Neuroprotective Effects of Naringenin: Pharmacological Targets,

Signaling Pathways, Molecular Mechanisms, and Clinical Perspective. *Biomolecules* **2019,** *9* (11). DOI: 10.3390/biom9110690

95. Paliwal, H.; Parihar, A.; Prajapati, B. G. Current State-of-the-Art and New Trends in Self-Assembled Nanocarriers as Drug Delivery Systems. *Front. Nanotechnol.* **2022,** *4*, 836674. DOI: 10.3389/fnano.2022.836674
96. Pardridge, W. M. Blood-Brain Barrier and Delivery of Protein and Gene Therapeutics to Brain. *Front Aging Neurosci.* **2019,** *11*, 373. DOI: 10.3389/fnagi.2019.00373
97. Pardridge, W. M. Treatment of Alzheimer's Disease and Blood-Brain Barrier Drug Delivery. *Pharmaceuticals (Basel)* **2020,** *13* (11). DOI: 10.3390/ph13110394
98. Pardridge, W. M. A Historical Review of Brain Drug Delivery. **2022,** *14* (6), 1283.
99. Parikh, H. R.; Patel, J. R. Nanoemulsions for Intranasal Delivery of Riluzole to Improve Brain Bioavailability: Formulation Development and Pharmacokinetic Studies. *Current Drug Deliv.* **2016,** *13* (7), 1130–1143. DOI: http://dx.doi.org/10.2174/1567201813666151202195729
100. Patel, R. J.; Patel, A. A.; Patel, H. P. Stabilized Amorphous State of Riluzole by Immersion-Rotavapor Method with Synthesized Mesoporous SBA-15 Carrier to Augment In Vitro Dissolution. *J. Drug Deliv. Sci. Technol.* **2021,** *61*, 102270. DOI: https://doi.org/10.1016/j.jddst.2020.102270
101. Patil, R. P.; Pawara, D. D.; Gudewar, C. S.; Tekade, A. R. Nanostructured Cubosomes in an In Situ Nasal Gel System: An Alternative Approach for the Controlled Delivery of Donepezil HCl to Brain. *J. Liposome Res.* **2019,** *29* (3), 264–273. DOI: 10.1080/08982104.2018.1552703
102. Pepe, G.; Calce, E.; Verdoliva, V.; Saviano, M.; Maglione, V.; Di Pardo, A.; De Luca, S. Curcumin-Loaded Nanoparticles Based on Amphiphilic Hyaluronan-Conjugate Explored as Targeting Delivery System for Neurodegenerative Disorders. *Int. J. Mol. Sci.* **2020,** *21* (22). DOI: 10.3390/ijms21228846
103. Raeisi Estabragh, M. A.; Hamidifar, Z.; Pardakhty, A. Formulation of Rivastigmine Niosomes for Alzheimer Disease. *Int. Pharm. Acta* **2018,** *1* (1), 104–104. DOI: 10.22037/ipa.v1i1.19964
104. Raiff, B. R.; Burrows, C. A.; Nastasi, J. A.; Upton, C. R.; Dwyer, M. J. Chapter 21—A Behavioral Approach to the Treatment of Chronic Illnesses. In: *Functional Analysis in Clinical Treatment*; Sturmey, P., Ed., 2nd edn.; Academic Press: San Diego, 2020; pp. 501–532.
105. Ramachandran, S.; Thangarajan, S. Thymoquinone Loaded Solid Lipid Nanoparticles Counteracts 3-Nitropropionic Acid Induced Motor Impairments and Neuroinflammation in Rat Model of Huntington's Disease. *Metabol. Brain Dis.* **2018,** *33* (5), 1459–1470. DOI: 10.1007/s11011-018-0252-0
106. Ray, S.; Sinha, P.; Laha, B.; Maiti, S.; Bhattacharyya, U. K.; Nayak, A. K. Polysorbate 80 Coated Crosslinked Chitosan Nanoparticles of Ropinirole Hydrochloride for Brain Targeting. *J. Drug Deliv. Sci. Technol.* **2018,** *48*, 21–29. DOI: https://doi.org/10.1016/j.jddst.2018.08.016
107. Rhea, E. M.; Banks, W. A. Role of the Blood-Brain Barrier in Central Nervous System Insulin Resistance. *Front. Neurosci.* **2019,** *13*, 521. DOI: 10.3389/fnins.2019.00521
108. Rinaldi, F.; Hanieh, P. N.; Chan, L. K. N.; Angeloni, L.; Passeri, D.; Rossi, M. et al. Chitosan Glutamate-Coated Niosomes: A Proposal for Nose-to-Brain Delivery. *Pharmaceutics* **2018,** *10* (2). DOI: 10.3390/pharmaceutics10020038

109. Rojas, P.; Ramírez, A. I.; Fernández-Albarral, J. A.; López-Cuenca, I.; Salobrar-García, E.; Cadena, M. et al. Amyotrophic Lateral Sclerosis: A Neurodegenerative Motor Neuron Disease With Ocular Involvement. *Front. Neurosci.* **2020,** *14*, 566858. DOI: 10.3389/fnins.2020.566858
110. Ross, C.; Taylor, M.; Fullwood, N.; Allsop, D. Liposome Delivery Systems for the Treatment of Alzheimer's Disease. *Int. J. Nanomed.* **2018,** *13*, 8507–8522. DOI: 10.2147/ijn.S183117
111. Sadegh Malvajerd, S.; Azadi, A.; Izadi, Z.; Kurd, M.; Dara, T.; Dibaei, M. et al. Brain Delivery of Curcumin Using Solid Lipid Nanoparticles and Nanostructured Lipid Carriers: Preparation, Optimization, and Pharmacokinetic Evaluation. *ACS Chem. Neurosci.* **2019,** *10* (1), 728–739. DOI: 10.1021/acschemneuro.8b00510
112. Sadegh Malvajerd, S.; Izadi, Z.; Azadi, A.; Kurd, M.; Derakhshankhah, H.; Sharifzadeh, M. et al. Neuroprotective Potential of Curcumin-Loaded Nanostructured Lipid Carrier in an Animal Model of Alzheimer's Disease: Behavioral and Biochemical Evidence. *J. Alzheimer's Dis.* **2019,** *69*, 671–686. DOI: 10.3233/JAD-190083
113. Sahinovic, M. M.; Struys, M. M. R. F.; Absalom, A. R. Clinical Pharmacokinetics and Pharmacodynamics of Propofol. *Clinical Pharmacokinetics, 57* (12), 1539–1558. DOI: 10.1007/s40262-018-0672-3
114. Sathe, S. Inherited Neurodegenerative Diseases. In: *Oxford Textbook of Medicine*; Oxford University Press, 2020. DOI: 10.1093/med/9780198746690.003.0606. https://doi.org/10.1093/med/9780198746690.003.0606
115. Sathya, S.; Shanmuganathan, B.; Devi, K. P. Deciphering the Anti-Apoptotic Potential of α-Bisabolol Loaded Solid Lipid Nanoparticles Against Aβ Induced Neurotoxicity in Neuro-2a Cells. *Colloids Surfaces B: Biointerfaces* **2020,** *190*, 110948. DOI: https://doi.org/10.1016/j.colsurfb.2020.110948
116. Sathya, S.; Shanmuganathan, B.; Manirathinam, G.; Ruckmani, K.; Devi, K. P. α-Bisabolol Loaded Solid Lipid Nanoparticles Attenuates Aβ Aggregation and Protects Neuro-2a Cells from Aβ Induced Neurotoxicity. *J. Mol. Liquids* **2018,** *264*, 431–441. DOI: https://doi.org/10.1016/j.molliq.2018.05.075
117. Sava, V.; Fihurka, O.; Khvorova, A.; Sanchez-Ramos, J. Enriched Chitosan Nanoparticles Loaded with siRNA Are Effective in Lowering Huntington's Disease Gene Expression Following Intranasal Administration. *Nanomed.* **2020,** *24*, 102119. DOI: 10.1016/j.nano.2019.102119
118. Savonenko, A. V.; Melnikova, T.; Li, T.; Price, D. L.; Wong, P. C. Chapter 21—Alzheimer Disease. In: *Neurobiology of Brain Disorders*; Zigmond, M. J., Rowland, L. P., Coyle, J. T., Eds.; Academic Press: San Diego, 2015; pp 321–338.
119. Sharifyrad, M.; Gohari, S.; Fathi, M.; Danafar, H.; Hosseini, M.-J.; Mostafavi, H.; Manjili, H. K. The Efficacy and Neuroprotective Effects of Edaravone-Loaded mPEG-b-PLGA Polymeric Nanoparticles on Human Neuroblastoma SH-SY5Y Cell Line as In Vitro Model of Ischemia. *J. Drug Deliv. Sci. Technol.* **2022,** *73*, 103378. DOI: https://doi.org/10.1016/j.jddst.2022.103378
120. Shupp, A.; Casimiro, M. C.; Pestell, R. G. Biological Functions of CDK5 and Potential CDK5 Targeted Clinical Treatments. *Oncotarget* **2017,** *8* (10), 17373–17382. DOI: 10.18632/oncotarget.14538
121. Silva, S.; Almeida, A. J.; Vale, N. Importance of Nanoparticles for the Delivery of Antiparkinsonian Drugs. *Pharm.* **2021,** *13* (4). DOI: 10.3390/pharmaceutics13040508

122. Singh, A. P.; Biswas, A.; Shukla, A.; Maiti, P. Targeted Therapy in Chronic Diseases Using Nanomaterial-Based Drug Delivery Vehicles. *Sign. Transduction Target. Therapy* **2019,** *4* (1), 33. DOI: 10.1038/s41392-019-0068-3
123. Sintov, A. C. AmyloLipid Nanovesicles: A Self-Assembled Lipid-Modified Starch Hybrid System Constructed for Direct Nose-to-Brain Delivery of Curcumin. *Int. J. Pharm.* **2020,** *588*, 119725. DOI: https://doi.org/10.1016/j.ijpharm.2020.119725
124. Solovyev, N.; Drobyshev, E.; Bjørklund, G.; Dubrovskii, Y.; Lysiuk, R.; Rayman, M. P. Selenium, Selenoprotein P, and Alzheimer's Disease: Is There a Link? *Free Radical Biol. Med.* **2018,** *127*, 124–133. DOI: https://doi.org/10.1016/j.freeradbiomed.2018.02.030
125. Soria Lopez, J. A.; González, H. M.; Léger, G. C. Chapter 13—Alzheimer's Disease. In: *Handbook of Clinical Neurology*; Dekosky, S. T., S. Asthana, S.; Eds., Vol. 167; Elsevier, 2019; pp 231–255.
126. Srinageshwar, B.; Peruzzaro, S.; Andrews, M.; Johnson, K.; Hietpas, A.; Clark, B. et al. PAMAM Dendrimers Cross the Blood-Brain Barrier When Administered through the Carotid Artery in C57BL/6J Mice. *Int. J. Mol. Sci.* **2017,** *18* (3). DOI: 10.3390/ijms18030628
127. Štětkářová, I.; Ehler, E. Diagnostics of Amyotrophic Lateral Sclerosis: Up to Date. *Diagnostics (Basel), 11* (2). DOI: 10.3390/diagnostics11020231
128. Sweeney, M. D.; Zhao, Z.; Montagne, A.; Nelson, A. R.; Zlokovic, B. V. Blood-Brain Barrier: From Physiology to Disease and Back. *Physiol. Rev.* **2019,** *99* (1), 21–78. DOI: 10.1152/physrev.00050.2017
129. Tan, J. P. K.; Voo, Z. X.; Lim, S.; Venkataraman, S.; Ng, K. M.; Gao, S. et al. Effective Encapsulation of Apomorphine Into Biodegradable Polymeric Nanoparticles Through a Reversible Chemical Bond for Delivery Across the Blood–Brain Barrier. *Nanomed.: Nanotechnol. Biol. Med.* **2019,** *17*, 236–245. DOI: https://doi.org/10.1016/j.nano.2019.01.014
130. Teixeira, M. I.; Lopes, C. M.; Gonçalves, H.; Catita, J.; Silva, A. M.; Rodrigues, F. et al. Formulation, Characterization, and Cytotoxicity Evaluation of Lactoferrin Functionalized Lipid Nanoparticles for Riluzole Delivery to the Brain. **2022,** *14* (1), 185.
131. Tello, J. A.; Williams, H. E.; Eppler, R. M.; Steinhilb, M. L.; Khanna, M. Animal Models of Neurodegenerative Disease: Recent Advances in Fly Highlight Innovative Approaches to Drug Discovery. *Front. Mol. Neurosci.* **2022,** *15*, 883358. DOI: 10.3389/fnmol.2022.883358
132. Terron, A.; Bal-Price, A.; Paini, A.; Monnet-Tschudi, F.; Bennekou, S. H.; Angeli, K. et al. An Adverse Outcome Pathway for Parkinsonian Motor Deficits Associated with Mitochondrial Complex I Inhibition. *Arch. Toxicol.* **2018,** *92* (1), 41–82. DOI: 10.1007/s00204-017-2133-4
133. Tran, M.; Reddy, P. H. Defective Autophagy and Mitophagy in Aging and Alzheimer's Disease. *Front. Neurosci.* **2020,** *14*, 612757. DOI: 10.3389/fnins.2020.612757
134. Verma, A. Clinical Manifestation and Management of Amyotrophic Lateral Sclerosis. In: *Department of Peripheral Nervous System Research*; *Amyotrophic Lateral Sclerosis*; Araki, T., Eds.,; Exon Publications, 2021; pp. 1–14.
135. Vickers, J. C.; Mitew, S.; Woodhouse, A.; Fernandez-Martos, C. M.; Kirkcaldie, M. T.; Canty, A. J. et al. Defining the Earliest Pathological Changes of Alzheimer's Disease. *Curr. Alzheimer Res.* **2016,** *13* (3), 281–287. DOI: 10.2174/1567205013666151218150322

136. Wang, G. Y.; Rayner, S. L.; Chung, R.; Shi, B. Y.; Liang, X. J. Advances in Nanotechnology-Based Strategies for the Treatments of Amyotrophic Lateral Sclerosis. *Mater. Today Bio.* **2020,** *6*, 100055. DOI: 10.1016/j.mtbio.2020.100055
137. Wang, Q.; Ma, R.; Liu, P.; Cheng, G.; Yang, Q.; Chen, X. et al. Efficient Sustained-Release Nanoparticle Delivery System Protects Nigral Neurons in a Toxin Model of Parkinson's Disease. **2022,** *14* (8), 1731.
138. Wanker, E. E.; Ast, A.; Schindler, F.; Trepte, P.; Schnoegl, S. The Pathobiology of Perturbed Mutant Huntingtin Protein–Protein Interactions in Huntington's Disease. *J. Neurochem.* **2019,** *151* (4), 507–519. DOI: https://doi.org/10.1111/jnc.14853
139. Wankhede, N. L.; Kale, M. B.; Upaganlawar, A. B.; Taksande, B. G.; Umekar, M. J.; Behl, T. et al. Involvement of Molecular Chaperone in Protein-Misfolding Brain Diseases. *Biomed. Pharmacother.* **2022,** *147*, 112647. DOI: https://doi.org/10.1016/j.biopha.2022.112647
140. Wareham, L. K.; Liddelow, S. A.; Temple, S.; Benowitz, L. I.; Di Polo, A.; Wellington, C. et al. Solving Neurodegeneration: Common Mechanisms and Strategies for New Treatments. *Mol. Neurodegen.* **2022,** *17* (1), 23. DOI: 10.1186/s13024-022-00524-0
141. Waris, A.; Ali, A.; Khan, A. U.; Asim, M.; Zamel, D.; Fatima, K. et al. S. Applications of Various Types of Nanomaterials for the Treatment of Neurological Disorders. **2022,** *12* (13), 2140.
142. Warren, K. E. Beyond the Blood:Brain Barrier: The Importance of Central Nervous System (CNS) Pharmacokinetics for the Treatment of CNS Tumors, Including Diffuse Intrinsic Pontine Glioma. *Front. Oncol.* **2018,** *8*, 239. DOI: 10.3389/fonc.2018.00239
143. Wilkaniec, A.; Gąssowska-Dobrowolska, M.; Strawski, M.; Adamczyk, A.; Czapski, G. A. Inhibition of Cyclin-Dependent Kinase 5 Affects Early Neuroinflammatory Signalling in Murine Model of Amyloid Beta Toxicity. *J. Neuroinflamm.* **2018,** *15* (1), 1. DOI: 10.1186/s12974-017-1027-y
144. Yasir, M.; Sara, U. V. S.; Chauhan, I.; Gaur, P. K.; Singh, A. P.; Puri, D.;, A. Solid Lipid Nanoparticles for Nose to Brain Delivery of Donepezil: Formulation, Optimization by Box–Behnken Design, In Vitro and In Vivo Evaluation. *Artif. Cells Nanomed. Biotechnol.* **2018,** *46* (8), 1838–1851. DOI: 10.1080/21691401.2017.1394872
145. Yazdani, S.; Jaldin-Fincati, J. R.; Pereira, R. V. S.; Klip, A. Endothelial Cell Barriers: Transport of Molecules Between Blood and Tissues. *Traffic, 20* (6), 390–403. DOI: https://doi.org/10.1111/tra.12645
146. Zhao, Y.; Xiong, S.; Liu, P.; Liu, W.; Wang, Q.; Liu, Y. et al. Polymeric Nanoparticles-Based Brain Delivery with Improved Therapeutic Efficacy of Ginkgolide B in Parkinson's Disease. *Int. J. Nanomed.* **2020,** *15*, 10453–10467. DOI: 10.2147/IJN.S272831
147. Zhou, X. X.; Jin, L.; Qi, R. Q.; Ma, T. pH-Responsive Polymeric Micelles Self-Assembled from Amphiphilic Copolymer Modified with Lipid Used as Doxorubicin Delivery Carriers. *R. Soc. Open Sci.* **2018,** *5* (3), 171654. DOI: 10.1098/rsos.171654
148. Zhu, J.; Chen, M. The Effect and Safety of Ropinirole in the Treatment of Parkinson Disease: A Systematic Review and Meta-Analysis. *Medicine* **2021,** *100* (46), e27653. DOI: 10.1097/md.0000000000027653

CHAPTER 7

Nano Approaches Toward CNS Drug Delivery

ASHWANI SHARMA[1], ANJALI SHARMA[2], GIRISH KUMAR[3], TARUN VIRMANI[3], and KAMLA PATHAK[4]

[1]Delhi Pharmaceutical Sciences and Research University (DPSRU), New Delhi, India

[2]Central Drugs Standard Control Organisation (CDSCO), FDA Bhawan, Kotla Road, New Delhi, India

[3]Amity Institute of Pharmacy, Amity University, Greater Noida Campus, Uttar Pradesh, India

[4]Faculty of Pharmacy, Uttar Pradesh University of Medical Sciences, Saifai, Etawah, Uttar Pradesh, India

ABSTRACT

Nanotechnology has emerged as a promising and intriguing new platform for treating neurological illnesses, demonstrating the considerable potential to address the issues associated with traditional therapeutic approaches. Nanotechnology is an innovative and promising state-of-the-art approach of delivering neurotherapeutic drugs across the blood–brain barrier (BBB). Nanotechnology has demonstrated tremendous potential for central nervous system (CNS) drug delivery in recent years due to its wide variety of nano-sizes, distinctive physicochemical features, and capacity to use surface-treated biodegradable and biocompatible nanomaterials. Nanotechnology-based methods for site-specific delivery of therapeutic agents and other substances throughout the BBB may be designed to perform specific tasks as needed. There are many different kinds of pharmaceutical nanocarriers that have been

Nanomedicine for Neurodegenerative Disorders: Selective Treatment Strategies. Rishabha Malviya, Kamla Pathak, & Swati Verma (Eds.)

developed, including nanoemulsions, polymeric nanoparticles (PNPs), solid lipid nanoparticles (SLNs), liposomes, nanostructured lipid carriers (NLCs), polymeric micelles, dendrimers, nanocrystals, metallic nanoparticles, carbon nanotubes, nanowires, and nanofibers. Molecules can be nano-engineered to perform some certain functions, such as crossing the BBB, targeting specific cells, or signaling pathways. This chapter details the delivery of various neurotherapeutic agents via nanocarrier systems such as nanoparticles, micelles, nanotubes, nanoemulsions, nanosensors, SLNs, liposomes, dendrimers, along with recent clinical trials, patents, and marketed formulations.

7.1 INTRODUCTION

The disorders of the central nervous system (CNS) provide a significant challenge to humanity and is the field that is attracting the most interest from researchers due to its rapid expansion. Neurological disorders are among the primary causes of death and disability in the modern world.[1] The diagnosis and treatment of CNS diseases such as epilepsy, Parkinson's disease, Alzheimer's disease, Huntington's disease, and head injuries remain difficult tasks as of this time. Numerous potential medications have been developed to treat various neurological illnesses, but their treatment efficacy is still constrained owing to a variety of difficulties. The difficulty of transporting substances such as medications, imaging agents, proteins, nucleic acids, and other macromolecules to the CNS throughout all peripheral obstacles, specifically the blood-cerebrospinal fluid barrier (BCSFB) and blood–brain barrier (BBB), is one of the most frequent challenges. The existing neurotherapeutics are connected with two key constraints, which are restricted entrance via BBB as an inadequate entry in the brain and limited access to immune cells to the brain, before entering into brain cells.[2] Alcohol and steroid hormones are examples of tiny lipophilic molecules that can pass through the BBB and enter cells via transcellular mechanisms, but the majority of medications used to treat neurological illnesses are lipophilic and have molecular weights of more than 400–500 Da which do not allow to pass through BBB in required quantity.[3] Furthermore, the availability of many, highly selective transporters on endothelial cells also restricts drug penetration. Additionally, the occurrence of tight junctions in the endothelial membranes results in cerebral microcapillaries exhibiting greater transendothelial electrical resistance (>1000 W cm^2).[4] The BBB endothelial cells prevent the entry or passage of endogenic or foreign substances. Endothelial cells include ATP-binding cassette (ABC) transporters, which prevent the entry of neurotoxic substances, metabolites, hormones, mediators, as well as therapeutic drugs. To move things across cell membranes, these membrane proteins designated as transporters require ATP. The BBB is composed of a monolayer of polarized endothelial cells coupled by intricate tight junctions whereas astrocytes, neurons, and pericytes are the cells that regulate its functioning. Drug entrance into the brain is restricted by the intricacy of the BBB and the availability of large quantities of efflux transport proteins such as the expression of metabolic enzymes, multidrug resistant protein-1 (MRP-1), and P-glycoproteins (P-gp).[5] Strong barriers separating the brain from other bodily parts prohibit the transmission of any pharmacological and diagnosing drugs or any other materials to the CNS. To conceptualize the physiological features of this BBB, techniques for the effective transport of medications and molecular imaging must be developed.[6] The BBB keeps the brain–blood supply separate from blood circulation. The human brain has roughly 100 billion neurons. The brain capillaries may have a diameter of only 7 to 10 μm.[7] The entrance channel from the environment to the brain is relatively constrained because the BBB lacks the intracellular and valvar gaps.[8] However, BBB may be circumvented and medication transport to the CNS made easier by the use of nanoparticles (NPs) and polymer coatings.[9] Multiple advancements in the detection and treatment of brain cancer, trauma, and nervous system problems have been made as a result of this technique.[10] To overcome this issue, some advancements were required in the formulation of drugs so that drugs can travel across BBB with significant bioavailability and are more specific to targets which were positively achieved by nanotechnology.

Nanotechnology refers to the application of nanoscience knowledge in research to make or modify formulations in nanomaterials. Nanoscience refers to the study of the special characteristics of nanomaterials having a size range in between 1 and 100 nm.[11] Nanomaterials can be produced due to atomic-scale structural manipulation.[12] Nanomaterials can be employed in a variety of applications, particularly medicines and electronics, since they exhibit special electrical, optical, and magnetic capabilities at the nanoscale. The word "nanomedicine" is used to describe the use of applications of nanotechnology in healthcare and medicine systems. In particular, illnesses can be prevented, detected, monitored, and treated using nanoscale technology and nano-enabled methods.[13] Nanotechnologies have the potential to significantly advance the field of medical, including imaging and diagnostic tools, pharmaceutical therapeutics, implants, drug delivery systems, and tissue-engineered constructs. They have also advanced the treatment of several diseases, such as diabetes, bacterial and viral infections, cancer, cardiovascular diseases, musculoskeletal conditions, and most importantly in CNS disorders.[14] Nanotechnology is a ground-breaking method for delivering neurotherapeutics through the BBB. Due to their wide variety of nanosized, distinctive physicochemical characteristics, and capacity to use surface-engineered biodegradable and biocompatible nanomaterials, nanomedicines have demonstrated tremendous potential for CNS drug delivery in recent years.[15] Target specific delivery and other substance distribution across the BBB has been formulated by using nanotechnology showing the potential to perform specific tasks as required. The drug or pharmacologically active ingredient to be delivered is one component of the nanoengineered complex, which is also made to carry out other essential functions like encapsulating the active ingredient, guarding it from enzymatic degradation, releasing the ingredient at a specific pH, being able to cross the BBB, and focusing on specific brain cells.[16] Liposomes, polymer NPs, solid lipid nanoparticles (SLNs), micelles, dendrimers, and other pharmacological nanocarriers have all are the types of nanoparticles which are developed for the CNS target drug delivery, which are discussed below.[17]

7.1.1 TRANSPORT OF SUBSTANCES ACROSS THE BBB

The BBB, which restricts entrance and shields the brain from viruses and dangerous substances, may prevent pharmaceutical substances from reaching the brain as they are circulated in the blood.[18] Even tiny substances cannot diffuse across the barrier into the brain. Even though many necessary molecules may get over this barrier, medicinal chemicals are frequently excluded due to their unique features.[19] The difficulty of medications to traverse the BBB emphasizes the requirement for creating NPs-based drug delivery systems. The BBB only permits a few substances to diffuse. These micro substances slip over this barrier and find various ways to get to neurons. For accessing the BBB, some NPs have been employed[20] and the medicine can cross the BBB due to the NPs ability to pierce via tight connections between the vessels of endothelial cells. Drug transport across the endothelial cell layer can also be facilitated by the transcytosis and endocytosis of NPs.[21]

Lipid NPs' lipophilic properties allow them to pass across the BBB and enter the brain via a variety of transport mechanisms, including receptor-mediated endocytosis, transcytosis, and the paracellular route.[22] Additionally, ligands can be conjugated or coated onto NPs to target specific cells and some ligands can be used to transport molecules from the circulation across the BBB via receptor-mediated transcytosis (RMT)[23] (Figure 7.1). Numerous receptors that can selectively bind to ligands and internalize into cells are expressed on the BBB. Over the mediation of

NPs, these ligands might be transported through the BBB. Because of the interaction between ligands and receptors, receptor-mediated transport has proven to be the most effective way to deliver NPs to the brain via the BBB.[24] Specific ligands, including lactoferrin, insulin, some antibodies, and transferrin, bind to the surface of NP during transcytosis that is mediated by receptors. The endothelium receptors present on the cell surface[25] are required for this binding. Other ligand molecules, including lipoprotein, can interact with certain receptors as well. Low-density lipoprotein receptors, which are abundantly expressed on the BBB, allow apolipoproteins, such as apolipoprotein A and apolipoprotein E, to enter the brain.[26] Because of this, NPs have a significant functional surface that may attach to and transport various substances, including medicines, probes, and proteins. There have been several attempts to alter proteins to make them more permeable to the BBB.[27] Proteins' ability to enter the nervous system through endocytosis is increased when they are conjugated with cations.[28] Based on the findings of several investigations, conjugation with pluronic copolymers boosted the distribution of proteins.[29] The fundamental drawback of these systems is the increased toxicity of these changed proteins.[30] In contrast to horseradish peroxidase polymer (HRP) alone, HRP binding to the P85 and L121 pluronic improves the permeability to the BBB.[31] Additionally, in vivo research has demonstrated that modified HRP diffuses to the brain at a rate four times higher than unmodified protein.[32] The interaction of proteins with fatty acids (such as palmitate or stearates) can also increase the transport of proteins to the CNS.[31] Although the hydrophobic terminals on this changed protein's molecule may even bind to highly hydrophilic proteins on the neuron cell's surface to increase cellular absorption, the molecule of this modified protein is still soluble in water.

7.2 NANO APPROACHES FOR CNS DRUG DELIVERY

Nanotechnology is a novel, ground-breaking, cutting-edge method for delivering drugs throughout the BBB. Due to their wide variety of nano-sized, distinctive physicochemical properties, and capacity to use surface-engineered biodegradable and biocompatible nanoformulations, these have demonstrated tremendous potential for CNS drug delivery in recent years.[33] The main obstacle in efficient drug delivery to CNS is BBB which prevents the entry of conventional therapeutic moieties into the brain. This obstacle can be overcome using various nanoformulations, namely liposomes, SLNs, dendrimers, nanostructured lipid carriers (NLCs), nanoemulsions, polymeric micelles, polymeric nanoparticles (PNPs), nanocrystals, metallic nanoparticles, carbon nanotubes (CNTs), nanowires, and nanofibers.[34] These nanoformulations are capable to surpass the BBB using various mechanisms including the transcellular pathway, paracellular pathway, the carrier-mediated pathway, the adsorptive transcytosis, and RMT. Moreover, the inability of nanoformulations to surpass the BBB is also affected by numerous physic-chemical properties like particle size, lipophilicity, hydrophilicity, surface charge, protein binding, hydrogen bonds, and shape.[35] The potentiation of a drug by surpassing the BBB using various nanoformulations has been illustrated in Figure 7.2. Nanoformulations designed to treat CNS disorders have been described in the preceding section.

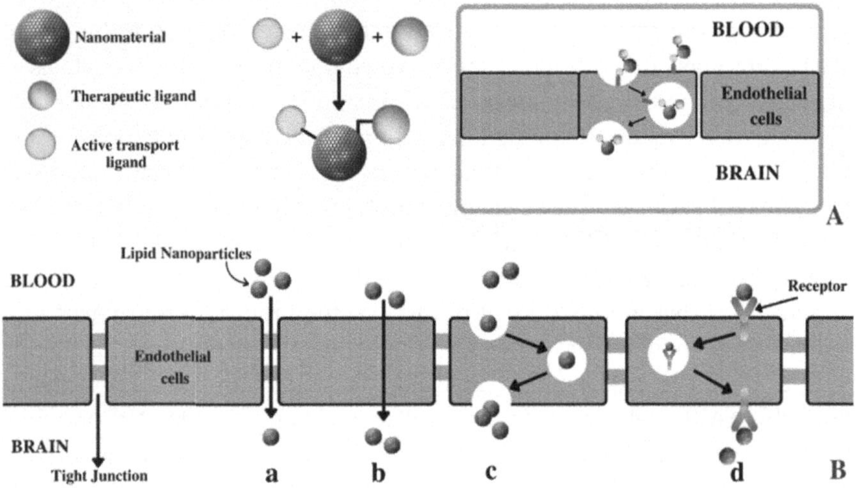

FIGURE 7.1 Main pathways for nanoformulations to penetrate through BBB—(A) Therapeutic ligands can be coupled to nanoparticles and subsequently delivered through the BBB to enable active transport, (B) A schematic depiction of the several routes used by NPs to penetrate the BBB and go to the brain, including—(a) the paracellular pathway, (b) transcellular pathway, (c) transcytosis, and (d) receptor-mediated endocytosis.

7.2.1 SOLID LIPID NANOPARTICLES (SLNS)

These are distinct lipid-based, biocompatible drug carrier system that primarily consist of modified lipid or lipid nanostructures (10–1000 nm in diameter range) capable to encapsulate hydrophilic as well as lipophilic drugs due to possession of a stable hydrophobic lipid core. These have drawn attention as a drug carrier to CNS due to various attributes of biocompatibility, improved drug loading capacity, avoidance of the use of

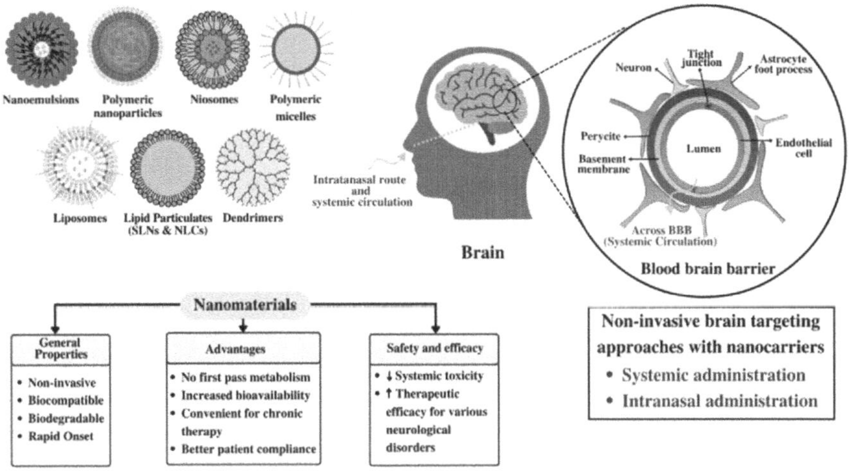

FIGURE 7.2 Potentiation of drug-loaded nanoformulations by surpassing the BBB and their general properties, benefits, safety, and efficacy.

organic solvents during preparation, controlled drug release, and improved stability.[36] Moreover, drugs encapsulated in SLNs can be targeted to the brain using coating with specific polymers and combining the legends to them. SLNs having a size range of 120–200 nm along with coating using hydrophilic polymers are not readily absorbed by the reticuloendothelial system (RES) of the BBB causing bypass of spleen infiltration and liver.[37] SLNs are enabled to cross the RES of BBB causing improved concentration of drug in the brain. The efficiency of SLNs to reach the drug in the brain can be further enhanced using modification with polyethylene glycol (PEG) as identified in a study in which comparison in between plain SLNs and PEG-modified SLNs having anticancer drug (doxorubicin and camptothecin) was done and PEG-modified SLNs were found having greater efficiency to deliver the drug in brain. Transcytosis and endocytosis, in which endothelial cells lining brain blood cells are taken up, are two ways that drugs might be delivered to the CNS via SLNs.[33] Various drugs have been encapsulated in SLNs to improve their delivery to CNS. Y. Mohammad et al. formulated piperine as SLN using polysorbate 80 for targeting brain to treat Alzheimer's disease and was evaluated for acetylcholenesterase enzymatic assays, forced swimming test, histopathology, and superoxide dismutase. It was found that piperine, in dose of 2 mg/kg body weight, reduced the superoxide dismutase levels by 504 ± 44.24 m units, increased the acetylcholenesterase enzyme levels by 29.24 ± 4.29 μg/mg, and decreased the immobility values to 41.36 ± 3.53 seconds. Histopathology studies demonstrated the decreased tangles and plaques. It suggested the superiority of piperine SLNs in dose of 2 mg/kg than donepezil as standard drug in dose of 5 mg/kg for delivery to the brain across the BBB.[38] For enhanced delivery to the brain in Alzheimer's disease, Sanju et al. created SLNs of quercetin utilizing compritol as a lipid and tween 80 as a surfactant. It was found that rats with aluminum-induced dementia showed a significant behavioral improvement in memory retention after receiving the optimized formulation. Additionally, the maintenance of glutathione, nitrite levels, lipid peroxidation, and rat brain homogenates indicated the efficient targeting of quercetin-loaded SLNs into the CNS. The considerable decrease in aluminum-induced neurotoxicity caused by the use of quercetin-loaded SLNs emphasizes the immense potential of SLNs as a platform technology to route various natural and synthetic chemicals to the brain and boost their efficacy in treating a range of CNS disorders.[39] Arora et al. prepared SLNs loaded with rivastigmine tartrate for intranasal delivery to treat Alzheimer's disease using glyceryl monostearate as solid lipid and polysorbate 80 as surfactant and found that drug-entrapped SLNs provided improved C_{max} of 73.99±5.66 ng/mL than drug solution administered by intranasal (65.24 ± 3.35 ng/mL) and intravenous (49.64 ± 5.58 ng/mL) route in brain. The $AUC_{0-24\,h}$ for drug entrapped SLNs was 20256.49 ± 30.60 ng.h/mL, while it was 9876.34 ± 11.62 ng.h/mL for intranasally administered solution and 6856.25 ± 14.46 ng.h/mL for intravenous solution suggesting improved accumulation of rivastigmine tartrate in brain using SLNs formulation.[40]

7.2.2 NANOSTRUCTURED LIPID CARRIERS (NLCS)

These are next-generation lipid nanocarriers that have paved the attention as an efficient carrier for delivering the drug to CNS due to various properties quick brain uptake, sustained and controlled drug release, biocompatibility, biodegradability, presence of lipids, improved stability, less toxicity, and enhanced drug transport in the brain using passive diffusion or transcellular transport across the BBB.[41] Moreover, it improves the dissolution of hydrophobic drugs by the formation of solubilized phases which provide rapid absorption of the encapsulated drug.[42] As a result of the pancreatic enzymes breaking down NLCs in the duodenum, monoglycerides and fatty acids are produced, which are combined with the bile salts to create micelles. Triglycerides are created in the intestinal cells as a result of these micelles reaching the enterocytes. These lipid elements aggregate with phospholipids and cholesterol to create the chylomicrons which are too big to pass through blood capillaries.[43] Then these are taken up by the lymphatic system first, then by the brain's glymphatic system, where NLC uses a mechanism called RMT.[44] The availability of concentration of drug through NLC depends on the factors namely permeability through BBB, plasma protein binding, efflux by the transporters, plasma drug concentration-time curve, and enzymatic metabolism of the drug. Various drug-encapsulated NLCs have proven their efficacy as a drug delivery system to the CNS. S.A. Khan et al. prepared NLCs of atazanavir and found higher C_{max} of 89.24±2.23 μg/mL and AUC of 1570.41 ±112.62 μg.h/mL than drug suspension having C_{max} of 32.46±1.49 μg/mL and AUC of 413.04 ±31.36 μg.h/mL. Drug-entrapped NLC provided 2.75-folds enhanced C_{max} in the brain and 4-fold improved brain bioavailability, demonstrating the concentration of 62.57±2.43 μg/mL, 7.54±1.68 μg/mL in brain by drug-loaded NLCs and drug suspension, respectively, suggesting that NLC is a superior carrier to improve the drug delivery to CNS.[45] Nair et al. prepared NLCs of phenytoin sodium composed of cholesterol, oleic acid as solid lipid and liquid lipid, respectively, and poloxamer 188 as surfactant using melt emulsification method followed by ultrasonication for the nose-to-brain delivery to treat epilepsy in efficient manner. It was found that phenytoin sodium laden nanoemulsion of size less than 50 nm provided C_{max} of 698.79±6.3 μg/mL and AUC of 466.44 ±4.8 μg.h/mL; drug-loaded NLCs of size more than 100 nm provided C_{max} of 347.33±4.9 μg/mL and AUC of 188.26 ±2.8 μg.h/mL; midazolam spray (commercialized preparation) provided C_{max} of 510.61 ±5.7 μg/mL and AUC of 43.30 ±2.2 μg.h/mL; commercialized injection provided C_{max} of 10.80±4.9 μg/mL and AUC of 9.15 ±2.1 μg.h/mL; and spray of drug-loaded NLCs having size less than 50 nm provided C_{max} of 712.53 ±7.6 μg/mL and AUC of 492.45 ±7.8 μg.h/mL—these improved drug concentration in the brain within 5 min of intranasal administration of NLCs as compared to drug solution as well as conventional intravenous drug formulation.[46]

7.2.3 NANOEMULSIONS

Various tremendous attributes of nanoemulsion, like cellular transport by transcellular or paracellular route, a colloidal solution of lipophilic drugs, prevention of hydrolysis of encapsulated drug, avoidance of enzymatic degradation, biocompatibility, biodegradability, and improvement of solubility, make it a potential drug carrier.[47,48] The arrival of a sufficient amount of drug in the brain is limited by biochemical and physiological restraints of BBB allowing only lipophilic substances to have a molecular weight of about

500 Da or lesser. Hence, the nanoemulsion could be a better drug carrier for lipophilic as well as hydrophilic drugs to overcome the BBB leading to arrival of drug in sufficient concentration in brain. Additionally, nanoemulsions can be used for drug targeting to the CNS using surface modification and particle engineering. Drug-encapsulated nanoemulsions can be delivered directly to the brain using intranasal route providing various benefits dose reduction, avoidance of first pass metabolism, quick onset of action, improved solubility, improved stability, lesser toxicity, and improved bioavailability.[49] Ashhar et al. prepared bromocriptine- and glutathione-loaded nanoemulsion using capmul PG-8 NF, PEG 400, and propylene glycol as excipients to ameliorate the oxidative stress in management of Parkinson's disease. The prepared nanoemulsion was evaluated for determining the depth of permeation using confocal laser microscopy, antioxidant activity, nasal cilio toxicity studies, and levels of superoxide dismutase, GSH, catalase, and pharmacokinetic properties. Depth of permeation of drugs-loaded nanoemulsion was higher than drug suspension; biocompatibility was proved by nasal cilio studies; levels of superoxide dismutase, GSH, and catalase were improved; levels of thiobarbituric acid were reduced on intranasal administration of nano-emulsion; and drugs-loaded nanoemulsion provided enhanced C_{max} of 10.37 ±2.59 μg/mL in the brain on intranasal administration than drug suspension administered by intranasal (5.93 ± 1.43 μg/mL) and intravenous (3.92 ± 0.98 μg/mL) route.[50] Song et al. prepared intranasal nanoemulsion of osthole (natural coumarin) to treat Alzheimer's disease and found that a low dose of osthole nanoemulsion provided neuroprotective effects like prevention of oxidative stress, apoptosis, and maintenance of the cholinergic system.[51] Jusril et al. prepared nanoemulsion having an ethanolic extract of *Centella asiatica* to enhance the BBB permeability and observed that nanoemulsion of ethanolic extract of *Centella asiatica* reduced anticholinesterase activity, level of pro-inflammatory mediators, as well as oxidative stress. In addition, it exhibited improved permeation through BBB having a higher value for experimentally calculated permeability.[52]

7.2.4 LIPOSOMES

Due to possession of distinctive characteristics of biocompatibility, less toxicity, biodegradability, improved peripheral circulation, enhanced stability, and easier attachment of ligands on their surface, liposomes are the choice as a carrier for delivering the medications to CNS.[53] Moreover, these enable to entrap hydrophobic as well as hydrophilic drugs. Hydrophilic drugs may be entrapped at the interface between the lipid bilayer and the exterior water phase or trapped within the watery core of the liposomes, while hydrophobic drugs are entirely trapped in the hydrophobic core of the lipid bilayers of the liposomes.[18] But conventional liposomes are unable to cross the BBB using simple diffusion due to larger size; hence, these are transported through BBB using various mechanisms, namely, RMT, adsorptive-mediated transcytosis (AMT), and carrier-mediated transcytosis (CMT).[55] These are also eliminated rapidly from the body due to possession of little circulation time within the body. Hence, to improve the circulation time in the body and efficient delivery of the drug to CNS, surface modification of liposomes is carried out.[33] Various modified liposomes for improved drug delivery to CNS have been depicted in Figure 7.3. Surface modification of liposomes leads to improvement in pharmacokinetics as well as biodistribution of drug-entrapped liposomes in the CNS just like the inclusion of PEG on the liposome's surface causes the prolongation of circulation time of liposomes and enables the penetration of it through the BBB.[56,57] PEG-modified liposomes can be targeted to CNS using more modification with many ligands like monoclonal antibodies. It has been shown that transferrin-modified liposomes preferentially carry the drug like 5-fluorouracil to the brain with the help of receptor-mediated endocytosis.[58] Immunoliposomes, also a modified category, improved the drug distribution within the brain tissues and have been used in gene therapy also to target CNS. Rajput and Butani prepared donepezil HCl-loaded liposomes using ethanol injection method and then formulated as in situ gel for better management of Alzheimer's disease. It was found that drug-loaded liposomes provided drug permeation of 80.11 ± 7.77% as compared to drug solution-based in situ gel, which permeated 13.12 ± 4.84 % drug through nasal mucosa of sheep. Pharmacokinetic studies demonstrated improved drug concentration of 1239.61 ± 123.60 pg/g in the brain on nasal administration.[59] Arumugum et al. prepared rivastigmine-entrapped liposomes to deliver into the brain using intranasal route and found five times improved area under the curve (AUC) for intranasal liposomes than orally administered drug solution and three times improved AUC than drug solution administered via intranasal route.[60] Al Asmari et al. prepared donepezil-loaded liposomes and found that donepezil-loaded intranasal liposomes exhibited significantly improved bioavailability than orally administered drug solution as well as intranasally administered drug solution.[61]

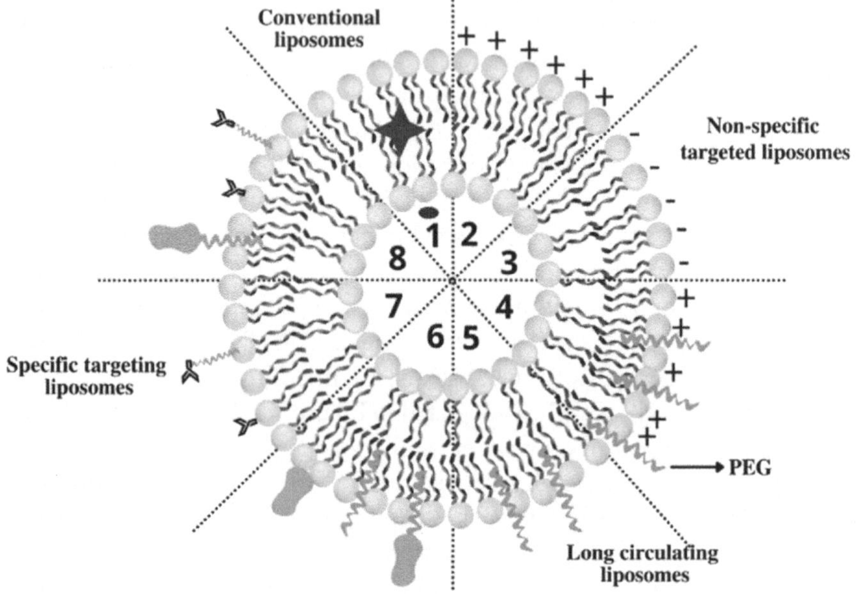

FIGURE 7.3 All in one feature of liposomes for CNS delivery. **(1)** Conventional liposome, **(2)** cationic liposome, **(3)** anionic liposome, **(4)** cationic PEGylated liposome, **(5)** long circulating liposome, **(6)** target liposome with single functional ligand like endogenous or cell penetrating liposome, **(7)** single functional ligand targeted liposome using antibodies, and **(8)** multifunctional ligands with targeted liposome.

7.2.5 DENDRIMERS

These are promising drug carriers due to possession of various properties, like, monodispersity, absence of immunogenicity, enhanced stability, ability to permeate through various biological barriers, regulation of concentration of drug in the required range, availability of various surface groups, and more importantly hyperbranched structure.[62] Various drug-entrapped dendrimers have been utilized for efficient drug delivery to the CNS which utilize the unique transport mechanisms expressed on the BBB for the delivery of drugs to the brain. These unique transport mechanisms expressed on BBB are transferrin receptors (TfRs), endocyticreceptor protein (PRP1 and LRP2), and glucose transport receptor (GLUT1).[63] Polyamidoamide (PAMAM) dendrimers have been prepared for delivery of drugs to the brain using TfR targeting. Xu et al. prepared G5 PAMAM dendrimers to deliver the doxorubicin modified using folic acid along with borneol to improve the

BBB permeability and was found that dendrimers provided increased half-life along with improved AUC as well as doxorubicin buildup the brain.[64] Gothwal et al. prepared G3 PAMAM dendrimers modified with lactoferrin for efficient delivery of rivastigmine to the brain and was found that the bioavailability of the rivastigmine improved 7.87 folds than simple drug and drug uptake by the brain was also enhanced on treating with GE PAMAM dendrimers than drug-entrapped dendrimers.[65]

7.2.6 POLYMERIC MICELLES

Researchers have focused their attention on polymeric micelles made using amphiphilic surfactants and amphiphilic copolymers as an effective drug carrier for CNS medication delivery. Polymeric micelles possessed a longer duration of action and improved biodistribution than conventional micelles.[66] They have a core shell-like structure having an external hydrophilic portion composed of PEG and an internal hydrophobic portion composed of molecules like propylene glycols, polycaprolactone, phospholipids, and fatty acids allowing the entrapment of lipophilic drugs.[67] The outer hydrophilic portion of the shell is responsible to exhibit stability in an aqueous environment and prolongation of circulation time in the blood which protects it from RES facilitating their deposition in specific areas with leaky vasculature.[33] Pluronic block copolymers are widely employed because of their capacity to inhibit efflux transporters and prevent P-gp efflux transporters from being expressed on BBB, which results in effective medication administration to the CNS.[68] Drug delivery to the CNS can be improved by modifying polymeric micelles, which can be done by attaching polyclonal antibodies to brain-specific antigens, insulin, or 2-glycoprotein for targeting at the luminal surface of the BBB.[69] In another way, the micelle can be conjugated directly to the drug molecule followed by targeting moiety to the amphiphilic segment of the micelle. Abourehab et al. prepared self-assembled polymeric micelles of dapoxetine to cross through BBB and found that AUC in brain tissues for the polymeric micelles entrapped with dapoxetine was 2571.35±118.6 ng h/mL, while it was 1337.63±99.21 ng h/mL for commercial tablet of dapoxetine suggesting the significantly improvement in bioavailability using polymeric micelles in brain.[70]. Liu et al. prepared polymeric micelles loaded with lamotrigine using Pluronic®P123 as polymer and was found that optimized nanoformulation provided accumulation of more drugs in the brain than free drugs on intravenous administration in animals.[71]

7.2.7 POLYMERIC NANOPARTICLES

Possession of distinctive characteristics improved biocompatibility and biodegradability. Low toxicity, nanosize, inimitable functionality, flexible surface properties, plasticity, and flexibility have made PNPs a viable approach for delivering medications to CNS.[72] Surface modification of PNPs can be performed using various ligands—apolipoprotein E, apolipoprotein B, and transferrin (Tf), which have proven their promising outcomes in delivering the drug carriers to the specific targeted site through various mechanisms. Ligands-attached PNPs can cross the BBB through endocytosis (receptor-mediated) enabling the drug targeting to brain.[73] Modification of PNPs with PEG enables the diffusion of drugs in the brain which is also termed brain-penetrating nanoparticles. PNPs for CNS drug delivery can be fabricated using various synthetic as well as natural polymers. The natural polymers does have sodium alginate, chitosan, and human serum albumin. Chitosan is a widely used polymer to prepare PNPs for brain targeting due to its possession of higher biocompatible and bioadhesive characteristics. Moreover, chitosan has a propensity to attract endothelial cells which enables improved permeation to the brain and cellular absorption as well.[74] The synthetic polymers used to fabricate the PNPs include polylactide-*co*-glycolide (PLGA), poly-alkyl-cyanoacrylate (PACA), PEG, and poly-ε-caprolactone, and have been approved by FDA.[75] A synthetic copolymer called PLGA has the ability to cross the BBB and provide prolonged medication release in the brain. The polymer PLGA-PEG-PLGA has been designed to deliver the medicine across the BBB and coated with polysorbate 80.[76] In a study, Krishna et al. prepared PNPs composed of methoxy poly(ethylene glycol)–polycaprolactone (mPEG–PCL) loaded with donepezil using nanoprecipitation method and was surface modified using polysorbate 80 and $ApoE_3$ to improve the bioavailability in brain. It was found that ApoE3-modified PNPs were stable in simulated gastric fluids along with sustained release pattern of the drug. ApoE3-modified PNPs exhibited improved donepezil levels of 84.97 ± 11.54 ng/mg in the brain after 24 h than pure drug.[77] Shah et al. created PLGA-based PNPs to deliver drugs more effectively into the brain for the treatment of epilepsy and found that PLGA nanoparticles provided delayed onset of time for seizure with drug-encapsulated nanoparticles than drug solution, provided prolonged drug release, improved bioavailability, and better targeting to brain.[78]

7.2.8 NANOCRYSTALS

Nanocrystals have proven their efficacy as drug carriers due to possession of various characteristics such as improved drug loading, improved stability, enhanced solubility, enhanced dissolution, enhanced bioavailability,[79] and more importantly ability to provide potent drug concentration required for achieving therapeutic action in brain disorders.[35] Nanocrystals are made completely of the drug; hence, the carrier's auxiliary function is no longer necessary. Moreover, surfactants are added to provide stability to the crystalline dispersion in the liquid phase.[80] Numerous drug-entrapped nanocrystals have been prepared for delivering the drugs efficiently in CNS. Xiong et al. prepared a nanocrystal formulation of resveratrol to improve oral bioavailability and efficacy in the brain tissues and was found that drug-loaded nanocrystals have C_{max} and AUC of 0.26 ± 0.02 μg/mL, 2.61 ± 0.21 μg.h/mL, respectively, while rol group have C_{max} and AUC of 0.11 ± 0.01 μg/mL and 1.12 ± 0.18 μg.h/mL in the brain. Additionally, $T_{1/2}$ of the nanocrystals formulation was 3.32 ± 0.14 h in the brain, while it was 1.45 ± 0.16 h in the plasma suggesting that drug elimination was delayed from brain than plasma.[81] In another study, Gol et al. fabricated nanocrystals of risperidone composed of polycaprolactone with pluronic F-68 combination using the lyophilization technique and found that % cumulative drug release of drug-entrapped nanocrystals was 90% in the initial 10 h, while it was about 11% for plain drug suspension. The drug-entrapped nanocrystals were found stable at 4°C for 3 months having particle size, zeta potential, and polydispersity index of 214 ± 3.4 nm, -10.2 ± 0.90, and 0.120 mV, respectively.[82]

7.2.9 CARBON NANOTUBES

Carbon nanotubes (CNTs) have a number of distinctive properties of good electronic properties, remarkably effective cell membrane penetration, thermal properties, high drug-loading, and pH-dependent therapeutic unloading capacities, large surface area, and ease of molecular modification which enable them an appropriate carrier for delivering the medication to CNS[83,84] When drugs are transported directly to the desired cells with the aid of CNTs, they can prolong drug survival in humans.[85] Single-wall CNTs (SWCNTs) and multi-wall CNTs are two forms that are available for these (MWCNTs). In an another study, Costa et al. prepared functionalized CNTs to improve the delivery of Pittsburgh B across the BBB to target the amyloid in brain tissues and found that conjugated Pittsburgh compound B is unable to cross the BBB; hence, the conjugation of Pittsburgh B derivatives namely Gd (L_3) and Gd (L_2) to functionalized MWCNTs provided improved accumulation in brain.[86] Han et al. reported that PEG functionalized MWCNTs conjugated with angiopep-2 were prepared to treat brain glioma successfully. Due to higher affinity among the angiopep-2 and LRP receptor, it is able to provide higher tumor suppression on C6 and BCEC cells.[87] Clinical research on CNTs reveal that they are toxic to the biological environment. Their exposure, dose, and route all affect both their efficacy and negative effects. CNTs can be coated with surfactants to lessen their toxicity to cells and break the bond between cells and CNTs.[88] However, the toxicity studies of CNTs must be addressed to guarantee their efficacy and safety as drug delivery system in CNS.

7.2.10 METALLIC NANOPARTICLES

Metallic nanoparticles (MNPs) have generated a great deal of interest due to their potential to transport therapeutic agents efficiently, prevent multidrug resistance, and improve the therapeutic index of medications through site specificity. Moreover, MNPs have many benefits for drug delivery systems including enhanced half-life and stability of drug carriers in circulation, needing passive or active targeting and biodistribution into the necessary target site.[89] Various MNPs have been employed as drug carrier to target the brain which include iron oxide nanoparticles (FeONPs), silver nanoparticles (AgNPs), zinc oxide nanoparticles (ZnONPs), gold nanoparticles (AuNPs), and platinum nanoparticles (PtNPs).[88] AgNPs can build up in the brain by surpassing the BBB followed by ingestion and inhalation.[90] AuNPs have a great potential to target the brain due to possession of various benefits improved solubility, targeting of drug molecules to brain endothelium, low toxicity, surpassing the brain parenchyma rapidly, low immunogenicity, minimal interaction with biological membrane, and easy to synthesize. AuNPs can be detected in brain within few minutes of infusion.[91] Zhang et al. prepared AuNPs laden with resveratrol and found that AuNPs provided suppression of tumor growth, promotion of tumor apoptosis, and reduction in expression of vascular endothelial growth factor (VEGF) in tumor tissues of brain.[92] Hou et al. prepared AuNPs laden with D and L glutathione which surpassed the BBB and prevented the Aβ42 without any toxicity.[93] In other study, Nathan et al. created iron oxide nanoparticles conjugated with anti-sauvagine-30 to cross the BBB effectively and observed that injection of nanoparticles decreased amphetamine withdrawal-induced anxiety without impairing movement, indicating that iron oxide nanoparticles conjugated with antisauvagine-30 provided anxiolytic effects which were sustained and its bioavailability was sufficient.[94] However, the MNPs are able to cross the BBB effectively but their long-term toxicities must be evaluated, which is a major issue with MNPs.

7.2.11 MISCELLANEOUS NANOFORMULATIONS

Nanowires fabricated as drug delivery system have a great potential in drug targeting and making neuronal communications rapid than other methods of nanotechnology prepared for same purpose. The nanowires are prepared mainly using titanium, silica, or copper coated with some adhesives to bind the drug followed by delivery to the biological system. These are less immunogenic than other nanoformulations but attached to the cell surface causing ingestion by cells and leads to cell toxicity, which restricts their use.[95] Nanofibers are another nanoformulation having enormous potential as drug delivery system to CNS due to various characteristics of microstructure, higher surface area, and great porosity having interconnectivity, which promotes cell adhesion, propagation and drug delivery. Benefits of nanofiber scaffold formulations include excellent stability, enhanced targeting, minimal toxicity, high drug-loading capacity, outstanding mechanical features, encapsulation of a wide range of drugs, and compatibility with thermolabile medications. It has long been difficult to administer medications to patients in the best way possible. Numerous biocompatible, biodegradable, and nonbiodegradable polymeric materials can be used as delivery matrices like chitosan.[96] Raddy et al. prepared chitosan coated nanofibers loaded with donepezil and found that chitosan-coated nanofiber exhibited higher AUC of 1860.5 ng/mL than chitosan nanofilm having AUC of 1450.3 ± 112.5 ng/mL.[97] Despite their utility, these nanoformulations are less explored as drug delivery system to CNS which need to be explored and toxicity studies must also be addressed for their clinical utility. A list of drug-entrapped nanoformulations for CNS delivery has been outlined in Table 7.1.

TABLE 7.1 A Collective List of Nanoformulations for CNS Delivery.

Nanocarrier	Drug moiety	Polymer	Method	Result outcomes	References
SLN	Donepezil	Tween 80, Glyceryl monostearate, poloxamer 188	Solvent emulsification diffusion	Drug entrapped SLN provided 2.61 fold improved AUC than an intravenous drug solution and 2.26 folds than intranasally administered solution in brain, scintigraphy pictures demonstrated the drug accumulation the brain	[98]
SLN	Rivastigmine tartrate	Glyceryl monostearate, polysorbate 80	Solvent emulsification diffusion	Drug-entrapped SLN provided improved C_{max} of 73.99 ± 5.66 ng/mL than solutions administered by intranasal (65.24 ± 3.35 ng/mL) and intravenous (49.64 ± 5.58 ng/mL) route in brain. The $AUC_{0-24\,h}$ for drug entrapped SLNs was 20256.49 ± 30.60 ng.h/mL whilst it was 9876.34 ± 11.62 ng.h/mL for intranasally administered solution and 6856.25 ± 14.46 ng.h/mL for intravenous solution	[40]
SLN, NLC	Ropinirole			Provided 2.1 and 2.7 folds improvement from drug-loaded SLNs and NLCs, respectively, in bioavailability on oral administration, hydrogel of drug-entrapped SLNs and NLCs demonstrated 3.0 and 3.3 folds improvement respectively in bioavailability on topical administration and hydrogel of drug entrapped SLNs and NLCs improved the bioavailability 1.4 and 1.2 times than drug-entrapped SLNs and NLCs	[99]

TABLE 7.1 *(Continued)*

Nanocarrier	Drug moiety	Polymer	Method	Result outcomes	References
SLN	Piribedil	Palmitic acid, polyvinyl alcohol	Hot homogenization and ultrasonication	Provided C_{max} of 245.83 ± 33.56 ng/g and AUC_{0-t} of 42046 ng/g.min by in situ gel of drug-loaded SLNs than drug-loaded suspension having C_{max} of 242.43 ± 45.84 ng/g and AUC_{0-t} of 10394 ng/g.min in brain	[100]
SLN	Temozolomide	Polyvinyl alcohol, sodium behenate	Coacervation	Provided improved effects in melanoma cells and neoangiogenesis than free drug also prevented the growth as well as vascularization of B16-F10 melanoma in C57/BL6 mice with the absence of toxic effects	[101]
SLN	Quercetin	Cetylpalmitate, polysorbate 80	Ultrasonication	LDH cytotoxicity studies in hCMEC/D3 cell line provided that at highest concentration of 30 μM, SLNs possessed no cytotoxicity after 4 hours of incubation, provided improved permeation through BBB using hCMEC/D3 cell monolayers and amyloid-beta studies provided that SLN-transferrin can prevent fibril formation	[102]
SLN	Camptothecin	Cetylpalmitate, polysorbate 80	Ultrasonication	Drug-loaded SLN caused cell death with the minimum maximal inhibitory concentration (IC50) values, Furthermore, improved brain deposition of the drug was observed in in vivo distribution studies	[103]

TABLE 7.1 *(Continued)*

Nanocarrier	Drug moiety	Polymer	Method	Result outcomes	References
NLC	Berberine	GMS, oleic acid, poloxamer 407, chitosan	Hot homogenization and ultrasonication	Drug-entrapped NLC coated with chitosan provided improved C_{max} of 1033 ng/mL than drug solution administered by intranasal (1000 ng/mL) and intravenous (780 ng/mL) route in the brain	[104]
NLC	Baicalin, salvianolic acid B	mPEG-MAL, Compritol® 888 ATO, MCT 812, mPEG-OH, lecithin, myrj 52	Emulsification and solvent evaporation method	OX26-modified NLCs having the combination of baicalin and salvianolic acid B have improved brain targeting ability than non-modified formulation and drug solution, OX26-modified NLCs exhibited significant improvement in baicalin amount in the brain, salvianolic acid B can be detected only at some time points in non-modified formulation and drug solution whereas OX26-modified NLCs can be detected within 4 h	[105]
NLC	Temozolamide	Gelucire, vitamin E, tween 80, transcutol	High pressure homogenization followed by ultrasonication	Drug-entrapped NLC exhibited improved C_{max} of 1189.1 ng/mL in the brain by intranasal route than the solution of drug administered by intranasal (263.1 ng/mL) and intravenous (2.96 ng/mL) route	[106]
NLC	Embelin	Cetylpalmitate, ctyldodecanol, poloxamer 188	Emulsification and ultrasonication	Drug-entrapped NLC provided an improved level of malondialdehyde (MDA), nitrite, and reduced level of glutathione in the brain	[107]

TABLE 7.1 *(Continued)*

Nanocarrier	Drug moiety	Polymer	Method	Result outcomes	References
Lipid nanoconstructs	Paliperidone	Capmul MCM, glycerylmonostearate, poloxamer 407, tween 20	Melt emulsification-probe sonication technique and high-pressure homogenization	Drug-entrapped formulation provided an improved C_{max} of 724.16±84.28 ng/mL in the brain than drug suspension having C_{max} of 275.87±51.93 ng/mL	[108]
NLC	Atazanavir	Precirol ATO, Lauroglycol 90, cremophor RH40	Probe sonication	Provided higher C_{max} of 89.24±2.23 µg/mL and AUC of 1570.41 ±112.62 µg.h/mL than drug suspension having C_{max} of 32.46±1.49 µg/mL and AUC of 413.04 ±31.36 µg.h/mL. Drug-entrapped NLC provided 2.75-folds enhanced C_{max} in the brain and 4-fold improved brain bioavailability, demonstrated the concentration of 62.57±2.43 µg/mL, 7.54±1.68 µg/mL in brain by drug-loaded NLCs and drug suspension, respectively	[106]
NLC	Curcumin			Curcumin entrapped NLC provided improved cytotoxicity than drug suspension to astrocytoma-glioblastoma cell line and improved levels of curcumin were found in the brain on intranasal administration of the formulation	[109]
NLC	Rivastigmine	Tween 80, Phospholipon® 90 G, Precirol ® ATO 5, vitamin E	High pressure homogenization and ultrasound method	Provided initial rapid drug release followed by prolonged release by drug-loaded NLCs, no significant changes in critical quality attributes were detected on storage at varying temperature for 90 days	[110]

TABLE 7.1 *(Continued)*

Nanocarrier	Drug moiety	Polymer	Method	Result outcomes	References
Nanoemulsion	Riluzole	Sefsol 218, tween 80, carbitol	Phase titration method	Provided significant higher brain uptake ($P < 4.10 \times 10^{-6}$) of riluzole on intranasal administration of drug-loaded nanoemulsion than oral administration, demonstrated absence of nasal ciliotoxicity, and stability for three months	[111]
Nanoemulsion	Rosemary oil with donepezil	PEG 400, tween 80, ethanol, diethyl glycol monoethyl ether	Phase titration method	Provided IC50 value of oil at 0.001 µL/min on in vitro anticholinesterase activity, safety, and permeation mechanism of rosemary oil-laden nanoemulsion were established using ex vivo nasal ciliotoxicity as well as permeation studies, in vitro permeation studies provided more permeation of drug from nanoemulsion as compared to plain drug and provided that drug-loaded nanoemulsion was stable for 3 months when stored at different conditions of temperature	[112]
Nanoemulsion	Bromocriptine and glutathione	Capmul PG-8 NF, PEG 400, propylene glycol	Ultrasonication	Provided higher depth of permeation of drugs-loaded nanoemulsion than drug suspension, biocompatibility was proved by nasal cilio studies, levels of superoxide dismutase, GSH, catalase were improved, and levels of thiobarbituric acid were	[50]

TABLE 7.1 *(Continued)*

Nanocarrier	Drug moiety	Polymer	Method	Result outcomes	References
				reduced on intranasal administration of nanoemulsion, drugs-loaded nanoemulsion provided enhanced C_{max} of 10.37 ±2.59 µg/mL in the brain on intranasal administration than drug suspension administered by intranasal (5.93 ± 1.43 µg/mL) and intravenous (3.92 ± 0.98 µg/mL) route	
Nanoemulsion	Donepezil	Capryol 90, labrasol, transcutol P	Sonication	Significant permeation of the drug was found via drug-laden nanoemulsion administered by an intranasal route along with improved bioavailability using bioadhesive polymers	[113]
Nanoemulsion	Resveratrol	Coconut oil, Cremophor EL, Pluronic P107	Ultrasonication	Drug-loaded nanoemulsion maximum drug concentration of 5762.30 ±316.9 ng/mL in the brain, while it was 3069.27 ±215.2 ng/mL for a drug suspension	[114]
Nanoemulsion	Rivastigmine	Capmul MCM, tween 80, transcutol P	Titration method	Maximum drug concentration for nanoemulsion formulation was 1112.24±12.5 ng/mL in the brain on intranasal administration while it was 393.32±4.6 ng/mL and 692.21±5.7 ng/mL for intravenous nanoemulsion and intravenous drug suspension, respectively	[115]

TABLE 7.1 *(Continued)*

Nanocarrier	Drug moiety	Polymer	Method	Result outcomes	References
Nanoemulsion	Letrozole	Triacetin, tween 80, PEG-400	Aqueous microtitration method	Enhanced onset time of status epilepticus was found and occurrence of status epilepticus was decreased on intranasal administration of formulation, nanoemulsion effectively reduced levels of 17-β estradiol while the levels of 5α-Dihydrotestosterone and 3α-androstanediol were significantly enhanced in the hippocampus	[116]
Nanoemulsion	Topiramate	Capmul MCM C8, tween 20, carbitol	Phase titration method	Improved bioavailability of drug-loaded nanoemulsion than drug suspension on administration by the intranasal route	[117]
Liposomes	Rivastigmine	Soya lecithin and cholesterol	Lipid layer hydration method	Liposomal formulation of the drug exhibited improved C_{max} of 1489.5±620.71 ng/mL than oral rivastigmine having C_{max} of 56.29±27.05 ng/mL	[118]
Liposomes	Donepezil		Ethanol injection method	Provided enhanced drug concentration of 1239.61 ± 123.60 pg/g in the brain on nasal administration	[59]
Liposomes	Aphanamixispolystachya leaf extract	Phospholipid and cholesterol	Solvent injection method	Provided significant enhancement in the memory function, locomotor activity, and ambulatory activity in dementia induced than the simple leaf extract	[119]
Liposomes	Allium cepa fraction	Phosphatidylcholine and cholesterol		Provided significant neuroprotective activity at 1/10th dose of the oral dose	[120]

TABLE 7.1 *(Continued)*

Nanocarrier	Drug moiety	Polymer	Method	Result outcomes	References
4.0 G PAMAM Dendrimers	Donepezil	Ethylenediamine		Provided 4-fold improved brain uptake in the case of the anocrysta-conjugated formulation	[121]
3.0 G PAMAM dendrimers	Rivastigmine	Lactoferrin (Lf)		Provided improved uptake of drug by brain on treatment with PAMAM-Lf-drug than drug and PAMAM encapsulated drug	[65]
Polymeric nanoparticle	Donepezil	Diblock copolymer methoxy poly(ethylene glycol)-polycaprolactone	Nanoprecipitation method	Drug-loaded polymeric nanoparticles surface modified with ApoE3 and polysorbate 80 provided improved maximum drug concentration of 484.61 ± 86.49 ng/mL than the pure drug	[7]
Polymeric nanoparticle	Rivastigmine	Eudragit, span 80, glutaraldehyde	Emulsion crosslinking method	Provided cumulative drug release of 97.59% and higher flux of 40.39 ± 3.52 µg.h/cm^2	[122]
Polymeric nanoparticle	Genistein and temozolomide	PLGA, Polyvinyl alcohol	Solvent evaporation method	Provided higher cytotoxicity on treating U87MG cells with drug-loaded polymeric with IC50 values of 35.2 µg/mL for 24 h and 8.7 µg/mL for 48 h	[123]
Polymeric nanoparticle	Lamotrigine	PLGA, poloxamer 407	Emulsification-solvent evaporation method	Provided delayed onset of time for seizure with drug encapsulated nanoparticles than drug solution, provided prolonged drug release, improved bioavailability, and better targeting to brain	[78]

TABLE 7.1 *(Continued)*

Nanocarrier	Drug moiety	Polymer	Method	Result outcomes	References
Polymeric nanoparticle	Ropinirole	PLGA, polyvinyl alcohol	Nanoprecipitation	Brain histology, immunochemistry, and behavioral testing provided the potential of drug-loaded nanoparticles for efficient delivery in Parkinson's disease	[124]
Polymeric nanoparticle	Withaferin-A	PLGA	Solvent evaporation method	Provided particle size of 121 ± 2 nm, drug entrapment efficiency was 54% at 500 μg/mL concentration of an entrapped drug.	[125]
Polymeric micelle	Lamotrigine	Pluronic®P123	Thin film hydration	Provided accumulation of more drugs in the brain than free drugs on intravenous administration in animals,	[71]
Polymeric micelles	Dapoxetine	PEG-PLGA copolymer		Drug-entrapped polymeric micelles exhibited AUC of 2571.35±118.6 ng h/mL in the brain whilst it was 1.337.63±99.21 ng h/mL for commercial tablet	[70]
Nanocrystals	Ginkgolide B	HPMC E5	Antisolvent precipitation technique	Provided improved drug concentration in plasma and neuronal tissues, provided improved behavior, decreased dopamine deficiency along with increased levels of the dopamine metabolite	[126]
Nanocrystals	Puerarin	HPMC E3	Antisolvent precipitation technique	Provided improved brain accumulation of drug via anocrystals formulation than drug suspension	[127]
Nanocrystals	Donepezil	D-α-Tocopherol polyethylene glycol 1000 succinate	High pressure homogenization	Provided that drug entrapped nanocrystals improved spatial memory learning on a single dose administered by intramuscular injection	[128]

TABLE 7.1 *(Continued)*

Nanocarrier	Drug moiety	Polymer	Method	Result outcomes	References
Nanocrystals	Resveratrol	Polyvinylpyrrolidone K90	Antisolvent precipitation technique	Provided C_{max} and AUC for drug-loaded nanocrystals of 0.26 ± 0.02 μg/mL, 2.61 ± 0.21 μg.h/mL, respectively, than 0.11 ± 0.01 μg/mL (C_{max}), 1.12 ± 0.18 μg.h/mL (AUC) for control group in the brain	[81]
Nanocrystals based orally disintegrating tablet	Ziprasidone	PVP K30	Microfluidization	Provided improved permeability value and % cumulative drug release on the cells with nanocrystals	[129]
Gold nanoparticles	Resveratrol			Provided suppression of tumor growth, promotion of tumor apoptosis and reduction in expression of vascular endothelial growth factor (VEGF) in tumor tissues of brain	[92]
Silver nanoparticles	L & D Glutathione			Surpassed the BBB and prevented the Aβ42 without any toxicity	[93]
Iron oxide nanoparticles	Antisauvagine-30			Provided that injection of nanoparticles decreased amphetamine withdrawal-induced anxiety without impairing movement, indicating that iron oxide nanoparticles conjugated with antisauvagine-30 provided anxiolytic effects which were sustained and its bioavailability was sufficient	[94]
Chitosan coated nanofiber	Donepezil			Exhibited higher AUC of 1860.5 ng/mL than chitosan nanofilm having AUC of 1450.3 ± 112.5 ng/mL	[97]

7.3 CLINICAL TRIALS AND PATENTS FOR NANOFORMULATIONS IN CNS DISORDERS

Clinical trials are investigations carried out on human subjects to ascertain if a therapeutic medicine or a therapeutic technology is suitable and effective for use by people. Before beginning, these investigations needed approval and they went through four steps before completing clinical trials. In recent years, a variety of nanoformulations for CNS delivery have been put through clinical studies, demonstrating the widespread acceptance of these formulations.[18]

Various nanoformulations for CNS delivery put for clinical trials have been summed up in Table 7.2.

A patent is an official privilege that the government grants to an inventor to authorize the exclusive manufacturing, sale, or use of a product for a specific amount of time.[131] In recent years, several patents for nanoformulations meant for CNS delivery have been granted, demonstrating the widespread acceptance of these formulations. Various patents issued for nanoformulations for CNS delivery have been summed up in Table 7.3.

7.4 COMMERCIALIZED NANOFORMULATIONS FOR CNS DELIVERY

Recently various drug-loaded nanoformulations have been effectively introduced in the market and are used by various patients on regular basis. These formulations have been manufactured by various pharmaceutical industries throughout the world and demonstrate the current and future success of nanoformulations as an effective therapeutic moiety. A variety of drugs used as treatment modalities for CNS disorders have been prepared as nanoformulation by various scientists out of which some have been introduced in the market. Various drugs formulated as nanoformulation for CNS disorders have been recapitulated in Table 7.4.[132,133]

7.5 NANOFORMULATIONS TOXICITY STUDIES

Tremendous growth has been achieved in nanotechnology-based drug formulations recently due to their surprising properties, including level of solubility and target specificity, improved solubility, systemic stability, controlled and sustained drug release, and minimal adverse effect which makes them unique than other type of drug formulations.[134] However, depending on the qualities in

TABLE 7.2 Summarized List of Nanoformulations for CNS Delivery Undertaking Clinical Trials.

Nanomaterial	Name	DISEASE	Route	Status	Clinical trial registration no.
Gold nanocrystals	CNM-Au8	• Multiple sclerosis	Oral	Phase 2	NCT03993171
Iron oxide NPs	Ferumoxytol	• Brain cancer • Brain injury • Brain tumors • Primary brain neoplasm • Hemorrhagic cerebrovascular accident • Central nervous system vascular malformation • Central nervous system degenerative disorder • Ischemic cerebrovascular accident • Central nervous system infectious disorder	Intravenous	Early phase 1	NCT02452216
Lipid-bases NPs	ARCT-810	• Ornithine transcarbamylase deficiency	Intravenous	Phase 1	NCT04442347
NPs albumin-bound rapamycin	ABI-009	• Epilepsy intractable	Intravenous	Phase 1	NCT03646240
Intranasal nanoparticles	APH-1105	• Alzheimer disease 1 • Alzheimer disease 2 • Alzheimer disease 3 • Dementia	Intranasal	Phase 2	NCT03806478
Cytarabine encapsulated in multivesicular liposomes	DepoCyt®	• Central nervous system metastases	Intravenous	Phase 2	NCT00992602

TABLE 7.2 *(Continued)*

Nanomaterial	Name	DISEASE	Route	Status	Clinical trial registration no.
Single dose liposomal amphotericin and fluconazole	AmBisome®	• Cryptococcal meningitis	Intravenous	Phase 2	NCT03945448
Liposomal fluconazole	AmBisome®	• Cryptococcal meningitis	Intravenous	Phase 3	NCT03945448
Polysiloxane gadolinium-chelates-based NPs	AGuIX	• Brain metastases	Intravenous	Phase I	NCT02820454
Pegylated Liposomal Doxorubicine	PEG-Dox	• Glioblastoma	Intravenous	Phase 2	NCT00944801
Polymer NPs	Copaxone®/ Glatopa (Teva)	• Multiple sclerosis	Subcutaneous injection	Phase 3	NCT01489254

TABLE 7.3 Summarized List of Patents Issued for Nanoformulations for CNS Delivery

Patent Number	NPs	Drug and disease	Outcomes
US20090148417A1	Carbon nanotubes	Parkinson Alzheimer's disease	Carbon nanotube serving as a stem cell scaffold without cytotoxicity. The carbon nanotube-based scaffold for stem cell transplantation has outstanding effects on networking between differentiated stem cells and tissues present in transplantation sites without cytotoxicity, demonstrating considerable cell therapy effectiveness.
US20100160299	Dendrimers	Psychotic disorders	Dendrimer linker composition claimed to cross the blood-brain barrier easily.
US20110027351	Liposome	Parkinson	The preferred liposomal formulation as per the invention claimed to penetrate through the BBB at a sufficient level.
US7659314	Micelles	Cancer	These mixed micelles help treat cancer, especially malignancies demonstrating multidrug resistance since the microenvironment of solid tumors (brain) is acidic. To improve medication delivery into cells, targeting ligands, such as folate, can also be added to the mixed micelles.
US10842755B2	NPs	Brain metastatic cancer	The nanoparticle has a core made of an active chemical and a core material like an inorganic or polymer, and it also has a shell made of a membrane taken from a brain cancer cell that has spread to other parts of the body. This cell helps the nanoparticle pass the blood–brain barrier.
US10307372B2	Polymeric nanoparticles	CNS disorders	A pharmaceutically approved excipient for distribution into the brain and effective dosage of a therapeutic, prophylactic, or diagnostic agent to diagnose or treat a brain ailment or illness.
WO2016090092A1	Nanoemulsions	Brain cancer	Compositions of nanoemulsions include a targeting agent, a drug delivery system, a therapeutic agent, an imaging agent, or a combination of these. Nanoemulsion formulation compositions and preparation techniques are also offered, as well as approaches for treating or detecting brain conditions including brain cancer.

TABLE 7.3 *(Continued)*

Patent Number	NPs	Drug and disease	Outcomes
US10028919B2	Lipid nanoparticle		Phospholipid nanoparticle compositions of cannabinoids made from phospholipids improve the bioavailability of the cannabinoid 2- to 8-fold. Short-term memory impairment is one of the main side effects of cannabis therapy in people.
US20210236542A1	Novel gold-based nanocrystals	Parkinson's disease	Parkinson's disease treatment involves giving a patient who needs it an effective dose of a pharmaceutically acceptable solution containing gold nanocrystals.
US11229705B2	Coated nanoparticles	Modulation of electrical polarization of neurons	The invention is related to medicine, more specifically to the control of neurons' electrical polarization. The current invention more especially pertains to a nanoparticle or aggregation of nanoparticles used to control the electrical polarisation of neurons in a person.

TABLE 7.4 List of Commercialized Nanoformulations to Treat CNS Disorders.

Trade name	Nanoformulation	Name of Drug	Indication	Manufacturer
Emend®	Nanocrystal	Aprepitant	Anti-emetic	Merck & Co., Inc., NJ, USA
AbilifyMaintena®	Nanocrystal	Aripiprazole	Schizophrenia	Otsuka
Aristada®	Nanocrystal	Aripiprazolelauroxil	Schizophrenia	Alkermes
Sublocade®	PLGA nanoparticles	Buprenorphine	Opioid use-related disorders	Indivior
InvegaSustenna®	Nanocrystal	Paliperidonepalmitate	Schizophrenia	Janssen
Focalin XR®	Nanocrystal	Dexmethylphenidate HCl	Psychostimulant	Novartis, East Hanover, NJ, USA
Ritalin LA®	Nanocrystal	Methylphenidate HCl	Psychostimulant	Basel, Novartis, Switzerland
Doxil®	Liposomes	Doxorubicin	Cancer	Alza, Pakistan
DaunoXome®	Liposomes	Daunorubicin	Cancer	Galen, Craigavon, UK
Marqibo®	Liposomes	Vincristine	Cancer	Talon therapeutics, CA, USA

various environments, it can be both advantageous and harmful emphasizing the significance of conducting nanotoxicology research before usage upon people. These nanoformulations interact with many biological processes and biomolecules in living things since they are entering the biological system. While special characteristics of nanoformulations make them suitable for drug delivery on the one hand, they can also present problems if they are not effectively tuned.[135] When present in a living organism, high surface-to-volume ratio of nanoformulation can boost drug-loading efficiency but can also increase the likelihood of interactions with other biomolecules. When employing nanoformulation as drug delivery systems, other characteristics such as their solubility, surface coating, charged surface, and particle size raise concerns among scientists.[136] The idea that nanoformulation can be a blessing or a curse is supported by several studies conducted over the years. The enormous benefits that nanoformulation provide are largely understood, but less is known about their toxicity, translocation to secondary target organs, non-specific protein interactions, etc.

Lipid-based nanocarriers (SLNs, NLCs) are made up of physiological lipids and surfactants which are considered safe (GRAS); hence, chances of toxicity are less which is main reason for availability of limited literature for toxicity profile of lipid-based nanocarriers. This holds great promise for oral and topical delivery while the parenteral drug delivery can cause toxic effect due to possession of surfactant which is responsible to activate the immune system. Hence, various toxicity studies upon cytotoxicity, hemocompatibility, and genotoxicity must be performed to assess the toxicity profile of the lipid-based nanocarriers.[137]

In a study, Tang et al. evaluated the distribution and deposition of the AgNPs in rats on subcutaneous injection and found that SNPs translocated to the systemic circulation and were dispersed in the form of particles in all of the major organs but particularly in the kidney, liver, spleen, brain, and lung. Findings from ultrastructural analysis suggest that SNPs that had accumulated in organs may have the ability to enter a variety of cell types, including liver and renal tubular epithelial cells. Additionally, astrocyte enlargement, BBB disruption, and neuronal degeneration were all brought on by SNPs.[138] Ma et al. demonstrated that brain damage could result from a high-dose infusion of anatase TiO_2 nanoparticles which can also transform some glia into filamentous cells and others into inflammatory cells.

The dosages of nanoparticles anatase TiO_2 used and the concentration of nanoparticles anatase TiO_2 in the brain were closely associated.[139] Superparamagnetic iron oxide nanoparticles (SPIONs) is safe at concentration less than 100 μg/mL due to absence of any toxic reaction but at concentration more than 100 µg/mL, it can cause various toxic reactions namely cytotoxicity, DNA damage, oxidative stress, and inflammatory processes.[140]

CNTs are able to cross the cell membranes during commuting the carrier biomolecule which insist to demonstrate the cytotoxicity of CNTs. CNTs have been linked to toxicity in the lungs, brain, immune system, genitalia, embryos, heart, liver, and ovaries. In a study, Gholamine et al. reported that toxicological profile of multi walled CNTs and single-walled CNTs and observed that both types of CNTs exhibited anxiogenic as well as depression effects along with impacting the gene expression of brain-derived neurotrophic factor (BNDF).[141] Norihiro et al. demonstrated the carcinogenicity and lung tumor causing ability of CNTs. It was found that long-term inhalation of CNTs caused lung gene damage, lung fibrosis, persistent inflammation, and lung cancer. CNTs also demonstrated great biopersistence in animal studies. Multi-walled CNTs were administered to mice and foetal malformations after intravenous, intraperitoneal, and intratracheal injections as well as foetal loss after intravenous injection, behavioral changes in offspring after intraperitoneal injection and a delay in the delivery of the first litter after intratracheal administration were reported.[142] Kavosi et al. studied the therapeutic and toxic effects of SWNCTs and MWCNTs on mice and observed that SWCNTs caused toxicity to various organs and lead to death at higher doses. Moreover, some liver cells also exhibited shrinkage.[143] In a study, G4 PAMAM dendrimers caused dose as well as time-dependent toxic effects and higher dose resulted in mortality due to arresting the embryonic growth.[140]

7.6 CONCLUSION AND FUTURE PERSPECTIVE

There is a group of CNS disorders which includes Alzheimer's disease, amyotrophic lateral sclerosis, Parkinson's disease, Huntington's disease, prion disease frontotemporal dementia, brain tumor, stroke, and spinal cord injury. Despite the availability of various drug moieties, these disorders are regarded as untreatable because of the unavailability of specific treatments to pass the BBB which ensures the low therapeutic concentration of the drug in CNS. In order to effectively treat CNS illnesses, it is imperative to create a unique drug carrier that can penetrate the BBB and assure efficient medication concentration in the brain. Substantial study in this paper provided that nanotechnology-based formulations like liposomes, SLNs, dendrimers, nanocrystals, NLCs, nanoemulsions, polymeric micelles, PNPs, metallic nanoparticles, CNTs, nanowires, and nanofibers can be an effective way to treat CNS disorders successfully. These nanoformulations surpass the BBB using various mechanisms namely the transcellular pathway, paracellular pathway, carrier-mediated pathway, adsorptive transcytosis, and RMT. Various nanoformulations for CNS disorders are under clinical trials, some have got patents and out of which some nanoformulations have been commercialized as a treatment option for CNS disorders. Despite of success of nanoformulations in CNS disorders, some nanoformulations like nanofibers, nanowires, and nanosponges for CNS delivery have limited literature which can be seen as future perspectives. Moreover, the long-term toxicity studies on metallic nanoparticles, CNTs, and nanowires must be addressed for their successful clinical use.

KEYWORDS

- **nanotechnology**
- **CNS drug delivery**
- **blood–brain barrier**
- **nanoformulations**
- **clinical trials**
- **patents**

REFERENCES

1. Feigin, V. L.; Nichols, E.; Alam, T.; Bannick, M. S.; Beghi, E.; Blake, N. et al. Global, Regional, and National Burden of Neurological Disorders, 1990–2016: A Systematic Analysis for the Global Burden of Disease Study 2016. *Lancet Neurol.* **2019,** *18* (5), 459–480.
2. Pandey, M.; Jain, N.; Kanoujia, J.; Hussain, Z.; Gorain, B. Advances and Challenges in Intranasal Delivery of Antipsychotic Agents Targeting the Central Nervous System. *Front. Pharmacol.* **2022,** *13*, 865590.
3. Kadry, H.; Noorani, B.; Cucullo, L. A Blood–Brain Barrier Overview on Structure, Function, Impairment, and Biomarkers of Integrity. *Fluids Barriers CNS* **2020,** *17* (1), 69.
4. Winkler, L.; Blasig, R.; Breitkreuz-Korff, O.; Berndt, P.; Dithmer, S.; Helms, H. C. et al. Tight Junctions in the Blood–Brain Barrier Promote Edema Formation and Infarct Size in Stroke – Ambivalent Effects of Sealing Proteins. *J. Cereb. Blood Flow Metab.* **2021,** *41* (1), 132–145.
5. Tajes, M.; Ramos-Fernández, E.; Weng-Jiang, X.; Bosch-Morató M, Guivernau, B.; Eraso-Pichot, A. et al. The Blood-Brain Barrier: Structure, Function and Therapeutic Approaches to Cross It. *Mol. Membr. Biol.* **2014,** *31* (5), 152–167.

6. Ceña, V.; Játiva, P. Nanoparticle Crossing of Blood–Brain Barrier: A Road to New Therapeutic Approaches to Central Nervous System Diseases. *Nanomedicine* **2018,** *13* (13), 1513–1516.
7. Pardridge, W. M. Drug and Gene Targeting to the Brain with Molecular Trojan Horses. *Nat. Rev. Drug Discov*. **2002,** *1* (2), 131–139.
8. Augustine, R.; Aqel, A. H.; Kalva, S. N.; Joshy, K. S.; Nayeem, A.; Hasan, A. Bioengineered Microfluidic Blood-Brain Barrier Models in Oncology Research. *Transl. Oncol*. **2021,** *14* (7), 101087.
9. Smith, W. R.; Hudson, P. W.; Ponce, B. A.; Rajaram Manoharan, S. R. Nanotechnology in Orthopedics: A Clinically Oriented Review. *BMC Musculoskelet Disord.* **2018,** *19* (1), 67.
10. Gendelman, H. E.; Anantharam, V.; Bronich, T.; Ghaisas, S.; Jin, H.; Kanthasamy, A. G. et al. Nanoneuromedicines for Degenerative, Inflammatory, and Infectious Nervous System Diseases. *Nanomed. Nanotechnol. Biol. Med.* **2015,** *11* (3), 751–767.
11. Joshi, M.; Pathak, K.; Dhaneshwar, S. Nanotechnology-Based Strategies for Effective Delivery of Phytoconstituents for the Management of Rheumatoid Arthritis. *Pharmacol. Res.—Modern Chinese Med.* **2022,** *2*, 100061.
12. Bayda, S.; Adeel, M.; Tuccinardi, T.; Cordani, M.; Rizzolio, F. The History of Nanoscience and Nanotechnology: From Chemical—Physical Applications to Nanomedicine. *Molecules* **2019,** *25* (1), 112.
13. Soares, S.; Sousa, J.; Pais, A.; Vitorino, C. Nanomedicine: Principles, Properties, and Regulatory Issues. *Front. Chem*. **2018,** *6*, 360.
14. Lombardo, D.; Kiselev, M. A.; Caccamo, M. T. Smart Nanoparticles for Drug Delivery Application: Development of Versatile Nanocarrier Platforms in Biotechnology and Nanomedicine. *J. Nanomater*. **2019,** *2019*, 1–26.
15. Kaur, I. P.; Bhandari, R.; Bhandari, S.; Kakkar, V. Potential of Solid Lipid Nanoparticles in Brain Targeting. *J. Controll. Release*. **2008,** *127* (2), 97–109.
16. Silva, G. A. Nanotechnology Approaches to Crossing the Blood-Brain Barrier and Drug Delivery to the CNS. *BMC Neurosci*. **2008,** *9* (S3), S4.
17. Teleanu, D. M.; Negut, I.; Grumezescu, V.; Grumezescu, A. M.; Teleanu, R. I. Nanomaterials for Drug Delivery to the Central Nervous System. *Nanomaterials* **2019,** *9* (3), 371.
18. Virmani, R.; Virmani, T.; Pathak, K. Chapter 17—Nanovesicles for Delivery of Central Nervous System Drugs. In: *Applications of Nanovesicular Drug Delivery*; Nayak, A. K., Hasnain, M. S., Aminabhavi, T. M., Torchilin, V. P., Eds.; Academic Press; 2022; pp 315–339. https://www.sciencedirect.com/science/article/pii/B9780323918657000043
19. Li, B.; Armstead. Nanomedicine as an Emerging Approach Against Intracellular Pathogens. *IJN*. **2011,** 3281.
20. Jain, K. K. Nanobiotechnology-Based Strategies for Crossing the Blood-Brain Barrier. *Nanomedicine* **2012,** *7* (8), 1225–1233.
21. Fischer, N. O.; Weilhammer, D. R.; Dunkle, A.; Thomas, C.; Hwang, M.; Corzett, M. et al. Evaluation of Nanolipoprotein Particles (NLPs) as an In Vivo Delivery Platform. *PLOS ONE* **2014,** *9* (3), e93342.
22. Gilmore, S. F.; Blanchette, C. D.; Scharadin, T. M.; Hura, G. L.; Rasley, A.; Corzett, M. et al. Lipid Cross-Linking of Nanolipoprotein Particles Substantially Enhances Serum Stability and Cellular Uptake. *ACS Appl. Mater. Interfaces* **2016,** *8* (32), 20549–20557.
23. Chen, Y.; Liu, L. Modern Methods for Delivery of Drugs Across the Blood-Brain Barrier. *Adv. Drug Deliv. Rev.* **2012,** *64* (7), 640–665.

24. Athira, S.; Prajitha, N.; Mohanan, P. Interaction of Nanoparticles with Central Nervous System and Its Consequences. *Am. J. Res. Med. Sci.* **2018,** *3* (1), 12.
25. Laron, Z. Insulin and the Brain. *Arch. Physiol. Biochem*. **2009,** *115* (2), 112–116.
26. De Jong, W. H.; Borm, P. J. A. Drug Delivery and Nanoparticles: Applications and Hazards. *Int. J. Nanomed*. **2008,** *3* (2):133–149.
27. Meyers, J. D.; Doane, T.; Burda, C.; Basilion, J. P. Nanoparticles for Imaging and Treating Brain Cancer. *Nanomedicine* **2013,** *8* (1), 123–143.
28. Malam, Y.; Loizidou, M.; Seifalian, A. M. Liposomes and Nanoparticles: Nanosized Vehicles for Drug Delivery in Cancer. *Trends Pharmacol. Sci.* **2009,** *30* (11), 592–599.
29. Tietze, R.; Zaloga, J.; Unterweger, H.; Lyer, S.; Friedrich, R. P.; Janko, C. et al. Magnetic Nanoparticle-Based Drug Delivery for Cancer Therapy. *Biochem. Biophys. Res. Commun.* **2015,** *468* (3), 463–470.
30. Harris, L. A.; Goff, J. D.; Carmichael, A. Y.; Riffle, J. S.; Harburn, J. J.; St Pierre, T. et al. Magnetite Nanoparticle Dispersions Stabilized with Triblock Copolymers. *Chem. Mater*. **2003,** *15* (6), 1367–1377.
31. Zhang, X.; Xie, Y.; Jin, Y.; Hou, X.; Ye, L.; Lou, J. The Effect of RMP-7 and Its Derivative on Transporting Evans Blue Liposomes into the Brain. *Drug Deliv.* **2004,** *11* (5), 301–309.
32. Batrakova, E. V.; Vinogradov, S. V.; Robinson, S. M.; Niehoff, M. L.; Banks, W. A.; Kabanov, A. V. Polypeptide Point Modifications with Fatty Acid and Amphiphilic Block Copolymers for Enhanced Brain Delivery. *Bioconjug. Chem.* **2005,** *16* (4), 793–802.
33. Naqvi, S.; Panghal, A.; Flora SJS. Nanotechnology: A Promising Approach for Delivery of Neuroprotective Drugs. *Front. Neurosci.***2020,** 14. https://www.frontiersin.org/articles/10.3389/fnins.2020.00494/full
34. Saeedi, M.; Eslamifar, M.; Khezri, K.; Dizaj, S. M. Applications of Nanotechnology in Drug Delivery to the Central Nervous System. *Biomed. Pharmacother*. **2019,** *111*, 666–675.
35. Zingale, E.; Bonaccorso, A.; Carbone, C.; Musumeci, T.; Pignatello, R. Drug Nanocrystals: Focus on Brain Delivery from Therapeutic to Diagnostic Applications. *Pharmaceutics* **2022,** *14* (4), 691.
36. Satapathy, M. K.; Yen, T. L.; Jan, J. S.; Tang, R. D.; Wang, J. Y.; Taliyan, R. et al. Solid Lipid Nanoparticles (SLNs): An Advanced Drug Delivery System Targeting Brain Through BBB. *Pharmaceutics* **2021,** *13* (8), 1183.
37. Gastaldi, L.; Battaglia, L.; Peira, E.; Chirio, D.; Muntoni, E.; Solazzi, I. et al. Solid Lipid Nanoparticles as Vehicles of Drugs to the Brain: Current State of the Art. *Eur. J. Pharm. Biopharm*. **2014,** *87* (3), 433–444.
38. Yusuf, M.; Khan, M.; Khan, R. A.; Ahmed, B. Preparation, Characterization, In Vivo and Biochemical Evaluation of Brain Targeted Piperine Solid Lipid Nanoparticles in an Experimentally Induced Alzheimer's Disease Model. *J. Drug Target*. **2013,** *21* (3), 300–311.
39. Dhawan, S.; Kapil, R.; Singh, B. Formulation Development and Systematic Optimization of Solid Lipid Nanoparticles of Quercetin for Improved Brain Delivery. *J. Pharm. Pharmacol*. **2011,** *63* (3), 342–351.
40. Arora, D.; Bhatt, S.; Kumar, M.; Verma, R.; Taneja, Y.; Kaushal, N. et al. QbD-Based Rivastigmine Tartrate-Loaded Solid Lipid Nanoparticles for Enhanced Intranasal Delivery to the Brain for Alzheimer's Therapeutics. *Front. Aging Neurosci.*. **2022,** 14. https://www.frontiersin.org/articles/10.3389/fnagi.2022.960246
41. Garg, J.; Pathania, K.; Sah, S. P.; Pawar, S. V. Nanostructured Lipid Carriers: A Promising Drug Carrier for Targeting Brain Tumours. *Future J. Pharm. Sci*. **2022,** *8* (1), 25.

42. Eleraky, E. N.; Omar, M. M.; Mahmoud, A. H.; Abou-Taleb, A. H. Nanostructured Lipid Carriers to Mediate Brain Delivery of Temazepam: Design and In Vivo Study. *Pharmaceutics* **2020,** *12* (5), 451.
43. Annu, Rehman, S.; Md, S.; Baboota, S.; Ali, J. Analyzing Nanotheraputics-Based Approaches for the Management of Psychotic Disorders. *J. Pharm. Sci.* **2019,** *108* (12), 3757–3768.
44. Clark, A. J.; Davis, M. E. Increased Brain Uptake of Targeted Nanoparticles by Adding an Acid-Cleavable Linkage Between Transferrin and the Nanoparticle Core. *Proc. Natl. Acad. Sci. USA* **2015,** *112* (40), 12486–12491.
45. Khan, S. A.; Rehman, S.; Nabi, B.; Iqubal, A.; Nehal, N.; Fahmy, U. A. et al. Boosting the Brain Delivery of Atazanavir through Nanostructured Lipid Carrier-Based Approach for Mitigating NeuroAIDS. *Pharmaceutics* **2020,** *12* (11), 1059.
46. Nair, S. C.; Vinayan, K. P.; Mangalathillam, S. Nose to Brain Delivery of Phenytoin Sodium Loaded Nano Lipid Carriers: Formulation, Drug Release, Permeation and In Vivo Pharmacokinetic Studies. *Pharmaceutics* **2021,** *13* (10), 1640.
47. Singh, S.; Virmani, T.; Kohli, K. Nanoemulsion System for Improvement of Raspberry Ketone Oral Bioavailability. *IGJPS* **2020,** *10* (01), 33–42.
48. Karami, Z.; Saghatchi Zanjani, M. R.; Hamidi, M. Nanoemulsions in CNS Drug Delivery: Recent Developments, Impacts and Challenges. *Drug Discov. Today* **2019,** *24* (5), 1104–1115.
49. Bahadur, S.; Pardhi, D. M.; Rautio, J.; Rosenholm, J. M.; Pathak, K. Intranasal Nanoemulsions for Direct Nose-to-Brain Delivery of Actives for CNS Disorders. *Pharmaceutics* **2020,** *12* (12).
50. Ashhar, M.; Vyas, P.; Vohora, D.; Sahoo, P.; Nigam, K.; Dang, S. et al. Amelioration of Oxidative Stress Utilizing Nanoemulsion Loaded with Bromocriptine and Glutathione for the Management of Parkinson's Disease. *Int. J. Pharm.* **2022,** *618*, 121683.
51. Song, Y.; Wang, X.; Wang, X.; Wang, J.; Hao, Q.; Hao, J. et al. Osthole-Loaded Nanoemulsion Enhances Brain Target in the Treatment of Alzheimer's Disease via Intranasal Administration. *Oxidative Med. Cell. Longevity* **2021,** *2021*, e8844455.
52. Jusril, N. A.; Abu Bakar, S. I.; Khalil, K. A.; Md Saad, W. M.; Wen, N. K.; Adenan, M. I. Development and Optimization of Nanoemulsion from Ethanolic Extract of Centella asiatica (NanoSECA) Using D-Optimal Mixture Design to Improve Blood-Brain Barrier Permeability. *Evid. Based Complement. Alternat. Med.* **2022,** *2022*, 3483511.
53. Pandian, S. R. K.; Vijayakumar, K. K.; Murugesan, S.; Kunjiappan, S. Liposomes: An Emerging Carrier for Targeting Alzheimer's and Parkinson's Diseases. *Heliyon* **2022,** *8* (6), e09575.
54. Virmani, T.; Kumar, G.; Virmani, R.; Sharma, A.; Pathak, K. Nanocarrier-Based Approaches to Combat Chronic Obstructive Pulmonary Disease. *Nanomedicine* **2022.**
55. Juhairiyah, F.; de Lange ECM. Understanding Drug Delivery to the Brain Using Liposome-Based Strategies: Studies that Provide Mechanistic Insights Are Essential. *AAPS, J.* **2021,** *23* (6), 114.
56. Vieira, D. B.; Gamarra, L. F. Getting into the Brain: Liposome-Based Strategies for Effective Drug Delivery Across the Blood–Brain Barrier. *Int. J. Nanomed.* **2016,** *11*, 5381–5414.
57. Misra, S.; Pathak, K. Functionalized Liposomes: A Nanovesicular System. In: 2022; pp 83–101.

58. Schmidt, J.; Metselaar, J. M.; Wauben, M. H. M.; Toyka, K. V.; Storm, G.; Gold, R. Drug Targeting by Long-Circulating Liposomal Glucocorticosteroids Increases Therapeutic Efficacy in a Model of Multiple Sclerosis. *Brain* **2003,** *126* (8), 1895–1904.
59. Rajput, A.; Butani, S. Donepezil HCl Liposomes: Development, Characterization, Cytotoxicity, and Pharmacokinetic Study. *AAPS PharmSciTech* **2022,** *23* (2), 74.
60. Arumugam, K.; Subramanian, G.; Mallayasamy, S.; Averineni, R.; Reddy, M.; Udupa, N. A Study of Rivastigmine Liposomes for Delivery into the Brain Through Intranasal Route. *Acta Pharm.* **2008,** *58* (3), 287–297.
61. Al Asmari, A. K.; Ullah, Z.; Tariq, M.; Fatani, A. Preparation, Characterization, and In Vivo Evaluation of Intranasally Administered Liposomal Formulation of Donepezil. *Drug Des. Devel. Ther.* **2016,** *10*, 205–215.
62. Gauro, R.; Nandave, M.; Jain, V. K.; Jain, K. Advances in Dendrimer-Mediated Targeted Drug Delivery to the Brain. *J. Nanopart. Res.* **2021,** *23* (3), 1–20.
63. Somani, S.; Dufès, C. Applications of Dendrimers for Brain Delivery and Cancer Therapy. *Nanomedicine* **2014,** *9* (15), 2403–2414.
64. Xu, X.; Li, J.; Han, S.; Tao, C.; Fang, L.; Sun, Y. et al. A Novel Doxorubicin Loaded Folic Acid Conjugated PAMAM Modified with Borneol, a Nature Dual-Functional Product of Reducing PAMAM Toxicity and Boosting BBB Penetration. *Eur. J. Pharm. Sci.* **2016,** *88*:178–190.
65. Gothwal, A.; Nakhate, K. T.; Alexander, A.; Ajazuddin null, Gupta, U. Boosted Memory and Improved Brain Bioavailability of Rivastigmine: Targeting Effort to the Brain Using Covalently Tethered Lower Generation PAMAM Dendrimers with Lactoferrin. *Mol. Pharm.* **2018,** *15* (10), 4538–4549.
66. Ghezzi, M.; Pescina, S.; Padula, C.; Santi, P.; del favero, E.; Cantu, L. et al. Polymeric Micelles in Drug Delivery: An Insight of the Techniques for Their Characterization and Assessment in Biorelevant Conditions. *J. Controll. Release* **2021,** *332*.
67. Virmani, R.; Pathak, K. Targeted Polymeric Micellar Systems for Respiratory Diseases. In: *Targeting Chronic Inflammatory Lung Diseases Using Advanced Drug Delivery Systems*; Elsevier; 2020; pp 411–39. https://linkinghub.elsevier.com/retrieve/pii/B9780128206584000200
68. Bawarski, W. E.; Chidlowsky, E.; Bharali, D. J.; Mousa, S. A. Emerging Nanopharmaceuticals. *Nanomed. Nanotechnol. Biol. Med.* **2008,** *4* (4), 273–282.
69. Kabanov, A. V.; Chekhonin, V. P.; Alakhov VYu, Batrakova, E. V.; Lebedev, A. S.; Melik-Nubarov, N. S. et al. The Neuroleptic Activity of Haloperidol Increases After Its Solubilization in Surfactant Micelles: Micelles as Microcontainers for Drug Targeting. *FEBS Lett.* **1989,** *258* (2), 343–345.
70. Abourehab, M. A.; Ahmed, O. A.; Balata, G. F.; Almalki, W. H. Self-Assembled Biodegradable Polymeric Micelles to Improve Dapoxetine Delivery Across the Blood–Brain Barrier. *Int. J. Nanomed.* **2018,** *13*, 3679–3687.
71. Liu, J. S.; Wang, J. H.; Zhou, J.; Tang, X. H.; Xu, L.; Shen, T. et al. Enhanced Brain Delivery of Lamotrigine with Pluronic® P123-Based Nanocarrier. *Int. J. Nanomed.* **2014,** *9*, 3923–3935.
72. Annu, Baboota, S.; Ali, J. Combination Antipsychotics Therapy for Schizophrenia and Related Psychotic Disorders Interventions: Emergence to Nanotechnology and Herbal Drugs. *J. Drug Deliv. Sci. Technol.* **2021,** *61*, 102272.
73. Annu, Sartaj, A.; Qamar, Z.; Md, S.; Alhakamy, N. A.; Baboota, S. et al. An Insight to Brain Targeting Utilizing Polymeric Nanoparticles: Effective Treatment Modalities for

Neurological Disorders and Brain Tumor. *Front. Bioeng. Biotechnol.* **2022,** 10. https://www.frontiersin.org/articles/10.3389/fbioe.2022.788128
74. Shakeri, S.; Ashrafizadeh, M.; Zarrabi, A.; Roghanian, R.; Afshar, E. G.; Pardakhty, A. et al. Multifunctional Polymeric Nanoplatforms for Brain Diseases Diagnosis, Therapy and Theranostics. *Biomedicines* **2020,** *8* (1), 13.
75. Zhao, Y.; Xiong, S.; Liu, P.; Liu, W.; Wang, Q.; Liu, Y. et al. Polymeric Nanoparticles-Based Brain Delivery with Improved Therapeutic Efficacy of Ginkgolide B in Parkinson's Disease. *IJN.* **2020,** *15*, 10453–10467.
76. Sardoiwala, M. N.; Kaundal, B.; Roy Choudhury, S. Development of Engineered Nanoparticles Expediting Diagnostic and Therapeutic Applications Across Blood–Brain Barrier. In: *Handbook of Nanomaterials for Industrial Applications*; Elsevier, 2018; pp 696–709. https://linkinghub.elsevier.com/retrieve/pii/B9780128133514000389
77. Krishna, K. V.; Wadhwa, G.; Alexander, A.; Kanojia, N.; Saha, R. N.; Kukreti, R. et al. Design and Biological Evaluation of Lipoprotein-Based Donepezil Nanocarrier for Enhanced Brain Uptake through Oral Delivery. *ACS Chem. Neurosci.* **2019,** *10* (9), 4124–4135.
78. Shah, P.; Dubey, P.; Vyas, B.; Kaul, A.; Mishra, A. K.; Chopra, D. et al. Lamotrigine Loaded PLGA Nanoparticles Intended for Direct Nose to Brain Delivery in Epilepsy: Pharmacokinetic, Pharmacodynamic and Scintigraphy Study. *Artif. Cells Nanomed. Biotechnol.* **2021,** *49* (1), 511–522.
79. Misra, S. K.; Pathak, K. Chapter 10 - Drug nanocrystals as Drug Delivery Systems. In: *Industrial Applications of Nanocrystals*; Mallakpour, S., Hussain, C. M., Eds.; Elsevier, 2022; pp 153–78. https://www.sciencedirect.com/science/article/pii/B9780128240243000269
80. Jahangir, M. A.; Imam, S. S.; Muheem, A.; Chettupalli, A.; Al-Abbasi, F. A.; Nadeem, M. S. et al. Nanocrystals: Characterization Overview, Applications in Drug Delivery, and Their Toxicity Concerns. *J. Pharm. Innov.* **2022,** *17* (1), 237–248.
81. Xiong, S.; Liu, W.; Zhou, Y.; Mo, Y.; Liu, Y.; Chen, X. et al. Enhancement of Oral Bioavailability and Anti-Parkinsonian Efficacy of Resveratrol Through a Nanocrystal Formulation. *Asian J. Pharm. Sci.* **2020,** *15* (4), 518–528.
82. Gol, D et al. Nanocrystal-Based Drug Delivery System of Risperidone: Lyophilization and Characterization. *Drug Dev. Ind. Pharm.*. **2018,** *44* (9). https://pubmed.ncbi.nlm.nih.gov/29619857/
83. Guo, Q.; Shen, X. T.; Li, Y. Y.; Xu, S. Q. Carbon Nanotubes-Based Drug Delivery to Cancer and Brain. *J. Huazhong Univ. Sci. Technol. Med. Sci.* **2017,** *37* (5), 635–641.
84. Pathak, K.; Kumar, M.; Misha, S.; Kaushal, N. Carbon Based Nanomaterials Potential Therapeutic applications. In: 2022; pp 1–23.
85. Murjani, B. O.; Kadu, P. S.; Bansod, M.; Vaidya, S. S.; Yadav, M. D. Carbon nanotubes in Biomedical Applications: Current Status, Promises, and Challenges. *Carbon Lett.* **2022,** *32* (5), 1207–1226.
86. Costa, P. M.; Wang, J. T. W.; Morfin, J. F.; Khanum, T.; To, W.; Sosabowski, J. et al. Functionalised Carbon Nanotubes Enhance Brain Delivery of Amyloid-Targeting Pittsburgh Compound B (PiB)-Derived Ligands. *Nanotheranostics* **2018,** *2* (2):168.
87. Han, H.; Mann, A.; Ekstein, D.; Eyal, S. Breaking Bad: The Structure and Function of the Blood-Brain Barrier in Epilepsy. *AAPS, J.* **2017,** *19* (4), 973–988.
88. Waris, A.; Ali, A.; Khan, A. U.; Asim, M.; Zamel, D.; Fatima, K. et al. Applications of Various Types of Nanomaterials for the Treatment of Neurological Disorders. *Nanomaterials (Basel)* **2022,** *12* (13), 2140.

89. Chandrakala, V.; Aruna, V.; Angajala, G. Review on Metal Nanoparticles as Nanocarriers: Current Challenges and Perspectives in Drug Delivery Systems. Emergent Mater. 2022. https://doi.org/10.1007/s42247-021-00335-x
90. Gonzalez-Carter, D. A.; Leo, B. F.; Ruenraroengsak, P.; Chen, S.; Goode, A. E.; Theodorou, I. G. et al. Silver Nanoparticles Reduce Brain Inflammation and Related Neurotoxicity Through Induction of H2S-Synthesizing Enzymes. *Sci. Rep.* **2017,** *7* (1), 42871.
91. Male, D.; Gromnicova, R.; McQuaid, C. Gold Nanoparticles for Imaging and Drug Transport to the CNS. In: *International Review of Neurobiology*; Elsevier, 2016; pp 155–98. https://linkinghub.elsevier.com/retrieve/pii/S0074774216301064
92. Zhang, D.; Zhang, J.; Zeng, J.; Li, Z.; Zuo, H.; Huang, C. et al. Nano-Gold Loaded with Resveratrol Enhance the Anti-Hepatoma Effect of Resveratrol In Vitro and In Vivo. *J. Biomed Nanotechnol.* **2019,** *15* (2), 288–300.
93. Hou, K.; Zhao, J.; Wang, H.; Li, B.; Li, K.; Shi, X. et al. Chiral Gold Nanoparticles Enantioselectively Rescue Memory Deficits in a Mouse Model of Alzheimer's Disease. *Nat Commun.* **2020,***11* (1), 4790.
94. Vinzant, N.; Scholl, J. L.; Wu, C. M.; Kindle, T.; Koodali, R.; Forster, G. L. Iron Oxide Nanoparticle Delivery of Peptides to the Brain: Reversal of Anxiety during Drug Withdrawal. *Front. Neurosci.* **2017,** *11.* https://www.frontiersin.org/articles/10.3389/fnins.2017.00608
95. Sharma, H. S.; Sharma, A. Nanowired Drug Delivery for Neuroprotection in Central Nervous System Injuries: Modulation by Environmental Temperature, Intoxication of Nanoparticles, and Comorbidity Factors. *WIREs Nanomed. Nanobiotechnol.* **2012,** *4* (2),184–203.
96. Singh, B.; Kim, K.; Park, M. H. On-Demand Drug Delivery Systems Using Nanofibers. *Nanomaterials (Basel)* **2021,** *11* (12), 3411.
97. AnjiReddy, K.; Karpagam, S. Chitosan Nanofilm and Electrospun Nanofiber for Quick Drug Release in the Treatment of Alzheimer's Disease: In Vitro and In Vivo Evaluation. *Int. J. Biol. Macromol.* **2017,** *105*, 131–142.
98. Yasir, M.; Sara, U. V. S.; Chauhan, I.; Gaur, P. K.; Singh, A. P.; Puri, D. et al. Solid Lipid Nanoparticles for Nose to Brain Delivery of Donepezil: Formulation, Optimization by Box–Behnken Design, In Vitro and In Vivo Evaluation. *Artif. Cells Nanomed. Biotechnol.* **2018,** *46* (8), 1838–1851.
99. Dudhipala, N.; Gorre, T. Neuroprotective Effect of Ropinirole Lipid Nanoparticles Enriched Hydrogel for Parkinson's Disease: In Vitro, Ex Vivo, Pharmacokinetic and Pharmacodynamic Evaluation. *Pharmaceutics* **2020,** *12* (5), 448.
100. Uppuluri, C. T.; Ravi, P. R.; Dalvi, A. V. Design, Optimization and Pharmacokinetic Evaluation of Piribedil Loaded Solid Lipid Nanoparticles Dispersed in Nasal In Situ Gelling System for Effective Management of Parkinson's Disease. *Int. J. Pharm.* **2021,** *606*, 120881.
101. Clemente, N.; Ferrara, B.; Gigliotti, C. L.; Boggio, E.; Capucchio, M. T.; Biasibetti, E. et al. Solid Lipid Nanoparticles Carrying Temozolomide for Melanoma Treatment. Preliminary In Vitro and In Vivo Studies. *Int. J. Mol. Sci.* **2018,** *19* (2), 255.
102. Pinheiro, R. G. R.; Granja, A.; Loureiro, J. A.; Pereira, M. C.; Pinheiro, M.; Neves, A. R. et al. Quercetin Lipid Nanoparticles Functionalized with Transferrin for Alzheimer's Disease. *Eur. J. Pharm. Sci.* **2020,** *148*, 105314.
103. Martins, S. M.; Sarmento, B.; Nunes, C.; Lúcio, M.; Reis, S.; Ferreira, D. C. Brain Targeting Effect of Camptothecin-Loaded Solid Lipid Nanoparticles in Rat After Intravenous Administration. *Eur. J. Pharm. Biopharm.* **2013,** *85* (3), 488–502.

104. Abo El-Enin, H. A.; Elkomy, M. H.; Naguib, I. A.; Ahmed, M. F.; Alsaidan, O. A.; Alsalahat, I. et al. Lipid Nanocarriers Overlaid with Chitosan for Brain Delivery of Berberine via the Nasal Route. *Pharmaceuticals (Basel)* **2022,** *15* (3), 281.
105. Wu, Y.; Song, X.; Kebebe, D.; Li, X.; Xue, Z.; Li, J. et al. Brain targeting of Baicalin and Salvianolic Acid B Combination by OX26 Functionalized Nanostructured Lipid Carriers. *Int. J. Pharm.* **2019,** *571*, 118754.
106. Khan, A.; Imam, S. S.; Aqil, M.; Ahad, A.; Sultana, Y.; Ali, A. et al. Brain Targeting of Temozolomide via the Intranasal Route Using Lipid-Based Nanoparticles: Brain Pharmacokinetic and Scintigraphic Analyses. *Mol. Pharm.* **2016,** *13* (11), 3773–3782.
107. Sharma, N.; Bhandari, S.; Deshmukh, R.; Yadav, A. K.; Mishra, N. Development and Characterization of Embelin-Loaded Nanolipid Carriers for Brain Targeting. *Artif. Cells Nanomed. Biotechnol.* **2017,** *45* (3), 409–413.
108. Rehman, S.; Nabi, B.; Javed, A.; Khan, T.; Iqubal, A.; Ansari, M. J. et al. Unraveling Enhanced Brain Delivery of Paliperidone-Loaded Lipid Nanoconstructs: Pharmacokinetic, Behavioral, Biochemical, and Histological Aspects. *Drug Deliv.* 29 (1):1409–22.
109. Madane, R. G.; Mahajan, H. S. Curcumin-Loaded Nanostructured Lipid Carriers (NLCs) for Nasal Administration: Design, Characterization, and In Vivo Study. *Drug Deliv.* **2016,** *23* (4), 1326–1334.
110. Cunha, S.; Costa, C. P.; Loureiro, J. A.; Alves, J.; Peixoto, A. F.; Forbes, B. et al. Double Optimization of Rivastigmine-Loaded Nanostructured Lipid Carriers (NLC) for Nose-to-Brain Delivery Using the Quality by Design (QbD) Approach: Formulation Variables and Instrumental Parameters. *Pharmaceutics* **2020,** *12* (7), 599.
111. Parikh, R. H.; Patel, R. J. Nanoemulsions for Intranasal Delivery of Riluzole to Improve Brain Bioavailability: Formulation Development and Pharmacokinetic Studies. *Curr. Drug Deliv.* *13* (7), 1130–1143.
112. Vasdev, N.; Handa, M.; Kesharwani, P.; Shukla, R. Rosemary Oil Low Energy Nanoemulsion: Optimization, µrheology, In Silico, In Vitro, and Ex Vivo Characterization. *J. Biomater. Sci.* **2022,** i (0), 1–23.
113. Espinoza, L. C.; Silva-Abreu, M.; Clares, B.; Rodríguez-Lagunas, M. J.; Halbaut, L.; Cañas, M. A. et al. Formulation Strategies to Improve Nose-to-Brain Delivery of Donepezil. *Pharmaceutics* **2019,** *11* (2), 64.
114. Kotta, S.; Mubarak Aldawsari, H.; Badr-Eldin, S. M.; Alhakamy, N. A.; Md, S. Coconut Oil-Based Resveratrol Nanoemulsion: Optimization Using Response Surface Methodology, Stability Assessment and Pharmacokinetic Evaluation. *Food Chem.* **2021,** *357*, 129721.
115. Haider, Md. F.; Khan, S.; Gaba, B.; Alam, T.; Baboota, S.; Ali, J. et al. Optimization of Rivastigmine Nanoemulsion for Enhanced Brain Delivery: In Vivo and Toxicity Evaluation. *J. Mol. Liquids* **2018,** *255*, 384–396.
116. Iqbal, R.; Ahmed, S.; Jain, G. K.; Vohora, D. Design and Development of Letrozole Nanoemulsion: A Comparative Evaluation of Brain Targeted Nanoemulsion with Free Letrozole Against Status Epilepticus and Neurodegeneration in Mice. *Int. J. Pharm.* **2019,** *565*, 20–32.
117. Patel, R. J.; Parikh, R. H. Intranasal Delivery of Topiramate Nanoemulsion: Pharmacodynamic, Pharmacokinetic and Brain Uptake Studies. *Int. J. Pharm.* **2020,** *585*, 119486.
118. Rompicherla, S. K. L.; Arumugam, K.; Bojja, S. L.; Kumar, N.; Rao, C. M. Pharmacokinetic and Pharmacodynamic Evaluation of Nasal Liposome and Nanoparticle

Based Rivastigmine Formulations in Acute and Chronic Models of Alzheimer's Disease. *Naunyn-Schmiedeberg's Arch Pharmacol.* **2021,** *394* (8), 1737–1755.

119. Shariare, M. H.; Rahman, M.; Lubna, S. R.; Roy, R. S.; Abedin, J.; Marzan, A. L. et al. Liposomal Drug Delivery of Aphanamixis Polystachya Leaf Extracts and Its Neurobehavioral Activity in Mice Model. *Sci. Rep.* **2020,** *10* (1), 6938.
120. Singh, V.; Krishan, P.; Shri, R. Amelioration of Ischaemia Reperfusion-Induced Cerebral Injury in Mice by Liposomes Containing *Allium cepa* Fraction Administered Intranasally. *Artif. Cells Nanomed. Biotechnol.* **2018,** *46* (sup3), S982–S992.
121. Singh, A. K.; Gothwal, A.; Rani, S.; Rana, M.; Sharma, A. K.; Yadav, A. K. et al. Dendrimer Donepezil Conjugates for Improved Brain Delivery and Better In Vivo Pharmacokinetics. *ACS Omega* **2019,** *4* (3):4519–4529.
122. Bhanderi, M.; Shah, J.; Gorain, B.; Nair, A. B.; Jacob, S.; Asdaq, S. M. B. et al. Optimized Rivastigmine Nanoparticles Coated with Eudragit for Intranasal Application to Brain Delivery: Evaluation and Nasal Ciliotoxicity Studies. *Materials (Basel).* **2021,** *14* (21), 6291.
123. Meteoglu, I.; Erdemir, A. Genistein and Temozolomide-Loaded Polymeric Nanoparticles: A Synergistic Approach For Improved Anti-Tumor Efficacy Against Glioblastoma. *Process Biochem.* **2021,** *110*, 9–18.
124. Barcia, E.; Boeva, L.; García-García, L.; Slowing, K.; Fernández-Carballido, A.; Casanova, Y. et al. Nanotechnology-Based Drug Delivery of Ropinirole for Parkinson's Disease. *Drug Deliv.* **2017,** *24* (1), 1112–1123.
125. Madhu, S.; Komala, M.; Pandian, P. Formulation Development and Characterization of Withaferin-A Loaded Polymeric Nanoparticles for Alzheimer's Disease. *BioNanoSci.* **2021,** *11* (2), 559–566.
126. Liu, Y.; Liu, W.; Xiong, S.; Luo, J.; Li, Y.; Zhao, Y. et al. Highly Stabilized Nanocrystals Delivering Ginkgolide B in Protecting Against the Parkinson's Disease. *Int. J. Pharm.* **2020,** *577*, 119053.
127. Xiong, S.; Liu, W.; Li, D.; Chen, X.; Liu, F.; Yuan, D. et al. Oral Delivery of Puerarin Nanocrystals To Improve Brain Accumulation and Anti-Parkinsonian Efficacy. *Mol. Pharma.* **2019,** *16* (4), 1444–1455.
128. Mittapelly, N.; Thalla, M.; Pandey, G.; Banala, V. T.; Sharma, S.; Arya, A. et al. Long Acting Ionically Paired Embonate Based Nanocrystals of Donepezil for the Treatment of Alzheimer's Disease: a Proof of Concept Study. *Pharm. Res.* **2017,** *34* (11), 2322–2335.
129. Tashan, E.; Karakucuk, A.; Celebi, N. Development of Nanocrystal Ziprasidone Orally Disintegrating Tablets: Optimization by Using Design of Experiment and In Vitro Evaluation. *AAPS PharmSciTech.* **2020,** *21* (3), 115.
130. Virmani, T.; Kumar, G.; Pathak, K. Non-Aqueous Nanoemulsions: An Innovative Lipid-Based Drug Carrier; Advancements in Controlled Drug Delivery Systems. IGI Global, 2022; pp 134–58. https://www.igi-global.com/chapter/non-aqueous-nanoemulsions/www.igi-global.com/chapter/non-aqueous-nanoemulsions/300404
131. Kumar, G.; Virmani, T.; Pathak, K.; Alhalmi, A. A Revolutionary Blueprint for Mitigation of Hypertension via Nanoemulsion. *BioMed Res. Int.* **2022,** *2022*, e4109874.
132. Joseph, A.; Nance, E. Nanotherapeutics and the Brain. *Annu. Rev. Chem. Biomol. Eng.* **2022,** *13*, 325–346.
133. Farjadian, F.; Ghasemi, A.; Gohari, O.; Roointan, A.; Karimi, M.; Hamblin, M. R. Nanopharmaceuticals and Nanomedicines Currently on the Market: Challenges and Opportunities. *Nanomedicine* **2019,** *14* (1), 93–126.

134. Patra, J. K.; Das, G.; Fraceto, L. F.; Campos, E. V. R.; Rodriguez-Torres M del, P.; Acosta-Torres, L. S. et al. Nano Based Drug Delivery Systems: Recent Developments and Future Prospects. *J. Nanobiotechnol.* **2018,** *16*, 71.
135. Sharma, S.; Parveen, R.; Chatterji, B. P. Toxicology of Nanoparticles in Drug Delivery. *Curr. Pathobiol. Rep.* **2021,** *9* (4), 133–144.
136. Pathak, K.; Raghuvanshi, S. Oral Bioavailability: Issues and Solutions via Nanoformulations. *Clin. Pharmacokinet.* **2015,** *54* (4), 325–357.
137. Dhiman, N.; Awasthi, R.; Sharma, B.; Kharkwal, H.; Kulkarni, G. T. Lipid Nanoparticles as Carriers for Bioactive Delivery. *Front. Chem.* 2021; p 9. https://www.frontiersin.org/articles/10.3389/fchem.2021.580118
138. Tang, J.; Xiong, L.; Wang, S.; Wang, J.; Liu, L.; Li, J. et al. Distribution, Translocation and Accumulation of Silver Nanoparticles in Rats. *J. Nanosci. Nanotechnol.* **2009,** *9* (8), 4924–4932.
139. Ma, L.; Liu, J.; Li, N.; Wang, J.; Duan, Y.; Yan, J. et al. Oxidative Stress in the Brain of Mice Caused by Translocated Nanoparticulate TiO_2 Delivered to the Abdominal Cavity. *Biomaterials* **2010,** *31* (1), 99–105.
140. Sarma, A.; Bania, R.; Devi, J. R.; Deka, S. Therapeutic Nanostructures and Nanotoxicity. *J. Appl. Toxicol.* **2021,** *41* (10), 1494–1517.
141. Gholamine, B.; Karimi, I.; Salimi, A.; Mazdarani, P.; Becker, L. A. Neurobehavioral Toxicity of Carbon Nanotubes in Mice: Focus on Brain-Derived Neurotrophic Factor Messenger RNA and protein. *Toxicol. Ind. Health.* **2017,** *33* (4), 340–350.
142. Kobayashi, N.; Izumi, H.; Morimoto, Y. Review of Toxicity Studies of Carbon Nanotubes. *J. Occup. Health.* **2017,** *59* (5), 394–407.
143. Kavosi, A.; Hosseini Ghale Noei, S.; Madani, S.; Khalighfard, S.; Khodayari, S.; Khodayari, H. et al. The Toxicity and Therapeutic Effects of Single-and Multi-Wall Carbon Nanotubes on Mice Breast Cancer. *Sci Rep.* **2018,** *8* (1), 8375.

CHAPTER 8

Current Trends in Drug-Nano Formulations Directed to the Brain

DIGNESH KHUNT[1], BRIJESH SHAH[2], SMIT NAYI[1], AKSHAY PARIHAR[3], and BHUPENDRA G. PRAJAPATI[4,5]

[1]*Graduate School of Pharmacy, Gujarat Technological University, Gandhinagar, Gujarat, India*

[2]*Postdoctoral Scholar at Anodyne Nanotech-Tufts University, Faculty of Technology, University College of Technology, Boston, Massachusetts, United States*

[3]*Faculty of Pharmaceutical Sciences, The ICFAI university, Himachal Pradesh*

[4]*Shree S.K. Patel College of Pharmaceutical Education and Research, Ganpat University, Mehsana, Gujarat, India*

[5]*Faculty of Pharmacy, Silpakorn University, Nakhon Pathom, Thailand*

ABSTRACT

The central nervous system (CNS) is one of the most essential and vital neurological systems, comprised of the brain and the spinal cord, which governs and maintains the body's basic functioning. After cardiovascular disease, treating neurological problems is the second-largest area of therapy. There is a unique membrane barrier known as the blood–brain barrier (BBB) that separates the sensitive brain from the circulating blood. This barrier inhibits the successful treatment of many serious and life-threatening neurological illnesses. Because of the BBB and the blood-cerebrospinal fluid barrier (BCSFB), it is challenging to get medications into the CNS to

Nanomedicine for Neurodegenerative Disorders: Selective Treatment Strategies. Rishabha Malviya, Kamla Pathak, & Swati Verma (Eds.)

treat neurological disorders. Nanotechnology has emerged as a fascinating and promising new paradigm for managing neurological disorders, and this technology has shown enormous promise in overcoming the limits associated with current therapeutic approaches. Nanotechnology allows for the customization of molecules to serve a wide variety of functions, including transporting genes, promoting neuron regeneration and cell survival, crossing the BBB, and targeting specific cells or signaling pathways in response to endogenous stimuli. The ability of nanocarrier systems such as microemulsion, liposomes, lipid nanoparticles (LNPs), polymeric micelles, dendrimers, etc. to transport a variety of neurotherapeutics to the brain has been highlighted in this book chapter.

8.1 INTRODUCTION

The central nervous system (CNS) is an important neurological system that is responsible for coordinating and sustaining the fundamental activities of the body. The CNS is composed of the brain and the spinal cord. More commonly referred to as neurological problems, diseases of the CNS and the brain, such as Alzheimer's disease (AD), Parkinson's disease, epilepsy, HIV infection of the brain, schizophrenia, mental disorders, etc., affect more than a hundred million people all over the world and are responsible for the requirement of prolonged therapy.[1,2] Neurological problem treatment is second only to cardiology. Despite substantial research, various aspects draw great attention to producing a viable neurological drug therapy for brain disorders and delivery methods. Due to the brain's complex physiology, which includes biological barriers at the blood-brain interface, drug transport to the CNS remains a mystery. These biological barriers govern ion and molecule flow into and out of the CNS. Due to these protective barriers, most neuropharmaceuticals cannot achieve therapeutic concentration at the brain interface.[3,4]

Being one of the most important, delicate, and intricate organs, the human brain is uniquely protected from the flow of blood by several layers of tissue. The brain acts as the body's control hub, orchestrating both conscious and unconscious activities. It also stores the data and sends out signals to the rest of the body.[5,6] It is still a mystery how drugs may be delivered directly to the CNS despite the number of technologies that are now available for brain targeting. There are many different biological barriers that act as a specialized interface between the systemic circulation and the parenchyma of the brain. These barriers are located throughout the body. Because of these obstacles, drugs cannot be transported properly to the CNS via the circulatory system. There are three barriers that exist between the blood and the brain. These barriers are referred to as the blood–brain barrier (BBB), the blood-cerebrospinal fluid barrier (BCSFB), and the blood–tumor barrier. In addition to these barriers, a variety of efflux transporter proteins, such as P-glyco protein (Pgp), multidrug resistance protein (MRP), and breast cancer-resistant protein (BCRP), also serve as a gatekeeper, which further inhibits the capability of drug molecules to reach the brain.[2,7–9]

When neurotherapeutics are given in a conventional manner to manage neurological disorders, they enter the brain through the systemic circulation. It is necessary to enhance the systemic drug levels by increasing the frequency of dosage or by administering the medication for a longer period of time to achieve effective therapeutic concentration at the target location. This frequently leads to a rise in the overall amount of toxicity.[10,11] As a result, there is a requirement for the development of techniques that can transport medications into the CNS without raising the amount of those drugs in the system. Therefore, researchers are focusing on developing innovative techniques, nanocarrier systems, and drug targeting systems that can deliver bioactives to the brain in an accurate manner either by circumventing the BBB or by using any other alternative route, such as intranasal drug-delivery systems.[7,10,12,13]

Nanoformulations are systems of the nanometer size, which can encapsulate both small and large molecules. To improve the therapeutic effectiveness and bioavailability of drugs across biological barriers such as the BBB, these colloidal formulations allow for the modification of their physicochemical characteristics and surface chemistry/functionality.[14] Drug nanocarriers have a wide range of applications, including drug stability, reduced toxic effects, the ability to overcome biological barriers, and enhanced targeting of the disease site.[9,15] Terms such as "nanoformulations," "nanocarriers," "nanoparticles," and "nanomedicines" are used interchangeably in this book chapter, although they all signify the same thing. At this point, the most important field of study is focused on increasing the adaptability of engineered nanomaterials by atomic-level manipulation of the size, shape, surface, and chemical characteristics of both organic and inorganic material. Nanomedicine is the designed nanomaterial that has been researched the most thoroughly, and it provides a wide range of benefits, including the delivery of genes, the treatment of cancer, biological imaging, the administration of drugs, and biosensing.[2]

Nanocarriers may be divided into three main categories: (1) Poymer-based nanocarriers [polymeric nanoparticles (NPs), polymeric micelles, dendrimer, and albumin nanoparticles], (2) Lipid-based nanocarriers [(liposomes, microemulsion, and lipid nanoparticles (LNP)], and (3) Nonpolymer-based NPs [gold nanoparticles (GNPs), carbon nanotubes (CNT), and quantum dots] which are illustrated in Figure 8.1. Apart from this antibody conjugate and viral NPs are also used for brain targeting.[7,15]

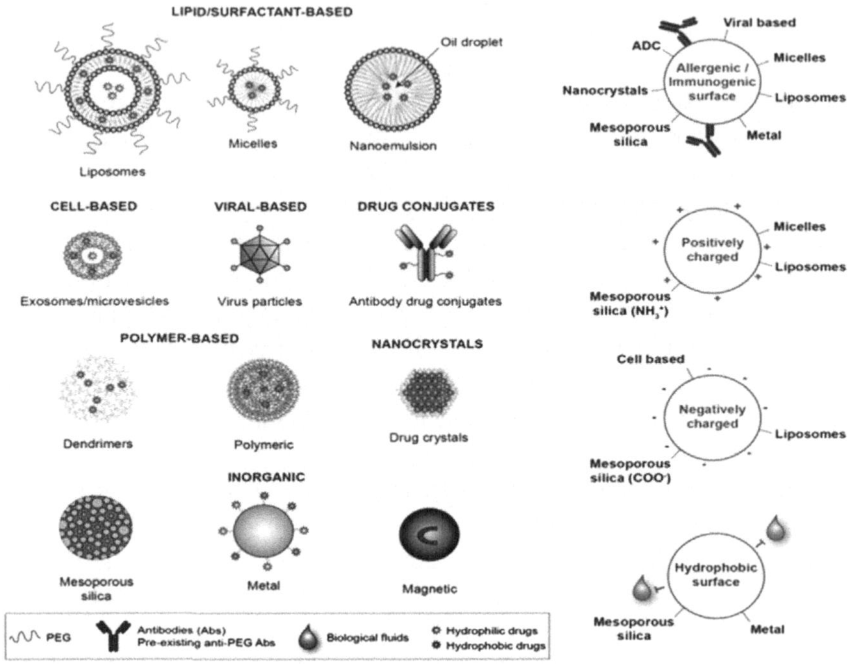

FIGURE 8.1 Graphical illustration of different type of nanoformulation.

Source: Reprinted with permission from Ref. [15]. Copyright © 2019 Elsevier B.V.

The current chapter briefly highlights the transport mechanism of drugs across the BBB. Different novel nanoformulations are also briefly discussed. The objective of the current book chapter was to give an idea about the current trend in drug nanoformulation for brain targeting.

8.2 TRANSPORT MECHANISMS FOR NANOCARRIERS TO CROSS THE BBB

The potential transport mechanism for crossing the BBB has facilitated diffusion, passive diffusion, transcellular diffusion, and active transport. Both active and passive diffusion of the material being transferred are involved in the process of transcellular transfer of substances. Macromolecules are transported by receptor-mediated transport, whereas Neurotransmitters, metabolites, amino acids, organic anions, and cations are transported via carrier proteins, and adenosine triphosphate binding cassette family proteins are involved in active transport across the BBB.[4,9]

P-glycoprotein and other members of the family of adenosine triphosphate binding cassette proteins are responsible for the impermeability of the BBB to drugs.[7] Drugs that can cross the BBB to treat CNS disorders remain an unmet need. It is imperative that the required concentration of the medicine accumulates in the appropriate area of the body and continues to be present there for the requisite amount of time to generate the desired therapeutic response. To lessen the severity of adverse effects, the medication concentration in all other organs and tissues must be kept to a bare minimum. In such a scenario, the existence of the BBB makes the process of medication transport into brain tissue substantially more difficult.[7]

Nanoformulation is one of the promising approaches in delivering drug to the brain by circumvention BBB which enhances the bioavailability and reduces side effects. There are primarily three methods through which NPs cross the BBB, namely, (1) opening of BBB, (2) adsorption of nanocarrier, and (3) transcytosis, endocytosis, and exocytosis of nanocarriers (Figure 8.2).[10,16]

In a nutshell, the absorption of NPs by cells can occur via one of three primary routes. Pinocytosis describes the initial step, and depending on the size of the nanocarrier and the kind of cell being targeted, it can be further classified into macropinocytosis and micropinocytosis. Alternative mechanisms for the uptake of nanotherapeutics into cells include clathrin-mediated and receptor-mediated endocytosis. This process is driven by clathrin-coated endocytic vesicles.[16,17] Caveolae-dependent endocytosis is the third method for loading NPs into cells. This method involves the production of calveolar vesicles. This particular kind of endocytosis is frequently observed in endothelial cells as well as muscle cells.[7]

Neurons, astrocytes, oligodendrocytes, and microglia are examples of the various types of neural cells that can exist in the human brain. Each of these cell types has the capability of acting as a target for the delivery of medicines. The capacity of nanotherapeutic agents to target a certain disease depends on the functioning of the NPs and, in some cases, the presence of particular molecules. When compared to glial cells, neurons do not possess the phagocytic nature required for delivery to individual neurons.[17,18] This makes neuron-specific administration relatively challenging. Numerous studies have used the loaded chemicals' connecting ability characteristics to target neurons specifically. Dopamine and rabies virus glycoprotein-containing ligands (RVG and RDP peptide) have been used as active strategies to improve neuronal targeting.[19] These ligands and peptides are examples of active strategies. Inducing neutron absorption of NPs often involves employing techniques that include receptor-mediated endocytosis. As an illustration, nanocarriers that are covered with apolipoprotein E have the potential to be taken in by neurons thanks to the presence of lipoprotein-binding receptors on the surface of neurons.[20]

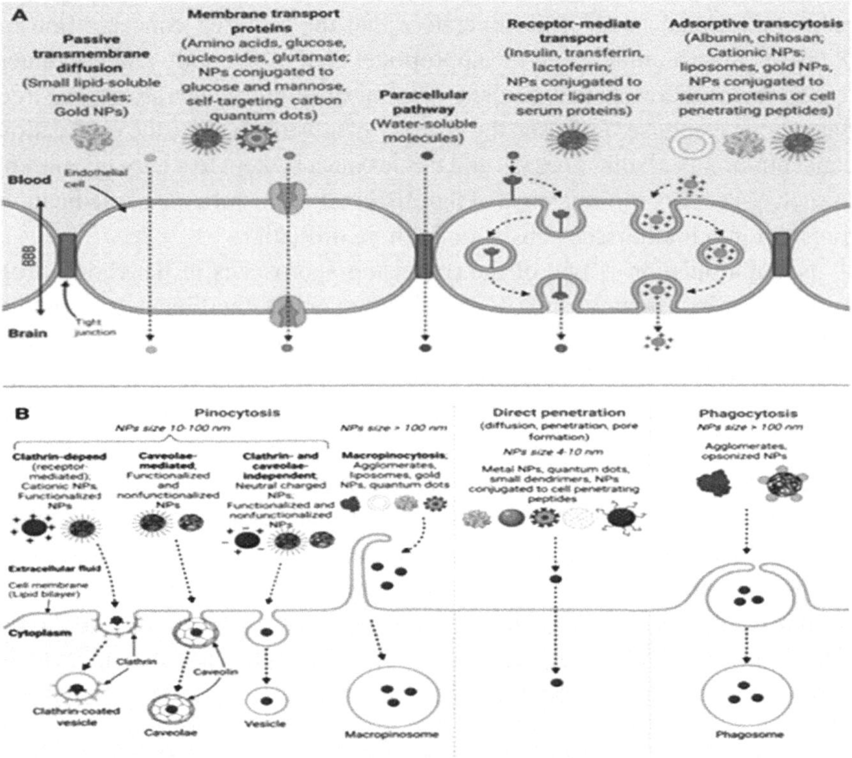

FIGURE 8.2 (A) Different mechanism for BBB crossing; (B) Major route of nanocarriers entry into the brain.

Source: Reprinted from Ref. [16]. Copyright © 2020 by the authors. Licensee MDPI, Basel, Switzerland. http://creativecommons.org/licenses/by/4.0/

Astrocytes are another kind of cells that have a lot of potential for use in nanomedicine. Phagocytosis is a common mechanism that may be utilized by NPs to gain entry into astrocytes. The release of glutamate, γ-aminobutyric acid, glycine, and histamine are all crucial for maintaining neuronal excitability, and their targeting can affect the release of these neurotransmitters.[21–24]

The myelination of axons in the CNS is facilitated by a kind of brain cell called an oligodendrocyte. Because of the properties of their surface, the distribution of medications through nanopreparations may be facilitated more easily. Specifically, oligodendrocyte progenitor cells express NG-2 chondroitin sulfate proteoglycans. Specifically targeting these cells with certain NPs, such poly(lactic-co-glycolic acid) (PLGA), can be highly efficient. When these nanocarriers loaded with leukemia inhibitory factor are utilized, it is conceivable for increased myelin repair to take place.[25–27]

Nanomedicine might potentially be used to target microglia or macrophages, which would be an exciting development. It is common knowledge that the primary mode through which microglia take in NPs is by a process called clathrin-mediated endocytosis. NPs with a greater surface area have a better absorption efficiency due to clathrin-mediated endocytosis. Studies indicated that microglial cells were able to absorb GNPs with a "urchin-mimicking" shape more efficiently than they were able to absorb spherical or rod-like GNPs.[28,29] This property was confirmed by the experiments. Absorption of nanocarriers by nonactivated microglia has been linked to many mechanisms, not just clathrin-mediated endocytosis.[30–32]

It has also been demonstrated that mannose receptors and macrophage scavenger receptors play a role in this process. There are primarily two ways that nanotherapy can have an effect on either microglia or macrophages. One study found that PLGA NP-encapsulated methylprednisolone administered locally resulted in a dramatic reduction in both macrophage and reactive microglial cell numbers.[33] The use of controlled cytokine release by the administration of NPs is the second method for modulating the actions of glial cells.[16]

Conjugation of ligands onto the surface of NPs is one method for functionalizing these particles. NPs are taken up by cells via binding to carrier or receptor-mediated transporters. Three-and-a-half percent of all studies examining the transport of medications to the brain involve the use of nanotechnology.[7] In spite of the fact that NPs have been developed over the past 30 years, there have only been a small number of NP formulations that have made it into CNS clinical drugs, and The use of nanoparticles in the treatment of brain disorders is not yet recognized by the US Food and Drug Administration (FDA).[34]

These nanocarriers are intricate entities that have the potential to injure the brain and result in neuropathologic disorders. However, these compounds have not been subjected to the rigorous preclinical good laboratory practice (GLP) safety pharmacology and toxicology investigations in two species required for an investigational new drug (IND) application due to the exceptionally low frequency of IND submissions for brain-targeted nanoparticles. A pharmaceutical product's cGMP manufacturing plant that has been validated and is scalable must be included in an IND submission.[7]

8.3 TYPE OF NANOCARRIERS

Different types of nanocarriers are shown in Figure 8.1.

8.3.1 POLYMERIC NANOCARRIERS

Polymeric NPs provide a potentially fruitful preference as a drug delivery platform for brain targeting because of their adaptable design (10–1000 nm), lack of toxicity, biocompatibility, and the ability to regulate the release of the medication. These polymeric NPs may be easily changed to add specialized ligands that target endothelial cell receptors, which allows for improved effectiveness of the transcytosis process (Figure 8.3).[34] By forming hydrophilic, hydrophobic, or electrostatic contacts, as well as responsive covalent connections, polymeric NPs can be used to deliver a number of neurotherapeutics.[7]

First time, polymeric nanoparticles (PNPs) were successfully used to transport medications through the BBB in 1995.[35] Dalargin loaded poly (ethylene glycol) (butyl cyanoacrylate) or poly(butyl cyanoacrylate (PBCA) was shown analgesia effect by tail-flick approach.[35]

Poly(alkyl cyanoacrylate), usually known as superglues, is a kind of polymer that has been utilized extensively in the medical field as a suture material.[30] In 1972, Couvreur et al. created the first PACA NPs.[30] After oral administration, pancreatic juice esterases in the intestines or blood serum esterases break them down, thus they pose no harm to the body.[30] Changing the length of the alkyl side chain affects the degradability time in hours. Longer side chains (like octyl) decay more slowly than shorter ones (like butyl) (PBCA).[36] In addition to this, the choice of side chain has an impact on the overall toxicity profile. It is possible for the cyanoacetic acid found in PACA NPs to be esterified with other compounds to form cyanoacetate esters, which may then be polymerized. These other substances include poly-ethylene glycol (PEG)-amine, folic acid, and medicines. PACA NPs may be functionalized in a number of different ways, including this technique. Both encapsulation and adsorption have been utilized as loading strategies for a vast range of medicines, including hydrophilic or poorly soluble drugs, as well as peptides, proteins, and nucleic acids.[30] PACA NPs are coated with PEG to inhibit macrophage absorption and polysorbate 80 to promote BBB crossing.[37] In a different experiment, mice with AD had their memories restored after being exposed to PACA NPs coated with anti-A1-42 antibody, which caused a dramatic rise in plasma Aβ level.[37]

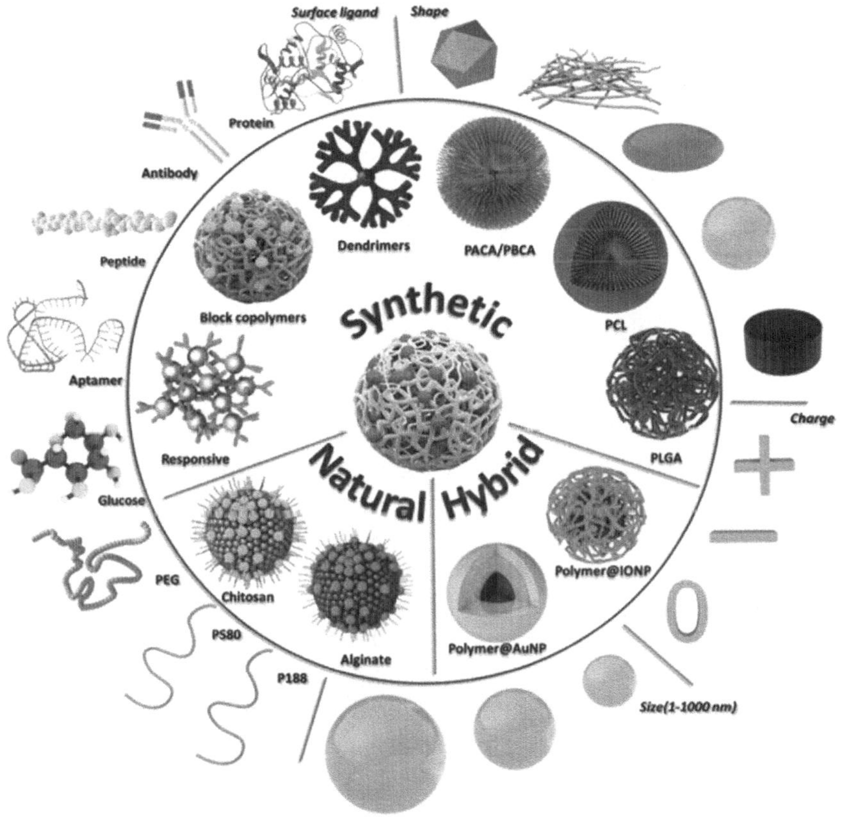

FIGURE 8.3 Graphical representation of the different types of polymeric nanocarriers for brain targeting. PACA: poly(alkyl cyanoacrylate); PBCA: poly(butyl cyanoacrylate; PCL: poly-ε-caprolactone; PLGA: poly(lactic-co-glycolic acid); Polymer@AuNP: polymer-coated GNP; Polymer@IONP: polymer-coated iron oxide NP; PEG: polyethylene glycol; PS80: polysorbate 80; and P188: poloxamer 188.

Source: Reprinted from Ref. [36]. Copyright © 2021 The Authors. Advanced Science published by Wiley-VCH GmbH. https://creativecommons.org/licenses/by/4.0/

The FDA has approved PLGA for sutures, medication-delivery systems, and biomaterials.[38] Glycolic and lactic acids may be mixed to generate PLGA, a linear copolymer with several uses (e.g., screws). PLGA copolymers are nontoxic and biodegradable after hydrolytic de-esterification (glycolate and lactate).[39] Changing a ratio of lactic acid to glycolic acid controls degradation rate, mechanical strength, crystallization, drug loading, and release kinetics. Due to its methyl sidechains, poly(lactic acid) (PLA) has little mechanical strength, while poly(glycolic acid) is stiff.[36] PLGA copolymers with a high PLA:PGA ratio are hydrophobic and impede drug release. In comparison to pure PLA, which can take up to 18 weeks to biodegrade, a 50:50 mixture biodegrades in about a week (also depending on molecular weight).[38-40] To modify the surface, such as when making diblock (PEG-b-PLGA) or triblock (PLGA-b-PEG-b-PLGA) copolymers, or to introduce targeted moieties like folic acid or antibodies, the terminal carboxylic acid groups can be used.[38] Alterations to the surface can also be introduced through the hydroxyl (OH) group that is found in the terminal carboxylic acid group. As a direct result of this, several various kinds of pharmaceutical compounds, including anti-cancer drugs, antibacterial, anti-inflammatory medications, and proteins, have been encased within PLGA NPs. These NPs have been used to treat a wide range of diseases.[41] Numerous formulations of PLGA have been investigated for their ability to traverse the BBB.[42] After coating PLGA NPs with a cyclic transferrin-targeting peptide and loading them with a generation inhibitor peptide and curcumin, transgenic mice showed enhanced spatial memory and recognition.[43]

Biodegradable polymer polycaprolactone (PCL) has been granted FDA approval.[44,45] It has been utilized in a variety of applications, including drug-delivery systems, contraceptive devices, sutures (in the form of Monocryl), and implants (in the form of 3D printed OsteoPlug for covering burr holes). PCL is made up of hexanoate units that repeat, and it may be broken down into 6-hydroxycaproic acid in the body through a process called hydrolysis. 6-hydroxycaproic acid, in turn, can be changed into adipate, which can then be catalyzed into carbon dioxide.[46] Nanoparticles derived from PCL have also been explored for use in the delivery of drugs to treat neurological illnesses.[47] Micelles composed of PEG-PCL functionalized with peptides enhanced transport ratios in an in vitro BBB model and accumulated in an in vivo model containing an intracranial glioma tumor.[48,49] PCL, on the other hand, degrades at a relatively slow rate, which is the fundamental reason why it cannot be used as a drug delivery route (up to 1 year). The disadvantage might be eliminated by changing the material's molar mass or encapsulating it with additional polymers, such as a copolymer that incorporates PLA.[36] To this day, there is not a single PCL-based NPs that has been granted clinical approval.[50]

Dendrimers are biocompatible, three-dimensional polymeric macromolecules that feature a central core that is surrounded by a corona that contains reactive functional groups. Dendrimers are also known as tree-like macromolecules. Because of the layer-by-layer construction process that is used to create them, their dimensions are expressed in terms of generations.[7,36] There are several unique types of dendrimers, the most well-known of which is based on polyamidoamine (PAMAM). By applying Michael addition reactions, which are subsequently followed by amidations, the synthesis of PAMAM may be carried out in either a divergent or convergent manner. PAMAM can be created in any of these two ways.[36] The amines are not the only surface functional groups that may be put into the material; OH and carboxylic acid (COOH) groups are other viable options.[50] The incorporation of these functional groups into PAMAM dendrimers may lead to improved water solubility, reduced clearance by the mononuclear phagocyte system, and decreased opsonization. PAMAM can load drugs either through the process of physically entrapping them in the hydrophobic cavities or through the process of conjugating them to the surface functional groups. Researchers have studied the prospect of employing PAMAM dendrimers as an alternate possible technique for the delivery of drugs to the brain due to the fact that their size is generally less than 15 nm (depending on generation).[50] The organ absorption of the cationic dendrimer was much greater than that of the neutral dendrimer. The lung was the organ that took in the most oxygen, while the brain was the organ that took in the least. Dendrimers by themselves are unable to pass through an undamaged BBB. Because of this, dendrimers have to be directed toward the brain.[7] Premade PAMAM-PEG-Tf and PAMAM-PEG-Lf conjugates were injected intravenously into mice. The uptake by both the heart and the brain was on the lower end of the scale. The largest uptake was found in the liver, followed by the lung, the spleen, and the kidney. It is not envisaged that exogenous Tf would function as a TfR-directed Trojan horse at the BBB in vivo. This is due to the huge quantity of endogenous Tf, which totally saturates the BBB TfR.[50] PAMAM dendrimers of the third generation coated with a streptavidin adaptor have also been shown to be able to transcytose across an intact BBB. In addition, 10% amine-containing G4 PAMAM dendrimers that were mildly protonated were able to cross the BBB and enter the brains of healthy mice.[50] In spite of the high medical expectations and research efforts, there has been a limited amount of clinical translation for dendrimers. The sole polylysine dendrimer-based antibacterial therapy that has been licensed for use in healthcare items is manufactured by Starpharma.[50] Regardless, researchers have been working to streamline the dendrimer production process and improve particle design. A greater drug loading has been accomplished using measures such as modifying numerous functional groups and introducing inner core functionalization.[36]

Polymer-based drug delivery methods have been studied for decades, but clinical use is restricted. This is due to the fact that polymers are notoriously difficult to work with. Recent research efforts have been centered on NP characteristics such as targeting, loading of drugs, and controlled release kinetics, with a particular emphasis given to a variety of polymer systems.[36] pH-responsive polymersomes constructed from POEGMA-b-PDPA can increase antibody transport to the brain. Other examples include polymersomes manufactured from poly(ethylene glycol) ethyl methacrylate block. For these polymersomes, block copolymer poly(ethylene glycol) ethyl methacrylate is employed. A conjugated version of a peptide that inhibits the low-density lipoprotein (LDL)-related protein was linked to the polymersomes (LRP-1).[51,52] The absence of endocytic sorting and, thus, pH-driven destruction during LRP-1-mediated transcytosis was an intriguing finding.[52] This made it possible to transfer the NPs in their natural state to the cells of the brain, where the protein was then liberated as a result of endocytic acidification.[51] One further option to increase the effectiveness of the process is to incorporate a wide range of different polymers into the drug-loading step of the technique. The NPs made of the diblock copolymer PLA-d-alpha-tocopheryl PEG 1000 succinate are examples of the countless block copolymers that have been investigated. These NPs were coated with transferrin and displayed a greater drug loading than PLGA NPs. PLGA NPs were utilized for this research project.[36]

An example of a natural polymer utilized to create a NP for drug delivery is Chitosan. It is one of the most frequent NPs since it is inexpensive, biodegradable, and available in a wide range of molecular weights.[53] In addition to this, it possesses a number of biological qualities that are wholly unique to itself, including anticancer, antibacterial, and antioxidant capabilities. Chitin is a natural polymer that may be obtained from crustaceans as well as fungi, and the production of Chitosan involves the partial N-deacetylation of chitin. Chitin is composed of-(1,4)-linked d-glucosamine and N-acetyl-d-glucosamine units that are randomly scattered throughout the molecule.[36] Chitosan consists of these two types of units. Chitosan possesses three distinct functional groups, which may be utilized for a wide variety of chemical changes. These functional groups include amine, primary and secondary OH.[36] Molecular weight, deacetylation, and chemical modifications can affect biodegradability. Their positive charge promotes cell absorption and renders them amenable to loading with negative-charged drugs.[12] Brown seaweed is the source of alginate, which is a straight, unbranched, anionic polymer (Phaeophyceae). It is a random copolymer that is made up of -d-mannuronic acid and -l-guluronic acid that are connected to one another by 1,4-glycosidic linkages. The Food and Drug Administration has granted alginate approval as a nonimmunogenic chemical.[36] New studies show that alginate NPs can make it to the brain. A neuroprotective steroid was successfully delivered to the brain in the form of alginate cholesterol micelles wrapped lactoferrin, while Chitosan cross-linked alginate NPs were revealed to improve CNS delivery of an antidepressant. We can confidently say that both of these presentations were effective.[36,53]

Amphiphilic block copolymers make up the structure of micelles. They are able to produce spheroidal nanostructures with a hydrophobic core and a hydrophilic surface that are stable in aqueous solutions. Micelles are a potentially promising carrier for transporting drugs to the brain. The solubility of molecules near the hydrophobic nucleus makes this possible, as does the ability to combine with specific target ligands.[16] Micelles consisting of block copolymers are often produced in an aqueous media by the self-assembly of amphiphilic molecules at concentrations that are higher than their critical micelle concentration into a nanoscopic supramolecular structure between 1 and 100 nanometers in size.[53] Since they are able to traverse the BBB and enter the parenchyma of the brain, polymeric micelles have garnered a great deal of interest in the field of brain-specific delivery. This is possible because of their nanosize, ability to increase membrane fluidity, and steric stabilization property that is caused by PEGylation.[53] Due to the fact that micelles on their own were unable to penetrate the BBB, lactoferrin was used to specifically target micelles (Lf). On the other hand, Lf is not an effective ligand for targeting the brain. D The LRP1 receptor is absent from the brain endothelium despite the fact that Lf is a ligand for this receptor. In addition, Lf does not meet the requirements to be considered a ligand for the TfR. The absorption of Lf-targeted micelles in the brain was modest, with 0.05% ID/g, suggesting they are exclusively in the brain's blood volume.[7] Micelles were generated using distearoylphosphatidylethanolamine-PEG2000-CREKA. The pentapeptide known as CREKA is able to bind fibrin deposits that are present in the vasculature of tumors. After being produced at a temperature of 80°C, the micelles were allowed to cool before being administered intravenously to mice. Micelles were cleared from the body through the liver and kidneys for the most part, and there was very little indication that they were able to pass the barrier that separates the blood from the brain.[7] Micelles (226 nm) were generated after incubating GM1 monosialogangliosides in water for 24 h. It was hypothesized that GM1 gangliosides would bind to serum albumin and that this combination would then assist RMT across the BBB via the gp60 albumin receptor produced in cultivated endothelial cells. This was one of the hypotheses that were tested. On the other hand, there is no evidence of albumin receptor activation on brain microvessels.[7]

Using a process that involves ethanol desolvation and the cross-linking of glutaraldehyde, human serum albumin (HSA) may be transformed into NPs.[7] Due to its numerous useful properties, including being nonimmunogenic, nontoxic, and biodegradable, albumin is frequently employed in the synthesis of nanocarriers.[53] Not only does it have a long half-life and a high conjugation capacity from its many binding sites, but its half-life also takes quite some time to reach zero (19 days). It tends to accumulate naturally in the areas surrounding tumors due to the various advantages connected with its integration. Because of its interaction with specific receptors on the surface of epithelial cells, albumin is actively transported through transcytosis.[54] Transcytosis contains endocytosis and exocytosis, therefore it's asymmetric. Glycoprotein 60, also known as Gp60, is a critical receptor that is shown to be elevated in the vascular endothelium cells that are responsible for supplying blood to tumors. Besides the brain, Gp60 is one of the most vital receptors. The presence of this receptor, together with the glycoprotein known as SPARC, facilitates albumin synthesis.[54,55] Combining the TGF-receptor I (TGFRI) inhibitor LY2157299 with the mammalian target of rapamycin (mTOR) inhibitor rapamycin inside of biomimetic BBB-penetrating albumin nanosystems led to successful codelivery of these two therapeutic agents (celastrol). By targeting BBB and glioma nAChRs with the albumin nanosystem, medication distribution into glioma can be improved, leading to better therapeutic results. By inhibiting the STAT6 pathway, biomimetic NPs were able to switch the phenotype of tumor-associated macrophages (TAMs) from M2 to M1; therefore, reversing the M2 to M1 transition. This resulted in a decrease in the amount of TGF-1 that was released, which ultimately led to the death of the cells. The TGF-/SMAD2 signaling pathway was likewise inhibited by the therapy. In an orthotopic glioma mouse model, both the targeting capacity and treatment effectiveness were validated. There was a marked improvement in survival time after treatment with biomimetic NPs; they decreased the percentage of M2-like TAMs, as well as TGF-1 and lactic acid levels in the glioma tissues. There is now a novel option for treating gliomas thanks to this delivery and treatment system.[56]

8.3.2 LIPIDIC NANOCARRIERS

Nanocarriers made of lipids and containing aqueous fluid on the inside are called liposomes. Solid lipid nanoparticles (SLNs), on the other hand, consist entirely of solid lipids within.[7] In 1990, researchers published the results of their initial experiment into using liposomes to carry drugs to the brain.[57] Liposomes comprised of phosphatidylcholine and cholesterol were formulated and then injected into the carotid artery of Fisher 344 rats that had an intracranial 9 L glioma. Liposomes were found to be incapable of crossing the BBB in healthy brain tissue. It's because they did not cross over into the tumor-free part of the brain. The liposomes entered both the primary tumor and the neighboring brain tumor in the 9 L glioma model due to the model's porous blood–tumor barrier.[57] Doxil, which is doxorubicin (Dox) that has been encapsulated in liposomes made from phosphatidylcholine/cholesterol/PEG1900, was given as an intravenous injection to rats that had an intracranial glioma. To treat the experimental glioma, Doxil liposomes were given to the tumor after it was found that this particular tumor had a leaky BBB.[58] Pegylated liposomes, according to the findings of this research, are unable to cross an unbroken BBB, a phenomenon that is analogous to the absence of BBB transport of pegylated HSA nanocarriers. Pegylated HSA nanocarriers are unable to cross an unbroken BBB.[7] Attempts have been made to use a geniposide–liposome conjugate (also known as GE–LP) for the treatment of cerebral ischemia–reperfusion damage (CIRI). These efforts have been followed by evaluations of the therapy's brain targeting, pharmacokinetics, and neuroprotection. Despite its great neuroprotective impact, GE has a short half-life in circulation and does not selectively act on the brain. A value of 223.8 nm was used to describe the formulation. Following that, the in vivo studies demonstrated that the GE-LP had a biodistribution and availability that was three times longer than that of the geniposide solution. The neuroprotective effect of geniposide in reducing CIRI-related damage was further evaluated in the middle cerebral artery occlusion (MCAO) rat model. This was done to examine the effect of MCAO on rats.[59,60] It has been demonstrated that PEGylated lipid nanoparticles (PLNs) containing fluorescent indocarbocyanine lipids (ICLs: DiD and DiI) may effectively penetrate and accumulate in glioblastoma (GBM). According to in vitro investigations utilizing GBM spheroids and organoids, the cellular penetration efficiency of PLN-synthesized ICLs was higher than that of liposomal ICLs. Within an hour of the systemic injection, more than 82% of the extravascular region of the tumor in the intracranial GBM model showed positive ICL fluorescence in the PLN group. On the other hand, in the liposomal group, only 13% of the extravascular area showed positive fluorescence. Within the first 48 h following delivery, ICLs that had been synthesized with PLN had accumulated in 95% of myeloid-derived suppressor cells and macrophages in the tumor, 70% of regulatory T cells in the tumor, 50% of microglia associated with the tumor, and 65% of cells that were not immune to the tumor. PEGylated liposomal Dox and fluorescent dextran were less successful in extravasation than ICLs made with PLN. Invasive tumor edges and brain-invading cells also gathered them more efficiently.[61]

In contrast to liposomes, which contain water inside their structure, SLNs are composed entirely of solid lipids on the inside. The amount of medicine that can be loaded into SLNs is not very large, but the amount that can be loaded into nanostructured lipid carriers (NLC) is significantly greater.[7,62] Liposomes, SLNs, NLCs, and cationic lipoplexes are all included in the category of LNP, which is a general word.[63] BBB transport was only studied in cell culture models in the earliest studies of SLNs for the brain. When it comes to administering pharmaceuticals that are not easily dissolved in water, SLNs are a fantastic delivery strategy. One use for SLNs was the incorporation of camptothecin, a medication that is insoluble in water, into cetyl palmitate SLNs with and without the use of PS80 for stabilization.[7] Almotriptan, a second-generation triptan, is used to treat acute migraines [99]. Youssef and his colleagues developed SLNs that contained almotriptan in their formulation. SLN was embedded into the in situ nasal mucoadhesive gel (composed of poloxamer 407 and sodium carboxymethyl cellulose) for nasal retention. Rapid brain targeting was also seen after intranasal administration of SLN gel to rats, with a T_{max} of 10 min. When comparing the DTE% values of the SLN gel and the free drug-loaded gel, it was found that the former had a value of 70.21 and the latter had a value of 60.80, indicating that both formulations were effective in reaching the brain.[64]

To improve active pharmaceutical ingredient (API) loading and avoid drug leakage during storage, NLC has been formulated. This has allowed for greater flexibility in targeting unique API release patterns while maintaining the same physicochemical features as SLN.[64] This was done to maximize API loading and avoid drug leakage while the SLN was being stored. With the help of solid and liquid lipids, NLC was formulated to improve the drug loading. This allows NLC to be used as a delivery vehicle for the API.[62,65]

This allows NLC to contain a higher concentration of the API. Because of this, when NLC particles are cooled, they become solid, but they do not recrystallize; instead, they maintain their amorphous form.[64] Because of the variations in the design of the lipid matrices, API ejection during lengthy storage is more unlikely to occur in NLC as opposed to SLN. This is owing to the fact that SLN.[65] The Chitosan-coated NLC of ceftriaxone that was produced by Padhi et al. was intended for use in brain targeting. For the formulation of ceftriaxone-loaded nanostructured lipid carriers [nanoliposomal carrier encapsulated factors (NLC-CEFs)], glyceryl monostearate and capryol 90 were mixed together. The resulting NLC-CEFs were coated with trimethyl Chitosan (NLC-CEFs-TMC) to enhance medication uptake by cells. The rat model was utilized to examine the drug's biodistribution in the brain and verify the viability of drug administration in NLC-CEFs-TMC carriers by means of the BBB. When compared to the pharmaceutical solution, it was seen to rise by a factor of 10.51 times when provided by IV and collected after an interval of 8 h. This was done after the drug had been in the patient's system for 8 h. After 8 h, NLC-CEFs and NLC-CEFs-TMC brain enhancement factors were 5.86 and 7.95. Both factors were similar. NLC-CEFs, NLC-CEFs-TMC, and CEF solution had brain targeting indices of 0.29, 0.50, and 0.029, respectively. NLC-CEFs-TMC had the greatest brain targeting index and enhancement ratio. The efficiency of lipid dosage forms may be connected to the lipophilic nature of NLCs, which is similar to the meninges. This idea may explain lipid dosage forms' success. The negatively charged CNS membrane may absorb more cationic NLCs, contributing to this success. It's possible that these two elements together led to his success.[64]

Lipospheres are solid spherical particles 0.2 to 100 μm in diameter. These particles have a hydrophobic fat core, such as triglycerides or fatty acid derivatives, and a phospholipid monolayer.[66] To investigate the possibility of improved medication delivery, a liposphere system was developed to administer quetiapine fumarate (QTF) via intranasal administration.[67] According to the findings of an in vivo tissue distribution study conducted with Wistar mice, the intranasal injection of QTF-loaded lipospheres demonstrated a shorter T_{max} in comparison to those of intranasal and oral solutions. The IN QTF lipospheres and IN QTF suspension, respectively, were found to have a higher percentage of DTE (228.36 vs 169.66) and a percentage of DTP (51.72 vs 48.82). The data on the percentage DTE, which was larger than 100, ensured that IN QTF lipospheres would transfer more drugs to the brain than oral dosage would. If the drug is in the form of a nanocolloidal lipophilic carrier and is administered intranasally, it can enter the brain via the olfactory and trigeminal nerves without having to cross the

BBB (BBB). In contrast, if the drug is in the form of a QTF suspension, it must first enter the bloodstream before it can reach the brain. The liposphere system is one that has the potential to be a successful approach for delivering QTF to particular areas of the brain.[67]

Colloidal dispersions of pharmaceuticals that have been complexed to lipids make up pharmacosomes, which are drug-delivery systems that are based on lipids. They are referred to as pharmacosomes since a drug (pharmakon) is linked to a carrier in the manufacturing process (soma). Phospholipids may form amphiphilic compounds, which carry an active hydrogen atom with them. It is possible for pharmacosomes to exist in the form of ultrafine vesicular aggregates, micellar aggregates, or hexagonal aggregates depending on the chemical nature of the API–lipid combination. Because of the covalent link that exists between the active ingredient (API) and the phospholipid, it is believed that they are more stable than liposomes.[64] The capacity of pharmacosomes to entrap both hydrophilic and hydrophobic medicines is one of the many ways in which they excel above more traditional methods of drug administration and bring with them a host of additional benefits. Pharmacosomes are capable of entrapping solutes and delivering APIs with varying degrees of solvability through the oral, parenteral, and topical administration routes. It is possible for pharmacosomes to have a unilamellar or multilamellar structure, and they are able to accept API in bilayer configurations.[64] Microemulsion/Nanoemulsion was also used for brain targeting via intranasal routes.[68]

8.3.3 NONPOLYMERIC NANOCARRIERS

Needles-like structures called CNT can be either single-walled nanotubes (SWNT) or multi-walled nanotubes (MWNT). Nanotubes with a single wall have sizes ranging from 0.4 to 2 nm, whereas nanotubes with multiple walls have diameters ranging from 10 to 100 nm [852]. The length of CNTs can range from 50 nm to over 1000 nm. CNTs are an allotrope of carbon; in contrast to fullerenes, which have a cage structure, graphene is two-dimensional and flat. CNTs may be produced using a number of different methods, including electric arc discharge, laser ablation, and the introduction of carbon-containing vapors to a preexisting metal-catalyzed furnace. All of these methods are viable options.[7] Because CNTs are insoluble in water, the carbon lattice needs to be functionalized by the application of chemical modifications before they can be used in biological applications. The 'needle' shape of CNTs is hypothesized to facilitate their translocation across cell membranes and into the intracellular space. Cancer-causing properties of CNTs have long been established.[7] Acetylcholine was adsorbed onto the walls of SWNTs and then administered IV into mice at a dosage of 20–50 mg/kg of SWNT, which is equivalent to a dose of 4–10 mg/kg of acetylcholine.[64] The findings of the research indicated that exposure of the mice to SWNTs resulted in a substantial increase in the quantity of acetylcholine that was taken up by the animals. As a result of improved performance in a shuttle box test by mice that had been genetically modified to have AD,[64] it was hypothesized that the SWCNTs may get across the BBB. Experiments carried out only in cell culture led researchers to conclude that SWCNTs were able to pass across the BBB.[64] The transport of MWCNTs over a monolayer of cultivated hCMEC/D3 endothelial cells was investigated.[64] These MWCNTs have either cationic, anionic, or nonionic groups added to their surfaces. The majority of MWCNTs, ionic or anionic, were found to be mostly localized within the glycocalyx of the cell. In cell culture, anionic MWCNTs showed the greatest rate of transport, although in vivo investigations of BBB transport of CNTs have not been undertaken.[69] CNTs, just like PNPs and SLNs, need to integrate surface ligands to induce endocytosis without causing harm to the cells.[7]

Graphene is a two-dimensional carbon nanosheet, and when it is oxidized, it produces graphene oxide (GO), where carboxyl and OH groups decorate the graphene surface. Graphene is a component of GO. Through a process known as "stacking," several medicines, including Dox, were able to form a noncovalent link with the GO sheet.[70] Dox-GO-PEG and free Dox were injected intravenously into rats. Binding Dox to GO-PEG had no effect on how much the brain absorbed. The scientists concluded that GO nanosheets must be modified with receptor ligands to improve BBB transit.[70]

Fullerenes are 60-carbon cages that are insoluble in water. Chemical coupling of water-soluble groups such as *tris*-malonic acid gives C3, a SOD-mimetic fullerene.[7] This fullerene has the chemical formula C3. Mice were given an intravenous injection of C3 fullerene, and the absorption of the fullerene in the brain appeared to be limited to the blood volume of the mouse, despite the fact that no adjustments were made for blood volume.[7]

GNPs, also known as Au NPs, have been the subject of a sizeable amount of the research that has been conducted in biomedical nanotechnological platforms ever since the birth of the field several decades ago.[71] Au NPs have distinctive chemical, physical, electrical, optical, and biological characteristics, all of which contribute to their exceptional use in the field of theranostic medicine. One of the many biological uses for Au NPs is the considerable potential for their use in applications involving targeted medication administration.[72] GNP-tagged resveratrol transferosomes and nanoemulsions have been developed (GNPs).[67] The water maze test was utilized to determine the effect on the recovery of spatial memory. Using computed tomography (CT) and histological examination using GNPs as a biomarker, the rats that had been given the treatment were analyzed for cellular uptake and bioaccumulation of the medication in the brain. Transferosomes demonstrated a greater penetration of up to 81.29 (2.64%) and a higher fluorescence intensity with a p-value of less than 0.05. This is in comparison to nanoemulsions. In comparison to the nanoemulsion formulation and the pure medication, the effects of transferosomes on the amnesic rats' behavioral acquisition and spatial memory function were dramatically improved. The buildup of GNPs was successfully verified by CT in the brains of all treated rats, although a much greater accumulation of GNPs was detected in the rats who were given the transferosome formulation. Both the transferosome-treated and the nanoemulsion-treated groups' brain tissues showed evidence of GNP accumulation in the nucleus and cytoplasm according to the histopathology findings. Because of this, the created transferosomes might be deemed a well-designed brain targeting system that could further be employed for targeting a variety of medications that will be used in the treatment of conditions that affect the CNS.[67]

In the late 1970s, the concept of using magnetic nanoparticles (MNPs) in the context of drug-delivery applications was initially explored.[67] Before being released into the bloodstream, therapeutic drugs may be encased within magnetic NPs or bonded to their surface. This allows for easier delivery of the agents. MNPs can be targeted using traditional active-targeting techniques (using RMT or AMT), or with the application of an external magnetic field that focuses on the target location. This can then localize the NPs at the desired spot to be employed in the treatment of illnesses of the CNS.[72] Using a T-junction device and bursting microbubbles, polyvinyl alcohol (PVA), PVA/bismuth ferrite ($BiFeO_3$), and polyvinyl alcohol/bismuth ferrite/donepezil hydrochloride (DO) monodisperse polymeric NPs was generated.[73] In this study, magnetic NPs made of $BiFeO_3$ and diatomaceous earth (DO) were loaded into PVA NPs. The $BiFeO_3$ NPs were created using the coprecipitation technique. According to the pictures obtained from the SEM, the structure of the NPs was uniform and smooth. In addition, the diameters of PVA NPs, PVA nanoparticles coated with $BiFeO_3$, and PVA NPs coated with DO were 148 nm, 159 nm, and 164 nm, respectively. The successful loading of $BiFeO_3$

magnetic NPs and DO into NPs generated with PVA was verified by X-ray diffraction and infrared spectroscopy, respectively. When healthy L929 cells were exposed to any of the NP samples, there was no harmful impact. To investigate the electrically controlled release behavior of PVA/$BiFeO_3$/DO NPs, a systematic electrical circuit has been established. The experimental conditions include 200 rpm, different values of voltages (0, 1.0, 0.5, +0.5, and +1.0 V), different values of currents (50, 100, and 200 A), and different voltages and currents. The application of an electric stimulus caused the release to rise, with the exception of when the voltage was +1.0. The release of DO increased with greater negative voltages, with a total release of 68.9% of DO after 15 stimulation with 1.0 V. The Higuchi model yielded higher R_2 values in virtually all situations, and the non-Fickian diffusion process ($0.45 \leq n \leq 1$) was responsible for the release of DO from NPs. Because it is possible to change the release of DO by adjusting the current and voltage when $BiFeO_3$ is present, the drug release that is used to treat AD is extremely controlled and can be finely tuned.[73]

8.4 CONCLUSION

Brain drug delivery technology is essential to the overall goal of developing medications for the CNS, given that the BBB is impermeable to all biologics (100%) and to 98% of small molecules (98%). When it comes to developing drugs for the CNS, the most difficult challenge to overcome is the BBB's inherent inability to transport drugs across its membrane. In spite of this, people who work in the field of drug development for the CNS adhere to two contradictory beliefs as they go about their work: (a) Drugs for diseases of the CNS can be developed, and (b) the BBB does not need to be taken into account when developing CNS drugs. Both of these beliefs are held by those who work in the field. Nanoformulation systems have the potential to solve the problems that are caused by the limitations of traditional medicines, which are currently being used for a variety of therapeutic reasons, including the treatment of neurodegenerative diseases. This is a very promising potential for the nanoformulation systems to solve these problems. However, these innovative systems are restricted in their capacity to target specific areas in an acceptable manner and have a poor capability of overcoming cellular barriers before releasing the medications that are contained within them. Both of these limitations make it difficult for these systems to be used. The many innovative nanocarriers that have been described up to this point are covered in the current chapter. In conclusion, the use of nanomedicines for drug delivery across the BBB has a significant amount of untapped potential.

KEYWORDS

- **central nervous system**
- **Alzheimer's disease**
- **Parkinson's disease**
- **nanoformulation**
- **blood–brain barrier**

REFERENCES

1. Khunt, D.; Misra, M. An Overview of Anatomical and Physiological Aspects of the Nose and the Brain. *Direct Nose-to-Brain Drug Deliv.* **2021,** 3–14.
2. Agrawal, M.; Saraf, S.; Saraf, S.; Dubey, S. K.; Puri, A.; Patel, R. J.; et al. Recent Strategies and Advances in the Fabrication of Nano Lipid Carriers and their Application Towards Brain Targeting. *J. Control Release.* **2020,** *321,* 372–415.
3. Costa, H. N.; Esteves, A. R.; Empadinhas, N.; Cardoso, S. M. Parkinson's Disease: A Multisystem Disorder. *Neurosci. Bull.* **2022,** 1–12.
4. Domingues, C.; Santos, A.; Alvarez-Lorenzo, C.; Concheiro, A.; Jarak, I.; Veiga, F.; et al. Where is Nano Today and where Is It Headed? A Review of Nanomedicine and the Dilemma of Nanotoxicology. *ACS Nano.* **2022,** *16* (7), 9994–10041.
5. Ghouri, M. D.; Saleem, J.; Ren, J.; Liu, J.; Umer, A.; Cai, R.; et al. Nanomaterials-Mediated Structural and Physiological Modulation of Blood–Brain Barrier for Therapeutic Purposes. *Adv. Mater. Interfaces* **2022,** *9* (1), 2101391.
6. Abbott, N. J. Anatomy and Physiology of the Blood–Brain Barriers. In *Drug Delivery to the Brain*; Springer, 2022; p 3–25.
7. Pardridge, W. M. A Historical Review of Brain Drug Delivery. *Pharmaceutics* **2022,** *14* (6), 1283.
8. Tian, T.; Qiao, S.; Tannous, B. A. Nanotechnology-Inspired Extracellular Vesicles Theranostics for Diagnosis and Therapy of Central Nervous System Diseases. *ACS Appl. Mater. Interfaces* **2022.**
9. Misra, A.; Ganesh, S.; Shahiwala, A.; Shah, S. P. Drug Delivery to the Central Nervous System: A Review. *J. Pharm. Pharm. Sci.* **2003,** *6* (2), 252–273.
10. Liu, T.; Xie, Q.; Dong, Z.; Peng, Q. Nanoparticles-Based Delivery System and Its Potentials in Treating Central Nervous System Disorders. *Nanotechnology* **2022,** *33* (45), 452001. http://dx.doi.org/10.1088/1361-6528/ac85f3
11. Keller, L.-A.; Merkel, O.; Popp, A. Intranasal Drug Delivery: Opportunities and Toxicologic Challenges During Drug Development. *Drug Deliv. Transl. Res.* **2022,** *12* (4), 735–757.

12. Shah, B.; Khunt, D.; Misra, M.; Padh, H. Application of Box-Behnken Design for Optimization and Development of Quetiapine Fumarate Loaded Chitosan Nanoparticles for Brain Delivery Via Intranasal Route*. *Int. J. Biol. Macromol.* **2016,** *89,* 206–218.
13. Khunt, D.; Shrivas, M.; Polaka, S.; Gondaliya, P.; Misra, M. Role of Omega-3 Fatty Acids and Butter Oil in Targeting Delivery of Donepezil Hydrochloride Microemulsion to Brain via the Intranasal Route: A Comparative Study. *AAPS Pharmscitech.* **2020,** *21* (2), 1–11.
14. Cheng, G.; Liu, Y.; Ma, R.; Cheng, G.; Guan, Y.; Chen, X.; et al. Anti-Parkinsonian Therapy: Strategies for Crossing the Blood–Brain Barrier and Nano-Biological Effects of Nanomaterials. *Nano-Micro. Lett.* **2022,** *14* (1), 105. https://doi.org/10.1007/s40820-022-00847-z
15. Agrahari, V.; Burnouf, P.-A.; Burnouf, T.; Agrahari, V. Nanoformulation Properties, Characterization, and Behavior in Complex Biological Matrices: Challenges and Opportunities for Brain-Targeted Drug Delivery Applications and Enhanced Translational Potential. *Adv. Drug Deliv. Rev.* **2019,** *148,* 146–180.
16. Zorkina, Y.; Abramova, O.; Ushakova, V.; Morozova, A.; Zubkov, E.; Valikhov, M.; et al. Nano Carrier Drug Delivery Systems for the Treatment of Neuropsychiatric Disorders: Advantages and Limitations. *Molecules* **2020,** *25* (22), 5294.
17. Adjei, I. M.; Sharma, B.; Labhasetwar, V. Nanoparticles: Cellular Uptake and Cytotoxicity. *Nanomaterial* **2014,** 73–91.
18. Siracusa, R.; Fusco, R.; Cuzzocrea S. Astrocytes: Role and Functions in Brain Pathologies. *Front Pharmacol.* **2019,** *10,* 1114.
19. Spencer, A. P.; Torrado, M.; Custódio, B.; Silva-Reis, S. C.; Santos, S. D.; Leiro, V.; et al. Breaking Barriers: Bioinspired Strategies for Targeted Neuronal Delivery to the Central Nervous System. *Pharmaceutics* **2020,** *12* (2), 192.
20. Hartl, N.; Adams, F.; Merkel, O. M. From Adsorption to Covalent Bonding: Apolipoprotein E Functionalization of Polymeric Nanoparticles for Drug Delivery Across the Blood–Brain Barrier. *Adv. Ther.* **2021,** *4* (1), 2000092.
21. Valenza, M.; Facchinetti, R.; Menegoni, G.; Steardo, L.; Scuderi, C. Alternative Targets to Fight Alzheimer's Disease: Focus on Astrocytes. *Biomolecules* **2021,** *11* (4), 600.
22. Lye, S.; Aust, C. E.; Griffiths, L. R.; Fernandez, F. Exploring New Avenues for Modifying Course of Progression of Alzheimer's Disease: The Rise of Natural Medicine. *J. Neurol. Sci.* **2021,** *422,* 117332.
23. Steardo, L.; Scuderi, C. Astrocytes and the Psychiatric Sequelae of COVID-19: What We Learned From the Pandemic. *Neurochem. Res.* **2022,** 1–11.
24. Scuderi, C.; Stecca, C.; Iacomino, A.; Steardo, L. Role of Astrocytes in Major Neurological Disorders: The Evidence and Implications. *IUBMB Life* **2013,** *65* (12), 957–961.
25. Mir, M.; Ahmed, N.; Ur Rehman, A. Recent Applications of PLGA Based Nanostructures in Drug Delivery. *Colloids Surf. B Biointerfaces* **2017,** *159,* 217–231.
26. Cunha, A.; Gaubert, A.; Latxague, L.; Dehay, B. PLGA-Based Nanoparticles for Neuroprotective Drug Delivery in Neurodegenerative Diseases. *Pharmaceutics* **2021,** *13* (7), 1042.
27. Rittchen, S.; Boyd, A.; Burns, A.; Park, J.; Fahmy, T. M.; Metcalfe, S.; et al. Myelin Repair In Vivo is Increased by Targeting Oligodendrocyte Precursor Cells with Nanoparticles Encapsulating Leukaemia Inhibitory Factor (LIF). *Biomaterials* **2015,** *56,* 78–85.
28. Hutter, E.; Boridy, S.; Labrecque, S.; Lalancette-Hébert, M.; Kriz, J.; Winnik, F. M.; et al. Microglial Response to Gold Nanoparticles. *ACS Nano.* **2010,** *4* (5), 2595–2606.

29. Zare, I.; Yaraki, M. T.; Speranza, G.; Najafabadi, A. H.; Haghighi, A. S.; Nik, A. B.; et al. Gold Nanostructures: Synthesis, Properties, and Neurological Applications. *Chem. Soc. Rev.* **2022.**
30. Rahmani, M.; Álvarez, S. E. N.; Hernández, E. B. The Potential Use of Tetracyclines in Neurodegenerative Diseases and the Role of Nano-based Drug Delivery Systems. *Eur. J. Pharm. Sci.* **2022,** 106237.
31. Papa, S.; Rossi, F.; Ferrari, R.; Mariani, A.; De Paola, M.; Caron, I.; et al. Selective Nanovector Mediated Treatment of Activated Proinflammatory Microglia/Macrophages in Spinal Cord Injury. *ACS Nano.* **2013,** *7* (11), 9881–9895.
32. Zhang, T.; Lin, F.; Liu, W.; Liu, Y.; Guo, Z.; Xiao, C.; et al. Reactive Oxide Species-Scavenging Lipid-Polymer Nanoparticles for Neuroprotection After Spinal Cord Injury. *Appl. Mater. Today* **2021,** *24,* 101109.
33. Kim, Y.; Caldwell, J.-M.; Bellamkonda, R. V. Nanoparticle-Mediated Local Delivery of Methylprednisolone After Spinal Cord Injury. *Biomaterials* **2009,** *30* (13), 2582–2590.
34. Mitchell, M. J.; Billingsley, M. M.; Haley, R. M.; Wechsler, M. E.; Peppas, N. A.; Langer R. Engineering Precision Nanoparticles for Drug Delivery. *Nat. Rev. Drug Discov.* **2021,** *20* (2), 101–124.
35. Kreuter, J.; Alyautdin, R. N.; Kharkevich, D. A.; Ivanov, A. A. Passage of Peptides Through the Blood–Brain Barrier with Colloidal Polymer Particles (Nanoparticles). *Brain Res.* **1995,** *674* (1), 171–174.
36. Zhang, W.; Mehta, A.; Tong, Z.; Esser, L.; Voelcker, N. H. Development of Polymeric Nanoparticles for Blood–Brain Barrier Transfer—Strategies and Challenges. *Adv. Sci.* **2021,** *8* (10), 2003937.
37. Andrieux, K.; Couvreur, P. Polyalkylcyanoacrylate Nanoparticles for Delivery of Drugs Across the Blood–Brain Barrier. Wiley Interdiscip. Rev. Nanomed. Nanobiotechnol. **2009,** *1* (5), 463–474.
38. Zeb, A.; Gul, M.; Nguyen, T.-T.-L.; Maeng, H.-J. Controlled Release and Targeted Drug Delivery with Poly (Lactic-Co-Glycolic Acid) Nanoparticles: Reviewing Two Decades of Research. *J. Pharm. Investig.* **2022,** 1–42.
39. Kumar, A.; Bhattacharya, S.; Singh, C.; Sharma, V. Poly (Lactic-Co-Glycolic Acid) & Tocopheryl Polyethylene Glycol Succinate Nanoparticles for the Treatment of Different Brain Cancer. *Anticancer Agents Med. Chem.* **2021.**
40. Caraway, C. A.; Gaitsch, H.; Wicks, E. E.; Kalluri, A.; Kunadi, N.; Tyler, B. M. Polymeric Nanoparticles in Brain Cancer Therapy: A Review of Current Approaches. *Polymers (Basel)* **2022,** *14* (14), 2963.
41. Rezvantalab, S.; Drude, N. I.; Moraveji, M. K.; Güvener, N.; Koons, E. K.; Shi, Y.; et al. PLGA-based Nanoparticles in Cancer Treatment. *Front. Pharmacol.* **2018,** *9,* 1260.
42. Hoyos-Ceballos, G. P.; Ruozi, B.; Ottonelli, I.; Da Ros, F.; Vandelli, M. A.; Forni, F.; et al. PLGA-PEG-ANG-2 Nanoparticles for Blood–Brain Barrier Crossing: Proof-of-Concept Study. *Pharmaceutics* **2020,** *12* (1), 72.
43. Huang, N.; Lu, S.; Liu, X.-G.; Zhu, J.; Wang, Y.-J.; Liu, R.-T. PLGA Nanoparticles Modified with a BBB-Penetrating Peptide Co-delivering Aβ Generation Inhibitor and Curcumin Attenuate Memory Deficits and Neuropathology In Alzheimer's Disease Mice. *Oncotarget* **2017,** *8* (46), 81001.
44. Atanase, L. I.; Salhi, S.; Cucoveica, O.; Ponjavic, M.; Nikodinovic-Runic, J.; Delaite, C. Biodegradability Assessment of Polyester Copolymers Based on Poly (Ethylene Adipate) and Poly (ε-Caprolactone). *Polymers (Basel)* **2022,** *14* (18), 3736.

45. Sinha, V. R.; Bansal, K.; Kaushik, R.; Kumria, R.; Trehan, A. Poly-ϵ-Caprolactone Microspheres and Nanospheres: An Overview. *Int. J. Pharm.* **2004,** *278* (1), 1–23.
46. Arif, Z. U.; Khalid, M. Y.; Noroozi, R.; Sadeghianmaryan, A.; Jalalvand, M.; Hossain, M. Recent Advances in 3D-printed Polylactide and Polycaprolactone-based Biomaterials for Tissue Engineering Applications. *Int. J. Biol. Macromol.* **2022.**
47. Madani, F.; Esnaashari, S. S.; Webster, T. J.; Khosravani, M.; Adabi, M. Polymeric Nanoparticles for Drug Delivery in Glioblastoma: State of the Art and Future Perspectives. *J. Control. Release* **2022,** *349,* 649–661.
48. Rabha, B.; Bharadwaj, K. K.; Pati, S.; Choudhury, B. K.; Sarkar, T.; Kari, Z. A.; et al. Development of Polymer-based Nanoformulations for Glioblastoma Brain Cancer Therapy and Diagnosis: An Update. *Polymers (Basel)* **2021,** *13* (23), 4114.
49. Xin, H.; Jiang, X.; Gu, J.; Sha, X.; Chen, L.; Law, K.; et al. Angiopep-Conjugated Poly (Ethylene Glycol)-Co-Poly (E-Caprolactone) Nanoparticles as Dual-targeting Drug Delivery System for Brain Glioma. *Biomaterials* **2011,** *32* (18), 4293–4305.
50. Anselmo, A. C.; Mitragotri, S. Nanoparticles in the Clinic: An Update. *Bioeng. Transl. Med.* **2019,** *4,* e10143.
51. Leite, D. M.; Seifi, M.; Ruiz-Perez, L.; Nguemo, F.; Plomann, M.; Swinny, J. D.; et al. Syndapin-2 Mediated Transcytosis of Amyloid-ß Across the Blood–Brain Barrier. *Brain Commun.* **2022.**
52. Tian, X.; Nyberg, S.; Sharp, P. S.; Madsen, J.; Daneshpour, N.; Armes, S. P.; et al. LRP-1-Mediated Intracellular Antibody Delivery to the Central Nervous System. *Sci. Rep.* **2015,** *5* (1), 1–14.
53. Shayganfard, M. A Review on Chitosan in Drug Delivery for Treatment of Neurological and Psychiatric Disorders. *Curr. Pharm. Biotechnol.* **2022,** *23* (4), 538–51.
54. Jiang, Y.; Wong, S.; Chen, F.; Chang, T.; Lu, H.; Stenzel, M. H. Influencing Selectivity to Cancer Cells with Mixed Nanoparticles Prepared from Albumin–Polymer Conjugates and Block Copolymers. *Bioconjug Chem.* **2017,** *28* (4), 979–985. https://doi.org/10.1021/acs.bioconjchem.6b00698
55. Begines, B.; Ortiz, T.; Pérez Aranda, M.; Martínez, G.; Merinero, M.; Argüelles-Arias, F.; et al. Polymeric Nanoparticles for Drug Delivery: Recent Developments and Future Prospects. *Nanomaterials (Basel)* **2020,** *10,* 1–41.
56. Zhu, S.; Sun, F.; Zhao, P.; Liang, G.; Sun, X.; Zeng, L.; et al. Brain-Targeting Biomimetic Nanoparticles for Codelivery of Celastrol and LY2157299 for Reversing Glioma Immunosuppression. *Int. J. Pharm.* **2022,** *619,* 121709. https://www.sciencedirect.com/science/article/pii/s0378517322002642
57. Shibata, S.; Ochi, A.; Mori, K. Liposomes as Carriers of Cisplatin into the Central Nervous System—Experiments with 9L Gliomas in Rats. *Neurol. Med. Chir. (Tokyo)* **1990,** *30* (4), 242–245.
58. Siegal, T.; Horowitz, A.; Gabizon, A. Doxorubicin Encapsulated in Sterically Stabilized Liposomes for the Treatment of a Brain Tumor Model: Biodistribution and Therapeutic Efficacy. *J. Neurosurg.* **1995,** *83* (6), 1029–1037.
59. Wan, J.; Long, Y.; Liu, S.; Zhang, Y.; Xiang, Y.; Li, D.; et al. Geniposide-Loaded Liposomes for Brain Targeting: Development, Evaluation, and In Vivo Studies. *AAPS Pharmscitech.* **2021,** *22* (7).
60. Pandian, S. R. K.; Vijayakumar, K. K.; Murugesan, S.; Kunjiappan, S. Liposomes: An Emerging Carrier for Targeting Alzheimer's and Parkinson's Diseases. *Heliyon* **2022,** *8* (6), E09575. https://www.sciencedirect.com/science/article/pii/s2405844022008635

61. Balyasnikova, I.; V.; Zannikou, M.; Wang, G.; Li, Y.; Duffy, J. T.; Levine, R. N.; et al. Indocarbocyanine Nanoparticles Extravasate and Distribute Better Than Liposomes in Brain Tumors. *J. Control. Release.* **2022,** *349,* 413–424. https://www.sciencedirect.com/science/article/pii/s0168365922004187
62. Shah, B.; Khunt, D.; Bhatt, H.; Misra, M.; Padh, H. Intranasal Delivery of Venlafaxine Loaded Nanostructured Lipid Carrier: Risk Assessment and QbD Based Optimization. *J. Drug Deliv. Sci. Technol.* **2016,** *33,* 37–50. http://www.sciencedirect.com/science/article/pii/s1773224716300806
63. Tenchov, R.; Bird, R.; Curtze, A. E.; Zhou, Q. Lipid Nanoparticles—from Liposomes to mRNA Vaccine Delivery, A Landscape of Research Diversity and Advancement. *ACS Nano.* **2021.**
64. Youssef, N. A. H. A.; Kassem, A. A.; Farid, R. M.; Ismail, F. A.; EL-Massik, M. A. E.; Boraie, N. A. A Novel Nasal Almotriptan Loaded Solid Lipid Nanoparticles in Mucoadhesive In Situ Gel Formulation for Brain Targeting: Preparation, Characterization and In Vivo Evaluation. *Int. J. Pharm.* **2018,** *548* (1), 609–624.https://www.sciencedirect.com/science/article/pii/s0378517318304824
65. Mehnert, W.; Mäder, M. Solid Lipid Nanoparticles: Production, Characterization and Applications. *Adv. Drug Del. Rev. Del. Rev.* **2001,** *47,* 165–196.
66. Domb, A. J. Lipospheres for Controlled Delivery of Pharmaceuticals, Pesticides and Fertilizers. *Nov. Pharm. Corp.***1990,** *79,* 8–11. https://cir.nii.ac.jp/crid/1570009750606141056.bib?lang=en
67. Zaki, R. M.; Aldawsari, M. F.; Alossaimi, M. A.; Alzaid, S. F.; Devanathadesikan Seshadri, V.; Almurshedi, A. S.; et al. Brain Targeting of Quetiapine Fumarate via Intranasal Delivery of Loaded Lipospheres: Fabrication, In-Vitro Evaluation, Optimization, and In-Vivo Assessment. *Pharmaceuticals* **2022,** *15,* 1083.
68. Khunt, D.; Polaka, S.; Shrivas, M.; Misra, M. Biodistribution and Amyloid Beta Induced Cell Line Toxicity Study of Intranasal Rivastigmine Microemulsion Enriched with Fish Oil and Butter Oil. *J. Drug Deliv. Sci. Technol.* **2020,** 101661. https://doi.org/10.1016/j.jddst.2020.101661
69. Gonzalez-Carter, D.; Goode, A. E.; Kiryushko, D.; Masuda, S.; Hu, S.; Lopes-Rodrigues, R.; et al. Quantification of Blood—Brain Barrier Transport and Neuronal Toxicity of Unlabelled Multiwalled Carbon Nanotubes as a Function of Surface Charge. *Nanoscale* **2019,** *11* (45), 22054–22069.
70. Liu, G.; Shen, H.; Mao, J.; Zhang, L.; Jiang, Z.; Sun, T.; et al. Transferrin Modified Graphene Oxide for Glioma-Targeted Drug Delivery: In Vitro and In Vivo Evaluations. ACS Appl. Mater. Interfaces **2013,** *5* (15), 6909–6914.
71. Zhang, J.; Yang, T.; Huang, W.; Yu, Y.; Sun, T. Applications of Gold Nanoparticles in Brain Diseases Across the Blood-Brain Barrier. *Curr. Med. Chem.* **2022,** *29* (39), 6063–6083.
72. Ayub, A.; Wettig, S. An Overview of Nanotechnologies for Drug Delivery to the Brain. *Pharmaceutics* **2022,** *14.*
73. Cesur, S.; Cam, M. E.; Sayin, F. S.; Gunduz, O. Electrically Controlled Drug Release of Donepezil and BiFeO3 Magnetic Nanoparticle-Loaded PVA Microbubbles/Nanoparticles for the Treatment of Alzheimer's Disease. *J. Drug Deliv. Sci. Technol.* **2022,** *67,* 102977. https://www.sciencedirect.com/science/article/pii/s1773224721006572

CHAPTER 9

Selection of an Appropriate Technique for Nano-Carrier Preparation: A Multi-Criteria Decision-Making Methodology

PANKAJ SHARMA

Department of Pharmaceutics, Shri Ram College of Pharmacy, Morena, Madhya Pradesh, India

ABSTRACT

Innovative scientific advances and engineering have advanced quickly in the direction of building nanocarriers to attain special qualities that are distinct from the properties of bulk materials. At a size below 100 nm, the particle exhibits intriguing characteristics. Using a multiple criteria decision making procedure, this study aims to choose the best way for creating nanocarriers. Future medical practice is being transformed by novel formulation strategies for medication delivery. Research and applications in various fields of nanotechnology have grown at an unparalleled rate in recent years. Even though they have the capacity to transport a wide variety of drugs to a variety of bodily regions, nanoparticles have emerged as a key topic of study in the area of medication delivery. Polymeric/non-polymeric nanocarriers are commonly employed to increase treatment effectiveness of medications despite substantial research and innovation. There are several methods available for creating polymeric/non-polymeric nanocarriers. The wrong technique choice might result in a waste of time, money, and materials. Analytical hierarchy process (AHP) was used to identify the best strategy as one option for overcoming these challenges. A decision hierarchy was built using the AHP, which included an aim, sub-criteria, criteria, and options.

Nanomedicine for Neurodegenerative Disorders: Selective Treatment Strategies. Rishabha Malviya, Kamla Pathak, & Swati Verma (Eds.)

The recommendation of experts program was then used to quantify overall importance of the criterion, sub-criteria, and possibilities after creating the AHP. The pair-wise number of interrelated is used in the analytical hierarchy process, a decision-making technique, to produce individualized judgments for qualitative criteria. An objective, conditions, and alternatives are used to build a decision hierarchy in AHP. The approach relies on three basic parameters. Instrument comes first, followed by process and output, then cost. Additionally, there are 11 possibilities and 11 alternatives. The total rating and essential weight for the choosing of the best approach are obtained using pair-wise evaluation matrices.

9.1 INTRODUCTION

Compounds with nanostructures have fascinated and challenged the worlds of science and engineering over the recent decades because of their astonishing ability to produce innovative forms, structures, and the strange occurrences connected with these substances.[1] According to Cientifica Ltd., the leading nanotechnology consulting firm located in London, the cost of developing nano-based medicine delivery systems was $3.4 billion in 2007, surged to $26 billion around 2012, and was predicted to reach $220 billion by 2015, underscoring the substantial growth and investment in this field during that period.[2] Manufacturing, nanoelectronics, nanopharmaceuticals, biotechnology, healthcare, information technology, and public safety are just a few of the industries where advances in nanotechnology are expected.[3] The phrase "nanopharmaceuticals" refers to the creation, design, and distribution of medications. About 90% of the active chemicals used in pharmaceutical product development are solid particles.[4] The advancement of nanotechnology may make it possible to create drug-loaded nanoparticles for use in a variety of unique purposes. A possible method for administering medications to treat neurodegenerative diseases and illnesses is nanopharmaceuticals.[5] For the pharmaceutical industry, developing an efficient system for a means of delivering drugs and distributing a medication accurately and treating a variety of ailments and conditions safely at the point of action is a key field of study.[6,7] Particle size has a direct impact on how well drugs are delivered to different parts of the body. The National Institutes of Health have lately alluded to the use of nanotechnology for the therapy, surveillance, diagnosis, and regulation of biological systems as "nanomedicine."[8] By decreasing the necessary dosages for successful therapy and improving the therapeutic parameters and low toxicity of the medication, nanotechnology plays a significant role in nanomedicine.[9,10] It has various benefits, including improving intracellular permeability and enhancing absorption into specific tissues while protecting the medicine from untimely destruction and interactions with the biological environment.[11,12]

The development of innovative nanotherapeutics has been helped by nanomedicine through the use of various nanomaterials. Many different kinds of nanoparticulate systems, such include lipid-based solid lipid nanoparticles (SLN); lipid carriers in nanostructures (NLC) and solid nanoparticles; inorganic nanoparticles like dendrimers; liposomes; magnetic nanoparticles like nanocrystals; lipid drug conjugates (LDC); quantum dots; and nanotubes, are still being researched for use in comfortable drug delivery.[13,14]

The delivery of medication to the brain for neurodegenerative illnesses via nanopharmaceuticals is a promising strategy.[5] Comprising 1–2% of the overall population, Parkinson's disease (PD) is the second-most common neurodegenerative condition with adult onset, behind Alzheimer's disease. A second-generation propargylamine drug called rasagiline (N-propargyl-1-R-aminoindan) mesylate (RM) is employed to treat PD.[15] RM is a brand-new anti-Parkinson medication that is also a subsidiary cyclic benzylamine and indane analogue of monoamine oxidase type B blocker.[16] The blood–brain barrier's special characteristics make delivering RM to the brain extremely difficult. An efficient solution to this problem has been offered by nanopharmaceuticals, which are presently employed to reduce the amount of drug loss after administration, increase the bioavailability and in vivo effectiveness of numerous substances, encourage cell selectivity, improve the stability of delicate agents, increase target efficacy, and control drug release.[2]

However, several factors must be taken into account while selecting a strategy. Therefore, finding a solution for choosing the best approach was a significant problem, since choosing the wrong one may result in a waste of time, money, and material resources.[17] A scientific methodology called multi-criteria decision making (MCDM) is required to meet the aim of choosing the best method for creating nanostrucured formulation loaded with drugs. In this sense, the analytical hierarchy process (AHP) might be useful. The AHP is an adaptable MCDM procedure that transforms a complicated question into a ranking system based on one or more elements. It was initially created by Saaty in 1980.[18] The AHP's ability to deal with circumstances where people's subjective judgments play a key part in the process of decision making is one of its advantages.

As a result, the AHP approach entails categorizing the multiple-choice factors, finding the proportional weights of the criteria, contrasting the options for putting a final priority weight on each criterion, and ranking the possibilities. The goal of this chapter is to use an analytical hierarchy approach to choose the best way among a variety of approaches for creating nanostructured formulation loaded with medication.

9.2 TECHNIQUES FOR DEVELOPMENT OF NANOCARRIER PREPARATION

9.2.1 HOMOGENIZATION UNDER HIGH PRESSURE

High-pressure homogenization is a stable and efficient method for producing SLN. In a nutshell, the medication is heated just above melting point of the solid lipid (stearic acid, palmitic acid, and glyceryl monostearate). To create the emulsion, a watery phase comprising surfactant (polysorbate 80 and polyethylene-polypropylene glycol) is added to the melting lipid drop-by-drop while being vigorously stirred. The heated emulsion would then be homogenized under increased pressure while maintaining the same temperature. To solidify the nanoparticles, the heated oil/water emulsion is immediately chilled in an ice bath.[19,20]

9.2.2 DESOLVATION METHOD

In order to create polymeric nanoformulation, desolvation process has been frequently employed. With the introduction of a desolvating chemical like ethanol or strong organic salt solution, this method may be applied for simply changing the charge and pH, a wide range of polymers. In a nutshell, the protein solution containing medicine is continually swirled while ethanol is added dropwise at a controlled rate of 1 mL/min. This process is repeated until the solution becomes turbid. By adding the cross-linking substance glutaraldehyde, the co-acervates generated are also strengthened. With response duration of 24 h, the lowest necessary glutaraldehyde content of roughly 40% is employed to create stable nanoparticles. Centrifugation is used to extract the free medicine and extra cross-linking agent from nanoparticulates after ethanol has been removed via pressure-induced evaporation.[26] A fine powder of nanocarrier is created by freeze-drying the created nanosuspension with 5% mannitol as a cryoprotectant.[22]

9.2.3 MICROEMULSION METHOD

Gasco was the first to develop the straightforward microemulsion technology for making SLN.[23] Drugs that are hydrophilic or lipophilic can be incorporated into microemulsions because they are transparent, thermodynamically stable, and have these qualities. In this technique, melted fat is combined with the medication (stearic acid and palmitic acid). To create a transparent microemulsion, the lipid phase is mixed with drops of the aqueous phase that contains the surfactant polyethylene-polypropylene glycol and the cosurfactant polysorbate 80. To harden the nanoparticles, a probe sonicator is used to distribute the heated o/w transparent emulsion into cold distilled water.[24]

9.2.4 DIALYSIS TECHNIQUE

A quick and efficient method for creating polymeric nanoparticles having restricted dispersion is the dialysis process. Briefly, after being dissolved in organic solvents that are water-soluble and have the appropriate molecular mass cutoff, the medication and polymers are put within a dialysis bag or membrane. The friction at the interface of the organic and aqueous phases is reduced as a result of the organic phase diffusing into the watery medium through the membrane or dialysis tube. Due to the lack of solubility, the polymer gradually aggregates as the solvent migrates within the membrane, resulting in the uniform suspension of the nanoformulation. Using 5% mannitol as a cryoprotectant, the resulting nanosuspension is freeze-dried to yield a fine powder of nanocarrier.[25,26]

9.2.5 SOLVENT EVAPORATION/EMULSIFICATION METHOD

The emulsification solvent migration process is used to create nanocarrier as well. This process involves dissolving the medication and the selected lipid in a water-immiscible organic solvent (such as cyclohexane, chloroform, or dichloromethane); the mixture is then mixed into a watery solution that includes a stabilizer. In a homogenizer with high pressure and decreasing pressure, the organic solvent is then vaporized. The nanocarrier is created via lipid precipitation in an aqueous environment. Avoiding any heat damage during the forming process is this technique's main benefit.[27]

9.2.6 IONIC GELATION TECHNIQUE

The use of chitosan and alginates as natural polymers in oral delivery systems rather than harmful chemical polymers improves the drug's capacity to permeate the mucosa, suppress enzyme activity, and adhere to mucous membranes. Depending on how soluble the drug and polymer are, they are first dissolved in water or a mildly acidic medium, and the resultant solution is then gradually added while vigorously stirring to the solution containing counter ions and stabiliser. The complexation of oppositely charged species causes gel formation and precipitation, resulting in the formation of spherical particles. By sonicating the end-product solution, the particle size is brought down to the nanometric range.[28]

9.2.7 DOUBLE EMULSION METHOD

In order to avoid drug segregation to the outer watery phase after external water phase evaporation in a w/o/w dual emulsion, stabilizers are added to hydrophilic pharmaceuticals before they are encapsulated and utilized in double emulsion techniques. In a nutshell, the medicine is dissolved in water before being emulsified with the help of a stabilizer in a water phase while being stirred. In order to create a double emulsion nanocarrier, the resultant pre-emulsion is stirred into an aqueous environment that contains hydrophilic emulsifier.[29]

9.2.8 NANOPRECIPITATION METHOD

Fessi invented the nanoprecipitation process in order to create polymeric nanocarrier. The precipitation and eventual solidification of polymers as a result of the ejection of semi-polar solvents miscible with aqueous from a lipophilic environment results in the production of particles. In a nutshell, the medication and polymer are diluted in an organic water-miscible liquid and introduced, while stirring, to the aqueous phase that includes the stabilizer. A decrease in the interfacial tension between the organic and aqueous phases is what leads to the rapid diffusion of the extraction liquid into the latter. At the time of immediate movement, diffusion, and interfacial tension at the extraction liquid-water phase interface, minute droplets of nanocarrier with well-defined sizes and characterized by a narrow size distribution are generated, generating turbulence.[30]

9.2.9 SOLVENT INJECTION TECHNIQUE

A fresh technique for creating nano-formulation and a process dependent on precipitation of soluble lipid in solutions is solvent injection. The liposome is dissolved using this approach in an aquatic miscible/immiscible extraction liquid (ethanol, acetone, or isopropanol), which would be delivered through with an injection into a water phase that is being stirred and contains surfactant, with or without. Using filter paper, the extra lipid is removed. By lowering the interfacial tension between aqueous and the solvent, the emulsifier-containing aqueous media aids in the formation of until solvent dispersion is achieved, lipid droplets at the injection site stabilize the formulation.[31]

9.2.10 SALTING OUT METHOD

A modified form of the emulsion procedure known as salting out is used to avoid using organic substances, for example, chlorinated solvents and surfactants may affect the environment and human health and the body's systems. In a nutshell, the salting out chemical and stabilizer are introduced to a water solution having the medication and the drug is soluble in a polymer, which is soluble in a water-soluble organic solvent. Calcium chloride, magnesium chloride, and magnesium acetate are the three most often utilized salting out chemicals. The development of an emulsion is prevented by the salting out chemicals, which stop the dispersibility of the extraction liquid in the aqueous environment. By diluting an emulsion with an excessive quantity of water, a reversal salting-out effect is produced. This causes polymer to precipitate, encasing the medication in the polymer matrices and creating nanoparticles. The cross flow filtration procedure is used to eliminate the leftover solvent and salting out compounds.[32]

9.2.11 SUPERCRITICAL FLUID METHOD

In order to produce polymeric nano-scaled carrier without using organic solvent, supercritical fluid science provides a fascinating and successful method. Environmentally friendly solvents, on the other hand, are employed in order to create very pure polymeric nano-scaled carrier free of any traces of organic solvent. A supercritical fluid is used to quickly expand a solution made of drugs and polymers past an aperture or a capillary nozzle and into the surrounding air. As a result of quick pressure drop during the expansions and a high level of super saturation, homogeneous nucleation and uniformly sized nanocarriers are produced.[33]

9.3 ANALYTICAL HIERARCHY PROCESS (AHP)

On the basis of the literature evaluation, the AHP was created. Figure 9.1 shows the multiple level hierarchy models that were used in this investigation. The following stages are covered in this model: developing a pair-wise comparison matrix, determining the overall priority ordering, computing the overall aim of the choice, identifying the pertinent criteria, and choosing the best option are all steps in the decision-making process.

This approach involves building a straightforward hierarchical model with a purpose, criteria, and options. Hierarchical organization, pair-wise comparisons, the eigen-vector approach for calculating values, and coherence concerns are just a few of the concepts and methods that make up AHP. Saaty claims that the process consists of three steps: decomposing, comparing, and synthesizing are the first three steps.[34]

The components of the decision issue are grouped in a hierarchy during the decomposing step. The best component of a hierarchy is the ultimate aim, followed by the criteria that directly affect the goal and the operational sub-criteria, by which the judgement alternative solutions at the smallest level of the hierarchy can be assessed. Each level's components are presumed to be independent of one another.[34]

The degree of an element's impact on an element at a subsequent greater level is evaluated pair-by-pair during the comparative judgement stage. Whenever comparing two components, Saaty suggests using a scale of 1–9, with 1 signifying a lack of distinction and 9 signifying a significant advantage for one element against the other. Pair-wise contrast matrix, which are the result of these comparisons, are supremacy matrices.[34]

The next step is to combine the objectives, a straightforward hierarchical model that compares options based on the main goal's requirements and sub-criteria. Calculations are made to assess the proportional weight assigned to each criterion for each potential. The pair-wise variety of related criteria are used to generate the overall priority ratings.[34] The AHP methodology's workflow is seen in Figure 9.1.

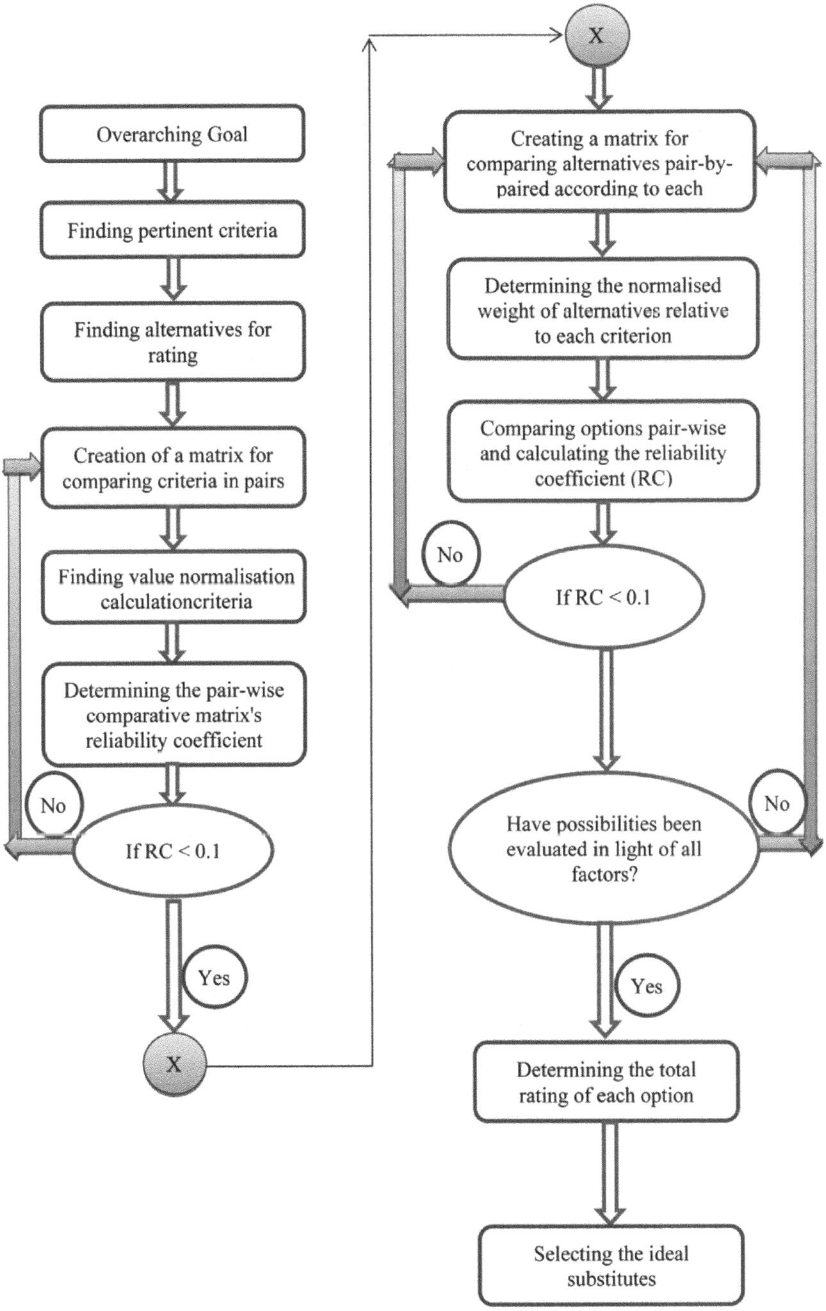

FIGURE 9.1 The AHP methodology's workflow.

9.4 HIERARCHY MODEL

The fabrication of medicament-loaded nanocarrier is shown in Figure 9.2 using the four-stages hierarchy model. The purpose of the issue is shown at the top stage. The model's purpose is broken down into four primary criteria—operational effectiveness, machinery details, procedure results, and nanocarrier development expense at the second stage. The third stage consists of various sub-criteria such as the capacity to measure performance, simplicity of use, erroneous diagnostic capacity, expand on, equipment accessibility, following protocol, equipment redundancy, precision, stability, value, and method of payment. Also, 11 potential alternatives/methods (Table 9.1) high-pressure homogenization (R1), desolvation method (R2), microemulsion method (R3), dialysis technique (R4), solvent evaporation/emulsification method (R5), ionic gelation technique (R6), double emulsion method (R7), nanoprecipitation method (R8), solvent injection technique (R9), salting out method (R10), and supercritical fluid method (R11) are presented in the suggested hierarchical model's final stage.[35]

9.4.1 PRIME CRITERIA AND SUB-CRITERIA

The four guidelines for creating safe nanocarrier serve as the foundation for choosing viable substitutes for creating medicaments-loaded nanocarrier as well as for choosing associated major criterion and sub-criteria (Table 9.2).[36] The key ideas, in further detail, are as described in the following: (1) Decreasing drug size to the nanoscale range without affecting the medicine's functionality. (2) Substituting acceptable harmless chemicals for the harmful ones that were employed in the production. (3) Atomic and molecular bonds to nanocarrier that preserve the required feature of the finished product while being non-toxic. (4) Encapsulating highly hazardous pharmaceuticals in harmless carriers to lessen their toxicity (5). When using dangerous substances cannot be prevented, just a little amount should be used.[36] For the creation of drug loaded nanocarrier, 11 distinct preparation techniques (R1, R2, R3, R4, R5, R6, R7, R8, R9, R9, R10, and R11) are being used.

9.4.2 RANKING AND PRIORITY WEIGHT CALCULATION

The hierarchy structure for choosing the best approach is shown in Figure 9.2, where primary objective is at the highest level. The picture also displays

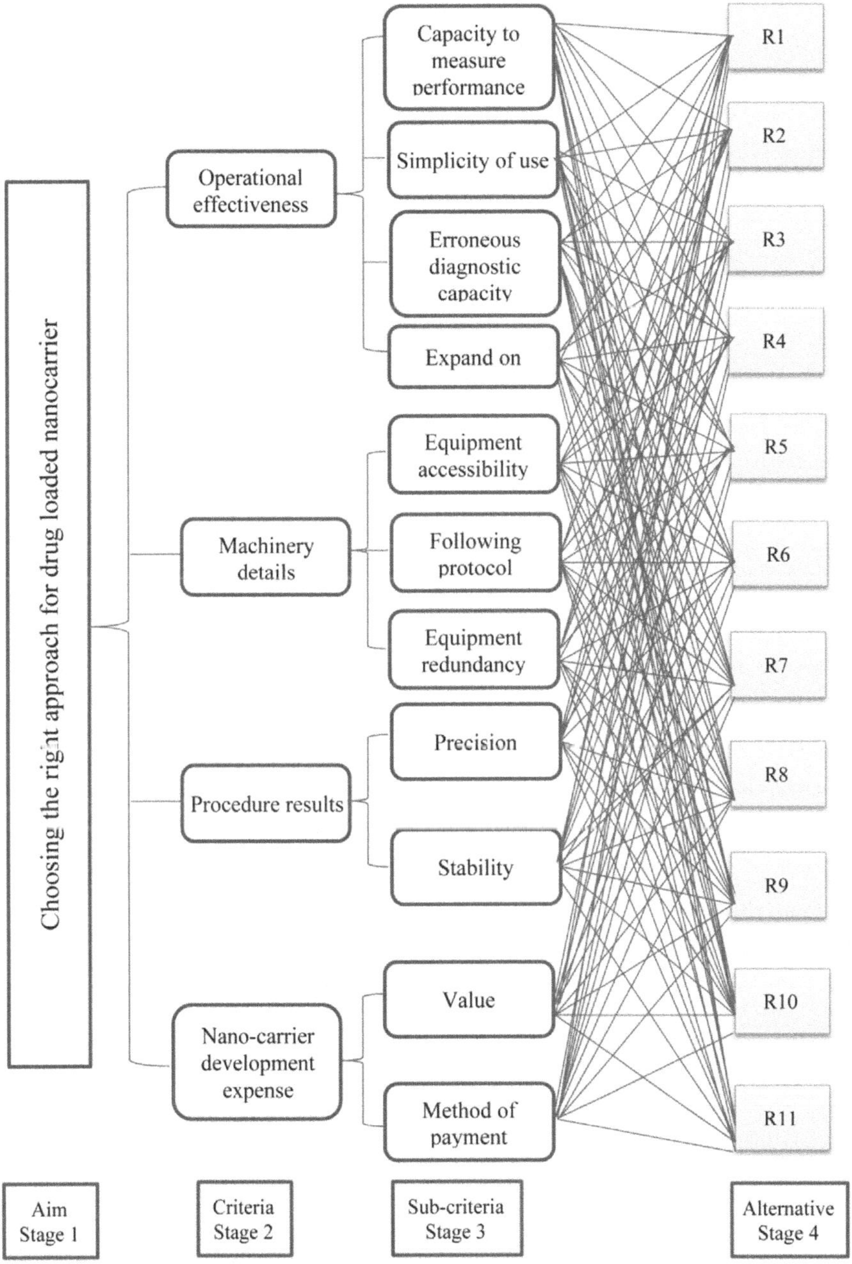

FIGURE 9.2 Model with four stages of hierarchy for choosing the optimum process for creating drug-loaded nanocarriers.

the third level's eleven options, the second level's three primary criteria and the third level's 11 supporting criteria. By employing pair-wise comparison, the criterion weights are evaluated.[37,38] The AHP approach compares items at each level in pairs with those at the level above it, producing a series of pair-wise comparison matrices. The Saaty's scale was used for the pair-wise comparisons (Table 9.3). The following is the assignment of the pair-wise comparative weights for the Ith and Jth criterion.

TABLE 9.1 Alternatives to Conventional Methods for Creating Drug Loaded Nanocarrier.

Possible substitutes or techniques	Code
High-pressure homogenization	R1
Desolvation method	R2
Microemulsion method	R3
Dialysis technique	R4
Solvent evaporation/emulsification method	R5
Ionic gelation technique	R6
Double emulsion method	R7
Nanoprecipitation method	R8
Solvent injection technique	R9
Salting out method	R10
Supercritical fluid method	R11

TABLE 9.2 The Primary and Supporting Criteria for Choosing an Appropriate Approach.

Prime criteria	Sub-criteria
Operational effectiveness	Capacity to measure performance
	Simplicity of use
	Erroneous diagnostic capacity
	Expand on
Machinery details	Equipment accessibility
	Following protocol
	Equipment redundancy
Procedure results	Precision
	Stability
Nano-carrier development expense	Value
	Method of payment

If both criteria I and J are significant, then

$$A_{IJ} = W_I/W_J = 1 \text{ and } A_{JI} = W_J/W_I = 1$$

Consequently, if criteria I is somewhat more significant than criteria J, then

$$A_{IJ} = W_I/W_J = 3 \text{ and } A_{JI} = W_J/W_I = 1/3$$

If factor I is significantly more essential than factor J, then

$$A_{IJ} = W_I/W_J = 9 \text{ and } A_{JI} = W_J/W_I = 1/9$$

For use with the AHP approach, the pair-wise comparability matrix A, that includes the relative weights assigned to the criteria, is needed.

$$A = \begin{bmatrix} W_1/W_1 & W_1/W_2 & \ldots/\ldots & W_3/W_n \\ - & - & - & - \\ - & - & - & - \\ - & - & - & - \\ W_I/W_1 & W_I/W_2 & \ldots/\ldots & W_I/W_n \\ - & - & - & - \\ - & - & - & - \\ - & - & - & - \\ W_n/W_1 & W_n/W_2 & \ldots/\ldots & W_n/W_n \end{bmatrix}$$

Where W_I represents the weighted significance of the ith criterion in relation to the aim, or the weighted significance of the Ith sub-criteria ($I = 1,\ldots, n$) in relation to the criterion, and so on. The following formula may also be used to determine the significance weights.

$$Aw = \lambda\text{max}W$$

Where $W = (W1,\ldots, Wn)$ is the appropriate Eigen-vector of A and λmax is the matrix's maximum Eigen-value. To determine the total priority weight of every possibility, intelligent selection software was employed. The best technique for creating medicaments loaded nanocarrier is one of the eleven possibilities with the greatest priority weight.[37,38]

9.4.3 RELIABILITY COEFFICIENT (RC)

To find discrepancies in the assessment, the reliability coefficient is determined. The values of all the pair-wise comparison matrices should be less than 0.1, indicating that the expert's ratings and weights were reasonable. Eigen-value λmax is taken from matrix A and used to determine the dependability coefficient. The below phrase can be used to assess the degree of consistency (CI).[39,40]

$$CI = \lambda max - n / n - 1$$

The relationship between the consistency index (CI) and the random consistency index (RI) may be used to compute the reliability coefficient (RC). The analytical hierarchy method yields the RI value, which is dependent on the value of n.[39,40]

$$CR = CI / RI$$

TABLE 9.3 Saaty's Pair-Wise Assessment Using a Nine-Point AHP Variables Studied.

Size of the problem	Meaning	Explanation
1	Equal significance	The goal is equally benefited by the two actions
2	Low or minimal	
3	Not terribly important	One activity marginally outweighs another in skill and intuition
4	Medium plus	
5	Powerful significance	One activity is greatly preferred over another by skill and intuition
6	Powerful plus	
7	Very potent or clearly important	A particularly strong preference for one activity over another is evident in practice
8	Extremely powerful	
9	Really significant	The strongest potential pattern of affirmation may be found in the data supporting one action over another
Reverse of above	As contrasted to action j, if action I has any of the non-zero integers listed above allocated to it, then J has the reversal value of I	A plausible presumption

9.5 CONCLUSION

The best approach for creating drug-loaded nanocarriers among all the options is determined via an analytical hierarchy methodology. The highest level of hierarchy was the focus of the choice problem's overarching goal. In this study, we looked at the issue of choosing the best technique for creating medication-loaded nanocarrier systems utilising a multi-criteria strategy to decision-making that utilised the analytical hierarchy process. In this chapter, a hierarchy structure with four primary criteria, 11 sub-criteria, and 11 options was suggested. The pair-wise criterion and sub-criteria were computed using the expert choice programme following the construction of the AHP. The created pairwise comparison matrices are all compatible with the chosen dependable coefficient value (≤ 0.10).

FUNDING

This work didn't receive any fund from any source.

ACKNOWLEDGMENTS

The authors acknowledge in particular Dr. Mukul Tailang (Professor, SOS in Pharmaceutical Sciences, Jiwaji University, Gwalior, Madhya Pradesh, India) and Dr. Vinay Jain for his kind support (Principal, Shri Ram College of Pharmacy, Banmore, Morena, Madhya Pradesh, India).

KEYWORDS

- **nanocarrier**
- **decision making**
- **analytical hierarchy process**
- **nanotechnology**
- **reliability coefficient**

REFERENCES

1. Ganguli, A. K.; Ahmad, T.; Vaidya, S.; Ahmed, J. Microemulsion Route to the Synthesis of Nanoparticles. *Pure Appl. Chem.* **2008,** *80* (11), 2451–2477.
2. Sosnik, A.; Amiji, M. Nanotechnology Solutions for Infectious Diseases in Developing Nations. *Adv. Drug Deliv. Rev.* **2010,** *62* (4–5).
3. Bhushan, B. *Handbook of Nanotechnology*, 1st ed.; Springer: Heidelberg, Germany, 2004.
4. Gupta, R. B.; Kompella, U. B.; Eds. *Nanoparticle Technology for Drug Delivery*; Taylor & Francis: New York, 2006.

5. Spuch, C.; Saida, O.; Navarro, C. Advances in the Treatment of Neurodegenerative Disorders Employing Nanoparticles. *Recent Pat. Drug Deliv. Formul.* **2012,** *6* (1), 2–18.
6. Sahoo, S. K.; Dilnawaz, F.; Krishnakumar, S. Nanotechnology in Ocular Drug Delivery. *Drug Discov. Today* **2008,** *13* (3–4), 144–151.
7. Faraji, A. H.; Wipf, P. Nanoparticles in Cellular Drug Delivery. *Bioorg. Med. Chem.* **2009,** *17* (8), 2950–2962.
8. Moghimi, S. M.; Hunter, A. C.; Murray, J. C. Nanomedicine: Current Status and Future Prospects. *FASEB J.* **2005,** *19* (3), 311–330.
9. Koo, O. M.; Rubinstein, I.; Onyuksel, H. Role of Nanotechnology in Targeted Drug Delivery and Imaging: A Concise Review. *Nanomedicine* **2005,** *1* (3), 193–212.
10. Kılıçay, E.; Demirbilek, M.; Türk, M.; Güven, E.; Hazer, B.; Denkbas, E. B. Preparation and Characterization of Poly (3-hydroxybutyrate-co-3-hydroxyhexanoate)(PHBHHX) based Nanoparticles for Targeted Cancer Therapy. *Eur. J. Pharm. Sci.* **2011,** *44* (3), 310–320.
11. Alexis, F.; Pridgen, E.; Molnar, L. K.; Farokhzad, O. C. Factors Affecting the Clearance and Biodistribution of Polymeric Nanoparticles. *Mol. Pharm.* **2008,** *5* (4), 505–515.
12. Kumari, A.; Yadav, S. K.; Yadav, S. C. Biodegradable Polymeric Nanoparticles based Drug Delivery Systems. *Colloids Surf. B: Biointerfaces* **2010,** *75* (1), 1–8.
13. Hamidi, M.; Azadi, A.; Rafiei, P. Hydrogel Nanoparticles in Drug Delivery. *Adv. Drug Deliv. Rev.* **2008,** *60* (15), 1638–1649.
14. Brigger, I.; Dubernet, C.; Couvreur, P. Nanoparticles in Cancer Therapy and Diagnosis. *Adv. Drug Deliv. Rev.* **2012,** *64,* 24–36.
15. Chen, J. J.; Swope, D. M.; Dashtipour, K. Comprehensive Review of Rasagiline, a Second-Generation Monoamine Oxidase Inhibitor, for the Treatment of Parkinson's Disease. *Clin. Ther.* **2007,** *29* (9), 1825–1849.
16. Fernandez, M.; Negro, S.; Slowing, K.; Fernandez-Carballido, A.; Barcia, E. An Effective Novel Delivery Strategy of Rasagiline for Parkinson's Disease. *Int. J. Pharm.* **2011,** *419* (1–2), 271–280.
17. Moorthi, C.; Kathiresan, K. Fabrication of Dual Drug Loaded Polymeric Nanosuspension: Incorporating Analytical Hierarchy Process and Data Envelopment Analysis in the Selection of a Suitable Method. *Int. J. Pharm. Pharm. Sci.* **2013,** *5* (2), 499–504.
18. Mohajeri, N.; Amin, G. R. Railway Station Site Selection Using Analytical Hierarchy Process and Data Envelopment Analysis. *Comp. Indus. Eng.* **2010,** *59* (1), 107–114.
19. Blasi, P.; Giovagnoli, S.; Schoubben, A.; Puglia, C.; Bonina, F.; Rossi, C.; Ricci, M. Lipid Nanoparticles for Brain Targeting I. Formulation Optimization. *Int. J. Pharm.* **2011,** *419* (1–2), 287–295.
20. Silva, A. C.; González-Mira, E.; García, M. L.; Egea, M. A.; Fonseca, J.; Silva, R.; Santos, D.; Souto, E. B.; Ferreira, D. Preparation, Characterization and Biocompatibility Studies on Risperidone-Loaded Solid Lipid Nanoparticles (SLN), High Pressure Homogenization Versus Ultrasound. *Colloids Surf. B Biointerfaces* **2011,** *86* (1), 158–165.
21. Weber, C.; Coester, C.; Kreuter, J.; Langer, K. Desolvation Process and Surface Characterisation of Protein Nanoparticles. *Int. J. Pharm.* **2000,** *194* (1), 91–102.
22. Elzoghby, A. O.; Samy, W. M.; Elgindy, N. A. Albumin-Based Nanoparticles as Potential Controlled Release Drug Delivery Systems. *J. Control. Release.* **2012,** *157* (2), 168–182.
23. Gasco, M. R. Method for Producing Solid Lipid Microspheres Having a Narrow Size Distribution. U.S. Patent 5,250,236, 1993.

24. Doijad, R. C.; Manvi, F. V.; Godhwani, D. M.; Joseph, R.; Deshmukh, N. V. Formulation and Targeting Efficiency of Cisplatin Engineered Solid Lipid Nanoparticles. *Indian J. Pharm. Sci.* **2008,** *70* (2), 203.
25. Liu, M.; Zhou, Z.; Wang, X.; Xu, J.; Yang, K.; Cui, Q.; Chen, X.; Cao, M.; Weng, J.; Zhang, Q. Formation of Poly (L, D-Lactide) Spheres with Controlled Size by Direct Dialysis. *Polymer* **2007,** *48* (19), 5767–5779.
26. Choi, S. W.; Kim, J. H. Design of Surface-modified Poly (D, L-Lactide-Co-Glycolide) Nanoparticles for Targeted Drug Delivery to Bone. *J. Control. Release* **2007,** *122* (1), 24–30.
27. Jun, H. U.; Zhou, S. W. New Research on Development of Solid Lipid Nanoparticles. *J. Med. Coll. PLA.* **2007,** *22* (6), 385–390.
28. Fan, W.; Yan, W.; Xu, Z.; Ni, H. Formation Mechanism of Monodisperse, Low Molecular Weight Chitosan Nanoparticles by Ionic Gelation Technique. *Colloids Surf. B Biointerfaces* **2012,** *90,* 21–27.
29. Wissing, S. A.; Kayser, O.; Müller, R. H. Solid Lipid Nanoparticles for Parenteral Drug Delivery. *Adv. Drug Deliv. Rev.* **2004,** *56* (9), 1257–1272.
30. Fessi, H. P.; Puisieux, F.; Devissaguet, J. P.; Ammoury, N.; Benita, S. Nanocapsule Formation by Interfacial Polymer Deposition Following Solvent Displacement. *Int. J. Pharm.* **1989,** *55* (1), R1–R4.
31. Yadav, N.; Khatak, S.; Sara, U. V. Solid Lipid Nanoparticles a Review. *Int. J. App. Pharm.* **2013,** *5,* 8–18.
32. Soppimath, K. S.; Aminabhavi, T. M.; Kulkarni, A. R.; Rudzinski, W. E. Biodegradable Polymeric Nanoparticles as Drug Delivery Devices. *J. Control. Release* **2001,** *70* (1–2), 1–20.
33. Sekhon, B. S. Supercritical Fluid Technology: An Overview of Pharmaceutical Applications. *Int. J. Pharmtech. Res.* **2010,** *2* (1), 810–826.
34. Murat, B. C.; Meral, S. The Analytic Hierarchy and Analytic Network Processes. *Hacet. J. Math. Stat.* **2003,** *32,* 65–73.
35. Yousefpour, M.; Rahimi, A. Characterization and Selection of Optimal Parameters to Achieve the Best Tribological Performance of the Electrodeposited Cr Nanocomposite Coating. *Mater. Des.* (1980–2015). **2014,** *54,* 382–389.
36. Morose, G. The 5 Principles of "Design for Safer Nanotechnology". *J. Clean. Prod.* **2010,** *18* (3), 285–289.
37. Saaty, T. L. *The Analytical Hierarchy Process: Planning, Priority Setting, Resource Allocation*; Mcgraw-Hill International Book Co: New York, 1980.
38. Saaty, T. L. Relative Measurement and its Generalization in Decision Making why Pairwise Comparisons are Central in Mathematics for the Measurement of Intangible Factors the Analytic Hierarchy/Network Process. In *RACSAM-Revista De La Real Academia De Ciencias Exactas, Fisicas Y Naturales. Serie, A. Matematicas*; Vol. 102 (2), 2008; pp 251–318.
39. Saaty, T. L. Decision Making with the Analytic Hierarchy Process. *Int. J. Serv. Sci.* **2008,** *1* (1), 83–98.
40. Velmurugan, R.; Selvamuthukumar, S.; Manavalan, R. Multi Criteria Decision Making to Select the Suitable Method for the Preparation of Nanoparticles Using an Analytical Hierarchy Process. *Pharmazie* **2011,** *66* (11), 836–842.

CHAPTER 10

Delivery of RNA/DNA to the Brain Using Nanoscience

AKANKSHA SHARMA[1], ASHISH VERMA[2], ADITI SINGH[3], and RISHABHA MALVIYA[4]

[1]*Monad College of Pharmacy, Monad University, Kastla, Kasmabad, Pilkhuwa, Uttar Pradesh, India*

[2]*Accurate College of Pharmacy, Greater Noida, Uttar Pradesh, India*

[3]*Ashoka Institute of Pharmacy, Ashoka Engineering Chauraha, Sarnath, Varanasi, Uttar Pradesh, India*

[4]*Department of Pharmacy, School of Medical and Allied Sciences, Galgotias University, Greater Noida, Gautam Buddha Nagar, Uttar Pradesh, India*

ABSTRACT

Brain is the most complicated organ of body. It plays a major role in controlling emotional, behavioral, and cognitive processes. Injuries, cancer, and neurodegenerative diseases are just a few of the diseases and disorders that attack the organ. Brain diseases are the main reasons of disability and death of individual. The development of medications that can target the intended region of the brain with minimum side effects while navigating physical—that is, blood–brain barrier—chemical, and electrical brain barrier has been a difficulty for researchers since long. Nanotechnology has recently become a significant method for molecularly altering and manipulating various objects to achieve desired properties. By facilitating drug distribution and enhancing its effectiveness, this approach has shown to be helpful in both treatment and diagnosis of brain-related illness and disorder. This chapter describes

Nanomedicine for Neurodegenerative Disorders: Selective Treatment Strategies. Rishabha Malviya, Kamla Pathak, & Swati Verma (Eds.)

the DNAs' and RNAs' delivery to the brain by using nanotechnology. It also describes the various dosages which are used in the treatment of brain diseases.

10.1 INTRODUCTION

Years ago, it was thought that DNA was translated into messenger RNA (mRNA), that was consequently transformed in a protein. Although, after discovery of RNA interference (RNAi), things grew more difficult. A conserved biological process known as RNAi occurs when small RNAs, such as microRNAs and synthetic small interfering RNAs (siRNAs), interact with protein compounds to repress expression of certain genes. Once bound, siRNAs target the mRNA for degradation or stop translation, depending on the sequence in which they bind to their respective target mRNAs. Due to this discovery, a lot more research has been done on RNAi-based therapies rather than the more conventional use of proteins and small molecules to treat diseases.

Small molecules or proteins that make up the majority of medications are now available in the market. Protein-based medications are frequently employed for the easy binding with target protein and substitute functioning target proteins; whereas small molecule-based therapies include typical competitive inhibitors of their own target proteins. The fact is that the maximum proteins are too large which cannot easily enter into the target cell; hence, it is only efficacious when their target molecule is extracellular or expelled, which is a severe problem with protein-based medicines.

Even while many diseases cannot be treated with either small molecules or proteins, it has been discovered that small molecule- and protein-based medications are often effective. For instance, a lot of diabetic people get insulin resistance, which means that giving them more insulin will no longer lower their level of blood sugar. Nevertheless, RNA-based therapies might be effective in treating conditions including Parkinson's disease, diabetes, cancer, Alzheimer's disease, Huntington's disease, and muscular dystrophies. In order to properly target pathophysiological mechanisms underlying these illnesses, RNA treatments may offer more effective therapeutic options. Additionally, a significant number of RNA therapies have now received FDA approval and few are undergoing different stages of clinical studies to show their efficacy for a range of diseases.[1–3] Figure 10.1 shows the RNA-based therapies used in treatment of different diseases.

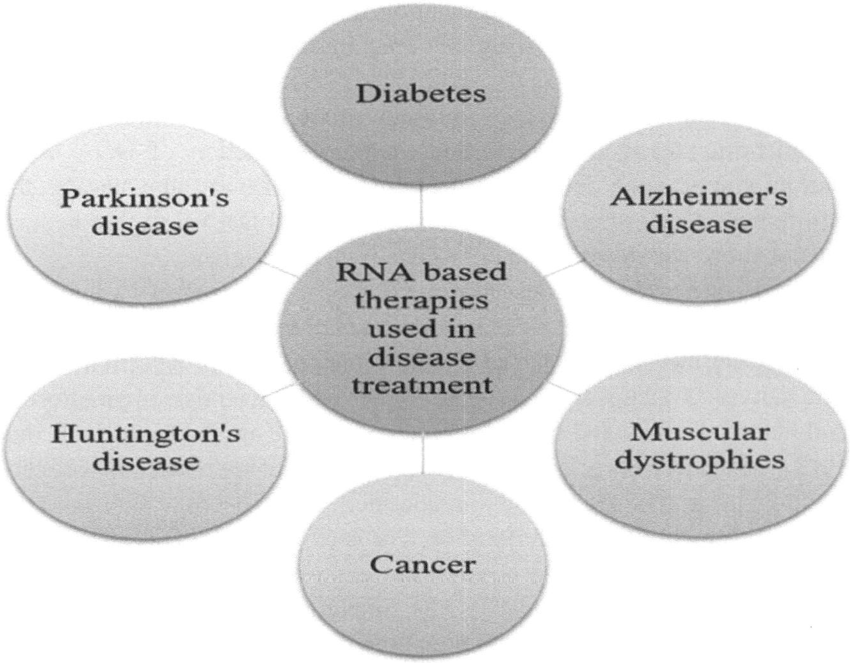

FIGURE 10.1 Schematic diagram shows the RNA-based therapies used in various disease treatment.

Gene therapy in human is the process to treat a sickness or illness by introducing genetically modified material inside the human cell, frequently through viral transduction. Meanwhile, science fiction has given an idea of viral gene transfer and its horrific ramifications have been played in the media. Non-viral methods of delivery of gene are constrained by efficiency of low gene transfer, but they have advantages, such as relative safety, production ease, low immunogenicity, and no restriction on insert size of DNA. Viral vectors can act as means of gene delivery and are also tuned to enable effective long-term treatment of both non-dividing and dividing cell, tissue-specific targeting and integration of site-specific chromosome.

Dr. James A. Wyngaarden, the Director of National Institutes of Health (NIH), gave his approval to the first clinical protocol to introduce a foreign or external gene inside cancer patients' immune cell on January 19, 1989. A four-year-old girl born with severe combined immunodeficiency (SCID) had the first-approved gene therapy treatment on September 14, 1990, thanks to W. French Anderson and co-workers at the NIH. Its original trial was also successful, which was also mentioned by a popular media. In 2004, it was observed that she is living a flourishing life as an 18-year-old girl at Suburban Cleveland.[4,5]

Because of relative safety, minimal toxicity and immunogenicity, administration ease and production, and no restriction of DNA insert size, polymeric gene delivery is preferred. The primary drawback is the requirement of post-uptake endosomal escape and DNA complex nuclear translocation, which results in poor gene transfer efficiency.

Viruses are a species-conserved method of transferring DNA into cells that have undergone millions of years of evolution, representing an ancient and intricate mechanism shaped by the forces of natural selection. These gene delivery systems are now being improved by scientists in an effort to treat human diseases and birth abnormalities. There are three standards that all viral gene therapy vectors must meet, regardless of approach. The delivery method must first be secure and immune-inert. It also needs to safeguard the genetic information from deterioration. The vector should encode therapeutic gene, which is efficient and consistently expressed at a designated target site. The packaged vector must also be simple-to-make process and have a reasonable shelf life for meaningful commercial applicability.[6]

When protein or pharmacokinetic therapy is ineffective for treating a single genetic defect in a patient, gene therapy is uniquely adapted to deliver a transgene over an extended time. This was the foundation of the first gene therapy-related clinical study, in which *ex vivo* genes get inserted into CD34+ cells to cure SCID patients. Amazingly, 12 years after treatment, peripheral blood leukocytes still carried the adenosine deaminase (ADA) transgene without any negative side effects. Genetic disorders such as muscular dystrophy, Leber congenital amaurosis, cystic fibrosis, Gaucher's disease, ornithine transcarbamylase deficiency, and hemophilia have all been treated clinically since 1990, with encouraging results that have been published.

The neurological and other chronic diseases treatment is another area where gene therapy is widely required. HIV/AIDS, angina pectoris, arthritis, solid tumors, Huntington's disease, Alzheimer's disease, Canavan disease, Batten disease, Parkinson's disease, and familial hypercholesterolemia have all been the subject of ongoing or finished clinical trials. Treatments for angina pectoris, prostate cancer, lung cancer, and neck and head cancer are currently approaching clinical trials phase III stage, despite the numerous obstacles.[4] Figure 10.2 shows the gene therapies used in treatment of different genetic disorders.

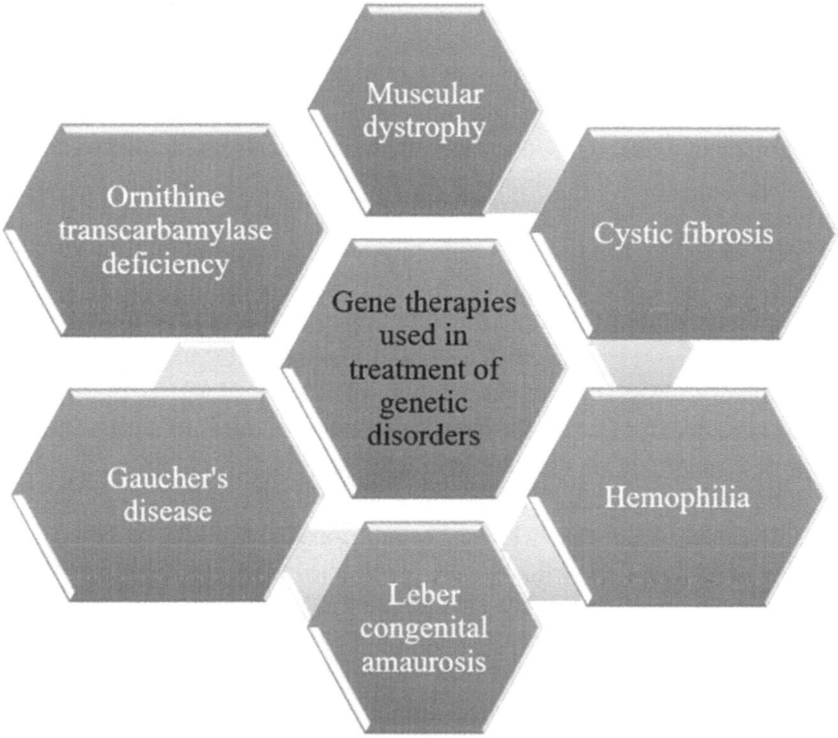

FIGURE 10.2 Schematic diagram shows the gene therapies used in various genetic disorders.

10.2 STRATEGIES FOR RNA BRAIN DELIVERY USING NANOTECHNOLOGY

Finding effective therapies is crucial since brain pathologies including neurodegenerative illnesses and brain cancer are becoming more common as the population ages. To cure diseases and their causes, drugs must be delivered to the central nervous system (CNS). The blood–brain barrier (BBB) is a foremost barrier in the treatments efficacy since it has the capacity to severely restrict the circulation of substances toward brain. Over years, various new strategies for defeating BBB and its efflux transporters have been proposed. siRNA, which can particularly target single gene and make it silent in post-transcriptional manner, is one of the methods discussed here. Different functional proteins in the BBB, such as those in charge of transport or simply for its tightness, may be potential targets for RNA. The method used to distribute RNA to its anatomical region of action is just as significant as effective silencing. Systems based on nanotechnology may be able to assist in this situation by safeguarding siRNA circulation, delivering RNA to certain cells or tissues, and targeting RNA intracellularly. This paper first provides a summary of the prevalence of brain-related diseases and the fundamental characteristics of BBB, CNS, and its efflux pumps before focusing on current RNA-based ways to enter into the brain and how to particularly target these methods to cure brain ailments.[7]

More than 1 billion people are currently affected by more than 1000 diseases of the CNS, but many of these lack appropriate treatments or medications, making CNS disorders one of the biggest risks to the health of human in the 21st century. While the pathway of RNA interference and its regulatory abilities were discovered, siRNA-based RNAi therapy has gained significant attention for treating a range of brain illnesses, including dementia, motor neuron diseases, and brain tumors.

First, unlike chemical medications, siRNA therapy can target any gene involved in disease, which accounts for its excellent specificity for pathogenic targets. Theoretically, siRNA are used to downregulate or silence any disease-related gene expression inside the body, comprising those that have historically been regarded as being "undruggable," far exceeding the potential of conventional small-molecule drug-based approaches. This is possible with rational sequence design. Traditional treatments (such as chemotherapy or surgery) are still ineffective for a significant share of brain illnesses, while siRNA medicines provide hopeful therapeutic options for conditions that were once thought to be untreatable.[8]

siRNA is quite effective. A single siRNA can only cleave a small number of mRNA targets because RNAi includes an enzyme-mediated method and siRNA activities are catalytic in nature. Brain is the most intricate and delicate organ; cytotoxicity could readily be brought in by the high dose or frequent administration of therapeutic medicines. For disease therapy, low-to-medium and relatively infrequent doses of siRNA are required, which enables the reduction of side effects related to current chemical medications.

It is quick and simple to develop siRNA drug candidates. Bioinformatic methods are used to filter sequences against mRNA target. SiRNA medications are simple to create and also ideal for orphan diseases treatment but it lacks the big market. Large market is required to attract funding resources for treatment research. So far, more than 20 RNAi clinical trial studies have either been finished or still being conducted. The majority are made to treat rare disorders. Alnylam Pharmaceuticals (Cambridge, MA, USA) has just demonstrated assuring outcomes with patisiran (ALN-TTR02), a drug for siRNA is being prepared to cure hereditary transthyretin-mediated (hATTR) amyloidosis with polyneuropathy. These results include neurological impairment amelioration, enhanced life quality, and decreased symptoms of disease and disability from Phase III analysis.

The high efficiency and specificity of RNAi process therefore suggests that siRNA drugs may assure to be a better candidate to treat brain diseases and disorders, including Huntington's disease, glioblastoma multiforme, amyotrophic lateral sclerosis, Alzheimer's disease, and spinal cord injury.

Even so, a number of biological hurdles that arise after systemic injection and before target mRNA is attained significantly limit the ability of siRNA therapies to effectively treat brain illnesses. These difficulties can be encountered during intracellular trafficking, cell endocytosis, blood circulation, brain entrance, and targeting targeted sites/tissues/cells. Thankfully, recent advances in nanotechnology have produced previously unheard of chances and techniques to mention these biological difficulties, making siRNA more suitable for cure of brain diseases.[9] Table 10.1 summarizes the FDA-approved RNA products which are used in treatment of diseases.

TABLE 10.1 FDA-Approved RNA Products Used in Treatment of Diseases.[1,10–12]

List of products	Disease treatment
Fomivirsen	Cytomegalovirus retinitis
Nusinersen	Spinal muscular atrophy
Inotresen	Familial amyloid polyneuropathy
Eteplirsen, Glodirsen, Casimersen	Duchenne muscular dystrophy
Givosiran	Acute hepatic porphyria
Inclisiran	Atherosclerotic cardiovascular disease
Pegaptanib	Neovascular age-related macular degeneration
Defibrotide	Veno-occlusive, a liver illness
BNT162b2, mRNA-1273	Corona virus

10.3 MECHANISM OF siRNA INTERFERENCE

RNA non-coding stretch regulates the action of multiple coding genes and silences the genes expression through a post-transcriptional process known as siRNA interference. In eukaryotic cells, siRNA, a brief dsRNA fragment, primarily facilitates homology-based gene expression regulation. This procedure is comparable to one that uses knockdown and miRNA replacement. A synthetic ssRNA, called as antagomirs/anti-miRs, is used as intrinsic miRNA antagonist by using an antisense method of suppression. Synthetic miRNAs are used in the replacement process, and they are delivered in vivo to imitate the endogenous miRNAs function. Gene silence and mRNA degradation/inhibition are the results of this RNA mimicking.

The RNAi initiation phase, which involves synthesis of effector molecule, is the first step of process. A complex enzyme, called Dicer, targets two main nucleotides at 3′-overhang of double-stranded molecules of RNA (dsRNA), which are around 21–22 base pairs lengthy in a homology-dependent manner to break identified mRNA. The longer dsRNA is broken down by the RNase III-like Dicer enzyme, which produces siRNAs through a homology-dependent procedure. In the cell cytoplasm, endonuclease Dicer converts dsRNA into siRNA structures.[13]

The execution stage starts when a complex of multiprotein binds with the effector molecules, which activate gene silencing after the synthesis of effector molecules. A multi-subunit group of specific protein is called RNA-induced silencing compound binds with siRNAs (RISC). Dicer, TRBP, and Argonaute 2 are the three proteins that make up the RISC complex. Each have a specific role for the complex. The siRNA–RISC binding is aided by the TAR–RNA binding protein (TRBP). The RISC complexes Ago-2 protein activates at a precise cleavage location in target mRNA molecules, between base 10 and 11, on the antisense siRNA strand 5′-terminal. Ago-2 protein detects and cuts mRNA strand that are virtually complementary for RNA strand which work as guide. The complementary siRNA-mRNA pair in the second case mimics miRNA bound to target sites on occasion. Drosha-DGCR8 complex processes miRNAs inside the nucleus, inhibiting translation or degrading the transcript.

The catalytic province of Ago-2 allows cleavage of the targeted mRNA area and Argonaute (Ago) protein are only members of RISC. The siRNAs implanted in RISC are duplex, and the passenger strand is one of the strands that Ago-2 proteins separate and remove from double-stranded siRNA linked to RISC. Guide RNA, the other single strand, is still a part of the RISC complex. Due to a unique intermolecular base pair interaction, the target is recognized by functionally active compound containing guide RNA. Three functional subunits of the ago-2 protein are PIWI, MID, and PAZ. PIWI domain, which belongs to this group, has a structural folding that is similar to RNase H and offers the RISC complex thermodynamic enthalpy for cleavage. In order to link to the RISC complex, Ago-2 proteins' PAZ component binds with two terminals of 3′-nucleotides. The core domain of the siRNA with staggered ends and the particular nucleotide are stacked at the base in a hydrophobic cavity made up of a variety of aromatic residues. Through a magnesium ion, the siRNA's 5′-phosphate group is attached to protein's carboxyl terminus in center of PIWI and MID domains. It has been noted that the Argonaute family also participates in the assortment of guide strand. As guide strand, argonaute protects the strand with the least thermodynamically stable 5′-terminal and cleaves a different strand to liberate the passenger strand. The choice of strand that stays anchored with RISC compound is governed by several fundamental criteria, like as the siRNA thermodynamic stability get end. Strand with lower terminal stability typically transforms to mRNA molecules, which Ago-2 may then detect and destroy. As a guide RNA, strand which is complementary to targeted mRNA is used.[14]

10.4 NANOTECHNOLOGY PLATFORMS FOR SIRNA DELIVERY

BBB is a major problem in growth of medications for CNS illnesses. A technique for delivering this novel treatment modality and another therapeutic compounds over BBB has been devised by delivery of target siRNA to CNS.

There is technique that allows rabies virus to penetrate neuron cell and disseminate all over brain, making it easier for siRNA to cross the BBB. Particular binding of nicotinic acetylcholine receptor (AchR) is found on vascular endothelium of BBB and neurons; a short peptide (29 amino acid) obtained from rabies virus glycoprotein (RVG) is demonstrated to work as a "key" for CNS, enabling transvascular delivery, most likely by receptor-mediated transcytosis.

By competitively inhibiting the binding of AchR of snake venom toxin, bungarotoxin, RVG peptide was discovered. A nonapeptide which is positively charged is made up of d-arginine (9R) which was attached to RVG peptide to link it with the siRNA, enabling the negatively charged siRNA to get attached through charge interactions. For control construct, peptide was obtained from rabies virus matrix protein; it was demonstrated in in vitro study that this construct facilitates the knockdown of siRNA-mediated gene in neuron cells.[15]

Mice were intravenously administered with fluorescent siRNA-RVG-9R peptide combination for in vivo investigation of siRNA delivery. No fluorescence was seen in spleen or liver, indicating that the uptake of the siRNA was entirely limited to the brain. Brain sections were examined under a microscope to confirm fluorescence. Transgenic mice with green fluorescent protein (GFP) were administered with siRNA particular to GFP which got binded to RVG-9R, which demonstrates the gene-specific silencing. The brain showed a considerable drop in GFP expression after three days of therapy (50%) but not in other tissues. When the endogenous gene superoxide dismutase 1 (SOD1), which is stated in a variety of brain cell types, was targeted, similar outcomes were attained. By employing these designs to administer an antiviral siRNA that had previously been shown to protect mice from lethal infection with the Japanese encephalitis virus (JEV) when administered intracranially, potential clinical utility was demonstrated. After JEV infection induced in immunocompromised mice, intravenous siRNA-RVG-9R medication was administered for three days and showed 80% survival as opposed to 100% death in control animals. The scientists excluded the role of immunological mediators by measuring the type I interferon levels.

Transvascular transport of siRNA to the CNS has now been proven to be safe and non-invasive thanks to these findings. The molecular specifics of the delivery mechanism are still unknown, and gene-silencing effectiveness may yet be enhanced. However, given the therapeutic potential of siRNA, this strategy may usher in a new wave of therapies for a variety of neurological conditions. Additionally, RVG-9R may not be a more assuring drug delivery method for siRNA and possibly another therapeutic agents, but also a robust method for comprehensively analyzing the function of gene in brain in an experimental setting. [15,16]

10.5 RNA-BASED TREATMENTS FOR BRAIN DISEASES

In theory, gene silencing might be utilized to cure or significantly decrease the progress of many neurological and neurodegenerative illnesses, but challenges with delivery have hampered development in comparison to siRNA administration in other organs, such as the liver. The only neurological treatment which received approval for systemic polyneuropathy or hTTR is Patisiran (Alnylam Pharmaceuticals). A lipid nanoparticle delivery method is used to intravenously administer patisiran. However, the BBB will decrease its usefulness for majority of brain conditions that call for efficient or direct delivery to the actual brain. Similar to other RNA drug-delivery systems, chemical alterations and conjugates are advancing the potential of siRNA treatments by enhancing the transport, stability, and longevity of the siRNA. Pharmaceutical companies have made significant investments and are strongly committed to advancing the brain-targeting siRNAs therapeutic development for a variety of neurological illnesses. The neurodegenerative disorders like Alzheimer's disease, Huntington's disease, and Parkinson's disease are among the goals of pre-clinical programmes. SiRNA-based treatments also offer a high ability to provide treatments for a comprehensive spectrum of neurological illnesses like brain tumors and stroke, in contrast to AONs, which is mostly concentrated on addressing particular genetic abnormalities.

Because siRNA only has a short-term effect on surrounding cells when directly administered inside brain; up until recently, regular administration was necessary. However, utilizing a divalent chemical scaffold (di-siRNA) administered through a single injection into CSF, robust and prolonged huntingtin gene silencing has now been accomplished in small and non-human primate animal models. Di-siRNAs are made up of two phosphorothioate siRNAs joined together by a linker; unlike research utilizing conventional siRNA, the number of PS modifications seems to be important. Alterman et al. found little proof of immunological stimulation, suggesting both its excellent tolerance and its few side effects. Alnylam Pharmaceuticals is developing novel conjugated-based delivery methods and has successfully targeted the liver using the sugar molecule N-acetylgalactosamine (GalNAc).[17]

A wide variety of RNAs are found in extracellular settings, and they are resistant to blood RNases. It is yet unclear how circulating RNAs maintain their stability, although it has been suggested that exosomes, which resemble extracellular vesicles, may be crucial to this stabilization. Due to their distinctive qualities, such as the ability to correlate miRNA levels with activity (because they are not translated) and their presence in peripheral biofluids, microRNAs are the species that is most explored for the diagnosis of AD. Recent research suggests that circulating miRNAs are a good indicator of tissues that are releasing their contents, providing insight into cellular processes. According to various studies, some miRNAs may be crucial in the aetiology of AD and show signs of being dysregulated in the blood of AD patients. Additionally, circulating miRNA profiles that are unique to AD have been identified in a study. These profiles can distinguish AD from controls with an accuracy of 93% and from other neurological illnesses including schizophrenia, depression, and bipolar disorder with an accuracy of roughly 76%.

A different study found that miRNA193b, an APP expression negative regulator, was considerably reduced in extracellular vesicles of AD murine serum when compared to wild-type mice. A panel of 15 miRNAs that are differently expressed in serum extracellular vesicles and are associated with APOE4 status have also been found. As a result, AD could be predicted with a sensitivity of 87%. These results demonstrate that miRNA could represent the next wave of AD biomarkers.[18]

The intricacy of neurodegenerative disorders possess an urgent obstacle to development of potent miRNA-based Parkinson's disease treatments. RNA interference has been used in the past with considerable success to reduce the amounts of certain PD-related proteins and to decrease expression of chosen target gene. For instance, protein levels were significantly reduced when small-hairpin RNA-specific lentiviral vector system or chemically modified siRNA were used to target synuclein. miRNAs is a superior choice for controlling endogenous gene expression in RNA-based treatments, which is strongly supported by the assumption that RNA-interference-based treatments will be the main classes of medications in future. MiRNA medications are gaining attention due to their unique ability in PD therapy because they do not seem to have same toxicity problems as small hairpin RNA-based therapies or siRNA-based therapies.

miRNA-based therapeutic techniques are studied in vivo and in vitro to modulate disease-related miRNAs expression levels with possibility of treating or delaying the onset of disease. On the one hand, it is possible to successfully downregulate the particular target proteins expression by introducing mature miRNA imitates, which is tiny RNA molecules that resemble miRNA precursors. Any gene implicated in the aetiology of the disease, or even the disease gene itself if it has undergone a gain-of-function pathogenic mutation, could be target protein. Before determining the effectiveness of this miRNA-based method in humans, there are two major obstacles that must be overcome. For starters, distribution of any medication through BBB acquire a unique technical challenge for peripheral administration to brain. Another drawback of modifying the function or amount particular miRNA is the off-target physiological effect. Prior to practical application, it is conceivable that proper dose optimization of miRNA imitate must be accomplished to provide long-lasting effect. [19]

10.6 DNA NANOPARTICLE IN BRAIN

With extremely high specificities, a variety of biomaterials and bio-functionalized nanomaterials have been demonstrated to interaction and regulations in biological systems at molecular and cellular levels. In order for cells and living organisms to function properly and to survive, complex, coordinated, and cross-linked actions are carried out by functional biological assemblies of nucleic acids, proteins, and another molecular components. Scientists have developed nanoscaled biodevices and DNA nanoparticle which can be employed as small programmable molecular robot for a variety of purposes by drawing inspiration from naturally occurring biological complexes and employing pattern specificity and molecular recognition. The application of DNA nanotechnology has expanded in many different ways. In terms of devices with the capability to cross BBB, neuronal cells differentiation and adhesion, imaging, and manipulating, DNA nanotechnology has developed nanomaterials to investigate systems of brain.[20] The majority of blood arteries supplying to brain contain the BBB, physical barrier with distinct characteristics. The BBBs' unmatched architecture is made up by a continuous layer of non-fenestrated endothelial cell ringed by smooth muscle cells, pericytes, and astrocyte projections which is essential for its ability to perform its role.[21] Table 10.2 summarizes the various types of nanoparticles which is utilized in brain disease treatment.

TABLE 10.2 Nanoparticles Used in Treatment of Brain Diseases.[22]

List of nanoparticles (NPs)	Brain disease treatment
Magnetic iron oxide NPs + reduced radiotherapy	Glioblastoma multiforme
Nano-curcumin + ω-3 fatty acids	Migraine
Silver nanoparticles	Acute occlusive hydrocephalus
Ultrasmall magnetic iron oxide	Ischemic stroke

10.7 WHY TO CHOOSE DNA NANOMATERIAL

Since DNA is a basic component of hereditary material and a common biomolecule, it has been used by various species to store genetic information. Due to its distinctive properties, such as great controllability according to Watson-Crick base-pairing precision, DNA materials have the potential to be used in nanofabrication.[23] The initial set of guidelines for the synthesis of DNA nanostructures were put forth by Seeman et al. in the 1980s, which set off an era of rapid progress for DNA nanotechnology.[24] A large range of structures, including two- and three-dimensional structures, were designed for DNA nanomaterials. Additionally, the architectures of synthetic DNA nanostructures contain multilayer and single-layer nanostructures that are categorized into circular, linear, and branching forms in accordance with the diverse molecular building-styles of functional DNA materials.[25] Numerous multipurpose polymeric DNA nanoparticles continue to have problems, such as being easily digested, lacking in targeting, and being unstable.[26–28]

There are various example of DNA nanoparticles which is used for brain targeting. Many illnesses of CNS, like neurodegenerative disease and brain tumor, are treated with gene therapy. However, both the BBB and brains extracellular matrix (ECM), which functions as adhesive and steric barriers, can obstruct the passage of systemically injected gene carriers which get delivered into the CNS.

DNA-bearing "brain penetrating" (DNA-BPN) nanoparticles with dense polyethylene glycol corona helps in the prevention of adhesion to ECM materials. Merging strategies could be used to regulate localized, strong, and long-lasting transgenic expression in brain of rat by systemically delivering DNA-BPN across BBB. Systemically administered DNA-BPN that was administered over BBB with focused ultrasound (FUS) resulted in expression of dose-dependent transgene that was present only in area that had received the FUS treatment and that became visible as soon as 24 h after administration and persisted for not less than 28 days. Finally, it is concluded that a safe and non-invasive approach for targeted gene therapy to brain is image-guided administration of DNA-BPN with micro bubbles combined with FUS. [29]

The most widespread, diverse, and challenging to treat physiological problems that doctors encounter are brain disorders. Numerous illnesses that are related to the brain's complexity and inaccessibility have inadequate treatment choices. However, strategies like DNA nanoparticle delivery have the ability to get over these obstacles. DNA nanoparticles frequently makes usage of DNA "gene segments" inserted into viral vectors to directly target defective or decreased amounts of proteins within cells.

Parkinson's illness has been treated with non-viral gene therapy vectors created at Copernicus. These vectors are packed into DNA (DNPs) nanoparticles that resemble rods by Dr Mark Cooper of Copernicus Therapeutics. DNPs are capable to safely and effectively diffuse to the nucleus across the nuclear membrane envelope in nuclease-rich settings.[30]

In general, the advantages of nanoparticles include their multifunctionality, capacity to transport drug payloads, ability to control release of drug, and ability to alter drugs pharmacokinetics. Additionally, enhanced permeability and retention (EPR) effect suggests that nanoparticles due to their nano size (200 nm) easily enter into tumor tissue that is "leaky" to help with medication administration.[31] Figure 10.3 shows the various nanoparticles used in CNS gene delivery.

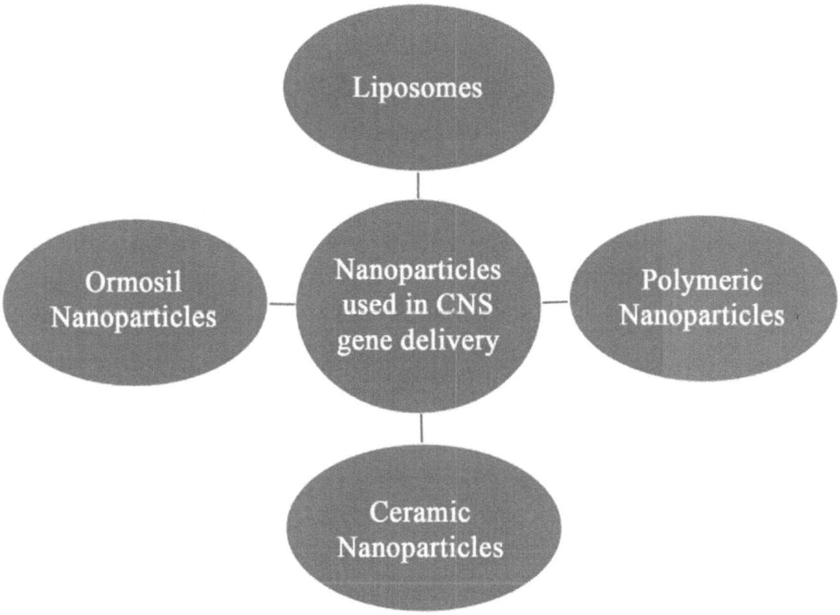

FIGURE 10.3 Schematic diagram shows the various nanoparticles used in gene delivery to CNS.

10.8 VARIOUS NANOPARTICLE USED IN DELIVERY OF GENE TOWARD CNS

10.8.1 LIPOSOMES IN GENE DELIVERY TO CNS

Beginning in the early 1990s, studies of gene transfer toward CNS by utilizing cationic liposomes started to be mentioned in literature. Holt et al. successfully injected liposome-DNA complexes directly into the Xenopus embryonic brain to transfect neurons.[32] Numerous labs subsequently documented CNS gene transfer utilizing various cationic liposome formulations like "lipofectins," which was mentioned early in the articles.[33] Imaoka et al. appealed to induce therapeutic changes in rats having an experimental form of Parkinson's disease by continuous and direct administration of a liposomal compound of a plasmid encoding tyrosine hydroxylase in 1998, which is likely the first report of effective liposome-mediated CNS gene therapy (TH).[34] Clinical acceptance of gene transfer toward CNS after systemic administration of DNA liposome compound would be higher. BBB which prevents macromolecules like circulating lipoplexes from reaching the brain, prevents this from being possible when using cationic liposomes for two reasons:

1. These liposomes are easily captured by the reticuloendothelial system because they are very unstable in biological fluids.
2. The BBB prevents macromolecular vehicles such as lipoplexes that circulate into blood and enters into the brain. Shi et al. has created neutral/anionic liposomes with polymer polyethylene glycol (PEG) to overcome this issue.[35]

10.8.2 POLYMERIC NANOPARTICLES IN DELIVERY OF GENE TO CNS

Due to its capacity to create stable compounds with genetic material, the cationic polymer polyethyleneimine (PEI) is perfect for delivering genes to the brain. Abdallah et al. made the very first evidence of effective PEI-mediated in vivo gene transport into brain by combining plasmid DNA with branching PEI (25 kDa) at an electrostatic charge near to neutral. Goula et al. were compressed DNA by using a linear 22-kDa polymer. For biological fluids, the compound was discovered to be extremely diffusible and stable and IV injection caused the complex to diffuse from the administration site to the whole space of brain.

10.8.3 CERAMIC NANOPARTICLES IN DELIVERY OF GENE TO CNS

A variety of cationic ceramic nanoparticles are investigated. Among these, carbon nanotubes, calcium phosphate nanoparticles, and cationic silica nanoparticles stand out. Although these nanoparticles demonstrated as great option for gene transfer in in vitro, there are no reports on their application in *in vivo*. A team has evaluated calcium phosphate nanoparticles condensed with the galactosidase. It is directly administered through injection at SN area of rat brain. One month after injection, the midbrain area showed moderate gene expression. As a result, their potential for CNS gene delivery with better formulations is highlighted. [36]

10.8.4 ORMOSIL NANOPARTICLES IN DELIVERY OF GENE TO CNS

Amino-terminated organically modified silica (ORMOSIL) nanoparticles carries condensed plasmid DNA inside of cell while also protecting it.

ORMOSIL nanoparticles contains cationic amino groups that electrostatically get stimulated to form a complex with the anionic plasmid DNA and the 30 nm is average diameter of the compounds. As a result of the plasmid nanoparticle complex destabilizing in acidic environment of intracellular compartments including lysosomes and endosomes, plasmid is anticipated to be release inside the cells. These nanoparticle complexes can get fluorescently marked to optically trace their movement both inside and outside of cell.[37] They investigated the potential for in vivo gene transfer in CNS by utilizing direct stereotaxic injection of ORMOSIL-DNA nanoparticle complexes (nanoplexes) inside the brain of mouse after successfully demonstrating their ability to transfer genes in vitro. In the beginning, the substantia nigra per compacta (SNc) area of brain was used to test a gene expression by using the plasmid encoding the enhanced green fluorescent protein (Pegfp), an area populated in neuronal cells and of considerable interest for its role in PD and other psychiatric diseases.[38,39] An efficient research method for *in vivo* testing of single gene and multiple gene therapy, the ORMOSIL nanoparticle-mediated transfection are utilized to represent hereditary brain illnesses in mice and also in other species.

10.9 DNA NANOPARTICLES IN PARKINSON'S DISEASE

The glial cell line-derived neurotrophic factor (GDNF) gene was successfully transfected to cells of the rat striatum to induce overexpression of the protein, measured at up to six months post-injection, according to Dr. Yurek's and Dr. Cooper's experiments assessing DNP performance and viability. It's interesting to note that GDNF has been found to reverse dopamine depletion in PD animal models, and it also significantly increases the effectiveness of embryonic dopaminergic cell grafts, another exciting PD treatment. Dr. Yurek and associates at Copernicus Therapeutics have researched the advantages of administering GDNF DNPs one week prior to administering striatal dopaminergic grafts to rats in order to develop this and the use of DNPs. These investigations found that transplanted dopaminergic cells performed better in terms of survival and function than when GDNF DNP was present in the transplanted treatment area.[30]

10.10 CHALLENGES FOR RNA-BASED TREATMENTS

As in the early days of gene-based medicine research, there was excitement around RNAi discovery, and it was expected that RNAi-based treatments can quickly enters in clinic. The prospect of early success has now been dampened by a number of problems that occurs by another nucleic acid based technology which is get experienced in past and have yet to solve. Strategies are being developed to get around natural delivery hurdles, prevent immune/non-immune toxicities, and track the delivery and therapeutic indices in real-time to get therapeutic effect of RNAi.

Due to BBB, it is hard to deliver inhibitory RNAs to CNS. As previously mentioned, our understanding of illness aetiology (such as its start, progression, and afflicted tissues or cell types) as well as the required length of gene silence will determine the most appropriate RNAi delivery mechanism. Non-viral nucleic acids (such as "naked" or complexed synthetic siRNAs) can enter to central nervous system by one of three main entry points: the vasculature, cerebrospinal fluid, or directly through the brain parenchyma. Stability of siRNA complexes and their ability to enter into target cells without inducing immune responses are the limiting variables in this. Initial attempts to overcome some of these difficulties centred on adding chemical alterations to the bases, backbone, or sugars of siRNA duplexes.

Increased stability is brought up by some modifications which effectively reduced the dose required to attain measurably and repeatedly gene silencing. Internal changes, however, did not enhance CNS entrance and uptake following systemic administration. Instead, new research has focused on exploring the potential of liposomes, cell-penetrating peptides, and nanoparticles to stabilize and transport siRNAs across brain. Researchers can also attached "brain homing" antibodies or peptides with nanoparticles and liposomes to improve brain uptake by following systemic administration.[40]

Future research will concentrates on finding ways to use disease-related epitopes to improve the potency, specificity, and efficacy of non-viral siRNA delivery to brain. Last but not least, the possibility of an unfavorable immune response to RNAi therapy is a crucial factor, especially in neurodegenerative disorders when the affected brain is already in a "heightened state of awareness" due to its response to persistent pro-inflammatory signaling cascades. These interactions are dose- and sequence-dependent and can take place during the internalization (lysosomal or endosomal compartments) or release of siRNA molecule intracellularly. The utilization of chemically altered or siRNA duplexes enclosed in nanoparticles prevents stimulation of these pathways. [41]

The development of RNAi-based therapeutics will continue to be guided by new findings in RNAi biology. The discovery that certain miRNAs are present in extracellular body fluids and plasma is one fascinating new discovery. According to latest research, miRNAs "secreted" can inhibit the gene expression after being taken up by nearby cell. The suggested pathway's individual components have been found by several research teams, but the mechanism and enzyme complexes responsible for miRNA trafficking from cell to cell are still mostly unknown. However, therapeutic potential of "secreted" RNAi-based approaches is proved important for additional research.

The recent inability to track in real-time, transport, specificity, and activity of an RNAi molecule inside brain is an another difficulty for neuroscientists to utilize RNAi. In contrast to skin conditions, infections, and many cancers, brain conditions make post-treatment sampling impractical. Therefore, model systems are needed to identify links between the effectiveness of gene silencing and dose specific toxicity. The easiest technique to track a concurrent response to therapeutic RNAi is through biomarkers specific to the neurodegenerative disease under investigation, albeit for various diseases accuracy of a given biomarker to denote a certain stage of disease is far from known. Finally, improvements in imaging methods that use quantum dots to follow RNA *in vivo* appear promising. [40,42]

10.11 LIMITATION FOR RNA-BASED TREATMENTS

While RNAi has potential therapeutic uses and also overcome the few drawbacks of traditional gene therapy, it can also have some limits. Delivery of drug is a great barrier in RNAi treatments while it is used in clinical application. Synthetic siRNA delivery can be improved through chemical stabilization and creation of targeting strategies, but in various other ways, these molecules are managed and improved in the same way as conventional pharmacological agents. Improved selection of siRNA sequence and inclusion of nucleotide changes to speed guide-strand loading into RISC have been made possible in recent years thanks to a better knowledge of the biology of RNA interference (RNAi). However, nonspecific off-target effects whether brought on by scant sequence homologies or miRNA-like effects remain a major source of worry. It is currently believed that particular chemical alterations to siRNAs may eliminate or mitigate these effects. For expressed siRNAs, vector capacity is not as important as it could be for traditional gene therapy; yet, these vectors' regulatory components still need to be improved. The majority of studies now use Pol III promoters, often H1 or U6, to activate expression of siRNA; however, these lack the ability to regulate time or space. Utilizing miRNA-like siRNAs will make it possible to evaluate Pol II promoters to drive tissue specific regulation more frequently.

Last but not least, while synthetic siRNAs have inflammatory issues, expressed siRNAs are anticipated to generate immune responses directed against vector components that are comparable to those described in conventional gene therapy research. Several investigations has documented siRNA-induced interferon responses that were initially believed to be related to longer dsRNAs. Immune system can be triggered by certain nucleotide motifs in dsRNAs via Toll-like receptors (TLRs), specifically TLR7, TLR3, TLR8, and TLR9. Such motifs are avoided in siRNA design when they have been characterized; however, it is now recognized that chemical alteration at particular nucleotides can eliminate TLR recognition and improve safety. [43]

10.12 CONCLUSION

Utilization of nanotechnology in the medical field aids in the improvement of disease detection and treatment by raising the sensitivity of diagnostic tools and altering pharmacological parameters, which increases the effectiveness of the drugs. The capacity of nanotechnologies to penetrate the BBB makes these substances a viable treatment option for brain disorders and diseases, which have been difficult to diagnose and treat for a long time. However, more research is required to ascertain their toxicity and bioaccumulation in clinical settings in order to guarantee the efficacy and efficiency of these particles.

ACKNOWLEDGMENTS

For the successful completion of this study, all of the writers of this publication are grateful to their respective universities/departments.

KEYWORDS

- **nanoscience**
- **RNA therapeutics**
- **DNA therapeutics**
- **disease**
- **brain delivery**

REFERENCES

1. Zogg, H.; Singh, R.; Ro, S. Current Advances in RNA Therapeutics for Human Diseases. *Int. J. Mol. Sci.* **2022,** *23* (5), 2736.
2. Winkle, M.; El-Daly, S. M.; Fabbri, M.; Calin, G. A. Noncoding RNA Therapeutics—Challenges and Potential Solutions. *Nat. Rev. Drug Discov.* **2021,** *20* (8), 629–651.
3. Bajan, S.; Hutvagner, G. RNA-based Therapeutics: From Antisense Oligonucleotides to miRNAs. *Cells* **2020,** *9* (1), 137.
4. Scheller, E. L.; Villa-Diaz, L. G.; Krebsbach, P. H. Gene Therapy: Implications for Craniofacial Regeneration. *J. Craniofacial Surg.* **2012,** *23* (1), 333.
5. Scheller, E. L.; Krebsbach, P. H. Gene Therapy: Design and Prospects for Craniofacial Regeneration. *J. Dental Res.* **2009,** *88* (7), 585–596.
6. Dewannieux, M.; Harper, F.; Richaud, A.; Letzelter, C.; Ribet, D.; Pierron, G.; Heidmann, T. Identification of an Infectious Progenitor for the Multiple-copy HERV-K Human Endogenous Retroelements. *Genome Res.* **2006,** *16* (12), 1548–1556.
7. Gomes, M. J.; Martins, S.; Sarmento, B. siRNA as a Tool to Improve the Treatment of Brain Diseases: Mechanism, Targets and Delivery. *Ageing Res. Rev.* **2015,** *21,* 43–54.
8. Haussecker, D.; Kay, M. A. Drugging RNAi. *Science* **2015,** *347* (6226), 1069–1070.
9. Zheng, M.; Tao, W.; Zou, Y.; Farokhzad, O. C.; Shi, B. Nanotechnology-based Strategies for siRNA Brain Delivery for Disease Therapy. *Trends Biotechnol.* **2018,** *36* (5), 562–575.
10. Scaglioni, D.; Catapano, F.; Ellis, M.; Torelli, S.; Chambers, D.; Feng, L.; Beck, M.; Sewry, C.; Monforte, M.; Harriman, S.; Koenig, E. The Administration of Antisense Oligonucleotide Golodirsen Reduces Pathological Regeneration in Patients with Duchenne Muscular Dystrophy. *Acta Neuropathol. Commun.* **2021,** *9* (1), 1–17.
11. Balwani, M.; Sardh, E.; Ventura, P., Peiró, P. A., Rees, D. C.; Stölzel, U.; Bissell, D. M.; Bonkovsky, H. L.; Windyga, J.; Anderson, K. E.; Parker, C. Phase 3 Trial of RNAi Therapeutic Givosiran for Acute Intermittent Porphyria. *New Engl. J. Med.* **2020,** *382* (24), 2289–2301.
12. Baden, L. R.; El Sahly, H. M.; Essink, B.; Kotloff, K.; Frey, S.; Novak, R.; Diemert, D.; Spector, S. A.; Rouphael, N.; Creech, C. B.; McGettigan, J. Efficacy and Safety of the mRNA-1273 SARS-CoV-2 Vaccine. *New Engl. J. Med.* **2020**.
13. Aagaard, L.; Rossi, J. J. RNAi Therapeutics: Principles, Prospects and Challenges. *Adv. Drug Deliv. Rev.* **2007,** *59* (2–3), 75–86.
14. Gupta, N.; Rai, D. B.; Jangid, A. K.; Pooja, D.; Kulhari, H. Nanomaterials-based siRNA Delivery: Routes of Administration, Hurdles and Role of Nanocarriers. In *Nanotechnology in Modern Animal Biotechnology*;Springer: Singapore, 2019; pp 67–114.
15. Flemming, A. siRNA: Brain Delivery Breakthrough. *Nat. Rev. Drug Discov.* **2007,** *6* (8), 601–601.
16. Kumar, P.; Wu, H.; McBride, J. L.; Jung, K. E.; Hee Kim, M.; Davidson, B. L.; Kyung Lee, S.; Shankar, P.; Manjunath, N. Transvascular Delivery of Small Interfering RNA to the Central Nervous System. *Nature* **2007,** *448* (7149), 39–43.
17. Anthony, K. RNA-based Therapeutics for Neurological Diseases. *RNA Biol.* **2022,** *19* (1), 176–190.
18. Riscado, M.; Baptista, B.; Sousa, F. New RNA-based Breakthroughs in Alzheimer's Disease Diagnosis and Therapeutics. *Pharmaceutics* **2021,** *13* (9), 1397.

19. Ma, L.; Wei, L.; Wu, F.; Hu, Z.; Liu, Z.; Yuan, W. Advances with microRNAs in Parkinson's Disease Research. *Drug Design, Dev. Ther.* **2013,** *7,* 1103.
20. Hivare, P.; Panda, C.; Gupta, S.; Bhatia, D. Programmable DNA Nanodevices for Applications in Neuroscience. *ACS Chem. Neurosci.* **2021,** *12* (3), 363–377.
21. Pinheiro, R. G.; Coutinho, A. J.; Pinheiro, M.; Neves, A. R. Nanoparticles for Targeted Brain Drug Delivery: What do we Know? *Int. J. Mol. Sci.* **2021,** *22* (21), 11654.
22. Ngowi, E. E.; Wang, Y. Z.; Qian, L.; Helmy, Y. A. S. H.; Anyomi, B.; Li, T.; Zheng, M.; Jiang, E. S.; Duan, S. F.; Wei, J. S.; Wu, D. D. The Application of Nanotechnology for the Diagnosis and Treatment of Brain Diseases and Disorders. *Front. Bioeng. Biotechnol.* **2021,** *9,* 629832.
23. Seeman, N. C. DNA Nanotechnology: From the Pub to Information-based Chemistry. *Methods Mol. Biol.* **2018,** *1811,* 1–9.
24. Seeman, N. C. DNA Nanotechnology: Novel DNA Constructions. *Annu. Rev. Biophys. Biomol. Struct.* **1998,** *27,* 225–248.
25. Roh, Y. H.; Ruiz, R. C.; Peng, S.; Lee, J. B.; Luo, D. Engineering DNA-based Functional Materials. *Chem. Soc. Rev.* **2011,** *40,* 5730–5744.
26. Seeman, N. C. Nucleic-acid Junctions and Lattices. *J. Theor. Biol.* **1982,** *99,* 237–247.
27. Seeman, N. C. DNA Engineering and its Application to Nanotechnology. *Trends Biotechnol.* **1999,** *17,* 437–443.
28. Seeman, N. C.; et al. Two Dimensions and Two States in DNA Nanotechnology. *J. Biomol. Struct. Dyn.* **2000,** *17,* 253–262.
29. Mead, B. P.; Mastorakos. P.; Suk, J. S.; Klibanov, A. L.; Hanes, J.; Price, R. J. Targeted Gene Transfer to the Brain via the Delivery of Brain-penetrating DNA Nanoparticles with Focused Ultrasound. *J. Control. Release* **2016,** *223,* 109–17.
30. https://researchfeatures.com/dna-nanoparticle-gene-therapy/
31. Dong, X. Current Strategies for Brain Drug Delivery. *Theranostics* **2018,** *8* (6), 1481.
32. Holt, C. E.; Garlick, N.; Cornel, E. Lipofection of cDNAs in the Embryonic Vertebrate Central Nervous System. *Neuron* **1990,** *4,* 203–14.
33. Ono, T.; Fujino, Y.; Tsuchiya, T.; Tsuda, M. Plasmid DNAs Directly Injected into Mouse Brain with Lipofectin can be Incorporated and Expressed by Brain Cells. *Neurosci. Lett.* **1990,** *117,* 259–63.
34. Imaoka, T.; Date, I.; Ohmoto, T.; Nagatsu, T. Significant Behavioral Recovery in Parkinson's Disease Model by Direct Intracerebral Gene Transfer Using Continuous Injection of a Plasmid DNA-liposome Complex. *Hum. Gene Ther.* **1998,** *9,* 1093–102.
35. Shi, N.; Pardridge, W. M. Noninvasive Gene Targeting to the Brain. *Proc. Natl. Acad. Sci. U. S. A.* **2000,** *97,* 7567–72.
36. Roy, I.; Stachowiak, M. K.; Bergey, E. J. Nonviral Gene Transfection Nanoparticles: Function and Applications in the Brain. *Nanomed.: Nanotechnol. Biol. Med.* **2008,** *4* (2), 89–97.
37. Roy, I.; Ohulchanskyy, T. Y.; Bharali, D. J.;, Pudavar, H. E.; Mistretta, R. A.; Kaur, N.; et al. Optical Tracking of Organically Modified Silica Nanoparticles as DNA Carriers: A Nonviral, Nanomedicine Approach for Gene Delivery. *Proc. Natl. Acad. Sci. U. S. A.* **2005,** *102,* 279–284.
38. Fisher, L. J.; Gage, F. H. Radical Directions in Parkinson's Disease. *Nat. Med.* **1995,** *1,* 201–203.
39. Wong, A. H.; Van, H.; Tol, H. Schizophrenia: From Phenomenology to Neurobiology. *Neurosci. Biobehav. Rev.* **2003,** *27,* 269–306.

40. Boudreau, R. L.; Rodríguez-Lebrón, E.; Davidson, B. L. RNAi Medicine for the Brain: Progresses and Challenges. *Hum. Mol. Genet.* **2011,** *20* (R1), R21–R27.
41. Robbins, M.; Judge, A.; MacLachlan, I. siRNA and Innate Immunity. *Oligonucleotides* **2009,** *19* (2), 89–102.
42. Hong, H.; Zhang, Y.; Cai, W. In vivo Imaging of RNA Interference. *J. Nucl. Med.* **2010,** *51* (2), 169–172.
43. Wood, M.; Yin, H.; McClorey, G. Modulating the Expression of Disease Genes with RNA-based Therapy. *PLoS Genet.* **2007,** *3* (6), e109.

CHAPTER 11

Application of Medicinal Plants and Their Phytoconstituents Used in the Management of Neurodegenerative Diseases

PADMINI SHUKLA and PRABODH SHUKLA

Faculty of Pharmacy, Uttar Pradesh University of Medical Sciences, Saifai, Etawah, Uttar Pradesh, India

ABSTRACT

Modern medicines that are based on psychoactive drugs are generally used for treatment purposes but unfortunately these medicines are limited. Ayurveda plays a very prominent role to overcome the current lifestyle diseases and is also helpful in disease management related to ageing processes. Ayurveda developed a separate branch known as Medhya Rasayanas to treat mental diseases. The Medhya Rasayan generally consists of four medicinal plants which can be used alone or in combination. The four drugs which are used in the Medhya Rasayana are *Centella asiatica* (Mandukaparni), *Glycyrrhiza glabra* (Yastimadhu), *Tinosporacardifolia* (Guduchi), and *Convolvulus pluricaulis* (Shankhpushpi). Apart from above-mentioned drugs, other drugs like *Bacopa monniera* (Aindri), *Celastruspanniculata* (Jyotishmati), *Acorus calamus* (Vach), *Benincasahispida* (Kushmanda), and *Nardostachys-jatamansi* (Jatamansi) also show prominent effect in novel drug delivery systems. Some secondary plant metabolites which are useful for the treatment of novel drug delivery systems are quercitin, epigenin, rosmarinic acid, epigallocatechin 3-galate, curcumin, resveratrol, shogaol, oleuropein, limonoids, ginkgolide, and ginsenoside. These secondary plant metabolites

Nanomedicine for Neurodegenerative Disorders: Selective Treatment Strategies. Rishabha Malviya, Kamla Pathak, & Swati Verma (Eds.)

have special ability to treat the novel drug delivery systems by targeting various mechanisms like protein misfolding and aggregation prevention, acetylcholinestrase inhibition, antithrombotic activity, monoamine oxidase inhibitors, antioxidant activity, anti-inflammatory activity, and neurotrophic and antiapoptotic activity. In this study, an attempt has been made to collect and compile the available information which will help the researchers and medical practitioners for further study.

11.1 INTRODUCTION

Neurodegenerative disorders (NDDs) indicate the progressive loss of structure as well as function of neurons. This occurs due to the deposition of abnormal proteins which causes inflammation and oxidative stress in the human central nervous system (CNS). The major diseases included in NDDs are amyotrophic lateral sclerosis (ALS), Parkinson's disease (PD), multiple sclerosis (MS), Huntington's disease, and Alzheimer's disease (AD).[1] In a rough estimate, around 26.6 million patients are suffering from AD worldwide, which may increase up to 106.2 million by 2050. Similarly, 6.3 million patients' are affected by PD.[2] The various factors which are responsible for NDDs are inflammation, oxidative and endoplasmic reticulum cellular stress, ischemia, injury of nervous system, toxic protein accumulation in neural tissues, infection through prions or viruses, and autoimmune-mediated neuronal loss.[3] Due to the loss of neurons, demyelination or gliosis can show the symptoms of behavioral disturbances, like motor deficiency and cognitive decline. NDDs are the most common disorder after headache. A great amount of energy is required when any neuron or immune cell comes in contact with toxic protein. This causes the stress. Due to the stress, mitochondria produces various mitochondrial proteins and cytochrome C which leads toward apoptosis. The high amount of protein affects the neuronal function and cellular signaling.[4,5]

The other causes which contribute in the neurodegeneration diseases are mentioned in the following sections.

11.2 GENETICS AND HEREDITARY

Lots of work is done on genetics in last few years. Genes and hereditary system are responsible for the progressive development of NDDs. In the case of AD, mutation occurs in three genes named presenilin protein-1 (PSEN1), presenilin protein-2 (PSEN2), and amyloid precursor protein (APP). These may be responsible for early arising of AD. Similarly, other eight different genes have been identified for PD.[6]

11.3 OXIDATIVE STRESS AND THEIR IMPACT

Oxidative stress is very common in today's day-to-day life and it is mainly responsible for generation of various neurodegenerative diseases like PD, Huntington's disease, AD, and others. The DNA can be damaged due to the oxidative stress which progresses the development of NDDs. Some enzymes like P_{450} present in mitochondria and endoplasmic reticulum are responsible for the generation of reactive oxygen species (ROS) along with various oxidative radicals which are promoted by the ageing process and develops NDDs.[7,8] Superoxide dismutase, glutathione, and catalase are some of the natural antioxidant mechanism which are present in our body; they neutralize the free radical oxidants which accelerates the ageing process.[9,10] Our human brain consists of rich amount of fatty acids which are unsaturated in nature. High oxygen demand is needed in our brain to function properly.[11] In the process of lipid peroxidation, the polyunsaturated fatty acids which are present in our brain gets oxidized and worsens the symptoms of NDDs.[12]

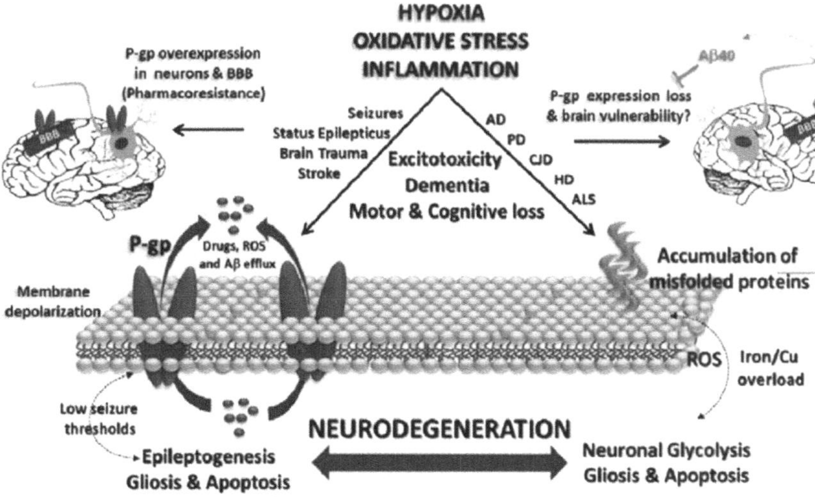

FIGURE 11.1 Causes of neurodegeneration.

11.4 ENVIRONMENTAL ROLE

Some of the toxic solvents and elements like manganese when they come in prolonged contact with human organs produce mitochondrial dysfunctions. Thus, alpha synuclein accumulates, which progresses PD. Similarly, the other elements like lead and mercury also increases the generation of tau protein and Aβ plaque, which accelerates the symptoms of AD. These microelements are important for various biological reactions in our body but sometimes it disturbs hemostasis from the free radicals.[13] Similarly, pesticides are also responsible for neuronal damage. The human dietary food should be rich in omega 3 fatty acids, vegetables, fish oil, and fruits, which can reduce the danger of NDDs.[14]

11.5 PROTEIN MISFOLDING AND AGGREGATION ROLE

Protein is very important for our body and plays various important roles. Generally, proteins are folded in 3D structures to perform its functions. If folding of protein is not proper, they form clump and hinder in functioning. The NDDs such as AD and PD are good examples of protein misfolding. Due to the deposition of misfolded abnormal proteins, the various cellular functions are disturbed. Molecular chaperons are helpful to protect these abnormal functions.[15] These molecular protein chaperons binds with synthesized proteins as well as unfolded proteins by the process of adenosin triphosphate (ATP) hydrolysis. This step contributes the overall completion process of mature protein confirmation through recruiting ubiquitin ligase to targeted misfolded proteins which are cleared by proteolytic process.[16,17] Sometimes the other factors like necrosis, inflammation, apoptosis, oxidative stress, ion imbalance, mitochondrial dysfunction, and altered blood–brain permeability occur in the case of injury which impedes the NDDs' process.[18]

Ayurveda plays a very prominent role in overcoming the current lifestyle diseases and is very helpful to treat diseases related to the ageing process, like AD, PD, trauma, injuries, etc. Ayurveda had developed a separate branch known as "Medhya Rasayanas" to treat mind-related diseases.

11.5.1 MEDHYA RASAYAN

Medhya Rasayan is derived from two words "Medhya" and "Rasayana." The literal meaning of Medhya is intellect and Rasayana means rejuvenation.

Various drugs used in Medhya Rasayan are generally helpful in improving the intellect. The entire Ayurveda is classified in eight branches known as "Astang." In this, *rasayanchikitsa* (rejuvenation therapy) is very prominent which plays crucial role in disease management. Ayurveda classifies mental disorders in eight different types like *Bhaya* (fear), *Unmada* (insanity), *Harsha* (excitation), *Udvega* (anxiety), *Shoka* (grief), *Avasada* (depression), *Apasmara* (epilepsy), and *Attavaabhinivesha* (obsessive disorder).

The Medhya Rasayan generally consists of four medicinal plants which can be used alone or in combination. These herbs are very helpful to increase the intellect, memory, retention power, and increase the cerebral metabolism. They provide relief from depression, stress, and anxiety. They are helpful in the regeneration of tissue after the disease so that they can treat diseases like Alzheimer's, age-related macular degeneration, PD, trauma, injuries, cardiac problems, etc. In Ayurveda, the idea of Rasayana is specifically connected to the regeneration of tissues and a particular Rasayana nourishes the corresponding tissue.[19] The important drugs which are used in the Medhya Rasayan are described below.

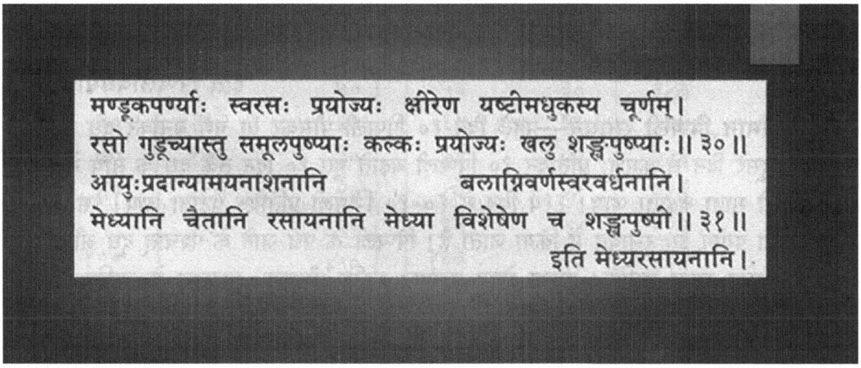
मण्डूकपर्ण्याः स्वरसः प्रयोज्यः क्षीरेण यष्टीमधुकस्य चूर्णम्।
रसो गुडूच्यास्तु समूलपुष्प्याः कल्कः प्रयोज्यः खलु शङ्खपुष्प्याः॥ ३०॥
आयुःप्रदान्यामयनाशनानि बलाग्निवर्णस्वरवर्धनानि।
मेध्यानि चैतानि रसायनानि मेध्या विशेषेण च शङ्खपुष्पी॥ ३१॥
इति मेध्यरसायनानि।

FIGURE 11.2 Description of Medhya Rasayana in ancient Vedas.

11.5.2 CENTELLA ASIATICA (MANDUKAPARNI)

Mandukaparni plays a vital role in enhancing memory and cognition. The accumulation of alpha synuclein is one of the main causes of PD. This aggregation of alpha synuclein can be stopped by the aqueous extract of *Centella asiatica* and it also disintegrates the formed fibrils. *Centella asiatica* plays a pivotal role as antioxidant and antiapoptopic mechanism. *Centella asiatica* shows the neuroprotective effect after the chronic exposure of aluminium.

Centella asiatica is a very good neuroprotective agent and acts against cognitive dysfunction, oxidative stress, and apoptosis.[20] It prevents the formation of amyloid plaque and is helpful to fight AD. The important constituents of *Centella asiatica* are asiatic acid (AA), which is a pentacyclic triterpene and shows prominent neuroprotective effect in different experimental models.[21]

11.5.3 GLYCYRRHIZA GLABRA (YASTIMADHU)

The important constituent of *Glycyrrhiza glabra* is glycyrrizin, which is present in roots and rhizomes. Glycyrrhizin shows neuroprotective action in mouse, which have administered kainic acid (responsible for neuronal cell death). The mechanism involved behind this is suppression of gliosis and enhancement of proinflammatory markers (TNF-α, iNOS, COX-2).[22] Trihydroxy charcoal, a component of *Glycyrrhiza glabra*, inhibits the beta site of the enzyme that breaks down APP, which improves memory in mice with cognitive impairment. The neuroprotective effect is also present in the other ingredient, glabridin, which was also isolated from *Glycyrrhiza glabra*. *Glycyrrhiza glabra*'s significance in improving learning and memory is mostly owing to its modification of the cholinergic transmission pathway.[23]

11.5.4 TINOSPORACARDIFOLIA (GUDUCHI)

Alcoholic extract of *Tinospora cardifolia* shows the prominent neuroprotective action in animal rat model of PD. The entire plant juice is therapeutically used to increase intellect. *Tinospora cardifolia*'s ameliorative and neuroprotective properties are brought on by its antioxidant activity and trace element content (like zinc and copper, which protects the cell from free radicals). It increases the cognitive effect by immune stimulation and promotion of acetylcholine formation.[24,25]

11.5.5 CONVOLVULUS PLURICAULIS (SHANKHPUSHPI)

This drug is used traditionally in Ayurveda to increase intellect and enhance memory.[26] It is a very important drug in Ayurveda to treat insomnia, anxiety, neurosis, and cerebral anomalies, and is also used as a memory enhancer and an effective nervine tonic.[27] The mechanism behind the above mentioned activity is the acetyl cholinesterase inhibitory and antioxidant properties.[28]

Aqueous extract shows neuroprotective effect on rat-induced neurotoxicity by feeding aluminium chloride.[29]

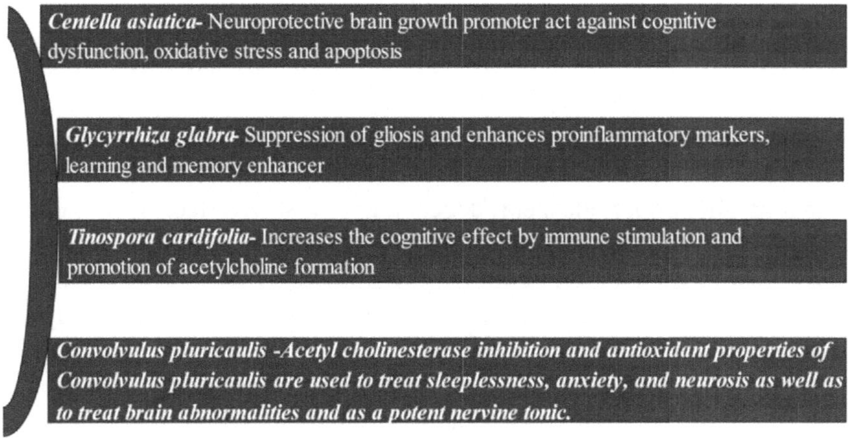

FIGURE 11.3 Medicinal plants used in Medhya Rasayan.

Apart from the abovementioned drugs, other drugs like *Bacopa monniera* (Aindri), *Celastruspanniculata* (Jyotishmati), *Acorus calamus* (Vach), *Benincasahispida* (Kushmanda), *Nardostachysjatamansi* (Jatamansi), etc., also show prominent effect treating neurodegenerative disorders.

TABLE 11.1 Medicinal Plants Used in NDDs.

S. no.	Medicinal plant	Phytoconstituent(s)	Used in disorder(s)	Reference(s)
1.	*Adhatodavasica*	Arachidic, cerotic, linoleicand oleic acids as well as vasicine, vasicol, and vasicinol	Parkinson and Alzheimer disease	30
2.	*Ginkgo biloba*	Biflavonoid amentoflavone	Neurodegenerative diseases like Parkinson	31
3.	*Panax ginseng*	Triterpene saponin ginsenoside	Neurodegenerative diseases like Parkinson	32
4.	*Rauwolfia serpentina*	Reserpine alkaloid	Neurodegenerative diseases like Schizophrenia	33
5.	*Withania somnifera*	Withanoside IV, Physagulin D, Withaferin A, Sitoindoside IX, and Viscosalactone B	Neurodegenerative diseases like Schizophrenia	33

11.6 PLANT SECONDARY METABOLITES

Various secondary plant metabolites play a crucial role in the treatment of NDDs. They have special ability to treat NDDs by targeting various mechanisms. Some of them are given in the following sections.

11.6.1 PROTEIN MISFOLDING AND AGGREGATION PREVENTION

Some of the important neurodegenerative diseases like Huntington's disease, AD, and PD can occur due to protein misfolding. In case of NDDs, like Alzheimer, the senile plaque formation occurs which is mainly assigned by the deposition of neurofibrillary tangles (NFT) and amyloid beta aggregate of tau proteins which are responsible for synaptic dysfunction, neuroinflammation, and neuronal loss.[34] During the natural and routine process tau proteins help in the stabilization of microtubules but in the case of Alzheimer ailment, tau protein is hyperphosphorylated, which results in aggregation and production of intracellular NFT. This causes the degeneration of axon and dendrites. Similarly, alpha synuclein aggregates are responsible for PD. This alpha synuclein aggregates have neurotoxic functions and affects the neurons. They are responsible for lysosome dysfunction, mitochondrial dysfunction, disturbance of axonal transport, and neuroinflammation. So, by treating this proteinopathies, we can target to treat NDDs.[35]

11.6.2 ACETYLCHOLINESTERASE INHIBITION ACTIVITY

The early stage of dementia can be treated by providing the acetylcholinesterase (AChE) inhibitor. It is an important neurotransmitter for memory processing but, in some NDDs, like Alzheimer's, it gets depleted. Since cholinergic neurons are being lost, impairment in cognition and memory loss occurs. So, by the use of selective AChE inhibitor dementia can be cured by increasing the acetylcholine (Ach) activity.[36,37]

11.6.3 ANTITHROMBOTIC ACTIVITY

Thrombosis is responsible for acute cerebral ischemia which causes obstruction in cerebral artery and hence the blood flow to a specific area of the brain gradually drops.[38] This causes hypoxia and low glucose level in neurons and hence the depletion of ATP causes the irreversible damage of neurons. By providing the antiplatelet or antithrombotic drug, we can reduce the chances of thrombosis and hence prevent ischemic stroke.[39]

11.6.4 MONOAMINE OXIDASE INHIBITOR (MAOS)

Some enzymes like monoamine oxidase (MAO) which are present in the mitochondria are responsible for amine neurotransmitter oxidative deamination. In general, two types of MAO inhibitors are present in humans: MAO-A and MAO-B. Furthermore, they metabolize the dopamine which causes PD.[40] Thus, MAO inhibitors finds application in curing NDDs and other diseases like anxiety, depression, and mood disorder because they are involved in the selective deamination of serotonin.[41]

11.6.5 ANTIOXIDANT ACTIVITY

One of the key factors in the onset and progression of neurodegenerative illnesses is oxidative stress. Because of its tremendous metabolic activity, the brain is particularly vulnerable to oxidative stress. Because cerebral ischemia produces nitric oxide (NO) and ROS, the brain is subjected to oxidative stress. ROS are produced in the cases of PD and AD. These ROS can be neutralized by antioxidants; so, the phytoconstituents which possess antioxidant activity have good neuroprotective effect.[42,43]

11.6.6 ANTI-INFLAMMATORY ACTIVITY

During cerebral ischemia, neuroinflammation performs a crucial character in neuronal loss as well as brain damage. Aggregation of the proteins like tau protein, Aβ, and α-synuclein are responsible for neuron damage and causes the activation of microglia. This produces inflammation. Reperfusion injury and cerebral ischemia are responsible for infiltrating the neutrophils and macrophiles and thus inflammatory response increases. Due to the increase in inflammatory response, production of inflammatory mediators, like cytokinin, increases. By inhibition of inflammatory response and regulation of inflammatory mediators, we can check chronic inflammation and cell death.[44]

11.6.7 NEUROTROPHIC AND ANTIAPOPTOTIC ACTIVITY

During the NDDs (like PD and AD), the cholinergic and dopaminergic neurons present in mid brain gets lost. The various complicated symptoms in NDDs like behavioral and movement deficits, and difficulty in cognition are the responses of neurodegeneration and neuron loss.[45] So, the primary therapies used to treat neurodegenerative diseases are stopping neuronal cell death, their regeneration, and promoting neuron survival. Various plants' secondary metabolites are used against oxidative stress to reduce inflammation; by protecting the neurons, they are also able to decrease apoptosis by impacting on neurotoxic agents and excitotoxicity. Plant secondary metabolite promotes the neurogenesis process by the upregulation of neurotrophic factor.[46]

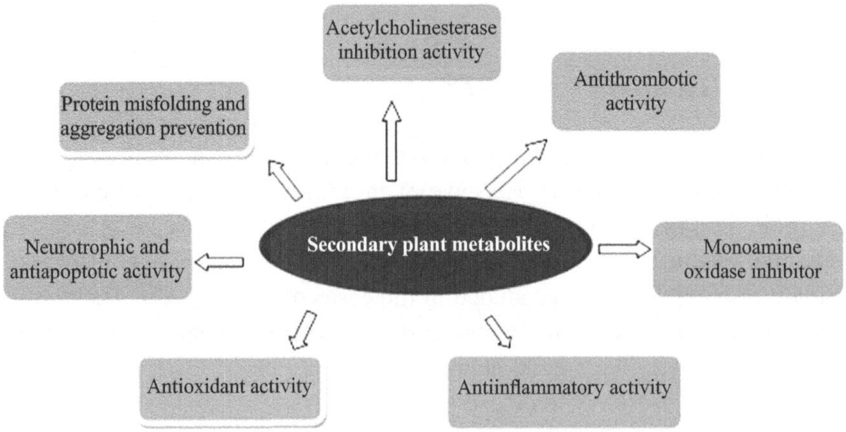

FIGURE 11.4 Various mechanisms of plant secondary metabolites contributing in neuro-degeneration disorders.

11.7 PHYTOCONSTITUENTS THAT REGULATE NDDS

Human beings are dependent on nature for healthcare benefits since the beginning of human civilization. Humans are using different parts of plants to cure various diseases. These different parts contain various types of plant secondary metabolites. Some secondary plant metabolites are also useful for the treatment of NDDs. Few of them are discussed below.

11.7.1 POLYPHENOLIC COMPOUNDS AND THEIR NEUROPROTECTIVE EFFECTS

11.7.1.1 QUERCETIN

It is an important secondary plant metabolite which is present in different plants like Mulberry fruits, grapes, broccoli, berries, and various other citrus fruits. It has anti-inflammatory, anti-ageing, and antioxidant activity.[47] Some studies show its beneficial effects in alcohol-induced neuron damage cell lines. Quercitin shows a good free radical scavenging activity and hence it is a good neuroprotective agent.[48] Quercetin nanoparticles (QNPs) have greater bioavailability, according to scientific studies. In this study, the preventive and therapeutic effects of QNPs were examined in an animal model of AD that was produced by aluminium trichloride ($AlCl_3$). Administration of QNPs significantly lowers the development of APs, NFTs, and other neuro-degenerative alterations in neurons (all $P \leq 0.05$). The study also revealed overexpression of TH and indications of regeneration (all $P \leq 0.05$). This amazing result was seen in the prophylactic group. According to studies, QNPs lessened $AlCl_3$'s harmful effects on hippocampus neurons at the molecular, subcellular, and cellular levels.

11.7.2 APIGENIN DERIVATIVES

The Brazillian folk medicine *Passiflora* is used as a tranquillizer and sedative agent. *Passiflora* contains various types of apigenin derivatives which are responsible for their antioxidant and anti-inflammatory activity.[50] These derivatives are responsible for reducing production of β-CTF, BACE, and β-amyloid deposition. By this mechanism, they improve the memory and synaptic plasticity. It plays a crucial role in NDDs. Apigenin shows prominent anti-inflammatory activity by preventing NO and PGE_2 production. Apigenin has the ability to penetrate the blood–brain barrier (BBB) and suppress a variety of neurotoxic agents. In a research investigation, in vitro models of neuroinflammation linked to AD were used to assess the neuroprotective and neuroimmunomodulatory potential of apigenin. From the cortex of neonatal and embryonic Wistar rats, a combined culture (co-culture) of neurons and glial cells were taken for this investigation. Following a 26-day period, the in vitro cultures were exposed to A oligomers (500 nM) for 4 h, or to lipopolysaccharide (LPS; 1 g/ml), IL-1 (10 ng/ml), or both. Then, for a further day, or for 24 h, this preparation was treated with apigenin (1 M). Following a 24-h observation period, it was found that apigenin therapy retained the integrity of the neurons and astrocytes.[52]

11.7.3 ROSMARINIC ACID

Rosmarinic acid (RA), present in *Melissa officinalis*, is also recognized as lemon balm in local communities. It is used traditionally as antioxidant as well as neuroprotective activity. The other constituents of *Melissa officinalis* are oleanolic acid, RA, and ursolic acid which are responsible for the promotion and increase in number of neuroblast by altering the level of carticosterone and gamma amino butyric acid (GABA) serum.[53] The other important constituents are citronellal, isogeranial, geraniol, geranic acetate, caryophyllene oxide, caryophyllene, germacrene, and carvacrol. Some studies that show these compounds inhibit hypoxia-induced proinflammatory cytokinin and prevent neuronal damage. The important constituents present in lemon balm (*Melissa officinalis*), like RA, have a very important role to enhance memory by impacting on cholinergic activity.[54] In scientific research, it was found that RA possesses the ability to combine with copper ions (Cu-II). Together with four oxygen donor atoms, it forms a bis-complex. By forming a mixed Cu (II) complex, RA also promoted the interaction between A and paramagnetic ions. Additionally, it was discovered through in vitro research that RA has the ability to destabilize and prevent the development of Aβ fibrils. RA medication inhibits the progression of AD in the Tg2576 mouse model, according to in vivo research. In the prevention of NDDs, RA plays a substantial positive influence.[55]

11.7.4 QUINIC ACID DERIVATIVES

A good source of caffeoylquinic acid is *Pimpinella brachycarpa*, which belongs to family Apiaceae. The plant is easily accessible in Europe, Africa, and Asia. It is used for the treatment of insomnia, GIT upset, asthma, and cough in Korean culture. Similarly, dicaffeoylquinic and dicaffeoylmucoquinic acids found in the plant of *Aster scaber* (family—Asteraceae), distributed widely in Eastern Asia especially in Korea, which is used for headache, bruises, and dizziness. Similarly, a Chinese medicine *Dipascus asper* (family—Dipsacaceae) contains 3, 4 dicaffeoylmucoquinic acid used to treat knee pain, anti-inflammatory effect, rheumatoid arthritis, abortion risk, and bone fracture. Quinic acid and their derivative help in the growth of neurite and protect them from Aβ toxicity in PC12 cells. They also protect neurodegenerative diseases by neutralizing free radicals.[56] A research has been done for the evaluation of neuroprotection study of D(-)Quinic acid on $AlCl_3$-induced animal rat model. The results have been observed on the basis of rats' neurobehavioral and metabolic alterations. In this study, rats received two oral doses of D-(-)-quinic acid at 200 and 400 mg/kg. The researcher observed and recorded the neurobehavioral deficits brought on by $AlCl_3$. In this study, the group of rats given D(-)-quinic acid showed a considerable suppression of MAO-B. According to histopathological tests, D-(-)-quinic acid significantly lessened the toxicity of $AlCl_3$ in the rat brain's cortex and hippocampus. This study came to the conclusion that D-(-)-quinic acid can prevent the negative effects of $AlCl_3$ and restore memory loss brought on by aluminum toxicity via lowering AChE activity.[57]

11.7.5 EPIGALLOCATECHIN-3-GALLATE

Epigallocatechin-3-gallate is a polyphenol which is mainly found in tea (*Camellia sinensis*, family—Theaceae). It is most commonly found in India and China and used as a beverage throughout world. Epigallocatechin-3-gallate shows the neuroprotective effect by increasing the concentration of NGF and promote the excretion of CREB.[58] Researchers looked at the pharmacological effects of the polyphenolic chemicals (-)-epigallocatechin (EGC) and (-)-epicatechin-3-gallate (ECG), which are obtained from tea. For this investigation, effects on the Cu^{2+}/Zn^{2+}-induced model were assessed. Numerous studies have been conducted, including those using immunohistochemistry, immunofluorescence tests, inductively coupled plasma mass spectrometry, UV-Visible spectroscopy, silver staining, and transmission electron microscopy. By weakly binding to Cu^{2+} and Zn^{2+}, the polyphenolic substances (-)-EGC and (-)-ECG inhibit Cu^{2+} or Zn^{2+}-induced or self-assembled A aggregation. By lowering the generation of ROS, EGC and (-)-ECG also modify the $Cu^{2+/}Zn^{2+-}$Aβ40-induced neurotoxicity on mouse neuroblastoma. According to the findings, green tea catechins such as EGC and (-)-ECG can lessen the toxicity of Aβ oligomers and fibrils. ECG, a phytoconstituent that may pass the BBB, reduces the Aβ plaques in the brains of APP/PS1 mice, and so guards against neuronal damage.[59]

11.7.6 CURCUMIN

Curcuma longa (family—Zinziberaceae) contain many phytoconstituents in which some phenolic phytoconstituents are demethoxycurcumin, curcumin, and bisdesmethoxycurcumin. *Curcuma longa* or turmeric is used widely in Indian food as a coloring and flavoring agent. In Indian traditional system, it is also used for hepatic disorder for the treatment of biliary disorder, rheumatism, cough, diabetes, etc. According to several studies, *Curcuma longa* active constituents control the levels of BDNF and CREB to control learning and spatial memory deficits brought on by dextrose. It also promotes formation of cell neurite. Curcumin decreases cisplatin-induced neuro differentiation. Curcumin also shows prominent neuroprotective activity by effecting 6-hydroxy dopamine. It also suppresses TNF-α and capase3 level. It increases the antioxidant level and show positive effect against memory impairment.[60] It was shown in a clinical trial investigation of a nanocurcumin formulation that levels of several miRNAs, including miR-132, miR-16, and miR-145, were decreased while levels of their targets, including sitrulin1, Sox2, Foxp3, and PDC1, respectively, were elevated. Additionally, it was shown that there was a considerable down-regulation in the expression of STAT1, NF-κB, AP-1, IL-1, IL-6, IFN, CCL2, CCL5, and TNF. Additionally, the group that received nanocurcumin treatment experienced a large drop in expanded disability status scale (EDSS) measurements.[61]

11.7.7 RESVERATROL

The good source of resveratrol is *Vitis venifera* (family—Vitaceae). The plant shows good anti-inflammatory, antioxidant, phytoestrogenic, cardioprotective, vasorelaxant, and anticarcinogenic pharmacological activity. The active phytoconstituents resveratrol inhibit chronic cerebral hypofusion. Resveratrol also reverses ethanol toxicity-induced apoptosis. Additionally, it inhibits the production of the transcription factors NF-κB and TNF-α, two pro-inflammatory mediators. It also increases the secretion of GDNF and BDNF, which include survival and growth of neuron.[62] In a study, two nanoformulations—nano emulsion and resveratrol-loaded transferosomes—were created and labeled with gold nanoparticles (AgNPs). In comparison to nano emulsions, the resveratrol-loaded transferosomes showed higher penetration (up to 81.29; 2.64%) and higher fluorescence intensity (P = 0.05). In amnesic rats, the transferosomes greatly improve behavioral acquisition and spatial memory performance. Comparing the transferomones to the nano emulsion formulation, the results were better.[63]

11.7.8 OLEUROPEIN

It is a polyphenolic compound found in the plant *Olea europea* (family—Oleaceae). The plant is traditionally used as herbal tea as well as also shows antioxidant, hypocholesterolemic, antihypertensive, hypoglycaemic, antiatherogenic, etc. Oleuropein is responsible for decreasing the level of GSH and enhances the secretion of NGF and BDNF in serum. Study reports that oleuropein aglycone prevents Aβ aggregation and reduces its cytotoxicity.[64] Through measuring the apoptotic response (caspase-3 activation) in rat models treated with colchicine, a study has been conducted to look at the protective effect of oleuropein. Comparing the treatment group to the control group, colchicine administration significantly ($P \leq 0.001$) increases caspase-3 activity. In comparison to the colchicine group, the tested groups of mice treated with oleuropein at doses of 10, 15, and 20 mg/kg displayed a substantial drop ($P \leq 0.001$) in caspase-3 activity. According to this study, oleuropein protects against the neuronal damage caused by colchicine by acting as an antioxidant.[65]

11.7.9 6-SHOGAOL

The phytoconstituent found in ginger (*Gingiber officinalis*, family—Zingiberaceae). It is a phenolic phytoconstituent and widely used as spices in India, Arab, Tibet, and China. A wide range of phytoconstituents are present in ginger like 6-gingerol, 8-gingerol, 10-gingerol, etc., which uses for the cure of nausea, motion sickness, vomiting, etc. 6-Shogaol shows prominent activity against AD, improves the antioxidant system, and enhances memory. The cognitive function in Aβ is improved by 6-Shogaol. It also minimizes apoptosis by decreasing ROS, caspase 3, Bax and enhances GDNF, BDNF, and NGNF-mediated signaling. 6-Shagoal imparts the neuroprotection by decreasing Bax and enhances BDNF, Bcl-2, and Bcl-xL. So, it is a very important phytoconstituent for the treatment and prevention of NDDs.[66] An academic investigation of 6-shogaol's neuroprotective properties against AD had been conducted. Additionally, studies on 6-shogaol's effects on the CysLT1R cysteinyl leukotriene 1 receptor were conducted. Both in vitro and in vivo models were used in this investigation. The study demonstrated that Aβ(1-42) enhanced CysLT1R and cathepsin B. The activation of the CysLT1R increases cathepsin B. Inhibition of CysLT1R/cathepsin B by 6-shogaol reduces the amount of Aβ deposited in the brain and improves behavioural impairments in APPSw/PS1-dE9 Tg mice. According to the findings, 6-shogaol inhibits the CysLT1R and cathepsin B. Thus, it represents a novel prospective therapeutic agent for the management of a variety of neurodegenerative diseases, including AD.[67]

11.7.10 GINKGOLIDE

The phytoconstituent present in the plant *Ginkgo biloba* (family—Ginkgoaceae) is frequently employed in China for the curing purpose of neurological disorders from thousands of years. Ginkgolide shows prominent neuroprotective effect by suppressing ethanol-mediated apoptosis. Its antioxidant effect decreases ROS-based endoplasmic reticulum and mitochondrial dysfunction. *Ginkgo biloba* shows protection from neurotoxicity brought on by oxidative stress. Ginkgolide crosses BBB and are helpful for the curing purpose of NDDs. Ginkgo biloba increases Krk-mediated axonal growth and protects neuron as well as decreases ROS production and apoptotic factors.[68] In a study, oxidative stress-induced SH-SY5Y cells were used as a model to assess the neuroprotective effect of ginkgolide extract-loaded chitosan nanoparticles (Gb-CsNPs). Results indicate that chitosan nanoparticles loaded with ginkgolide extract (Gb-CsNPs) had an average size of 104.4 nm, a zeta potential of 29.3 mV, and a polydispersity index (PDI) value of 0.09. The loading capacity and encapsulation efficacy were 97.4% and 40%, respectively. The outcomes demonstrated the biocompatibility of Gb-CsNPs. Gb-CsNPs increased cell survival from 60% to 92.30%, demonstrating neuroprotective action.[69]

11.7.11 LIMONOIDS

The phytoconstituent is used as an antifeedant, insecticide, and growth regulator in insects. It also shows various activities like antifungal, anticarcinogenic, antimalarial, antiviral, and neuroprotective effect. The phytoconstituent found in the plant *Melia toosendan* (family—Meliaceae). The plant potentially induced neuronal differentiation and increased neurite outgrowth as well as increased NGF secretion and thus are helpful in neurodegenerative diseases.[70] Hesperidin and limonoids had their neurological effects examined in a study. Hesperidin at doses of 125 and 250 mg/kg and limonoids at dose of 100 mg/kg both improved psychological state in this study. In comparison to the positive control group, there was a considerable rise in the frequency of ambulation in the tested group. Low doses of limonoids have positive effects on beta-amyloid (amyloid) and AChE levels.[71]

11.7.12 LIGRAMINOL E4-B-D XYLOSID

Ligraminol E4-β-D xyloside occurs in *Abies holophylla* (family—Pinaceae). It is widely found in China, Korea, and Russia. It contains six different types of lignans which inhibit LPS-induced NO production. Some lignans of them increase NGF level. The plant also contains two novel sesquiterpene which are responsible to inhibit LPS-activated microglial NO production.[72]

11.7.13 CLERODANE DITERPENOID

The phytoconstituent belongs to the plant *Ptychopatalum olacoides* (family—Olacaceae). The plant contains seven different types of diterpenoids in which two enhances the neurite outgrowth. The methanolic extract of the plant contains clerodane diterpenoid which potentiates NGF secretion and enhance neurite outgrowth.[73]

11.7.14 GINSENOSIDE

The phytoconstituent found in Ginseng plant (*Panax ginseng*, family—Araliaceae). The various varieties of ginseng are famous like Chinese, Korean, Japanese, Russian, etc. The important phytoconstituents of the ginseng is saponins (steroidal and triterpenoidal).[74] The ginseng extract shows prominent role in apoptotic-related neurodegenerative diseases. Ginsenoside and other such constituents from ginseng passes the BBB and shows the prominent role in the cure of neurodegenerative diseases. Ginsenosides increases neuritogenesis and cholinergic markers level through NGF-TrkA signaling trail.[75] Ginseng contains ginsenoside Rg1, which is an active phytoconstituent. In the literature, it is now accessible on ginsenoside Rg1; it is stated that this compound acts on the neurological system to treat AD in older people. Given that Rg1 is easily destroyed by intestinal bacteria when administered orally, the parenteral route may be more advantageous. Its bioavailability ranges from 1% to 20%, and the blood eliminates it swiftly. In a study, Rg1 was administered intraperitoneally for 90 days to transgenic AD mice (aged six and nine months) over-expressing APP/A and their non-transgenic littermates. The outcome demonstrates a change in the mice's behavior, neuropathology, and amyloidosis, demonstrating that Rg1 had significant and varied neuroprotective benefits in AD mouse models. The outcome demonstrates a change in the mice's behavior, neuropathology, and amyloidosis, demonstrating that Rgl had significant and varied neuroprotective benefits in AD mouse models. According to observations, Rgl improves amyloid pathology, stops the production of APPs, improves cognition, and increases hippocampal-dependent protein kinase/hippocampal respond element binding protein (PKA/CREB) signaling, which enhances neuroprotection. These findings demonstrate the possibility of ginsenoside Rgl for usage in novel medication classes for the treatment of AD. It was discovered in another investigation that nasal delivery of ginsenoside Rgl has greater distribution and transport efficiency (5.05 times and 2.50 times, respectively). Less time is needed for complete transportation of drug in brain. The greater observed Rgl distribution and transport efficiency (11.80 and 3.35 times, respectively). Additionally, the area under curve also increases from of the above study, it can be said that nasal spray is a superior dosage form for the treatment of neurodegenerative illnesses.[76]

11.7.15 3,4-SECOCYCLOARTENE TRITERPENOID

The phytoconstituent found in the plant *Schisandra chinensis* (family—Schisandraceae) used traditionally for insomnia, antitussive, tranquilliser, increase memory function, fatique, and as sedative. The constituent present in the plant decreases NO production and enhances BDNF expression. It also induces neuritogenesis. It has potential neuroprotective effect.[77]

11.7.16 HUPERZINE

Huperzine is mainly a sesquiterpene alkaloid which is chiefly found in the plant *Huperzia serrata* (family—Lycopodiaceae). The plant has been in use in Chinese traditional system from ancient time and shows prominent reversible acetylcholinestrase inhibitor activity. The active phytoconstituent present in the plant, huperazine, shows prominent neuroprotective effect by Aβ peptide processing inhibiting AchE and reducing oxidative stress. It also promotes the expression of NGF and antiapoptopic protein. The NGF level decreased by H_2O_2-induced oxidative stress can be reversed by huperzine. It also enhances neurite outgrowth by decreasing AchE and enhancing the expression level of NGF.[78] For effective intranasal transport of huperzine A to the brain for the treatment of AD, a study was conducted using huperzine A-loaded mucoadhesive and targeted polylactic co glycolic acid (PLGA) nanoparticles with surface modification by lactoferrin-conjugated N-trimethylated chitosan.

The nanoparticles demonstrated effective targeting, sustained release, and outstanding adherence. These results indicate that huperazine has a broad potential for use as a nasal drug delivery system.[79]

11.7.17 BERBERINE

It is an important isoquinoline alkaloid mainly occurs in various plants of Berberidaceae family. The phytoconstituent found in *Coctis chinensis*. The *Coctis* plant widely uses for the treatment and cure of diarrhoea, liver problems and microbial infection. The active constituent berberine shows the prominent neuroprotective activity by enhancing NGF expression. It decreases ROS level and enhance NGF mediated neurite outgrowth. Additionally, berberine maintains the levels of BDNF and CREB while lowering the expression of the cytokines COX 2 and TNF-α.[80] Serotonin levels rise by 47%, dopamine levels rise by 31%, and norepinephrine levels rise by 29% in the CNS after berberine (5–10 mg/kg) administration, which helps treat depression.[81]

11.7.18 GENIPOSIDIC ACID

The phytoconstituent found in the plant *Eucommia ulmoides* (Family-Eucommiaceae) is a folk medicine and used traditionally to control blood pressure, strengthen muscle and lungs, avoids miscarriages, arthritis, enhances stamina, and improves kidney and liver functions. It shows neuroprotective effect by increasing the expression of BDNF and decreases AchE activity by increasing cholinergic signaling. It also protects brain from Aβ-induced impairment of cognitive deficits.[82] Geniposidic acid (GPA) administration reduces Aβ deposition and neuronal apoptosis in AD animal mice model. It reduces inflammation and axonal injury of Aβ1-42-induced neurons. Hence, it showed significant improvement in the cognitive function. As per available literature, geniposidic acid (GPA) mainly targets on GAP43 in AD. GPA is mainly oppressed on tranquillity of GAP43 which shows neuroprotective activity of GPA in AD mice model. To reduce nerve damage in AD mice, GPA activates the PI3K/AKT pathway and enhances GAP43 expression. GPA medication on cognitive function has been studied to determine its efficacy. GPA was given to 6–7-month-old APP/PS1 mice for three months as part of this investigation. The neurobehavioral studies were conducted to assess mice's memory and spatial learning capacities. Research has concentrated on amyloid-deposition, microglia and astrocyte activation, and neuroinflammation to understand the mechanism of GPAs neuroprotective action. The outcomes demonstrated a significant improvement in the mice's capacity for spatial learning and memory. In APP/PS1 mice, geniposidic acid therapy also reduces the amount of amyloid deposition in the brain.[83]

11.7.19 HONOKIOL AND MAGNOLOL

The lignin compounds named Honokiol and Magnololare isolated from the plant *Magnolia officinalis* (family—Magnoliaceae) which mainly found in China. It shows prominent anti-inflammatory, anticancer, and anxiolytic effect. The lignins deceases the generation of ROS and prevents Aβ-induced neuronal cell death. It also enhances NGF and BDNF secretions.[84,85] The phytoconstituents honokiol and magnolol have been shown in scientific studies to considerably lessen the Aβ-induced cell damage. Additional research revealed that the principal mechanism by which Honokiol and Magnolol exert their neuroprotective benefits by reducing the generation of ROS. In addition, it inhibited caspase-3 activity and reduced intracellular calcium levels.[86]

Note: Through the Ras/MAPK, PI3K/AKT, and PL-C pathways, neurotrophin signaling promotes cell survival, proliferation, and differentiation by attaching to the Trk receptor. Bidirectional cell survival and death are triggered by NGF-p75NTR receptor interaction through the NF-κB and JNK pathways. External stress stimuli also cause the formation of ROS while antioxidative enzyme levels are suppressed. NADPH stands for nicotinamide adenine dinucleotide phosphate, PI3K stands for phosphatidylinsoitol-3-kinase, mTOR stands for mammalian target of rapamycin, MEK stands for mitogen-activated protein kinase, MAPK stands for mitogen activated protein kinase, ERK stands for extracellular signal-regulated kinases, NF-κB stands for nuclear factor kappa B, JNK stands for Jun N-terminal kinase, IκB stands for inhibitory kappa B, and CREB stands for cyclic adenosine monophosphate response element binding protein, Glucose Synthase Kinase 3 (GSK3) and Calcium-Calmodulin Kinase II/IV (CaMKII/IV)

Phytoconstituents involved are:

(a) Quercetin, (b) Apigenin, (c) RA, (d) Quinic acid derivatives (e) Epigallocatechin-3-galate (f) Curcumin, (g) Resveratrol (h) Oleuropini) 6-shogaol (j) Ginkgolide B, (k) Limonoid, (l) Ligraminol (m) Clerodane diterpenoids (n) Ginsenosides (o) 3, 4- Secocycloartene triterpenoid (p) Huperzine (q) Berberine, (r) Geniposidic acid (s) Honokiol and magnolol

TABLE 11.2 Phytoconstituents Which Affects Neutrophins.

Medicinal plant	Phytoconstituent	Pharmacological activity	Therapeutic use
Aster scaber	(-)3, 5-dicaffeoyl mucoquinic acid	Activates neurogenesis mediated by Trk/ERK1/2/PI3K	Neurodegenerative disease, neuroinflammation, neuroprotection
Abies holophylla	Ligraminol E4-O-β d xyloside	Increases NO production, Trk-mediated NGF production	Neurodegenerative disease, neuroinflammation
Camellia sinensis	Epigallocatechin 3 gallate	Increase in Trk mediated signaling pathway, inhibits ROS level	neuroinflammation, neuroprotection, neuritogenesis
Coptis chinensis	Berberine	Increase in cholinergic activity-mediated neurite outgrowth and AKT/GSK 3/Nrf 2-mediated regulation	Neuroinflammation, neuroprotection, neuritogenesis
Curcuma longa	Curcumin	Induce BDNF secretion, increase AKT/GSK 3-mediated regulation	Neuroinflammation, neuroprotection, neuritogenesis
Eucommia ulmoides	Geniposidic acid	PI3/AKT, cleavage caspage 3, MMPs, and cytochrome C, AChE inhibition	Neuroprotection, anti-apoptopic
Ginkgo biloba	Ginkgolide B	Enhances proapoptopic factors such ROS, LDH, caspase 3, neurite outgrowth mediated by Trk/Ras/MAPK	Dementia, nootropic, neuritogenesis, neuroinflammation
Huperzia serrata	Huperzine A	Increases Trk/MAPK/ERK-mediated neuronal growth, induces NGF and BDNF secretion	Neuritogenesis, neuroinflammation, neuroprotection
Magnolia officinalis	Honokiol, magnolol	Induces BDNF and NGF secretion, inhibit ROS level	Neuritogenesis, neuroinflammation, neuroprotection
Melissa officinalis	Rosmarinic acid	Improves cholinergic activity, NF-κβ pathway	Cognitive disorder, neuritogenesis, neuroinflammation, neuroprotection
Melia toosendan	Limonoids	PKA/ERK2/2-mediated neurite outgrowth	Neuritogenesis, neuroinflammation, neuroprotection
Morus alba	Quercetin	Induces PI3K/ERK1/2-mediated CREB activation	Cognitive disorder, neuritogenesis, neuroinflammation, neuroprotection

TABLE 11.2 *(Continued)*

Medicinal plant	Phytoconstituent	Pharmacological activity	Therapeutic use
Olea europea	Oleuropein	Induces NGF, BDNF secretion	Neuroinflammation, neuroprotection
Passiflora edulis	Apigenin	Inhibit NO, iNOS, PGE_2-mediated modulation of ERK	Neuritogenesis, neuroinflammation, neuroprotection
Panax ginseng	Ginsenoside	Induces neuritogenesis through cAMP/MAPK Trk-mediated pathway	Neuritogenesis, neuroinflammation, neuroprotection
Ptychopetalumolacoides	Clerodane diterpenoid	Neurite outgrowth mediated by neutrophic mimetic activity	Neuritogenesis, neuroinflammation, neuroprotection
Vitis vinifera	Resveratrol	Activates ERK-mediated CREB regulation, inhibits caspase 3	Neuritogenesis, neuroinflammation, neuroprotection
Zingiber officinale	6-shogaol	Induces Trk-mediated neurite outgrowth, Accelerates BDNF, NGF, GDNF secretion	Neuritogenesis, neuroinflammation, neuroprotection

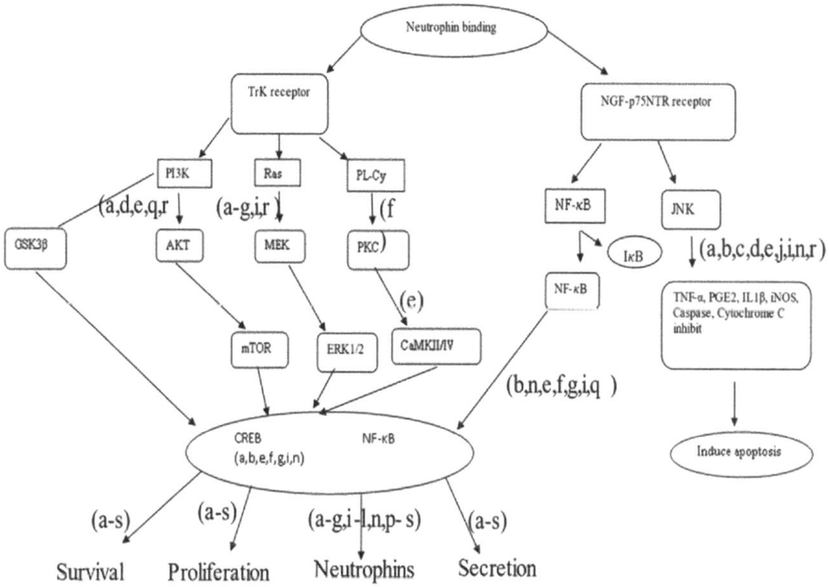

FIGURE 11.5 Neurotrophin-related mechanisms of phytoconstituents.

11.8 CONCLUSION

Although the modern treatment pattern of neurodegenerative diseases is very advanced but their accomplishment is very low due to their multifactorial nature. There are so many numbers of medicines in the modern era which shows neurotonic potential and uses in various neurological disorders. The ayurvedic system of medicine particularly for neurological problems named as "Medhya Rasayana" has established and is practicing from long time which shows prominent effect in the treatment of mental patients. Due to their anti-inflammatory, antioxidant, and anti-cholinesterase properties, medicines employed in Medhya Rasayana and other plant secondary metabolites or phytochemicals may be used as promising therapeutic agents for neurodegenerative diseases in the future. At the molecular and subcellular levels, neurodegenerative diseases including AD, PD, and Huntington's diseases share comparable characteristics. Apart from these, apoptosis, necrosis, and inflammation are caused by shared molecular signaling pathways. Therefore, plant secondary metabolites or phytochemicals provide intriguing alternatives to existing medicines for the treatment of neurodegenerative illnesses by acting on numerous cellular levels and signaling pathways.

KEYWORDS

- **neurodegenerative disorders**
- **Medhya Rasayana**
- **medicinal plants**
- **phytoconstituents**
- ***Centella asiatica***
- ***Glycyrrhiza glabra***
- ***Tinospora cardifolia***

REFERENCES

1. Rasool, M.; Malik, A.; Qureshi, M. S.; Manan, A.; Pushparaj, P. N.; Asif, M.; Qazi, M. H.; Qazi, A. M.; Kamal, M. A.; Gan, S. H.; Sheikh I. A. Recent Updates in the Treatment of Neurodegenerative Disorders Using Natural Compounds. *Evid. Based Complementary Altern. Med.* **2014,** *2014,* 979730, 7.
2. Venkatesan, R.; Ji, E.; Kim, S. Y. Phytochemicals that Regulate Neurodegenerative Disease by Targeting Neurotrophins: Acomprehensive Review. *Biomed. Res. Int.* **2015,** *2015,* 814068, 22.
3. Winner, B.; Kohl, Z.; Gage, F. H. Neurodegenerative Diseases and Adult Neurogenesis. *Eur. J. Neurosci.* **2011,** *33* (6), 1139–1151.
4. Finkel, T. Signal Transduction by Reactive Oxygen Species (ROS). *J. Cell Biol.* **2011,** *194* (1), 7–15.
5. Nakamura, T.; Lipton, S. A. S-Nitrosylation and Uncompetitive Fast Offrate (UFO) Drug Therapy in Neurodegenerative Disorders of Protein Misfolding. *Cell Death Differ.* **2007,** *14* (7), 1305–1314.
6. Seyed, M. A.; Ayesha, S.; Azmi, N.; Alrabae, F. M.; Alalawy, A. I.; Alzahrani, O. R.; Hawsawi, Y. The Neuroprotective Attribution of *Ocimumbasilicum*: A Review on Prevention and Management of Neurodegenerative Disorders. *Future J. Pharm. Sci.* **2021,** *7* (139), 2–14.
7. Fischer, R.; Maier, O. Interrelation of Oxidative Stress and Inflammation in Neurodegenerative Diseases: Role of TNF. *Oxid. Med. Cell. Longev.* **2015,** *2015,* 1–18.
8. Harman, D. Aging: A Theory based on Free Radical and Radiation Chemistry. *J. Gerontol.* **1956,** *11* (3), 298–300.
9. Mattson, M. P. Apoptosis in Neurodegenerative Disorders. *Nat. Rev. Mol. Cell Biol.* **2000,** *1,* 120–129.
10. Uttara, B.; Singh, A. V.; Zamboni, P.; Mahajan, R. T. Oxidative Stress and Neurodegenerative Diseases: A Review of Upstream and Downstream Antioxidant Therapeutic Options. *Curr. Neuropharmacol.* **2009,** *7* (1), 65–74.
11. Cobb, C.; Cole, M. Oxidative and Nitrative Stress in Neurodegeneration. *Neurobiologicaldisorder* **2015,** *84,* 4–21.

12. Gandhi, S.; Abramov, A. Y. Mechanism of Oxidative Stress in Neurodegeneration. *Oxid. Med. Cell. Longev.* **2012,** 428010.
13. Breydo, L.; Wu, J. W.; Uversky, V. N. α-Synuclein misfolding and Parkinson's Disease. *Biochim. Biophys. Acta* **1822,** *2,* 261–285.
14. Baldi, I.; Lebailly, P.; Mohammed, B.; Letenneur, L.; Dartigues, J. F.; Brochard, P. Neurodegenerative Diseases and Exposure to Pesticides in the Elderly. *Am. J. Epidemiol.* **2003,** *157* (5), 409–414.
15. Qiu, C.; Kivipelto, M.; von Strauss, E. Epidemiology of Alzheimer's Disease: Occurrence, Determinants, and Strategies Toward Intervention. *Dialogues Clin. Neurosci.* **2009,** *11,* 111–128.
16. Morimoto, R. I. Roteotoxic Stress and Inducible Chaperone Networks in Neurodegenerative Disease and Aging. *Genes Dev.* **2008,** *22* (11), 1427–1438.
17. Pegoraro, G.; Voss, T. C.; Martin, S. E.; Tuzmen, P.; Guha, R.; Misteli, T. Identification of Mammalian Protein Quality Control Factors by Highthroughput Cellular Imaging. *PLoS One* **2012,** *7* (2):e31684.
18. Dobson, C. M. Protein Aggregation and Its Consequences for Human Disease. *Protein Peptide Lett.* **2006,** *13* (3), 219–227.
19. Upadhyay, S. D.; Lodha, S.; Ahmad, Y.; Kohli, S.; Sharma, R. K. A Review on MedhyaRasayanas: A Brain Bracer. *Pharmacognosy Commun.* **2021,** *11* (4), 182–185.
20. Gray, N. E.; Magana, A. A.; Lak, P.; Wright, K. M.; Quinn, J.; Stevens, J. F.; Maier, C. S. Soumyanath, A. *Centella asiatica*—Phytochemistry and Mechanisms of Neuroprotection and Cognitive Enhancement. *Phytochem. Rev.* **2018,** *17* (1), 161–194.
21. Gupta, S.; Saxena, A. Histological Study of Action of Alcohol on Hippocampal Region of Brain and Use of Mandukaparni as a Brain Rejuvenator. *Int. J Eng. Technol. Sci. Res.* **2017,** *4* (6), 301–306.
22. Shajahan, M. A.; Hameed, A. S. Yashtimadhu (*Glycyrrhiza glabra*)—A Review. *Indian J. Appl. Res.* **2020,** *23* (9), 1–12.
23. Ishtiyaq, A.; Alam, A.; Siddiqui, J. I.; Kazmi. M. H. Therapeutic Potential of Widely Used Unani Drug Asl Us Soos (*Glycyrrhiza glabra*linn.): A Systematic Review. *J. Drug Deliv. Ther.* **2019,** 25 (9), 765–773.
24. Pansare, T. A.; Pranita, D.; Archana B. Review on MEDHYA (Intellect Promoting) action of GUDUCHI [*Tinospora cordifolia* (wild) Miers]. *Psychology* **2018,** Corpus ID 212609630.
25. Bhardwaj, M. Review on Phytochemical and Pharmacological activities of *Tinospora cordifolia* Linn. *J. Gujarat Res. Soc.* **2019,** *1* (21), 1934–1954.
26. Kizhakke, P. A.; Olakkaran, S.; Antony, A.; Tilagul, K. S.; Hunasanahally, P. G. *Convolvulus pluricaulis* (Shankhapushpi) Ameliorates Human Microtubule-associated Protein tau (hMAPτ) Induced Neurotoxicity in Alzheimer's DISEASE Drosophila Model. *J. Chem. Neuroanat.* **2019,** *1* (95), 115–122.
27. Batra, P. Impact of Shankhapushpi (*Convolvulus pluricaulis*) on Attention. *Indian J. Health Wellbeing* **2018,** *9* (2), 188–192.
28. Bai, D. L.; Tang, X. C.; He, X. C. Huperzine A, A Potential Therapeutic Agent for Treatment of Alzheimer's Disease. *Curr. Med. Chem.* **2000,** *7,* 355–374.
29. Tiwari, K.; Joshi, S. C.; Sharma, O. P. Exploring the Effects of *Convolvulus pluricaulis* Extract on Memory in Albino Rats. *Indian J. Health Wellbeing* **2017,** *8* (9), 1–9.
30. Hussain, I.; Khan, N.; Khan, H.; et al. Screening of Anti-oxidant Activities of Selected Medicinal Plants. *World Appl. Sci. J.* **2010,** *11* (3), 338–340.

31. Jeyam, M.; Karthika, G. R. R.; Poornima, V.; Sharanya, M. Molecular Understanding and In Silico Validation of Traditional Medicines for Parkinson's Disease. *Asian J. Pharm. Clin. Res.* **2012,** *5* (4), 125–128.
32. Bagchi, P.; Kar, A.; Vinobha, C. S. Establishing an In-Silico Ayurvedic Medication Towards Treatment of Schizophrenia. *Int. J. Syst. Biol.* **2009,** *1* (2), 46–50.
33. Mahdy, K.; Shaker, O.; Wafay, H.; Nassar, Y.; Hassan, H.; and Hussein, A. Effect of Some Medicinal Plant Extracts on the Oxidative Stress Status in Alzheimer's Disease Induced in Rats. *Eur. Rev. Med. Pharmacol. Sci.* **2012,** *16* (3), 31–42.
34. Kovacs, G. G. Current Concepts of Neurodegenerative Diseases. *Eur. Med. J. Neurol.* **2014,** *2,* 78–86.
35. Rocha, E. M.; De Miranda, B.; Sanders, L. H. Alpha-synuclein: Pathology, Mitochondrial Dysfunction and Neuroinflammation in Parkinson's Disease. *Neurobiol. Dis.* **2018,** *109,* 249–257.
36. Dos Santos, T. C.; Gomes, T. M.; Pinto, B. A. S.; Camara, A. L.; Paes, A. M. A. Naturally Occurring Acetylcholinesterase Inhibitors and their Potential Use for Alzheimer's Disease Therapy. *Front. Pharmacol.* **2018,** *9,* 1192.
37. Francis, P. T.; Palmer, A. M.; Snape, M.; Wilcock, G. K. The Cholinergic Hypothesis of Alzheimer's Disease—A Review of Progress. *J. Neurol. Neurosurg. Psychiatry* **1999,** *66,* 137–147.
38. Huang, L.; Wang, S.; Ma, F.; Zhang, Y.; Peng, Y.; Xing, C.; Feng, Y.; Wang, X.; Peng, Y. From Stroke to Neurodegenerative Diseases: The Multi-target Neuroprotective Effects of 3-n-butylphthalide and Its Derivatives. *Pharmacol. Res.* **2018,** *135,* 201–211.
39. Wojciechowski, V. V.; Calina, D.; Tsarouhas, K.; Pivnik, A. V.; Sergievich, A. A.; Kodintsev, V. V.; Filatova, E. A.; Ozcagli, E.;D ocea, A. O.; Arsene, A. L. A Guide to Acquired Vitamin K Coagulophathy Diagnosis and Treatment—The Russian Perspective. *Daru* **2017,** *25* (1), 10.
40. Finberg, J. P.; Rabey, J. M. Inhibitors of MAO-A and MAO-B in Psychiatry and Neurology. *Front. Pharmacol.* **2016,** *7,* 340.
41. Larit, F.; Elokely, K. M.; Chaurasiya, N. D.; Benyahia, S.; Nael, M. A.; Leon, F.; Abu-Darwish, M. S.; Efferth, T.; Wang, Y. H.; Belouahem-Abed, D. Inhibition of Human Monoamine Oxidase A and B by Flavonoids Isolated from Two Algerian Medicinal Plants. *Phytomedicine* **2018,** *40,* 27–36.
42. Wang, X.; Michaelis, E. K. Selective Neuronal Vulnerability to Oxidative Stress in the Brain. *Front. Aging Neurosci.* **2010,** *2,* 12.
43. Padureanu, R.; Albu, C. V.; Mititelu, R. R.; Bacanoiu, M. V.; Docea, A. O.; Calina, D.; Padureanu, V.; Olaru, G.; Sandu, R. E.; Malin, R. D. Oxidative Stress and Inflammation Interdependence in Multiple Sclerosis. *J. Clin. Med.* **2019,** *8,* 1815.
44. Sharifi-Rad, M.; Lankatillake, C.; Dias, D. A.; Docea, A. O.; Mahomoodally, M. F.; Lobine, D.; Chazot, P. L.; Kurt, B.; Tumer, T. B.; Moreira, A. C.; Sharopov, F.; Martorell, M.; Martins, N.; Cho, W. C.; Calina, D.; Sharifi-Rad, J.; Impact of Natural Compounds on Neurodegenerative Disorders—From Preclinical to Pharmacotherapeutics. *J. Clin. Med.* **2020,** *9,* 1061.
45. Kumar, G. P.; Khanum, F. Neuroprotective Potential of Phytochemicals. *Pharmacogn. Rev.* **2012,** *6,* 81–90.
46. Xu, J.; Lacoske, M. H.; Theodorakis, E. A. Neurotrophic Natural Products: Chemistry and Biology. *Angew. Chem. Int. Ed.* **2014,** *53,* 956–987.
47. Ercisli, S.; Orhan, E. Chemical Composition of White (*Morus alba*), Red (*Morus rubra*) and Black (*Morus nigra*) Mulberry Fruits. *Food Chem.* **2007,** *103* (4), 1380–1384.

48. Rifaai, R. A.; Mokhemer, S. A.; Saber, E. A.; El-Aleem, S. A. A.; El-Tahawy, N. F. G. Neuroprotective Effect of Quercetin Nanoparticles—A Possible Prophylactic and Therapeutic Role in Alzheimer Disease. *J. Chem. Neuroanat.* **2020,** *107,* 101795.
49. Peng, C. H.; Liu, L. K.; Chuang, C. M.; Chyau, C. C.; Huang, C. N.; Wang, C. J. Mulberry Water Extracts Possess an Anti-obesity Effect and Ability to Inhibit Hepatic Lipogenesis and Promote Lipolysis. *J. Agric. Food Chem.* **2011,** *59* (6), 2663–2671.
50. Barbosa, P. R.; Valvassori, S. S.; Bordignon, C. L. The Aqueous Extracts of *Passiflora alata* and *Passiflora edulis* Reduces Anxietyrelated Behaviors Without Affecting Memory Process in Rats. *J. Med. Food* **2008,** *11* (2), 282–288.
51. Zhao, L.; Wang, J. L.; Liu, R.; Li, X. X.; Li, J. F.; Zhang, L. Neuroprotective, Antiamyloidogenic and Neurotrophic Effects of Apigenin in an Alzheimer Disease Mouse Model. *Molecules* **2013,** *18* (8), 9949–9965.
52. Dourado, N. S.; Souza, C. D. S.; de Almeida, M. M. A.; Bispo da Silva, A.; Santos, B. L. D.; Silva, V. D. A. Neuroimmunomodulatory and Neuroprotective Effects of the Flavonoid Apigenin in *in vitro* Model of Neuroinflammation Associated with Alzheimer Disease. *Front. Aging Neurosci.* **2020,** *15* (12), 119.
53. Pereira, R. P.; Fachinetto, R.; Prestes, A. S. Antioxidant Effects of Different Extracts from *Melissa officinalis*, *Matricariarecutita* and *Cymbopogon citratus*. *Neurochem. Res.* **2009,** *34* (5), 973–983.
54. Kola, A.; Hecel, A.; Lamponi, S.; Valensin, D. Novel Perspective on Alzheimer Disease Treatment—Rosmarinic Acid Molecular Interplay with Copper (II) and Amyloidβ. *Life* **2020,** *10,* 118. doi:10.3390/life10070118.
55. Yoo, D. Y.; Choi, J. H.; Kim, W. Effects of *Melissa officinalis* L. (Lemon Balm) Extract on Neurogenesis Associated with Serum Corticosterone and GABA in the Mouse Dentate Gyrus. *Neurochem. Res.* **2011,** *36* (2), 250–257.
56. Liu, L.; Liu, Y.; Zhao, J.; Zhang, X. X. C.; Meng, H. Neuroprotective Effects of D(-) Quinic Acid on Aluminum Chloride-Induced Dementia in Rats. *Evid. Based Complement. Altern. Med.* **2020,** *2020,* 5602597. doi: 10.1155/2020/5602597
57. Ahn, S.; Kim, M.; Jung, I.; Sohn, H.; Antibacterial, Antioxidative and Anti-proliferative Activity Against Human Colorectal Cell of *Pimpinella brachycarpa*. *Korean J. Food Preserv.* **2011,** *18* (4), 590–596.
58. Zhang, Z. J.; Qian, Y. H.; Hu, H. T.; Yang, J.; Yang, G. D. The Herbal Medicine *Dipsacus asper* Wall Extract Reduces the Cognitive Deficits and Overexpression of β-amyloid Protein Induced by Aluminum Exposure. *Life Sci.* **2003,** *73* (19), 2443–2454.
59. Chen, T.; Yang, Y.; Zhu, S.; Lu, Y.; Zhu, L.; Wang, Y.; Wang, X. Inhibition of Aβ Aggregates in Alzheimer's Disease by Epigallocatechin and Epicatechin-3-gallate from Green Tea. *Bioorg. Chem.* **2020,** *105,* 104382. doi: 10.1016/j.bioorg.2020.104382.
60. Hoppe, J. B.; Coradini, K.; Frozza, R. L. Free and Nano Encapsulated Curcumin Suppresses β-amyloidinduced Cognitive Impairments in Ratsinvolvement of BDNF and Akt/GSK-3β Signaling Pathway. *Neurobiol. Learn. Memory* **2013,** *106,* 134–144.
61. Yavarpour, B.; H.; Ghasemi-Kasman, M.; Pirzadeh, M. Curcumin-Loaded Nanoparticles: A Novel Therapeutic Strategy in Treatment of Central Nervous System Disorders. *Int. J. Nanomed.* **2019,** *14,* 4449–4460. doi: 10.2147/IJN.S208332.
62. Zhang, F.; Lu, Y. F.; Wu, Q.; Liu, J.; Shi, J. S. Resveratrol Promotes Neurotrophic Factor Release from Astroglia. *Exp. Biol. Med.* **2012,** *237* (8), 943–948.
63. Salem, H. F.; Kharshoum, R. M.; Heba, A.; Taleb, A.; Naguib, D. M. Brain Targeting of Resveratrol through Intranasal Lipid Vesicles Labelled with Gold Nanoparticles:

In-vivo Evaluation and Bioaccumulation Investigation Using Computed Tomography and Histopathological Examination. *J. Drug Target.* **2019,** *27* (10), 1127–1134.

64. Kostomoiri, M.; Fragkouli, A.; Sagnou, M. Oleuropein, an Anti-oxidant Polyphenol Constituent of Olive Promotes α-secretase Cleavage of the Amyloid Precursor Protein (AβPP). *Cell. Mol. Neurobiol.* **2013,** *33* (1), 147–154.
65. Pourkhodadad, S.; Alirezaei, M.; Moghaddasi, M.; Ahmadvand, H.; Karami, M.; Delfan, B.; Khanipour, Z. Neuroprotective Effects of Oleuropein Against Cognitive Dysfunction Induced by Colchicine in Hippocampal CA-1 Area in Rats. *J. Physiol. Sci.* **2016,** *66,* 397–405.
66. Na, J.-Y.; Song, K.; Lee, J.-W.; Kim, S.; Kwon, J. 6-Shogaol has Anti-amyloidogenic Activity and Ameliorates Alzheimer Disease via CysLT1R-mediated Inhibition of Cathepsin B. *Biochem. Biophys. Res. Commun.* **2016,** *477* (1), 96–102.
67. Shim, S.; Kim, S.; Kwon, Y B.; Kwon, J. Protection by [6]-shogaol Againstlipopolysaccharideinduced Toxicity in Murine Astrocytes is Related to Production of Brainderived Neurotrophic Factor. *Food Chem. Toxicol.* **2012,** *50* (3–4), 597–602.
68. Xiao, Q.; Wang, C.; Li, J. Ginkgolide B Protects Hippocampal Neurons from Apoptosis Induced by beta-amyloid 25–35 Partly via Up-regulation of Brain-derived Neurotrophic Factor. *Eur. J. Pharmacol.* **2010,** *647* (1–3), 48–54.
69. Karavelioglu, Z.; CakirKoc, R. Preparation of Chitosan Nanoparticles as Ginkgo Biloba Extract Carrier: In Vitro Neuroprotective Effect on Oxidative Stress-Induced Human Neuroblastoma Cells (SH-SY5Y). *Int. J. Biol. Macromol.* **2021,** *192,* 675–668.
70. Zhang, Q.; Li, J. K.; Ge, R.; Liang, J. Y.; Li, Q. S.; Min, Z. D. Novel NGF-potentiating Limonoids from the Fruits of *Melia toosendan*. *Fitoterapia* **2013,** *90,* 192–198.
71. . Baker, D. H. A.; Ibrahim, B. M. M.; Hassan, N. S.; Yousuf, A. F.; El Gengaihi, S. Exploiting *Citrus aurantium* Seeds and their Secondary Metabolites in the Management of Alzheimer Disease. *Toxicol. Rep.* **2020,** *7,* 723–729.
72. Kim, C. S.; Kwon, O. W.; Kim, S. Y.; Lee, K. R. Bioactive Lignans from the Trunk of *Abies holophylla*. *J. Nat. Prod.* **2013,** *76* (11), 2131–2135.
73. Tang, W.; Kubo, M.; Harada, K.; Hioki, H.; Fukuyama, Y. Novel NGF-Potentiating Diterpenoids from a Brazilian Medicinal Plant, *Ptychopetalumolacoides*. *Bioorganic Med. Chem. Lett.* **2009,** *19* (3), 882–886.
74. Huang, X.; Li, N.; Pu, Y.; Zhang, T.; Wang, B. Neuroprotective Effects of Ginseng Phytochemicals-Recent Perspectives. *Molecules* **2019,** *24* (16), 2939–2945.
75. Kang, K. A.; Kang, J. H.; Yang, M. P. Ginseng Total Saponin Enhances the Phagocytic Capacity of Canine Peripheral Blood Phagocytes in-vitro. *Am. J. Chinese Med.* **2008,** *36* (2), 329–341.
76. Kim, M. S.; Yu, J. M.; Kim, H. J. Ginsenoside Re and Rd Enhance the Expression of Cholinergic Markers and Neuronal Differentiation in Neuro-2a Cells. *Biol. Pharmaceut. Bull.* **2014,** *37* (5), 826–833.
77. Hu, D.; Yang, Z.; Yao, X. Dibenzocyclooctadiene Lignans from *Schisandra chinensis* and their Inhibitory Activity on NO Production in Lipopolysaccharide-Activated Microglia Cells. *Phytochemistry* **2014,** *104,* 72–78.
78. Wang, Z. F.; Tang, L. L.; Yan, H.; Wang, Y. J.; Tang, X. C. Effects of Huperzine A on Memory Deficits and Neurotrophic Factors Production after Transient Cerebral Ischemia and Reperfusion in Mice. *Pharmacol. Biochem. Behav.* **2006,** *83* (4), 603–611.
79. Meng, Q.; Wang, A.; Hua, H.; Jiang, Y.; Wang, Y.; Mu, H.; Wu, Z.; Sun, K. Intranasal Delivery of Huperzine A to the Brain Using Lactoferrin-Conjugated N-Trimethylated

Chitosan Surfacemodified PLGA Nanoparticles for Treatment of Alzheimer Disease. *Int. J. Nanomed.* **2018,** *13,* 705.

80. Asai, M.; Iwata, N.; Yoshikawa, A. Berberine Alters the Processing of Alzheimer Amyloid Precursor Protein to Decrease Aβ Secretion. *Biochem. Biophys. Res. Commun.* **2007,** *352* (2), 498–502.
81. Mohiuddin, R.; Hassan, R.; Wani, T. U.; Shah, A. J. Berberine in the Treatment of Neurodegenerative Diseases and Nanotechnology Enabled Targeted Delivery. *Comb. Chem. High Throughput Screen.* **2021,** *24* (4), 616–633.
82. Zhou, Z.; Hou, J.; Mo, Y.; Ren, M.; Yang, G.; Qu, Z.; Hu, Y. Geniposidic Acid Ameliorates Spatial Learning and Memory Deficits and Alleviates Neuroinflammation via Inhibiting HMGB-1 and Downregulating TLR4/2 Signaling Pathway in APP/PS1 Mice. *Eur. J. Pharmacol.* **2020,** *869,* 172857. doi: 10.1016/j.ejphar.2019.172857.
83. Chen, Q. Y.; Yin, Y.; Li, L.; Zhang, Y. J.; He, W.; Shi, Y. Geniposidic Acid Confers Neuroprotective Effects in a Mouse Model of Alzheimer's Disease through Activation of a PI3K/AKT/GAP43 Regulatory Axis. *J. Previous Alzheimer Dis.* **2022,** *9* (1), 158–171. doi: 10.14283/jpad.2021.60.
84. Kwon, S. H.; Lee, H. K.; Kim, J. A. Neuroprotective Effects of *Eucommia ulmoides* Olivbark on Amyloid beta(25-35)-induced Learning and Memory Impairments in Mice. *Neurosci. Lett.* **2011,** *487* (1), 123–127.
85. Li, L. F.; Lu, J.; Li, X. M. Antidepressant-like Effect of Magnolol on BDNF Up-regulation and Serotonergic System Activity in Unpredictable Chronic Mild Stress Treated Rats. *Phytother. Res.* **2012,** *26* (8), 1189–1194.
86. Wang, H.; Liao, Z.; Sun, X. Intravenous Administration of Honokiol Provides Neuroprotection and Improves Functional Recovery After Traumatic Brain Injury Through Cell Cycle Inhibition. *Neuropharmacology* **2014,** *86,* 9–21.

CHAPTER 12

Molecular Mechanisms Underpinning Neuroprotection of Nutritional Polyphenols

JOHNSON O. OLADELE[1], ISAAC O. BABATUNDE[2], and OLUWASEUN T. OLADELE[2]

[1]*Department of Chemical Sciences, Faculty of Science, Kings University, Ode-Omu, Osun State, Nigeria*

[2]*Phytomedicine and Toxicology Laboratories, Department of Biochemistry, Faculty of Basic and Applied Sciences, Osun State University, Osogbo, Nigeria*

ABSTRACT

Polyphenols are one of the most notable phytochemicals present abundantly in fruit, vegetables, and other nutritional sources. A number of therapeutic significances have been attributed to this phytochemical which include antioxidant, anti-inflammatory, antiapoptotic, modulatory effects, and so on. This therapeutic importance has also been reported in polyphenols' neuroprotective actions such as enhancement of memory, learning, and cognitive performances, neuronal detoxification and repairment, downstream modulation of signaling pathways of neuronal oxidative stress, neuro-inflammation, and necrosis which are all implicated in neurodegenerative diseases as well as transcription, translation, amyloid congestion, and neuronal disruption pathways within the nerve cells. This article presents the molecular mechanisms underpinning neuroprotective action of polyphenols via Nrf-2, neurotropic pathways, NF-kB/MAPK, c-JUN, c-FOS, p53 pathway, anti-apoptotic, and anti-neuro-inflammatory signaling pathways. Considering the

Nanomedicine for Neurodegenerative Disorders: Selective Treatment Strategies. Rishabha Malviya, Kamla Pathak, & Swati Verma (Eds.)

deteriorating effects of apoptosis, protein misfolding, neuroinflammation, and oxidative stress in the pathogenesis of neurodegenerative diseases, modification of these key neurodegenerative pathological mediators at the molecular level may offer promising treatment approaches to slow down neurodegeneration and mitigate associated symptoms. Polyphenols pose promising therapeutic candidates to halt/mitigate/reverse the pathogenesis of these neuronal degenerative diseases via signaling pathways discussed in this article.

12.1 INTRODUCTION

The role of phytochemicals in maintenance of structural components; integrity of nerve cell and tissues, neuronal homeostasis, and disease prevention presently cannot be undervalued. Most notable among the phytochemicals are polyphenols, which are larger polymeric hydroxyl-containing substances which acts as secondary metabolites. Plant sources like fruit and vegetables are rich in polyphenols. They are majorly classified as flavonoid and non-flavonoids-based polyphenols which selectively cross through the blood–brain barrier to exact their therapeutic roles in neuronal detoxification and repairment in order to enhance memory, learning, and cognitive performances.[1,2]

Polyphenols have many therapeutic roles in combating many cellular and neuronal oxidative damages and inflammation which are all stack development of neurodegenerative diseases. Review on these groups of compound shows that they possessed antioxidant via free radicals scavenging and metal chelating potentials. Dietary polyphenols are either natural bioactive or considered to be xenobiotics within but, upon biotransformation by gut microbiota, they tend to be made biologically therapeutically and pharmacological active.[1–3]

Polyphenols currently are of major discussion among the populace of researchers due to their neuroprotective therapeutic role in prevention of neurological and cognitive decline disorders and age-related cognitive malignancies.[1,4] Molecular mechanism of neuroprotective action of polyphenols in neuronal damage and disorders occurs via downstream modulation of signaling pathways of oxidative stress, inflammation, and necrosis which are all implicated in neurodegenerative diseases as well as transcription, translation, amyloid congestion, and neuronal disruption pathways within the nerve cells.[1,2,4–5]

Inhibition of expression pro-oxidant biological catalyst and some molecules associated with and susceptible to oxidative attack such as nuclear factor-kB, direct ROS scavenging, down regulation of Bcl-2, and other molecules associated with apoptotic pathways are all involved in the molecular mechanism associated with polyphenols. Modulation of mitogen-activated protein kinase (MAPK) activity, dissociation of nuclear factor erythroid 2–related factor 2 (Nrf2) associated complexes and other signaling pathway involved in developmental protective mechanism against neuronal damages processes.[6,7]

Neuronal damages, amyloid congestion, and impairment of nerves cell are major causes of developmental neuronal losses of functions and structure which leads to degenerative diseases such Parkinson disease, Alzheimer's, Huntington, and so on. The prevalence of these pathological conditions has been increasing yearly; presently over 50 million people worldwide are suffering from these pathological conditions, and statistical prediction has shown that numerical values might increase to 115 million by 2025.[8]

Although the uses of polyphenols in neurodegenerative research are limited due to its reduced bioavailability and low ability to pass through the blood–brain barriers, the advent of nanotechnology in drug delivery and structural modification strategy have help in delivering the polyphenols-containing compound in the brain. Exploiting the role of these phyto-polyphenols is paramount in prevention and treatment of these neurodegenerative diseases. Therefore, in exploiting their therapeutic and pharmacological functions, the molecular mechanism underpinning their neuroprotective mechanisms must be understood clearly for their effective use and in their drug design. Hence, in this paper, the discussion on the polyphenol's neuroprotective mechanism down to the molecular level will be done explicitly.

12.2 NEURODEGENERATIVE DISEASES

The continuous loss of neuronal structure and functions collectively are clinically referred to as neuronal degenerative diseases.[4,9] These progressive degenerative disorders are still incurable; they effectually result in complete loss of nerve cell's biological functions and death at final stage. These diseases affect the brain at both molecular, cellular, and systemic levels. Apoptosis, neuro-inflammation, and oxidative destruction of nerve cells are major-known contributory factors which have been implicated in the onset and progression of degenerative diseases.[9,10]

Alzheimer, multiple atrophy and sclerosis, Parkinson, Huntington, and amyotrophic lateral sclerosis diseases are all most-notable known neurodegenerative disorders. These pathological conditions result in formation of protein assembly, misfolding, and aggregation, which eventually leads to total cell death.[9,11] Research in this field is growing but still need more focus as longevity is ultimate desired by everyone.

12.2.1 PARKINSON'S DISEASE

Parkinson's disease is the most popular degenerative disease after Alzheimer's. This disease was earlier called shaking palsy disease. Parkinson disease is a slow onset degenerative condition which affects nerves cell at the substantial nigra compacta of the mid-brain region. Continuous loss of function and death of the dopaminergic neurons at this region of the brain occurred in Parkinson.[4,12] Bradykinesia, instability of posture, involuntary slow motor of hands (tremor), and rigidity of body parts are major cardinal motor symptoms of Parkinson while language speaking and memory defaults, inability to recall and recapture, and slowness in thinking and action are part of neurological psychology symptoms.[4,12,13]

Oxidative destruction of neuronal cells and its components, mitochondria cellular malfunctioning, neuronal inflammation, and default in protein clearance, which result in Lewis bodies build up (due continuous accumulation of misfolded alpha synucleins proteins) within and outside the brain interacting with other cellular and extracellular components, are all involved in the pathogenesis of the Parkinson disease.[4,12] Although its etiology is multifactorial, genetic, or environmental, exposure to agrochemicals and heavy metals, caffeine, and cigarettes smoking are all environmental factors that have been implicated in the development of the disease while changes in nucleotides of DNA coding for alpha synucleins, Tau proteins, and many others, which have been identified, encompassed the genetic factors (Figure 12.1). These genes are collectively called *PARK* genes.[4,14,15]

The prevalence of this degenerative disease is about less than 1% in age range of 65–69 years and 4% in those at 80 years and above.[4,16] The prevalence has been suggested to raise statistically to more than 30% by year 2030.[17] This has shown a need to arrest this slow-killing deadly disorder.

Several molecular mechanisms have been reported to implicate in the disease pathogenesis.[4,9] Building of misfolded alpha synucleins proteins is part of these molecular mechanisms.[9] In native form, alpha synucleins exhibit alpha helical structure or unfolded form but in diseased state, it (Parkinson) exhibits beta sheet helical amyloid structure due to conformation changes through the processes of ubiquitination, phosphorylation of its serine 129, or terminal carbon distortion.[18,19] Accumulation of these over a long time combined with reduce efficiency or default in protein clearance system of the cell bring about formation of insoluble oligomeric protein call Lewis bodies which is the cause of loss and death of dopaminergic neurons.[20]

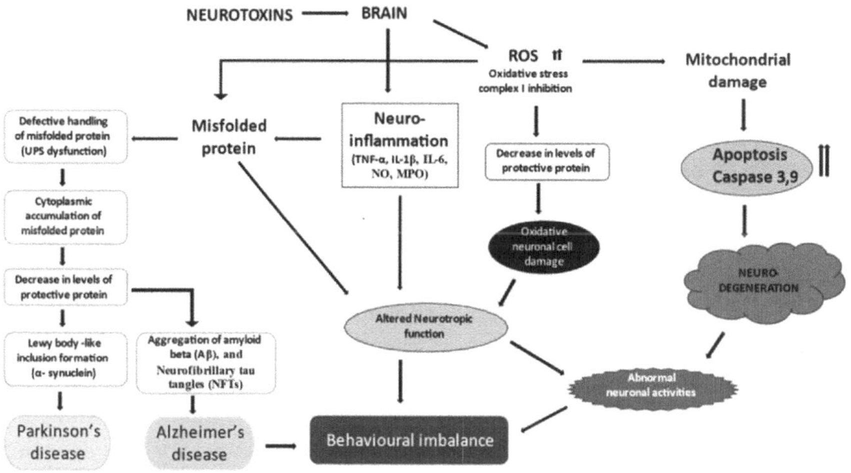

FIGURE 12.1 Molecular mechanisms underlying pathogenesis of Parkinson's disease and Alzheimer's disease.

Source: Modified from Ref. [9]

These oligomeric proteins block and suppress the activities of mitochondria complex 1 activity, leading to reduction in activities of the complex resulting in mitochondria dysfunction which eventually leads to exposure of the brain and nerve cells to oxidative attack and depletion in ATP generation. In addition to this, exposure of cell to neurotoxins like pesticide and heavy metals combined with depletion in antioxidant capacity of cell due to oxidative attack results in imbalance in free radicals/reactive oxygen species generation and antioxidants levels.[21,22]

Presently, there is no true cure for Parkinson disease; the disorder is being managed based on symptoms presented by the patients. Levodopa is still the current precious method of treatment of Parkinson disease and has been used over decades.[4,23] Besides this, there are other methods used currently in addition to or following the uses of Levodopa, some of these include monoamine oxygenase-B inhibitor, dopamine antagonist, and dopa decarboxylase inhibitor.[24] The advent and choice of use of these other drugs in preference to, after, and in combination with levodopa are due to its clinical complications like dyskinesias, nauseas, vomiting, and low blood pressure.[23] Fluctuations in its effectiveness due to on-off effect of the drug and low bioavailability due to blood–brain barrier and many more are notable factors that limits its usage. Others drugs used in combination still shown side effects like hallucination and insomnia to mention a but few. Stem cell transplants, surgery, and gene therapy are alternative means but these are very expensive.[25]

12.2.2 ALZHEIMER'S DISEASE

Alzheimer's disease is another neurodegenerative disease that people mistakenly confuse with aging symptomatically, due to some similar features and process and about 20% are diagnosed wrongly.[26] Loss of functional neurons and nerves synapses within brain cerebral cortex and extending to some part of the subcortical are major characteristic features of this disease.[27] Alzheimer's disease is most common and rampant degenerative diseases in terms of number of sufferers in the world. The disease was named after the scientist who first gives public description about this clinical condition back then in 1906.[28] The disease is basically referred to as memory loss disorder. The disease is also slow in onset and continues to worsen progressively over years. In fact, this disease accounted for over 60% of medical cases reported and linked to dementia worldwide.[29] The disease primarily affects that part of the brain that caters to memory, which is known as hippocampus, and affects or alters the physio-anatomical function of this region resulting in loss of memory attributed to brain impairment.

Although memory loss is the most paramount and most identifiable symptoms in Alzheimer's, language problem, apraxia, difficulties in perception, writing, dressing, and other fine motor activities as well as movement coordination are clinically identified as early-stage symptoms.[30] Detrimental damages to long time memory which is affected in early stage, difficulties in patient speech most notable paraphasia, failure to recognize relatives, untailored aggressiveness, loss of courtesy in urination, and other neuropsychiatric-behavioral alteration have been identified diagnostically as middle-stage symptoms while at severe stage, complete reliance of care giver and absolute loss of speech exist.[31]

The prevalence of Alzheimer's disease is about 6% in adults of age 65 and above;[4,32] this disease affects woman more in terms of number and over 50 million of people were affected globally. The pathogenesis of this disease has been attributed protein misfolding due to larger gathering together in place of folded amyloid beta proteins in neurons and brain tissues. In homeostatic state, the amyloid beta proteins are subparts of transmembrane protein called amyloid beta precursor which function upon transport via neuron's membrane to promote growth and repair of nerve cell, but when largely gathers thus ravel them to fold randomly so as to associate together leading to abnormal folding within the cell as neurofibrillary tangles and outside the cell as amyloid plaques and Tau proteins.[33]

These plaques are insoluble deposits which are named proteopathy. Also, the Tau proteins aids transport of nutrients and other vital nutrients and are further subjected to phosphorylation leading to formation of paired thread-like structure called neurofibrillary tangles.[34] All these results in neuronal toxicity, then coupled with oxidative stress, decreased protein clearances of the system and neuro-inflammation response in eliminating, these plagues results in neuronal functions loss and death, disruption of calcium homeostasis, induction of apoptosis, mitochondria malfunctioning, and energy depletion.[35]

The etiology of this disease is also multifactorial like Parkinson disease, as this is linked to genetic and environmental factors. In term of genetic factors, Alzheimer's disease can be inherited when any of these autosomal dominant gene's *APP, PSEN1/2* which codes for amyloid precursor proteins and presenilins are inherited[36] or when there is mutation of gene *APOE4* which codes for apolipoproteins E.[37] Environmental factors include exposure to traffic exhaust and burning, excessive consumption of alcohol, poor sleeping lifestyle, and high cholesterol intake and are channels toward development of Alzheimer's disease.

Like Parkinson disease, the Alzheimer's disease is being managed based on symptoms presented by the sufferers. There is no true cure for Alzheimer's diseases; medicinal intervention made so far on it was on way of reducing the onset and the disease progression. The use of drug that could enhance memory and cognitive function such as tacrine (an acetylcholinesterase inhibitor) and memantine which function as the N-Methyl-D-aspartate receptor antagonist,[38] as well as other drug which could lower depression, inflammation, hypertension, and cholesterol level are usually employed depending on the pronounce symptom in individuals.[39,40] Also, physical exercise, educational engagement, abstinent from smoking, adequate sleep, and living less stressful are life style changes that could help in management this disease.

12.2.3 HUNTINGTON DISEASES

The disease pathogenesis has been linked to inclusion bodies' neuronal toxicity which present itself similar to amyloid plaque protein deposit which exist in other neurodegenerative diseases. The inclusion bodies exist due to cellular cleavage of polyglutamine chains into smaller fragments, which are misfolded and build up to form beta strand amyloid deposit with the help of hydrogen bonds interaction between the amino acids of the short polypeptide chains.[41]

The inclusion bodies are not useful to the cell and present neuronal toxicity. They further interact and impair activities of other proteins like chaperone and caspases, thereby exacerbating the neuronal toxicity level. Mitochondria malfunctioning is present after due interaction with the nerve cell membrane metabolic processes. This leads to oxidative stress, ROS release, and energy depletion which finally causes cell death.[42]

Like other types of neurodegenerative diseases, there is no true cure for Huntington disease. Medications available so far for treatment are all for the symptoms associated with these diseases in order to improve the healthy living in such patient. Psychotic combating drug like benzodiazepines is used to treat Huntington-related psychology symptoms, tetrabenazine is used for treatment of chorea-related symptoms, while the used of eicosapentanoic acid is for improvement in the motor and cognitive problems.[43,44] Physical and speech therapies are also part of the multidisciplinary caregiving in the disease management.

12.2.4 OTHER KINDS OF NEURODEGENERATIVE DISEASES

Other neuronal function degenerative disorders include multiple sclerosis, a disease whose pathogenesis has been attributed to inflammation response due to autoimmune attack leading to migration on nerve cell signaling molecules such as myelin proteins and glycoprotein, proteolipids, and other antigen-related responses, moving to the blood–brain barrier of the myelin layer of the neuronal cell.[45] Other forms of neuronal function degenerative disorders like Amyotrophic lateral sclerosis, progressive nuclear palsy, ataxia, and others diseases have their pathogenic mechanisms from either amyloid protein formation or fibrillary aggregates in case of synucleino-or TDP-43 proteinopathy or prion proteins build up or shared any of its combination.[46]

12.3 CHEMISTRY AND BIOLOGICAL SIGNIFICANCE OF POLYPHENOLS

The relevance of polyphenols in biomedical research cannot be underestimated due to their ability to combat diseases whose origin of molecular pathology can be traced to oxidative stress and free radicals' attacks, inflammation, protein misfolding and amyloid aggregation, unregulated growth, and mitochondria malfunctioning; these include diseases like cancer, cardiovascular and neurodegenerative diseases to mention but few.[1,47,48]

In term of structural overview, polyphenols belongs to compound having more than one phenol moiety in their structure, many thousands of them have been analytical identified and classified. Some of these compounds are edible while the rest are not.

Polyphenols exist abundantly and are largely derived from plants and this is the major reason they were classified as phytochemicals. They exist naturally as the nutritional component of plants like fruits, vegetables, cereal red wine, etc.[1,49] Polyphenols have minimum of 15 carbon skeletons in its structure which are surrounded by hydroxyl moieties, the phenol moiety are linked together by ester or through carbon-to-carbon bonds. This ester connection is hydrolysable tannins whereas the carbon-to-carbon connection is nonhydrolysable but condensed tannins like linked.

Because of their structural diversification and wide distribution in natural products, polyphenols are classified in different ways based on the chemical structure, biological roles, and sources. Of all the chemical structural classification, the most common and widely used are discussed in this article.

Polyphenols can be grouped two categories—flavonoids and non-flavonoids polyphenols. The non-flavonoid polyphenols include the simple and free phenol such as gallic acid which are benzoic acid derivatives having C1 to C6 backbone and coumaric acids which are cinnamic derivatives having C3 to C6 backbone. Others non-flavonoids polyphenols include hydrolysable tannins, lignans, phenylacetic acids, etc.[50]

The flavonoids polyphenols group are the most abundant categories and most commonly studied due to the antioxidant and counter inflammatory potentials. In term of structural skeleton, they have two benzyl moeities tagged rings A and B linked together by three carbon C3 skeleton tagged ring C in their structure. These comprises of the following:

1. Those having their ring B attached to carbon-3 position of ring C in open or closed ring form as found in isoflavones (genistein), neoflavonoids (dalbergin), and chalcones.[51]
2. Those having their three carbon skeletons forming a ring chain with ring A and the last carbon of the three carbon skeletons attached to the ring C as found inflavanones (furanoflavanones), flavones (nobiletin), flavonols (quercetin), and flavanonols (taxifolin).[52]
3. Flavanols and proanthocyanidins which are structurally similar to the group of flavonols except that there is no double bond between

the carbon 2 and 3 of the ring C. Flavanols includes catechin and epicatechin while proanthocyanidins includes tannins.

4. Polyphenolic amides are polyphenols having N-containing functional substituent. This includes capsaicinoids in chili peppers.

Other polyphenols include resveratrol, curcumin, rosmarinic acid, and others which are complex polyphenols but have been reported to have crucial antioxidative, anti-inflammatory, and neuroprotective roles.[1,51]

The physiological roles of polyphenols to healthy living are diverse ranging from chemopreventive, treatment and management of diseases like cancer, diabetes, cardiovascular diseases, and degenerative diseases.[1,53] They play their health beneficial roles either directly or indirectly by modulation; the signal pathways and its components which have been implicated to play role in disease development. Research on physiology of polyphenols is increasing nowadays because of their multifunctional therapeutic and pharmacological importance. In promoting healthy brain, polyphenols have been reported to help scavenging reactive chemical species generated in the brain due to metabolic processes or due to exposure to xenobiotics, thus exhibiting antioxidant role which help in lowering the risk of developing neurodegenerative disorder.[1,54]

Polyphenol such as curcumin of turmeric, flavonoids, and carotenoids has reported to be useful cytoprotective and chemoprotective agent which promote tissue generation and repair of the lining of the digestive tracts as well as suppressing of inflammation. In preventing stress on cardiovascular vessel, polyphenols have been reported to help inhibiting the oxidation of low-density lipoprotein cholesterol in the blood and blood vessels and also promote blood conveying process by increasing the vasodilation of the blood channels.[55,56] In ensuring healthy bone function and structure, polyphenols show protective effects against deterioration of bone, which occurs via oxidative attack on the bone components, thus helping prevention and management of bone conditions like osteoporosis and arthritis.[57]

Another most distinct physiological function of polyphenols is therapeutic role in combating cancer via anti-oxidative and anti-inflammatory effects. Antioxidant potential of curcumin and flavonoids against DNA damages by free radicals' attacks has been reported via direct free radical scavenging action, as this act triggers and promotes cancer cell development.[58] Polyphenols also act indirectly via the signaling pathway of some transcriptional factors whose alteration have implicated in oxidative stress, inflammation, and cancer. Such factors includes p53, c-Jun, Nrf-2, COX-2, and MAPK.[59]

The dietary polyphenols also help in promoting healthy digestion of food and in control of the metabolic activities of gut microbiota, by favoring the growth of beneficial bacteria and fending off the system of the harmful pathogens. Evidence of these was reported for green tea polyphenols in an in vitro study using bifidobacteria. The available research evidences support the nutritional and microbial regulatory roles of dietary polyphenols by promoting the survival of probiotics and improving the symptomatic features of inflammatory bowel diseases and peptic ulcer.[60,61] Furthermore, compositional modulation of the gut microbiota and function, quorum bacterial sensing interfering, sensitizing of the gut bacteria to xenobiotics, and membrane permeability were also reported as the beneficial roles of polyphenols.[61,62]

12.4 MECHANISMS OF NEUROPROTECTIVE EFFECT OF NUTRITIONAL POLYPHENOLS

Among the most notable ways by which polyphenols demonstrated neuronal protection against neurological damages and brain ageing is via modulation of signaling pathway which are directly or indirectly involved in the molecular and pathological events of these diseases such as oxidative stress, inflammation, protein misfolding, mitochondria malfunctioning, and many more. Some of these signaling pathways are Nrf-2, neurotropic pathways, NF-kB/MAPK, c-JUN, c-FOS, p53 pathway, anti-apoptotic, anti-neuro-inflammatory pathways, and others.[1,4,63] Studies have elucidated the physiological role of polyphenols in modulating these pathways; some of which will be discussed here.

12.4.1 NEUROPROTECTIVE MECHANISM OF POLYPHENOLS VIA NF-KB SIGNALING PATHWAY

Nuclear factor kappa-light-chain-enhancer of activated B cells (NF-κB) is an ubiquitous transcriptional factor hosted in nearly all types of animal cell. NF-κB major roles involve modulating the genetic expression of cytokines and chemokines which includes interferons, interleukins, lymphokines, and tumor necrosis factors[64] (Figure 12.2). These factors play wide roles in inflammatory and immune responses; survival of cells as well as promoting integrity of signaling pathway in nervous system involve in learning, plasticity, and memory.[65] Likewise, its role in management of cancerous cell has been linked with down line suppression of tumor necrosis factors cellular cytosol toxicity via apoptotic route and suppression of c-Jun pathway via the N-terminal enzymatic kinase activities.[66]

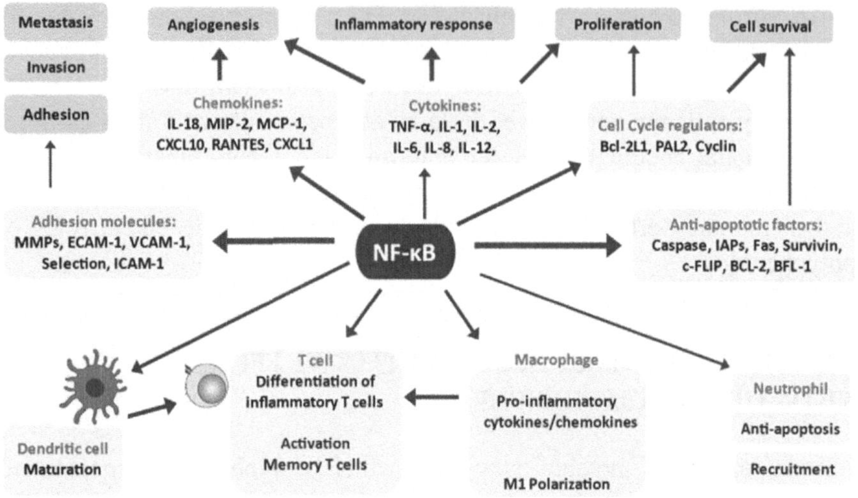

FIGURE 12.2 NF-κB target genes which are linked to inflammation development and progression being an inducible transcription factor.

NF-kB undergoes either canonical or non-canonical route which are both dependent on the structural oligomeric dimerized components. The p50 and p65 (RelA) subunits play role in the canonical route while RelB and p52 play role in non-canonical route.

In homeostatic state, the NF-kB exist as an inactive hetero-dimer forms composing of p50 and p65 (RelA) subunits, complexing with an inhibitory proteins IkB-α or IkB-β and mask with the cytoplasm, but upon stimulation by microglia, expression of the membranes receptor like toll-like receptors (TLRs) and their associate which recognized the pathogen-associated molecules like and damage-associated molecules of bacteria, virus, fungal, and other parasites as pro-inflammatory ligands are initiated.[67,68] The signaling response results in activation of the IκB protein kinases which phosphorylate the inhibitory protein for its dissociation from the complexes to free NF-kB for nuclear transport in order to bind with its nuclear receptor for expression and recruitment of expression of chemokines, inflammatory enzymes: COX-2 and iNOS, pro-inflammatory cytokines, and tissues adhesion cytokine molecules[69,70] (Figure 12.3). These molecules are collectively markers for cellular or tissues or neuronal inflammatory responses.

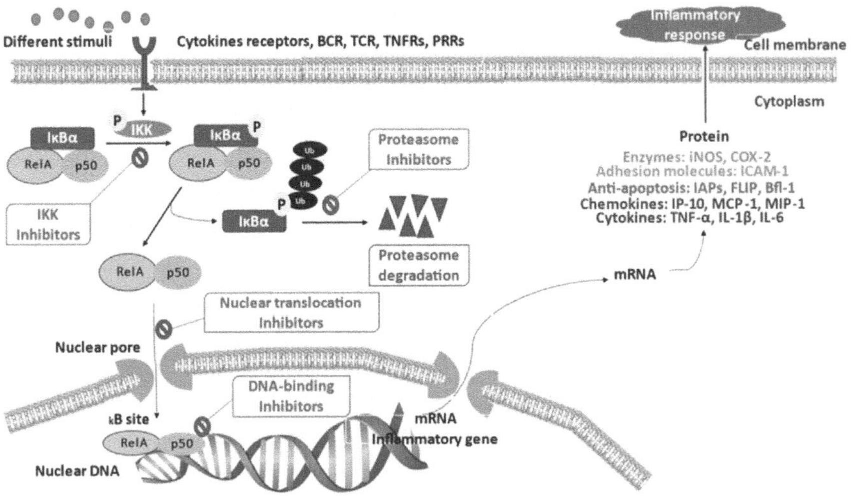

FIGURE 12.3 Mechanistic approaches in NF-κB-mediated intervention in inflammatory diseases.

Suppression of the active level of NF-KB could be therapeutic tool in prevention of cancer, cardiovascular, and degenerative diseases. Research have shown that polyphenols exhibit anti-inflammatory potential in neuronal cells via these mechanism: (i) by inhibiting the activity of the enzyme IκB protein kinases, thereby halting the phosphorylation and ubiquitination processes which are essential for liberation of IkB moiety from the NF-kB complexes;[71] (ii) by inhibiting the productive interaction of the NF-κB subunits even after translocation into the nucleus with the targeted DNA;[71] and (iii) polyphenols also interfere directly with arachidonic acid (AA) dependent pathways by inhibiting the expression of the enzyme which promote progression of inflammatory process (cyclooxygenase-2) and AA independent pathways indirectly as this depends on it counterpart pathway.[72]

Among the reported polyphenols which have been shown to exhibit these neuronal anti-inflammatory mechanisms are curcumin, quercetin, epigallocate catechin, and resveratrol.[73–75]

12.4.2 NEUROPROTECTIVE MECHANISM OF POLYPHENOLS VIA NRF2 SIGNALING PATHWAY

Many dietary polyphenols have been identified to participate actively in the activation of the heterodimer's transcription factor: nuclear factor-erythroid factor 2-related factor 2 (Nrf2) in mediating neuronal protection against oxidative destruction/stress and inflammation.[76,77]

Nrf2 is a transcription factor which belongs to Cap "n" Collar family of basic leucine zipper (bZip) which are located in the cytoplasm to regulates the main genes for antioxidant and cellular protection.[78] It interacts under physiological conditions with Kelch-like ECH-associated protein 1(Keap 1) to enhance proteasomal degradation via interaction with ubiquitin ligase. This complex, Nrf2-Keap1 is essential for passage of Nrf2 in to the nuclear for associative interaction with other leucine zipper (bZip) transcription factors and to the non-coding region of DNA which plays role in pleiotropy of many neighboring genes called Cis-acting element, specifically the anti-oxidant response element (ARE) (Figures 12.4 and 12.5).

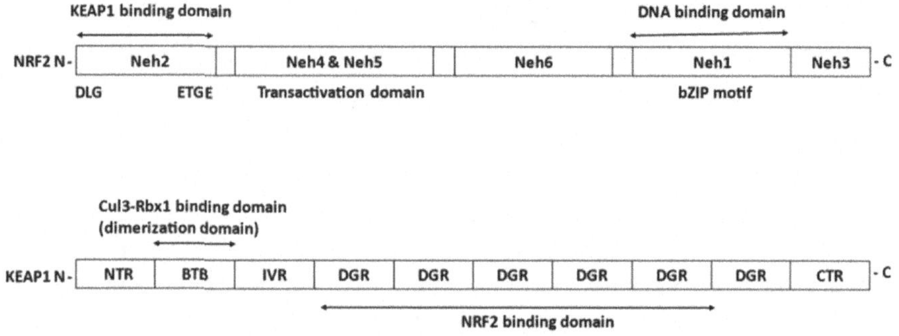

FIGURE 12.4 NRF2 and KEAP1 proteins. DGR, double glycine repeat (=Kelch); IVR, intervening region; NTR, N-terminal region; BTB, broad complex, Tramtrack, and Bric-a-Brac; bZIP, basic leucine zipper; and CTR, carboxyl terminal region.

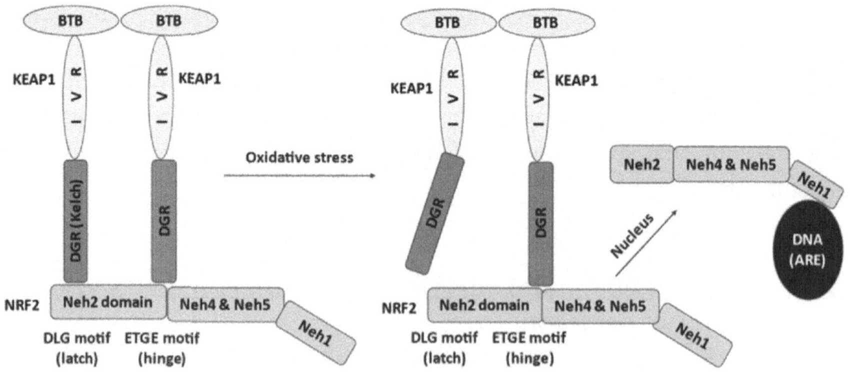

FIGURE 12.5 Reaction between NRF2 and KEAP1: latch and hinge model.

Under cellular oxidative stress, the condition serves as signal for the Nrf2 to dissociate from the Nrf2-Keap1 complex and for its activation, which further translocate into nuclear through E3 ubiquitin ligase catalytic action. ARE responses give rise to induction of inducible cytoprotective biological proteins like hemeoxygenase-1 (HO-1), glutathione-s-transferase, and other associated enzymes complexes which all play roles in detoxification of xenobiotics and removal of endogenously generated toxic molecules[79] (Figure 12.6). The Nrf2-ARE interaction is the major target for polyphenols enhanced neuroprotective signaling. Polyphenols promote NrF2 and ARE interaction as this interaction activates HO-1 (regulatory enzymes) and activate of xenobiotics/drug detoxifying enzymes complexes. Likewise, the end products of HO-1 catalyzed reaction results in generation of carbon monoxide and bilirubin.[80] These end products enable HO-1 to demonstrate its immuno-modulatory and neuronal anti-inflammation role via end products regulatory actions which includes regulation of neuronal vessel tone, platelets aggregation prevention, neuronal tissue injury prevention, neuronal tissue congestion, and neuro-inflammation prevention.[80,81]

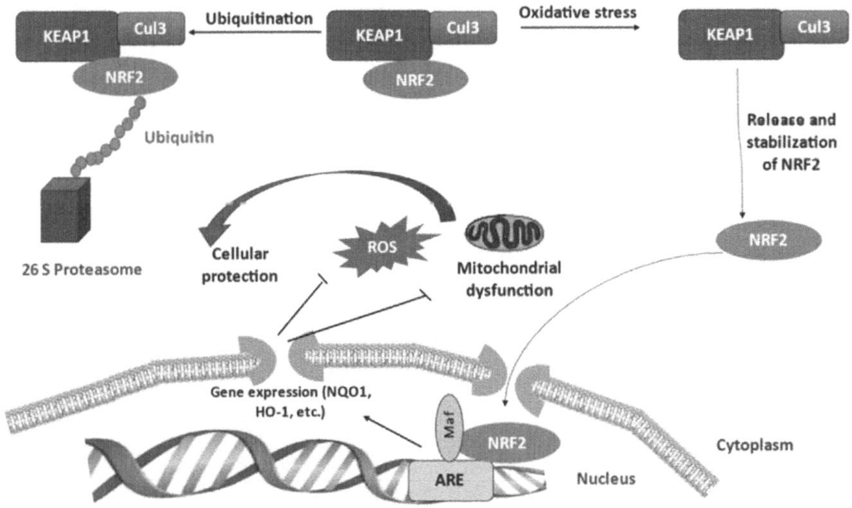

FIGURE 12.6 KEAP1 regulates NRF2 stability.

Asides from the direct free radicals and lipid peroxides quenching potentials, polyphenols via Nrf2 pathways exhibited neuroprotection through phase II detoxifying enzymes system, HO-1 expression and Nrf2-ARE signaling complex activation. Curcumin, caffeic acid phenethylester, and green tea catechins have been shown to exhibit this neuroprotective role via HO-1 expression and Nrf2-ARE signaling routes.[82,83] Curcumin rich diet have been reported to enhance memory, learning, and cognitive functions through decreased amyloid protein aggregation, suppression of inflammation responses, reversing of brain lipid peroxidation and lipid modifications, and increased glutathione levels in Alzheimer and Parkinson patient. Likewise, the green tea catechins had been shown to possess anti-inflammation in addition to its neuroprotective actions, its daily intake has been reported to help in delaying the occurrence of ageing and age-related diseases. Furthermore, neuronal vessel formation and inhibition of the spread of cancerous are other beneficial roles accounted for its intake.[84]

The health benefits of polyphenols have been linked to its direct antioxidant and anti-inflammatory role due to their ability to scavenge free radicals through their hydroxyl functional group present in its structure, but an underlined indirect neuroprotective mechanism not well study is their role in modulation of signaling pathway within the cells. Curcumin, green tea catechins, cinnamic acid of ferulic acid source, and caffeic acid phenethyl ester are all polyphenols which modulate Nrf2 signaling pathway, specifically by enhancing Nrf2-ARE interaction which activates and promotes the expression of the phase II detoxifying enzymes and expression of HO-1 gene which accounted for their powerful antioxidant, neuroprotective, and anti-inflammatory capacities.[83] Additionally, the Nrf2 pathway also helps in moderating the levels and effect principal neurotransmitters including norepinephrine, dopamine, and glutamate. This underlined mechanism of action could be another significant therapeutic tool for treatment of cancer and neurodegenerative diseases.

12.4.3 NEUROPROTECTIVE MECHANISM OF POLYPHENOLS VIA MAPK PATHWAY

Among the important pathway which helps in signal transduction from the extracellular components of the cell to the intracellular or target region is MAPK pathway. MAPK pathway comprises of cascade of events which plays role in modulating signaling event which is vital for mammalian cells proliferation, development and differentiation, inflammatory responses, and apoptosis.[85] The pathway comprises of many proteins which transfer signal via phosphorylation of their tyrosine, serine or threonine amino acids containing moiety in their structure of the neighboring proteins in order to send signal to the DNA for transcription purposes.

The phosphorylation process caused conformational changes in their protein structure enabling them to activate neighboring proteins. Mutation is gene expression of any of these proteins results in development of cancer. C-Jun N-terminal kinases (JNK), extracellular signal-regulated kinases (ERKs), and p38 MAPKs are major MAPK subfamilies of popular discussions, although other subfamilies like Nemo-like kinase exist.[86] In general, each cascade event is activated by binding of ligand to the extracellular receptor sites which pronounce three sequential kinases event where MAPK kinase kinase (MAPKKK) stimulates MAPK kinase (MAPKK) which finally turn on MAP kinase (MAPK).

The ligand type determines which cascade among the subfamilies will activate within the enzymatic complexes. The canonical ERKs is activated by growth factor and cytokines while oxidative stress, cytokines, lipopolysaccharide, and infections turn on the p38 and JNK signaling routes.[85]

MAPK pathway play crucial roles in mitigating oxidative stress and oxidative damages which occurs as a consequence of destructive effect of free radicals and reactive nitric oxides species. This occurs via activation and expression of transcriptional factor for regulation of apoptosis and inflammatory processes. When the cell is under oxidative stress irrespective of the causative agent either ROS or iNOS, this serves as effector ligand that binds the extracellular receptor components causing activation of the MAPK upstream regulatory proteins thioredoxin which is a classical component of apoptosis signal-regulating kinase 1 (ASK1).[87] The ROS caused dissociation of the thioredoxin from the complexes converting it to active form, where its kinases activity catalyzed phosphorylation of the MEKs component i.e., MAPKs and proceed further to the phosphorylate JNK and p38 of MAPK. Likewise, the causative agent, ROS, can also directly activate MAPK via inhibition of its phosphatase's components. This cascade event caused expression of transcriptional factor the regulates apoptosis and inflammation.[85,87] With respect to inflammation, MAPK pathway plays roles in turning on of transcriptional factor gene NF-κB which is essential in the induction of pro-inflammatory cytokines, cyclooxygenase-2, and the inducible nitric oxide synthase, which are all promoters of inflammation response.[85]

From this point of view, inhibition of the signal transduction of MAPK vis ERKs, JNK, and p38 pathway either at transcriptional level should be the major target of therapeutic drug for promoting neuroprotection against oxidative and inflammation. Many reports have shown that polyphenols exhibit neuroprotective role via this mechanism. They regulate the MAPK pathway by inhibiting the activation processes at each step. For example, report from research conducted using activated human THP1 monocyte cell line showed that the polyphenol catechins regulates MAPK pathway by inhibiting activity the p38 and JNK of MAPK and their phosphorylated form, while quercetin demonstrated its inhibition on ERK, JNK, and their phosphorylated forms, thereby preventing further signaling transduction via phosphorylation process catalyzed by kinases.[88] Likewise, research conducted using lipopolysaccharide activated macrophages in mouse showed that polyphenol (quercetin) displayed its regulatory role against expression of TNF-α by inhibiting the prevention production of TNF-α protein synthesis via inhibiting the phosphorylation ERK1/2 and activity of p38 MAPK as well as TNF-α expression by halting the phosphorylation.[89]

Furthermore, the green tea catechins displayed its neuroprotective mechanism by inhibiting the expression of the gene for cyclooxygenase-2, an enzyme that promote inflammatory response by suppressing its expression via phosphorylation of the p38 MAPK pathway and it binding to DNA of NF-κB.[75]

12.4.4 NEUROPROTECTIVE MECHANISM OF POLYPHENOLS VIA P^{53} PATHWAY

P^{53} pathway is another signaling pathway of great significant to the cell. This pathway and its transcriptional products participate in stress response signaling processes like cell cycle arrest, senescence and apoptosis and most importantly the pathway helps in expression and synthesis of p53 protein which act as tumor suppressor protein preventing development of cancer.[90] Additionally, p53 helps in the process of inhibition of angiogenesis, metastasis, and IGF-1/mTOR pathway, and facilitates exosomes secretion and in DNA damage repair.

Damaged DNA via ROS and radiation, activated oncogenes, nitric oxide, cold and heat shock, hypoxia, damage spindle are stress signals that activate *p53* genes which result in expression of p53, in same way the Murine double minute 2 (MDM-2) are degraded in response to these stress signals via MDM-2 ubiquitin ligase.[91,92] P53 response genes upstream mediating follows a ND, the activated p53 proteins caused transcription of many genes, among which are GADD-45, MDM-2, cycling G, and p21 which play role in cell cycle arrest; secreted protein fas and killer/DR5 which works in conjunction with PIDD to activate caspases 8 and Bid to release cytochrome c in extrinsic apoptotic pathway; Bax, p53AIP, and PIGs in intrinsic apoptotic pathway; p48, GADD-45, and p53R2 which play role in DNA damage repair mechanism; BAI-1, KAI, and Maspin which play role as inhibitors of protease which degrades extracellular matrix and surface; and PTEN/IGF-BP3 genes which gene products IGF-1R, IGF 1 and others inhibit the activation of growth response signal transduction routes thereby regulating cell growth negatively after stress signals are triggered with cell.[93,94]

Available evidence proved that the p53 cross the nucleus and acting directly on mitochondria and its protein components BCL-2 to enhance the liberation of cytochrome c and apoptotic p53 also play role in communication between neighboring cell by inducing the TSAP-6 gene which enhances production of exosome for cell-cell communication. However, the p53 protein level is regulated by MDM-2 via ubiquitin ligase enzyme like constitutively photomorphogenic 1(COP1) and Pirh2 (p53-induced RING-H2 domain protein) and catalytic turn over.[90]

Polyphenols help in activation of p53 transcriptional activity in order to mediated increase synthesis of p53 protein which suppresses neuronal tumors and neurological cancer via initiation of apoptosis, cell arrest, ROS generation and cell senescence with the neurological tumor.[95,96] Furthermore, polyphenols caused up-regulation of p53 dependent target like p21, Bax, and DR5.[95]

12.5 CONCLUSION

Neurodegenerative diseases affect the brain at both molecular, cellular, and systemic levels. Apoptosis, neuro-inflammation, and oxidative destruction of nerve cells are majorly known contributory factors which have implicated in the onset and progression of the degenerative diseases. Polyphenols are one of the most notable phytochemicals present abundantly in fruit, vegetables, and other nutritional sources. A number of therapeutic significances have been attributed to this phytochemical which include antioxidant, anti-inflammatory, antiapoptotic, modulatory effects, and so on. This therapeutic importance has also been reported in polyphenols neuroprotective actions such as enhancement of memory, learning, and cognitive performances, neuronal detoxification and repairment, downstream modulation of signaling pathways of neuronal oxidative stress, neuro-inflammation, and necrosis which are all implicated in neurodegenerative diseases as well as transcription, translation, amyloid congestion, and neuronal disruption pathways within the nerve cells. The molecular mechanisms underpinning neuroprotective actions of polyphenols involved signaling pathways such as Nrf-2, neurotropic pathways, NF-kB/MAPK, c-JUN, c-FOS, p53 pathway, anti-apoptotic, and anti-neuro-inflammatory. Polyphenols pose to be a potential therapeutic candidate to halt or mitigate the pathogenesis of these neuronal degenerative diseases due to its multi-signaling modulatory properties.

KEYWORDS

- **polyphenols**
- **phytochemicals**
- **neurodegenerative diseases**
- **Parkinson disease**
- **Alzheimer's disease**
- **oxidative stress**
- **neuro-inflammation**

REFERENCE

1. Oladele, J. O.; Oladele, O. T.; Oyeleke, O. M. Possible Health Benefits of Polyphenols in Neurological Complications Associated with COVID-19. *Acta Fac. Med. Naiss.* **2021,** *38,* 294–309.
2. Oladele, J. O.; Oladele, O. T.; Oyeleke, O. M.; Oladiji, A. T. Neurological Complications in COVID-19: Implications on International Health Security and Possible Interventions of Phytochemicals. In *Contemporary Developments and Perspectives in International Health Security*; 2021, Vol. 2. doi: 10.5772/intechopen.96039
3. Deprez, S.; Mila, I.; Huneau, J. F.; Tome, D.; Scalbert, A. Transport of Proanthocyanidin Dimer, Trimer, and Polymer Across Monolayers of Human Intestinal Epithelial Caco-2 Cells. *Antioxid. Redox. Signal.* **2001,** *3,* 957–967.
4. Oladele, J. O.; Oyeleke, O. M.; Oladele, O. T.; Olaniyan, M. D. Neuroprotective Mechanism of *Vernonia Amygdalina* in a Rat Model of Neurodegenerative Diseases. *Toxicol. Rep.* **2020,** *7,* 1223–1232.
5. Smolensky, D.; Rhodes, D.; McVey, D. S.; Fawver, Z.; Perumal, R.; Herald, T.; Noronha, L. High-polyphenol Sorghum Bran Extract Inhibits Cancer Cell Growth through ROS Induction, Cell Cycle Arrest, and Apoptosis. *J. Med. Food* **2018,** *21,* 990–998.
6. Gupta, S.; Hastak, K.; Afaq, F.; Ahmad, N.; Mukhtar, H. Essential Role of Caspases in Epigallocatechin-3-Gallate-Mediated Inhibition of Nuclear Factor Kappa B and Induction of Apoptosis. *Oncogene* **2004,** *23,* 2507–2522.
7. Bhakkiyalakshmi, E.; Dineshkumar, K.; Karthik, S.; Sireesh, D.; Hopper, W.; Paulmurugan, R.; Ramkumar, K. M. Pterostilbene-mediated Nrf2 Activation: Mechanistic Insights on Keap1: Nrf2 Interface. *Bioorg. Med. Chem.* ***2016,*** *24,* 3378–3386.

8. Livingston, G; Huntley, J; Sommerlad, A. Dementia Prevention, Intervention, and Care: 2020 Report of the Lancet Commission. *Lancet* **2020,** *396* (10248), 413–446.
9. Oladele, J. O.; Oladiji, A. T.; Oladele, O. T.; Oyeleke, O. M. Reactive Oxygen Species in Neurodegenerative Diseases: Implications in Pathogenesis and Treatment Strategies [Online First]. *IntechOpen* **2021**. doi: 10.5772/intechopen.99976
10. Singh, A.; Kukreti, R.; Saso, L.; Kukreti, S.; Oxidative Stress: A Key Modulator in Neurodegenerative Diseases. *Molecules* **2019,** *24* (8).
11. Bredesen, D. E.; Rao, R. V.; Mehlen, P. Cell Death in the Nervous System. *Nature* **2006,** *443* (7113), 796–802.
12. Kouli, A.; Torsney, K. M.; Kuan, W. L. Parkinson's Disease: Etiology, Neuropathology, and Pathogenesis. In *Parkinson's Disease: Pathogenesis and Clinical Aspects*; Stoker, T. B., Greenland, J. C., Eds.; Codon Publications: Brisbane (AU), 2018; Chapter 1. doi: 10.15586/codonpublications.parkinsonsdisease.2018.ch1
13. Jankovic, J. Parkinson's Disease: Clinical Features and Diagnosis. *J. Neurol. Neurosurg. Psychiatry* **2008,** *79* (4), 368–376.
14. Deng, H.; Wang, P.; Jankovic, J. The Genetics of Parkinson Disease. *Ageing Res. Rev.* **2018,** *42,* 72–85.
15. Schulte, C.; Gasser, T. Genetic basis of Parkinson's Disease: Inheritance, Penetrance, and Expression. *Appl. Clin. Genet.* **2011,** *4,* 67–80.
16. De-Lau, L. M.; Breteler, M. M. Epidemiology of Parkinson's Disease. *Lancet Neurol.* **2006,** *5,* 525–535.
17. Chen, R. C.; Chang, S. F.; Su, C. L.; Chen, T. H.; Yen, M. F.; Wu, H. M. Prevalence, Incidence, and Mortality of PD: A Door-to-door Survey in Ilan County, Taiwan. *Neurology* **2001,** *57* (9), 1679–1686. doi: 10.1212/WNL.57.9.1679
18. Eliezer, D.; Kutluay, E.; Bussell, R.; Browne, G. Conformational Properties of α-synuclein in its Free and Lipid-associated States 11 Edited by P. E. Wright. *J. Mol. Biol.* **2001,** *307* (4), 1061–1073.
19. Fujiwara, H.; Hasegawa, M.; Dohmae, N.; Kawashima, A.; Masliah, E.; Goldberg, M. S. Alpha-Synuclein is Phosphorylated in Synucleinopathy Lesions. *Nat. Cell Biol.* **2002,** *4* (2), 160–164. doi: 10.1038/ncb748
20. Winner, B.; Jappelli, R.; Maji, S. K.; Desplats, P. A.; Boyer, L.; Aigner, S. In Vivo Demonstration that α-Synuclein Oligomers are Toxic. *Proc. Natl Acad. Sci.* **2011,** *108* (10), 4194–4199. doi: 10.1073/pnas.1100976108
21. Devi, L.; Raghavendran, V.; Prabhu, B. M.; Avadhani, N. G.; Anandatheerthavarada, H. K. Mitochondrial Import and Accumulation of alpha-synuclein impair complex I in human dopaminergic neuronal cultures and Parkinson disease brain. *J. Biol. Chem.* **2008,** *283,* 9089–9100.
22. Liu, G.; Zhang, C.; Yin, J.; Li, X.; Cheng, F.; Li, Y.; Yang, H.; Uéda, K.; Chan, P.; Yu, S. alpha-Synuclein is differentially expressed in mitochondria from different rat brain regions and dose-dependently down-regulates complex I activity. *Neurosci. Lett.* **2009,** *454,* 187–192.
23. The National Collaborating Centre for Chronic Conditions, Ed. (NCCCC) Symptomatic Pharmacological Therapy in Parkinson's Disease. In *Parkinson's Disease*; Royal College of Physicians: London, 2006; pp 59–100. ISBN 978-1-86016-283-1.
24. Connolly, B. S.; Lang, A. E. Pharmacological Treatment of Parkinson Disease: A Review. *JAMA* **2014,** *311* (16), 1670–1683.
25. Poewe, W.; Seppi, K.; Tanner, C. M. Parkinson Disease. *Nat. Rev. Dis. Primers* **2017,** *3* (1), 17013. doi: 10.1038/nrdp.2017.13

26. Hamilton, R. L.; Lewy Bodies in Alzheimer's Disease: A Neuropathological Review of 145 Cases Using alpha-Synuclein Immunohistochemistry. *Brain Pathol.* **2000,** *10* (3), 378–384.
27. Wenk, G. L. Neuropathologic Changes in Alzheimer's Disease. *J. Clin. Psychiatry* **2003,** *64* (Suppl. 9), 7–10. PMID 12934968.
28. Berchtold, N. C.; Cotman, C. W. Evolution in the Conceptualization of Dementia and Alzheimer's Disease: Greco-Roman Period to the 1960s. *Neurobiol. Aging* **1998,** *19* (3), 173–189.
29. Simon, R. P.; Greenberg, D. A.; Aminoff, M. J. *Clinical Neurology*, 10th ed.; McGraw Hill: New York, 2018; p 111. ISBN 978-1-259-86173-4. OCLC 1012400314
30. Bäckman, L.; Jones, S.; Berger, A. K.; Laukka, E. J.; Small, B. J. Multiple Cognitive Deficits during the Transition to Alzheimer's Disease. *J. Intern. Med.* **2004,** *256* (3), 195–204.
31. Taler, V.; Phillips, N. A. Language Performance in Alzheimer's Disease and Mild Cognitive Impairment: A Comparative Review. *J. Clin. Exp. Neuropsychol.* **2008,** *30* (5), 501–556. doi: 10.1080/13803390701550128
32. Burns, A.; Iliffe, S. Alzheimer's Disease. *BMJ* **2009,** *338,* b158. doi: 10.1136/bmj.b158
33. Tackenberg, C.; Kulic, L.; Nitsch, R. M. Familial Alzheimer's Disease Mutations at Position 22 of the Amyloid β-peptide Sequence Differentially Affect Synaptic Loss, tau Phosphorylation and Neuronal Cell Death in an Ex Vivo System. *PLoS One* **2020,** *15* (9).
34. Sun, W.; Samimi, H.; Gamez, M.; Zare, H.; Frost, B. Pathogenic tau-induced piRNA Depletion Promotes Neuronal Death through Transposable Element Dysregulation in Neurodegenerative Tauopathies. *Nat. Neurosci.* **2018,** *21* (8), 1038–1048.
35. Sinyor, B.; Mineo, J.; Ochner, C. Alzheimer's Disease, Inflammation, and the Role of Antioxidants. *J. Alzheimer Dis. Rep.* **2020,** *4* (1), 175–183. doi: 10.3233/ADR-200171. PMC 7369138
36. Atri, A. The Alzheimer's Disease Clinical Spectrum: Diagnosis and Management. *Med. Clin. North Am.* **2019,** *103* (2), 263–293. doi:10.1016/j.mcna.2018.10.009
37. Mahley, R. W.; Weisgraber, K. H.; Huang, Y. Apolipoprotein E4: A Causative Factor and Therapeutictarget in Neuropathology, Including Alzheimer's Disease. *Proc. Natl Acad. Sci. U. S. A.* **2006,** *103* (15), 5644–5651.
38. Weller, J.; Budson, A. Current Understanding of Alzheimer's Disease Diagnosis and Treatment. *F1000 Res.* **2018,** *7,* 1161. doi: 10.12688/f1000research.14506.1
39. Chu, C. S.; Tseng, P. T.; Stubbs, B.; et al. Use of Statins and the Risk of Dementia and Mild Cognitive Impairment: A Systematic Review and Meta-analysis. *Sci. Rep.* **2018,** *8* (1), 5804.
40. Yu, J. T.; Xu, W.; Tan, C. C.; et al. Evidence-based Prevention of Alzheimer's Disease: Systematic Review and Meta-analysis of 243 Observational Prospective Studies and 153 Randomised Controlled Trials. *J. Neurol. Neurosurg. Psychiatry* **2020,** *91* (11), 1201–1209. doi: 10.1136/jnnp-2019-321913
41. Rubinsztein, D. C.; Carmichael, J. Huntington's Disease: Molecular basis of Neurodegeneration. *Expert Rev. Mol. Med.* **2003,** *5* (20), 1–21. doi: 10.1017/S1462399403006549
42. Liu, Z.; Zhou, T.; Ziegler, A. C.; Dimitrion, P.; Zuo, L Oxidative Stress in Neurodegenerative Diseases: From Molecular Mechanisms to Clinical Applications. *Oxid. Med. Cell Longev.* **2017,** *2017,* 2525967.
43. Coppen, Emma, M.; Roos, R. A. C. Current Pharmacological Approaches to Reduce Chorea in Huntington's Disease. *Drugs* **2017,** *77* (1), 29–46.

44. Morsy, S.; Khalil, S. M.; Doheim, M. F.; Kamel, M. G.; El-Basiony, D. S.; Ahmed Hassan, H. I.; et al. Efficacy of ethyl-EPA as a Treatment for Huntington Disease: A Systematic Review and Meta-analysis. *Acta Neuropsychiatr.* **2019,** *31* (4), 175–185.
45. Stys, P. K.; Tsutsui, S. Recent Advances in Understanding Multiple Sclerosis. *F1000 Res.* **2019,** *8,* 2100.
46. Dugger, B. N.; Dickson, D. W. Pathology of Neurodegenerative Diseases. *Cold Spring Harb. Perspect. Biol.* **2017,** *9* (7), a028035.
47. Milner, J. A. Reducing the Risk of Cancer. In *Functional Foods: Designer Foods, Pharmafoods, Nutraceuticals*; Goldberg, I., Ed.; Chapman & Hall: New York, NY, USA, 1994; pp 39–70.
48. Duthie, G. G.; Brown, K. M. Reducing the Risk of Cardiovascular Disease. In *Functional Foods: Designer Foods, Pharmafoods, Nutraceuticals*; Goldberg, I., Ed.; Chapman & Hall: New York, NY, USA, 1994; pp 19–38.
49. Ajayi, E. I. O.; Molehin, O. R.; Adefegha, S. A.; Fakayode, A. E.; Oladele J. O. Adewumi, S. O. Nutritional Regulation of Metabesity. In *Nutrition, Food and Diet in Ageing and Longevity*; Healthy Ageing and Longevity, 2021; p 14. doi: 10.1007/978-3-030-83017-27
50. Adom, K. K.; Liu, R. H. Antioxidant Activity of Grains. *J. Agric. Food Chem.* **2002,** *50,* 6182–6187.
51. Bravo, L. Polyphenols: Chemistry, Dietary Sources, Metabolism, and Nutritional Significance. *Nutr. Rev.* **1998,** 56, 317–333. doi: 10.1111/j.1753-4887.1998.tb01670.x
52. Valant-Vetschera, K. M.; Wallenweber, E. Flavones and Flavonols. In *Flavonoids: Chemistry, Biochemistry and Applications*; Anderson, O. M., Markham, K. R., Eds.; CRC Press/Taylor & Francis Group: Boca Raton, FL, USA, 2006; pp 618–748.
53. Hunter, P. The Inflammation Theory of Disease. *EMBO Rep.* **2012,** *13* (11), 968–970. doi: 10.1038/embor.2012.142
54. Vauzour, D. Dietary Polyphenols as Modulators of Brain Functions: Biological Actions and Molecular Mechanisms Underpinning their Beneficial Effects. *Oxid. Med. Cell Longev.* **2012,** *2012,* 914273. doi: 10.1155/2012/914273
55. Tangney, C. C.; Rasmussen, H. E. Polyphenols, Inflammation, and Cardiovascular Disease. *Curr. Atheroscler Rep.* **2013,** *15* (5), 324. doi: 10.1007/s11883-013-0324-x
56. Potì, F.; Santi, D.; Spaggiari, G.; Zimetti, F.; Zanotti, I. Polyphenol Health Effects on Cardiovascular and Neurodegenerative Disorders: A Review and Meta-Analysis. *Int. J. Mol. Sci.* **2019,** *20* (2), 351. doi: 10.3390/ijms20020351
57. Hubert, P. A.; Lee, S. G.; Lee, S. K.; Chun, O. K. Dietary Polyphenols, Berries, and Age-related Bone Loss: A Review based on Human, Animal, and Cell Studies. *Antioxidants* **2014,** *3,* 144–158. doi: 10.3390/antiox3010144
58. Zhang, P. H.; Tsao, R. Dietary Polyphenols, Oxidative Stress and Antioxidant and Anti-inflammatory Effects. *Curr. Opin. Food Sci.* **2016,** *8,* 33–42.
59. Graef, J. L.; Rendina-Ruedy, E.; Crockett, E. K.; Ouyang, P.; Wu, L.; King, J. B.; et al. Osteoclast Differentiation is Downregulated by Select Polyphenolic Fractions from Dried Plum via Suppression of MAPKs and Nfatc1 in Mouse C57BL/6 Primary Bone Marrow Cells. *Curr. Dev. Nutr.* **2017,** *1,* e000406. 10.3945/cdn.117.000406
60. Oladele, J. O.; Anyim, J. C.; Oyeleke, O. M.; Olowookere, B. D.; Bamigboye, M. O.; Oladele, O. O.; Oladiji, A. T. *Telfairia Occidentalis* Mitigates Dextran Sodium Sulphate-Induced Ulcerative Colitis in Rats via Suppression of Oxidative Stress, Lipid Peroxidation and Inflammation. *J. Food Biochem.* **2021.** doi: 10.1111/jfbc.13873

61. Pacheco-Ordaz, R.; Wall-Medrano, A.; Goñi, M. G.; Ramos-Clamont-Montfort, G.; Ayala-Zavala, J. F.; González-Aguilar, G. A. Effect of Phenolic Compounds on the Growth of Selected Probiotic and Pathogenic Bacteria. *Lett. Appl. Microbiol.* **2018,** *66* (1), 25–31. doi: 10.1111/lam.12814
62. Lee, H. C.; Jenner, A. M.; Low, C. S.; Lee, Y. K. Effect of Tea Phenolics and their Aromatic Fecal Bacterial Metabolites on Intestinal Microbiota. *Res. Microbiol.* **2006,** *157* (9), 876–884. doi: 10.1016/j.resmic.2006.07.004
63. Kim, J.; Lee, H. J.; Lee, K. W. Naturally Occurring Phytochemicals for the Prevention of Alzheimer's Disease. *J. Neurochem.* **2010,** *112* (6), 1415–1430.
64. Karunaweera, N.; Raju, R.; Gyengesi, E.; Münch, G. Plant Polyphenols as Inhibitors of NF-κB Induced Cytokine Production—A Potential Anti-inflammatory Treatment for Alzheimer's Disease? *Mol. Neurosci.* **2015,** *8,* 24.
65. Mattson, M. P.; Meffert, M. K. Roles for NF-kappaB in Nerve Cell Survival, Plasticity, and Disease. *Cell Death Differ.* **2006,** *13* (5), 852–860. doi: 10.1038/sj.cdd.4401837. PMID 16397579.
66. Papa, S.; Bubici, C.; Knabb, J. R.; Dean, K.; Franzoso, G. The NF-kappaB-Mediated Control of the JNK Cascade in the Antagonism of Programmed Cell Death in Health and Disease. *Cell Death Diff.* **2006,** *13* (5), 712–729. doi: 10.1038/sj.cdd.4401865. PMID 16456579.
67. Figuera-Losada, M.; Rojas, C.; Slusher, B. S. Inhibition of Microglia Activation as a Phenotypic Assay in Early Drug Discovery. *J. Biomol. Screen.* **2014,** *19,* 17–31. doi: 10.1177/1087057113499406
68. Mogensen, T. H. Pathogen Recognition and Inflammatory Signaling in Innate Immune Defenses. *Clin. Microbiol. Rev.* **2009,** *22,* 240–273. doi:10.1128/CMR.00046-08
69. Ghosh, S.; Karin, M. Missing Pieces in the NF-kappaB Puzzle. *Cell* **2002,** *109* (Suppl.), S81–S96. doi: 10.1016/S0092-8674(02)00703-1
70. Perkins, N. D. Integrating Cell-signalling Pathways with NF-kappaB and IKK Function. *Nat. Rev. Mol. Cell Biol.* **2007,** *8,* 49–62. doi: 10.1038/nrm2083
71. Ruiz, P. A.; Haller, D. Functional Diversity of Flavonoids in the Inhibition of the Proinflammatory NF-kappaB, IRF, and Akt Signaling Pathways in Murine Intestinal Epithelial Cells. *J. Nutr.* **2006,** *136,* 664–671.
72. Yoon, J. H., Baek, S. J. Molecular Targets of Dietary Polyphenols with Anti-inflammatory Properties. *Yonsei Med. J.* **2005,** *46,* 585–596. doi: 10.3349/ymj.2005.46.5.585
73. Endale, M.; Park, S. C.; Kim, S.; Kim, S. H.; Yang, Y.; Cho, J. Y.; et al. Quercetin Disrupts Tyrosine-phosphorylated Phosphatidylinositol 3-kinase and Myeloid Differentiation Factor-88 Association, and Inhibits MAPK/AP-1 and IKK/NF-kappaB-induced Inflammatory Mediators Production in RAW 264.7 Cells. *Immunobiology* **2013,** *218,* 1452–1467. doi: 10.1016/j.imbio.2013.04.019
74. Jobin, C.; Bradham, C. A.; Russo, M. P.; Juma, B.; Narula, A. S.; Brenner, D. A.; et al. Curcumin Blocks Cytokine-mediated NF-kappa B Activation and Proinflammatory Gene Expression by Inhibiting Inhibitory Factor I-kappa B Kinase Activity. *J. Immunol.* **1999,** *163,* 3474–3483.
75. Kundu, J. K.; Surh, Y. J. Epigallocatechingallate Inhibits Phorbol Ester-induced Activation of NF-kappa B and CREB in Mouse Skin: Role of p38 MAPK, *Ann. N. Y. Acad. Sci.* **2007,** *1095*, 504–512.
76. Nakatani, N. Phenolic Antioxidants from Herbs and Spices. *Biofactors* **2000,** *13,* 141–146.
77. Van Dyk, K.; Sano, M. The Impact of Nutrition on Cognition In the Elderly. *Neurochem. Res.* **2007,** *32,* 893–904.

78. Sun, Z.; Zhang, S.; Chan, J. Y.; Zhang, D. D. Keap1 Controls Postinduction Repression of the Nrf2-Mediated Antioxidant Response by Escorting Nuclear Export of Nrf2. *Mol. Cell Biol.* **2007,** *27* (18), 6334–6349. doi: 10.1128/MCB.00630-07.
79. Ma, Q. Xenobiotic-activated Receptors: From Transcription to Drug Metabolism to Disease. *Chem. Res. Toxicol.* **2008,** *21,* 1651–1671.
80. Pamplona, A.; et al Heme Oxygenase-1 and Carbon Monoxide Suppress the Pathogenesis of Experimental Cerebral Malaria. *Nat. Med.* **2007,** *13* (6), 703–710.
81. Scapagnini, G.; Vasto, S.; Abraham, N. G.; Caruso, C.; Zella, D.; Fabio, G. Modulation of Nrf2/ARE Pathway by Food Polyphenols: A Nutritional Neuroprotective Strategy for Cognitive and Neurodegenerative Disorders. *Mol. Neurobiol.* **2011,** *44* (2), 192–201. doi: 10.1007/s12035-011-8181-5
82. Yang, C.; Zhang, X.; Fan, H.; Liu, Y. Curcumin Upregulates Transcription Factor Nrf2, HO-1 Expression and Protects Rat Brains Against Focal Ischemia. *Brain Res.* **2009,** *1282,* 133–141.
83. Scapagnini, G.; Foresti, R.; Calabrese, V.; Giuffrida Stella, A. M.; Green, C. J.; Motterlini, R. Caffeic Acid Phenethyl Ester and Curcumin: A Novel Class of Heme Oxygenase-1 Inducers. *Mol. Pharmacol.* **2002,** *61* (3), 554–561. doi: 10.1124/mol.61.3.554
84. Khan, N.; Mukhtar, H. Tea Polyphenols for Health Promotion. *Life Sci.* **2007,** 81, 519–553.
85. Behl, T.; Rana, T.; Alotaibi, G. H.; Shamsuzzaman, M.; Naqvi, M.; Sehgal, A.; Singh, S.; Sharma, N.; Almoshari, Y.; Abdellatif, A. A. H.; Iqbal, M. S.; Bhatia, S.; Al-Harrasi, A.; Bungau, S. Polyphenols Inhibiting MAPK Signalling Pathway Mediated Oxidative Stress and Inflammation in Depression. *Biomed. Pharmacother.* **2022,** *146,* 112545. doi: 10.1016/j.biopha.2021.112545
86. Yu, J.; Sun, X.; Goie, J.; Zhang, Y. Regulation of Host Immune Responses against Influenza A Virus Infection by Mitogen-Activated Protein Kinases (MAPKs). *Microorganisms* **2020,** *8* (7), 1067. doi: 10.3390/microorganisms8071067
87. Matsuzawa, A.; Saegusa, K.; Noguchi, T.; Sadamitsu, C.; Nishitoh, H.; Nagai, S.; Koyasu, S.; Matsumoto, K.; Takeda, K.; Ichijo, H. ROS-dependent Activation of the TRAF6-ASK1-p38 Pathway is Selectively Required for TLR4-mediated Innate Immunity. *Nat. Immunol.* **2005,** *6,* 587–592.
88. Huang, S. M.; Wu, C. H.; Yen, G. C. Effects of Flavonoids on the Expression of the Pro-Inflammatory Response in Human Monocytes Induced by Ligation of the Receptor for AGEs, *Mol. Nutr. Food Res.* **2006,** *50,* 1129–1139.
89. Wadsworth, T. L.; McDonald, T. L.; Koop, D. R. Effects of Ginkgo Biloba Extract (EGb 761) and Quercetin on Lipopolysaccharide-induced Signaling Pathways Involved in the release of Tumor Necrosis Factor-alpha. *Biochem. Pharm.* **2001,** *62,* 963–974.
90. Levin, A. J.; Hu, W.; Feng, Z. The P53 Pathway: What Questions Remain to be Explored? *Cell Death Differ.* **2006,** *13,* 1027–1036. doi:10.1038/sj.cdd.4401910
91. Vogelstein, B.; Lane, D.; Levine, A. J. Surfing the p53 Network. *Nature* **2000,** *408,* 307–310.
92. Zhao, R.; Gish, K.; Murphy, M.; Yin, Y.; Notterman, D.; Hoffman, W. H.; Tom, E.; Mack, D. H.; Levine, A. J. The Transcriptional Program Following p53 Activation. *Cold Spring Harb. Symp. Quant. Biol.* **2000,** *65,* 475–482.
93. Moll, U. M.; Wolff, S.; Speidel, D.; Deppert, W. Transcription-independent Pro-apoptotic Functions of p53. *Curr. Opin. Cell Biol.* **2005,** *17,* 631–636.
94. Chipuk, J. E.; Kuwana, T.; Bouchier-Hayes, L.; Droin, N. M.; Newmeyer, D. D.; Schuler, M.; Green, D. R. Direct Activation of Bax by p53 Mediates Mitochondrial Membrane Permeabilization and Apoptosis. *Sciencem* **2004,** *303,* 1010–1014.

95. Khan, H.; Reale, M.; Ullah, H.; Sureda, A.; Tejada, S.; Wang, Y.; Zhang, Z. J.; Xiao, J. Anticancer Effects of Polyphenols via Targeting p53 Signaling Pathway: Updates and Future Directions. *Biotechnol. Adv.* **2020,** *38,* 107385. doi: 10.1016/j.biotechadv.2019.04.007.
96. Sheikh, M. S.; Fornace, A. J., Jr. Death and Decoy Receptors and p53-mediated Apoptosis. *Leukemia* **2000,** *14,* 1509–1513. doi: 10.1038/sj.leu.2401865.

CHAPTER 13

Implication of Herbal Nano-Formulations in the Treatment of Neurological Disorders

SUNNY R. SHAH[1], VIJAY R. CHIDRAWAR[2], PRASHANT L. PINGALE[3], SUDARSHAN SINGH[4], BHUPENDRA G. PRAJAPATI[5,7], and DEVANG SHETH[6]

[1]*B. K. Mody Government Pharmacy College, Gujarat Technological University, Rajkot, India*

[2]*Department of Pharmacology, Raghavendra Institute of Pharmaceutical Education and Research, Andhra Pradesh, India*

[3]*GES's Sir Dr. M. S. Gosavi College of Pharmaceutical Education and Research, Nashik, India*

[4]*Faculty of Pharmacy, Chiang Mai University, Chiang Mai, Thailand*

[5]*Shree S. K. Patel College of Pharmaceutical Education and Research, Ganpat University, Kherva, India*

[6]*L. M. College of Pharmacy, Gujarat Technological University, Ahmedabad, India*

[7]*Faculty of Pharmacy, Silpakorn University, Nakhon Pathom, Thailand*

ABSTRACT

As per WHO, neurological and psychiatric diseases are a significant and growing cause of morbidity around the world. That is why it is inlcuded recently in the Global Burden of Diseases. Alzheimer's and other dementias, PD, MS, epilepsy, and headache disorder make up 3% of all diseases in the globe. Complementary and alternative medicine has grown in popularity in the

Nanomedicine for Neurodegenerative Disorders: Selective Treatment Strategies. Rishabha Malviya, Kamla Pathak, & Swati Verma (Eds.)

treatment of a variety of chronic diseases, including neurological disorders, in recent decades. Several synthetic drugs such as tacrine, memantine, donepezil, rivastigmine, metrifonate, etc., have been developed for the treatment of neurodegenerative disorders. Furthermore, a lack of proper clinical knowledge in disease identification delays treatment even more. Natural remedies have been linked to considerable improvements in both human and animal health and illness prevention. These natural compounds offer a variety of biological qualities that have been experimentally proven, including antioxidant, anti-inflammatory, and apoptotic activity. Natural products (NP), which include a range of bioactive compounds, offer potential opportunities in transformation within novel or targeted drug delivery in various preclinical or clinical models of neurodegenerative disorders (NDDs). These bioactives may conceivably inhibit neurodegeneration (ND) and enhance brain functioning including memory with the prevention and cure of different neurodegenerative diseases, including Alzheimer's, epilepsy, Parkinson's, anxiety, insomnia, migraines, and related neuronal disorders. In this chapter, treatment strategies for NDDs with the implication of herbs in novel drug delivery systems have been emphasized.

13.1 INTRODUCTION

Humans have the greatest developed and dynamic brain that makes us the most powerful creature on the planet. The fundamental feature of mental activity is reasoning, reactions, and perception. The important action of the brain activity is constant change in response to the external stimuli or/and even a constant environment.[50] Compared to other organ systems, the human brain has the highest metabolic rate and high energy demand. 20% of the total blood supply is used by this organ, which weighs about 2% of the total body weight. Any small change in the energy supply produces profound effects including psychological and physical changes. This may be due to primary and/or secondary failure of the other organ system including the cardiovascular system and renal system. Further, cerebral blood flow is important for the delivery of oxygen and taking away waste products. The brain neurons have inadequate capacity for anaerobic respiration, i.e., $\approx 92\%$ of ATP (adenosine triphosphate) is produced in the brain by the oxidative phosphorylation of glucose. Moreover, both hypoperfusion and hyperperfusion can cause damage in the form of ischemic brain injury and hemorrhage respectively which give rise to conditions like epilepsy, headaches, and encephalopathy.[8]

Broadly, neurological disorders can be classified into central and peripheral disorders. Central disorders further are of many kinds, i.e., trimers, seizers disorders, cerebrovascular accidents, disorders of development, neurological developments, NDs, headaches, and facial pain. Psychological disorders are due to an imbalance between neurotransmitter levels and their function in the neuronal circuit. Among all neurological disorders, NDs are the most prevalent type of disability worldwide.[49]

NDD is described as an irreversible disorder and leads to progressive loss of neurons as well as intellectual capacities.[23] Alzheimer's disease (AD), Parkinson's disease (PD), and amyotrophic lateral sclerosis (ALS) are three of the major NDs (multiple sclerosis (MS) and Huntington's disease are less common) which is the growing cause of morbidity and mortality, particularly among the elderly. This is of particular interest as the world population is getting older and, in many countries, the average life expectancy has increased by more than 6 years.[59] As per the statement by UN, Department of Economic and Social Affairs 2019, by 2050, 1 in every 6 people in the world will be over the age of 65, up from 1 in 11 in 2019.[41]

Among all cases of dementia, AD contributes nearly 50% of the cases. The occurrence of AD is around 30% among the population over 85 years and the prevalence is infrequent below the age of 50 years except in the cases of familial dementia.[27] PD is second numbered movement NDs characterized by the motor (termers and micro termers at rest, hypokinesia, rigidity, stooped posture, decreased arm swing, and postural instability) and non-motor (memory impairment, disturbed thought process, insomnia, and pain) complications.[79] PD is generally affected after the age of 50 years and is rare before 50 years of age, but rises sharply from the age of 50–80 years (the prevalence is the same as AD). Men have 20–30% more incidence of PD than women and the yearly incidence rates of 10-15/100,000 have been noted.[26] As per the report published by WHO 2022, worldwide, PD-related disability and death rates are rising more quickly than those of any other ND. In 2019, worldwide over 8.5 million people were diagnosed with PD and the occurrence of PD has folded twice in the last two decades.

The most common cause of NDs is the imbalance between oxidative/nitrosative stress and the antioxidant defence system, excite-toxicity, mitochondrial dysfunction, protein mis-folding and/or aggregation, synapse loss, and apoptosis.[66] Any pathological process that causes the death of the neurons has permanent effects as the dead neurons in the developed mammalian nervous system are not substituted and nor do their axons redevelop.[66] Due to the irreversible loss of the neurons at the first glance, it looks irrational to use pharmacological interventions for its repair and revegetate, except in the case of PD. However, in recent years, massive research is being conducted to overcome these challenges by understanding the detailed pathology of neuronal death. Neuronal death is the major cause of disability in many ND disorders.

13.2 GENERAL MECHANISM OF NEURONAL DEATH

Many common characteristics exist in various types of NDs viz rise in the prevalence with age, slow and progressive nature, loss of the neurons in the specific anatomical region of the brain, injury to the neuronal network, and selective brain mass loss.[78] Neuronal death may be because of many reasons including protein mis-folding, oxidative stress, excite-toxicity, etc. A few of the major mechanisms of neuronal death are explained here.

13.2.1 PROTEIN MISFOLDING

Protein folding (PF) is one of the major biological functions that make the protein function. During the PF mechanism, the nascent protein is transformed into a final form called the native protein. Nascent protein is nonfunctional in nature while the native protein is functional. The nascent protein is arranged linearly and is one-dimensional while the native protein is nonlinear and it is three-dimensional in nature. The function of the protein is determined by its 3D structure. If the PF does not occur or the proteins got misfolded it rendered nonfunctional and sometimes it may cause diseases. In the mammalian nervous system protein misfolding and its aggregation is the first step in many NDs.[89]

Misfolded proteins form large insoluble aggregates due to the execution of uncharacteristic shapes by some normally expressed proteins. During the translation process, the ribosome forms the linear amino acid chain, and later gets folded correctly to form the functional proteins. The functional proteins have compact conformation with the specific amino acids placed suitably on their surface. This complicated sequential multistep process of conversion of nascent protein to native protein may sometimes go wrong and misfolded protein variants may form. During the process, the misfolded proteins could not correct themselves self-back to the native protein. The formed misfolded proteins do not function normally for what it was coded for; instead they disturb the function of surrounding proteins and start aggregating to nearby neurons. The aggregation of misfolded proteins is due to its exposure of the hydrophobic portion on its surface which has the strong propensity to stick to the cell membrane of the surrounding neurons initially as a monomer, slowly self-propagate to the oligomer, and eventually as insoluble microscopic aggregates, which cause the death of the neurons. The formation of such specific but abnormal conformation of the protein may be due to the mutation and/or infection by the prions.[60]

Aggregation of a large number of misfolded proteins in the brain does not generally happen suddenly; instead, it is a gradual and spontaneous process that may begin in middle age and accrue with time. In the brain, misfolded proteins (protein aggregates) may be present in distinct forms called an amyloid deposit, which is the characteristic feature of NDs. For instance, AD is due to the accumulation of β-Amyloid (Aβ) and Tau proteins, in PD α-Synuclein and Lewy bodies are involved whereas superoxide dismutase aggregates are observed in ALS. Despite distinct protein aggregates involved in different NDs but the process of protein misfolding, involvement of intermediates, final product, and core features are much similar.[84] All the misfolded proteins do not have all the similarities though they are formed through the same sequence of events. Diseases associated with misfolded proteins vary in terms of amino acid sequence, structure, size, and function. However, in the diseased brain, the misfolded proteins are formed from their native states and turn into intermolecular β-sheet-rich structures extending from the oligomer to the large insoluble aggregates. In particular, amyloid proteins are highly organized of 100–200 Å in size compared to intermolecular β-sheet. Earlier, large insoluble protein aggregates were considered the main cause of the NDs but later it was clear that the main culprits are small misfolded oligomers and their precursors.[85]

To tackle this problem brain is armed with many protective mechanisms to avoid protein aggregates. One such important mechanism is the formation of chaperon proteins which bind to the misfolded proteins and boost them to fold suitably. Another protective mechanism is to destroy the misfolded protein in the cells by ubiquitination reaction. The misfolded protein accumulates when these proactive mechanisms are overwhelmed or saturated.[94]

13.2.2 APOPTOSIS AND NECROSIS

Apoptosis and necrosis are the two major pathways of neuronal death. Apoptosis is well organized, active, program process of cellular dismantling without provoking any inflammatory response while necrosis is considered a passive, accidental death due to some environmental effects. Necrotic cells release their inflammatory cellular contents to the surroundings electing an inflammatory response. Chronic inflammation is a hallmark of many NDs and anti-inflammatory drugs play a role in therapeutic interventions.[29] Both apoptosis and necrosis are inevitable processes that neuronal cells may pass through in acute (stroke, head injury) and chronic (AD and PD) ND disorders. The difference between apoptosis and necrosis is the extent of stress the neurons tolerate. For example, in the case of excitotoxicity and oxidative/nitrosative stress, both these processes may kill the cell directly (necrosis), if the stress is less intense neurons may undergo apoptosis.[97] A variety of signaling pathways are involved to initiate the program cell death mechanism which ultimately ends up by activating the caspases. Caspase deactivates many intracellular organelles and causes neuronal death. Neurons in the brain normally survive by preventing apoptosis by some growth factors including nerve growth factors and brain-derived neurotrophic factors. These growth factors are involved in the regulation of two sets of gene products, i.e., Bax and Bcl-2. The Bax is proapoptotic while Bcl-2 is antiapoptotic in nature. Suppression of Bax and activation of Bcl-2 will be a good strategy to prevent neuronal death.[97]

13.2.3 EXCITOTOXICITY AND OXIDATIVE STRESS

The neuronal circuit is finely balanced by excitatory and inhibitory neurons. Excitatory neurons are involved in the spreading of neuronal information in and out of the circuit, while inhibitory neurons provide strong control over the excitatory response. Excitotoxicity is considered one of the primary reasons of neuronal death; basic cause is the imbalance in the excitatory and inhibitory neurotransmitters. The principle excitatory neurotransmitters are glutamate and aspartate while norepinephrine and dopamine are other excitatory neurotransmitters that are controlled by powerful inhibitory neurotransmitters like GABA (γ-Aminobutyric acid), glycine, and serotonin. Glutamate is present in more than half of nervous tissues and has also been used by the brain for the synthesis of GABA. One of the major roles of glutamate is memory and learning which appears to be by modulating synaptic plasticity. Glutamate shows its action by inotropic (NMDA, kainite, and AMPA receptors) and metabotropic receptors (mGluR1 to mGluR8). Ionotropic receptors are faster in spreading the information while metabotropic receptors produce more prolonged stimulation. GABA executes its effects via $GABA_A$ (ion channels) and $GABA_B$ (G protein-coupled receptors, GPCRS) receptors. Excitotoxicity happens when there is an imbalance between excitatory and inhibitory neurotransmitters.[20]

Stimulation of NMDA receptors is a complex phenomenon, as NMDA not only requires glutamate to bind but also another inhibitory neurotransmitter like glycine concurrently binds to a separate binding site on the same receptor. The stimulation has been affected by the voltage across the membrane due to Zn^{++} and Mg^{+} binding in the pores. Further, the entry of the Ca^{2+} ions through the NMDA receptors changes the membrane current and also acts as a second messenger.[20]

Calcium ions and glutamate are the two most important messengers that perform many vital functions to maintain neuronal homeostasis but the rise in the levels of these messengers causes many toxic effects so their levels must be adequate. In the neurons, Ca^{2+} is stored in the specialized intracellular organelles like mitochondria and endoplasmic reticulum which dynamically participates in Ca^{2+} homeostasis and also in buffering the excess of Ca^{2+} ions entering the cytoplasm through various sources like Na^{+}- Ca^{2+} exchanger, voltage-gated Ca^{2+} channels, and activation of NMDA receptors by glutamate. The rise of Ca^{2+} level in the intracellular calcium storage organelles controls the availability of intracellular Ca^{2+} release and hence generates a mechanism in neuronal activity.[92] The extra amount of intracellular calcium can be expelled out of the neuronal cell by the Ca^{2+} efflux pump powered by the mitochondrial ATP molecules. In certain conditions overstimulation of NMDA receptors by glutamate causes massive entry of Ca^{2+} ions in the cells and beyond the buffering capacity of mitochondria and endoplasmic reticulum. This massive amount of intracellular Ca^{2+} disrupts the mitochondrial function and declines the ATP synthesis and eventually reduces the energy required to expel out the Ca^{2+} by the Ca^{2+} pump and Ca^{2+} start accumulating in the endoplasmic reticulum. The extra amount of Ca^{2+} in the mitochondria affects adversely the functioning of the electron transfer chain leading to the formation of reactive oxygen species (ROS).[93] Apart from this, an increased amount of Ca^{2+} affects many other processes, the important effects relevant to the neurotoxicity include activation of calpains and lipases which causes membrane damage and boosts the production of nitric oxide in larger quantities. A small quantity of nitric oxide (NO) has neuroprotective effects. In the presence of ROS, a high amount of NO produces peroxynitrite and hydroxyl-free radicals which digest neuronal membrane lipids, proteins, and DNA. Further, intracellular excess Ca^{2+} causes a rise in arachidonic acid production, rise in free radical levels also inhibits glutamate reuptake and triggers inflammatory mediators' production.[63] Defence against excitotoxicity has prime importance, mitochondrial ATP production is the first line of defence as discussed, weakened mitochondrial function in the neurons makes them prone to excitotoxicity-induced neuronal death which is an important factor in many NDs. Lastly, diminished mitochondrial function causes apoptosis by releasing cytochrome C in the cytosol.[12]

13.3 ROLE OF NATURAL PRODUCTS AND THEIR BIOACTIVE IN THE MANAGEMENT OF NEUROLOGICAL DISORDER

Herbal-based nano formulations for PD treatment have been researched in preclinical models,[74,101] and can be used to restore dopamine levels in the brain. ALS is a neurological illness that causes motor neurons in the central nervous system to die.[64] Herbal nano-formulations are currently being tested in clinical studies and may be used to treat the condition. These medications have the potential to improve the survival rate of motor neurons, which regulate the muscles. The medications that are currently available are mostly intended to provide brief symptom alleviation.[46] As a result, there is a strong need for the creation of innovative treatments and neuroprotective substances to halt and delay the disease's course. Moreover, the majority of traditional herbal medicines are made from raw materials, raising issues regarding their specific therapeutic effects and repeatability, mode of action, and active components. However, these natural phytochemicals are also less hazardous than modern synthetic medicines. As a result, many active chemicals from medicinal plant extracts have been extracted and identified. These include tannins lignans, polyphenols, triterpenes, sterols, and alkaloids. It has been demonstrated that these substances have a number of advantageous pharmacological properties, including those that are anti-inflammatory, anti-amyloidogenic, anti-cholinesterase, antioxidant, which inhibit protein misfolding, lessen neuroinflammation, and are anti-apoptotic, neurotrophic. Natural products including *Valeriana officinalis*, *Bacopa monnieri*, *Clitoria ternatea*, *Piper betle, Evolvulus alsinoides, Crocus sativus L., Ocimum gratissimum, Gingko Biloba, Convolvulus pluricaulis, Cassia occidentalis, Mucuna pruriens, Curcuma longa*, *Lantana camara, Rauwolfia vomitoria, Khaya senegalensis, Ageratum conyzoids, Withania somnifera,* and *Panax quinquefolius, L.* (Ginseng) are widely used in the treatment of neurodegenerative disorders, which has been briefly elaborated in the chapter (Figure 13.1).

13.3.1 VALERIANA OFFICINALIS

Valeriana officinalis is a perennial flowering plant found in the European and Asian habitat. It has been utilized for its sedative characteristics as well

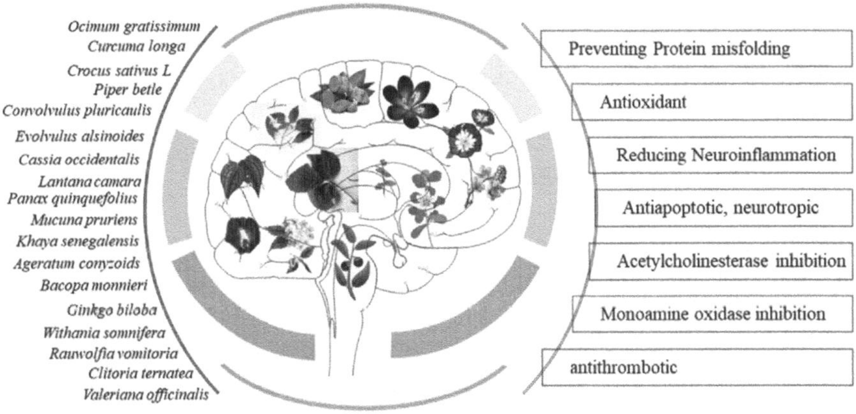

FIGURE 13.1 Natural products widely used in the treatment of neurodegenerative disorders.

as its potential influence on neurological illnesses like AD, PD, and HD. *V. officinalis* includes valerenic acids, which have been found to have an effect on the GABA receptor in the brain.[46] While there has been substantial research on *V. officinalis* calming characteristics, there has also been fresh research on the potential neuroprotective effects of the component Valeriana acid on the neurological system. When *V. officinalis* is consumed, the plant's valerenic acid is absorbed into the bloodstream via the gastrointestinal tract. It is subsequently delivered to the brain, where it interacts with the GABA receptor.[102] The GABA receptor is in charge of controlling neurotransmission in the brain. This regulation is being investigated in order to better understand *V. officinalis* possible neuroprotective properties. *Valeriana officinalis* has been shown in preliminary investigations to block GABA receptors. GABA is in charge of controlling excitatory impulses in the central nervous system. Excitatory impulses are diminished when GABA receptors are blocked. This has been shown in animal models to have neuroprotective properties against both acute and chronic stresses.[51] Because *V. officinalis* main goal is to calm the central nervous system, it might cause a condition known as benign positional vertigo. When older individuals change positions from laying down to sitting up, they are more likely to develop this syndrome. While *V. officinalis* is not known to cause nausea, it can occur as a side effect when combined with other drugs such as antidepressants. *V. officinalis* used in excess might produce restlessness, shivering, and insomnia and dry mouth.[16] *Valeriana officinalis* is a plant that has been used medicinally since antiquity. When valerenic acid is taken, it can alter the GABA receptors in the brain, which have been shown in preliminary research to have neuroprotective benefits.

There has been substantial research on *V. officinalis* sedative characteristics, as well as fresh studies on the potential neuroprotective effects of valerenic acid on the neurological system.

13.3.2 BACOPA MONNIERI

Bacopa monnieri, also known as Brahmi from Scrophulariaceae family, is native to the Indian subcontinent, where it grows in humid, muddy environments with moist soil.[1] The plant flourishes lavishly in moist soil close to aquatic areas. It has oblong leaves, purple blooms, and a height range of 6 inches to 3 feet. Both the roots and the entire plant can be utilized medicinally. It is well known for its use in Ayurveda as a nootropic drug known as a Medhya Rasayana. It is also known for its antidepressant, revitalizer of sensory organs, diuretic, brain tonic, and anticonvulsant activities.[13] Several major constituents are reported such as Bacoside A (consisting of Bacoside A3, Bacopaside II, Bacopaside X, and Bacopasaponin C5), which is primarily responsible for the neuro-pharmacological action of *B. monnieri*.[34] Additionally, it also contains apigenin, cucurbitacin, the alkaloids brahmine, monnierin, hersaponin, monnierasides I–III, plantain side B, d-mannitol, herpestine, and nicotine. Numerous in vitro and animal investigations have established the antioxidant and free radical scavenging properties of *B. monnieri*.[43] Early research indicated that in the rat prefrontal brain, hippocampus, and striatum, *B. monnieri* prevents lipid peroxidation.[81]

Brahmi's antioxidant and iron chelating properties have been recognized in the treatment of AD. It is noteworthy that *B. monnieri* demonstrate a significant effect on neuropsychological tests in older patients. Several studies have been conducted to investigate how *B. monnieri* impacts elderly adults with memory or cognitive difficulties. Animal models of a variety of disorders have been employed in an extensive study on *B. monnieri* extract and its constituents. A previous study found that Bacoside A can reduce oxidative stress in the brain by increasing the activity of catalase, glutathione peroxidase, superoxide dismutase, and glutathione reductase.[14] Furthermore, *B. Monnieri* has made significant contributions to the treatment of memory impairment and cognitive defects. AD is characterized by amnesia and cognitive deficits. Brahmi has been shown in numerous studies on people and animals to increase memory performance and cognitive function. Aside from that, *B. Monnieri* has been demonstrated to improve cerebral blood flow, neuronal and glial plasticity, and amyloid, all of which aid in the treatment of AD.[10]

13.3.3 CLITORIA TERNATEA

A traditional Ayurvedic plant of the Fabaceae family, *C. ternatea*, sometimes known as butterfly pea, originated in tropical Asia and has subsequently spread to South and Central America, China, and India, where it has since become a naturalized species. All components of the plant are used for therapeutic reasons, including the roots, seeds, and leaves. The plant extracts are utilized as a part of Ayurvedic 'Medhya Rasayana', which is consumed as a brain tonic to boost memory and intelligence. Meanwhile, the blooms of *C. ternatea* are exploited widely as gorgeous flowers and have traditionally been employed as a source of natural food color and antioxidants.[68] The primary phytochemicals reported are delphindin-3,5-diglucoside, flavanol 3-O-D-glucoside, genistein, kaempferol, kaempferol-3,7-diglucoside, clitorin, linolenic acid, oleic acid, palmitic acid, taraxerol, and taxaxeron.[91] The leaves, roots, flowers, seeds, and even roots of this plant are useful. The many biological activities of its phytochemicals make it relevant for investigation. The strong reactivity of the phytochemicals might be read as high polarizabilities. *C. ternatea* shows remarkable potential as an anti-neuroinflammatory drug without acute toxicity in mice in *in vitro* and *in vivo* studies.

13.3.4 PIPER BETLE

A tiny shrub called *P. betle* was first employed for therapeutic purposes by north-east Indian traditional healers. The thicket-growing piper betel is indigenous to tropical Asia. It is widely cultivated in tropical and subtropical areas, particularly in South-East Asia, India, and the Philippines.[25] The betel pepper vine may be grown in a short amount of time roughly 100 days and it grows quite swiftly. The *P. betel* vine is cultivated for its leaves, immature fruits (betel nuts), ripe fruits, and roots. *P. betel's* leaves and unripe fruits are dried and used as an herbal medicine. The roots are used in Ayurvedic medicine and as a spice, and the ripe fruits are used as a mouth refresher. Researchers have discovered that the plant possesses antiviral, antimicrobial, and anti-inflammatory effects. Piperine, Piperoside A, Alkamides, Lippic Acid, and Piperazin are a few of the ingredients found in *P. betle*.[44] For its potential advantages in treating neurodegenerative conditions including AD and PD, *P. betle* has been the subject of substantial research.[6] The alkamides found in *P. betle's* roots and leaves have demonstrated potential for reducing certain diseases' symptoms. Small shrubs in the pepper family include *P. betel.*

The alkamides found in *P. betle's* roots and leaves have demonstrated potential for reducing AD symptoms.[53] The acetylcholinesterase inhibition caused by the alkamides has been successfully reversed, and it has also been established that they have neuroprotective properties.[77] In animal models of AD, *P. betel* leaves have been proven to have anti-amnesic effects. Additionally, antioxidant and anti-inflammatory effects of the leaves have been discovered. It has also been discovered that the alkamides found in the *P. betle's* roots and leaves are useful in easing PD symptoms. A neurodegenerative ailment called PD is characterized by a decline in dopamine levels. Researchers have discovered that the alkamides have anti-inflammatory and antioxidant effects. The generation of alpha-synuclein, which is in charge of the aggregation of proteins linked to PD, has been discovered to be effectively inhibited by the alkamides.[86]

13.3.5 EVOLVULUS ALSINOIDES

In today's environment, neurodegenerative disorders are growing more common. Scientists have been looking for remedies to these terrible illnesses and have discovered that particular plants may hold the key. *Evolvulus alsinoides* (Linn.) Linn. (Convolvulaceae), also known as Vishnukranti, is a prostrate perennial herb native to tropical and subtropical marshy regions of India. The plant extracts revitalize the neurological system, improve sexual vigor, expel phlegm and humor from the body, and promote sleep.[62] The entire plant was employed in Ayurvedic medicine as a brain tonic and hepatoprotective,[31] as well as for amnesia and asthma. Furthermore, the herb has also been used to cure anemia, increase breast milk flow, and reduce fever. Several studies suggest that Indian physic may be beneficial for neurological disorders such as AD and (HD). The principal phytochemicals reported in the plant extract are *β*-sitosterol, scopolin, scopoletin, umbelliferon, triacontane, shankpushpine, and betaine which are chemicals that inhibit the breakdown of acetylcholine, a neurotransmitter important for learning and memory.[31] AD and HD are both incurable ND that deteriorate memory and cognitive function over time. While further research is needed to discover whether Indian goosefoot can help people with AD and HD, eating it may help prevent or delay the onset of these diseases, as well as the associated loss of memory and cognitive function. Strong antioxidants in *E. alsinoides* prevent oxidative stress, which can harm cells and lead to ND.

Dementia is a broad term that refers to cognitive deterioration caused by a wide range of diseases and ailments, including Alzheimer's. The frequency of dementia is predicted to rise as the population ages. While some drugs are available to treat dementia symptoms, there is no cure. *E. alsinoides* may also help people suffering from cognitive degeneration caused by other illnesses. In a study of patients with moderate cognitive impairment (MCI),[30] a precursor to AD, those who ingested *E. alsinoides* for eight weeks had increased blood flow to the brain and neuronal activity.[61] If *E. alsinoides* are shown to be as good for people with dementia as they are for those with MCI, they could be employed as a preventive and therapeutic treatment to boost mental health in both healthy and cognitively impaired individuals.

13.3.6 *CROCUS SATIVUS L.*

Crocus sativus L., generally referred to as saffron, is a spice obtained from the purple-blue stigmas of the saffron crocus flower. The saffron crocus bloom is a perennial plant that is native to Southwest Asia, notably Iran, Turkestan, and the Caucasus region.[75] This plant is cultivated in many other countries of the world as well, including Spain, Greece, Italy, and China. Saffron is commonly used for culinary applications. It is also used for dyeing clothes, cosmetics, and pharmaceuticals.[7] It has been used for ages in cooking and medicinally. Saffron is also referred to as "red gold" or "the king of spices" because of its high cost. It is one of the costliest spices by weight, coming in only after black pepper, cinnamon, and cardamom. *Crocus sativus* has been discussed recently with reference to potential implications for neuro-degenerative illness and its possible implications for the treatment of AD, PD, ALS, HD, and other associated disorders.[17] Saffron is most notably used to help alleviate symptoms of mood disorders such as anxiety and sadness. Saffron is also used to treat various illnesses such as hay fever, autoimmune diseases, and infertility.

Saffron contains small amounts of beta carotene, essential fatty acids, linoleic and linolenic acid, as well as some essential vitamins. Campesterol, stigmasterol, and bsitosterol, as well as oleanolic, ursolic, palmitoleic, palmitic, and oleic acids, have all been identified. Terpenes, terpene alcohols, and their esters make up the majority of the volatile chemicals. Picrocrocin safranal, crocetin, crocins, and flavonoids (quercetin and kaempferol) are nonvolatile chemicals, with safranal being the most abundant. Picrocrocin is a carotenoid (a sort of orange-red pigment) that is also responsible for the orange-red hue of saffron. Safranal is an aroma component that gives saffron its characteristic smell.[11]

There are various pathways that are hypothesized to be responsible for the neuroprotective benefits of saffron. One way is via its antioxidant effects. Saffron includes significant levels of vitamin A, vitamin C, and carotenoids. These chemicals help scavenge damaging oxygen radicals and minimize oxidative stress. Oxidative stress is believed to play a role in the progression of several neurodegenerative disorders such as AD, PD, and ALS. Anti-oxidants property of saffron has been demonstrated to lower oxidative stress and have neuroprotective effects. Saffron also contains anti-inflammatory effects, suggesting that it could have significance in the treatment of AD, PD, ALS, and other associated diseases.[99] Not only has saffron been proven to decrease levels of pro-inflammatory cytokines, but it has also been shown to decrease levels of the COX-2 enzyme that is responsible for creating these cytokines.[9] AD is a neurological illness that is the most frequent cause of dementia. The condition is characterized by a progressive deterioration in cognitive ability, aberrant brain pathology, and the deposition of amyloid-beta (A) plaques. Although the specific etiology of AD is uncertain, it is likely to be tied to both genetic and environmental factors. Saffron has been found to have preventive benefits against AD. Studies have revealed that saffron can decrease the levels of the plaques that are prevalent in patients with AD.[98] Saffron has also been demonstrated to lessen oxidative stress and inflammation, which are both known to be involved in the advancement of AD.[65]

13.3.7 OCIMUM GRATISSIMUM

Ocimum gratissimum is a well-known South Asian medicinal herb. It is also referred to as "the gooseberry" or "the great Indian sanitary leaf." For generations, the plant has been a key element of traditional medicine practises in India, Sri Lanka, and Nepal, with its leaves being utilized as a natural cure for a variety of maladies.[76] Historically, *O. gratissimum* has been used to alleviate stress, sleeplessness, nausea, and high blood pressure, among other things.[56] Researchers have become interested in its potential significance in neurodegenerative illnesses such as AD, PD, HD, and ALS.[83] While the exact etiology of these disorders is unknown, it is thought that central nervous system malfunctions caused by oxidative stress and chronic inflammation, among other things, may be to blame. When there is an imbalance between free radical generation and the body's ability to detoxify the toxic metabolites, oxidative stress arises. Oxidative stress is thought to play a role in the pathogenesis of many ND. Chronic inflammation, on the other hand, is caused by an excessive immune response to infections, poisons, or other foreign substances. Neurodegeneration caused by oxidative stress and persistent inflammation can result in major health issues, including death. *O. gratissimum* includes a high concentration of essential oils such as ocimol, gratissimin, -sitosterol, flavonoids, linolenic acid, and polyphenolic substances. According to animal studies, *O. gratissimum* has antioxidant, anti-inflammatory, antimicrobial, antifungal, antimutagenic, immunomodulating, smooth muscle contraction actions of lipid-soluble principles, hepatoprotective, antimycobacterial, and antidiarrheal properties.[55] Several studies have demonstrated that *O. gratissimum* can increase cognitive function as well as learning and memory. The authors discovered that *O. gratissimum* reduced cognitive impairment and apoptosis (programmed cell death) in a mouse model of AD. Another in vitro study discovered that *O. gratissimum* enhanced the levels of critical chemicals related to learning and memory. The study also discovered that *O. gratissimum* boosted neuronal communication and increased neurons' ability to expand and make new connections. This shows that *O. gratissimum* could be beneficial in treating memory loss and increasing cognitive function in people suffering from ND.

As previously stated, oxidative stress and chronic inflammation are thought to be involved in the pathogenesis of many neurodegenerative disorders. *Ocimum gratissimum* possesses antioxidant and anti-inflammatory effects, which could explain why it could be employed as a neuroprotective agent against various disorders. Rosmarinic acid, a bioactive component found in *O. gratissimum*, is known for its antioxidant effects. Furthermore, *O. gratissimum* leaves are high in vitamins C, E, and B. Vitamins C and E are well-known antioxidants, but vitamin B is responsible for mood and cognitive function regulation. OG has been found in studies to reduce the level of malondialdehyde, a sign of oxidative stress, in the neurological system. This shows that *O. gratissimum* may be beneficial in the treatment of oxidative stress-related conditions such as neurodegenerative diseases. *O. gratissimum* has been demonstrated to have anti-inflammatory qualities in addition to antioxidant capabilities. *O. gratissimum* has been found in studies to prevent the activation of microglia, central nervous system immune cells that are responsible for the inflammatory response. This shows that *O. gratissimum* leaves may be effective in the treatment of neurological illnesses.

Ocimum gratissimum leaves are high in antioxidants. Rosmarinic acid, caffeic acid, ursolic acid, oleanolic acid, ferulic acid, and vitamin C are the primary antioxidants contained in OG leaves. These chemicals have antioxidant characteristics and can neutralize the damaging by-products of oxidative stress. They can also protect the neurological system from oxidative stress by inhibiting the oxidation of lipids and proteins in the body. This shows that *O. gratissimum* leaves may be beneficial in the treatment of oxidative stress-related conditions such as ND.

13.3.8 GINGKO BILOBA

Ginkgo biloba has been used for centuries as a natural treatment for many diseases. It has been found to be effective in the treatment of ND such as AD and PD. *Ginkgo biloba* extract contains flavonoids, terpenes, and ginkgolides that are responsible for its therapeutic effects. It is also known to possess antioxidant and anti-inflammatory properties, which make it an excellent candidate for treating neurodegenerative disorders.[42] The use of natural products in the field of medicine is becoming more popular. They are often considered safer than synthetic drugs because they have fewer side effects, and they can be more effective than traditional treatments. One example is *Ginkgo biloba*, which has been used by ancient civilizations to treat many ailments, including Alzheimer's.[82]

13.3.9 CONVOLVULUS PLURICAULIS

The Convolvulaceae family of plants, which includes morning glory, contains more than 1000 different plant species. *Convolvulus pluricaulis* Choisy, a perennial wild prostrate herb that seems like morning glory, mostly found in Northern India, is another member of the Convolvulaceae family.[57] It has blue flowers and branches that are 30 cm long. It contains branches, flowers, and elliptical leaves arranged in an alternating pattern. It is commonly referred to as shankhpushpi and is used in the Ayurvedic medical system as a nervine tonic to enhance memory and intellect. Alkaloids (shankhpushpine and convolamine), volatile oils (cinnamic acid, palmitic acid, and linoleic acid), favanoid-kampferol, phytosterols, amino acids, fatty acids (ceryl alcohols), scopoletin, squalene, and β-sitosterol are the main chemical components.[2] Ascorbic acid, maltose, rhamnose, sucrose, starch, flavonoids, terpenoids, rivastigmine, vitamin E, and steroids are other active ingredients. In addition to neutralizing free radicals, it also aids in stabilizing muscarinic receptors.

13.3.10 CASSIA OCCIDENTALIS

Cassia occidentalis L. of the family Caesalpiniaceae is widely used in traditional medicine around the world, particularly in several African nations, to cure a variety of illnesses. *Cassia occidentalis* is a plant having significant therapeutic properties. It has been discovered that occidentalis possesses important pharmacological activities, including antibacterial, antifungal, antimalarial, anti-inflammatory, laxative, analgesic, choleretic, and diuretic qualities.[58] *Cassia occidentalis* contains bundle of phyto-constituents such as achrosin, aloe-emodin, emodin, anthraquinones, anthrones, apigenin, aurantiobtusin, campesterol, cassiollin, chryso-obtusin, chrysophanic acid, chrysarobin, chrysophanol, chrysoeriol, emodin, essential oils, funiculosin, galactopyranosyl, helminthosprine, islandicine, kaempferol, lignoceric acid, linoleic acid, mannitol, mannopyranosyl, mateucinol, obtusifolin, obtusin, oleic acid, physcrion, quercetin, rhamnosides, rhein, rubrofusarin, sitosterols, tannins, and xanthorine.[96]

13.3.11 MUCUNA PRURIENS

Mucuna pruriens (Fabaceae) is a well-known traditional annual climbing legume that grows 3–18 m in height, native to India and southeast region of Asia, with significant pharmacological importance including antioxidative, antineoplastic, analgesic, antiepileptic, and anti-inflammatory. Moreover, *M. pruriens* have been widely explored for the treatment of neurological disorders, treatment of arthritis, and male infertility in varied ages. In addition, several reports indicated plant exhibits antimicrobial and cognitive improvement property. *Mucuna pruriens* is infused with various phyto-compounds that majorly belong to Tannins, polyphenols, amino acids, and alkaloids such as mucunadine, mucunine, prurienidine, prurienine enables its various parts such as stem, seed, and root-rich reservoir of bioactives. Furthermore, *M. pruriens* is reported to contain major compound such as L-dopa, abundant in seeds.[38] According to ethnobotanical database *M. pruriens* contains diverse bioactives including 1-methyl-3-carboxy-6, 7-dihydroxy-1,2,3,4-tetrahydroisoquinolone, 5-hydroxy tryptamine, 5-methoxy-n, n-dimethyl tryptamine-n-oxide, 5-oxyindole-3-alkylammine, 6-methoxyharman, alanine, arachidic acid, arginine, aspartic acid, behenic acid, leucine, linoleic acid, myristic acid, n,n-dimethyltryptamine, n,n-dimethyltryptamine-n-oxide, nicotine, oleic acid, palmitic acid, palmitoleic acid, phenylalanine, phosphorous, proline, protein, saponins, serine, stearic acid, threonine, tryptamine, tyrodine, valine, and vernolic acid. Although traditionally *M. pruriens* has been known for various pharmacological effects, however the usage as nerve tonic for nervous system is widely accepted due to rich L-dopa content. The highest percentage of L-dopa is reported to be present in the seed extract. Several in vivo studies on human and animals have been conducted and reported the significant efficacy of *M. pruriens* in the treatment of PDs with neuroprotective effect.[21] Recently, several studies reported fortification of *M. pruriens* L-dopa rich-extract such as ethanolic, hexane, aqueous, etc., in novel drug delivery including nanogel, phytosome, green synthesized nanomaterials using *M. pruriens* extract, scaffold, etc., for their enhanced pharmacological response.[15]

13.3.12 CURCUMA LONGA

Curcuma "the golden spice" is well known for therapeutic potential, genus Curcuma includes approximately 80 species and is regarded as one of the largest genera of the Zingiberaceae family. Among several species of *Curcuma,* the *Curcuma longa* Linn. (Harida), *Curcuma aromatics* Salisb (Vana Haridra), *Curcuma amada* Roxb (Amaragandhi Haridra), *Curcuma angustifolia* Roxb, *Curcuma caesia* Roxb (Kali Haridra), and *Curcuma zedoaria* Rossc (Zedoary) grow in different parts of world known for pharmacological efficacy and widely employed as adjuncts to impart flavor and aroma or piquancy to food. Curcumin (1,7-bis(4-hydroxy-3-methoxyphenyl)-1, 6 heptadiene-3, 5 dione) is a principal lipophilic polyphenol active compound of popular *Curcuma longa* Linn. with analogue of desmethoxycurcumin and bis-desmethoxycurcumin, yellow in color have been significantly investigated for pharmacological properties. In addition, a less known curcumin derivative tetrahydrocurcumin and its analogue tetrahydrodemethoxy curcumin and tetrahydobisdemethoxy curcumin white in color are widely investigated as an alternative to major compound curcumin due to high biocompatibility and similar efficacy. Curcumin can exist in at least two tautomeric forms, keto and enol. The enol form is more stable in solid phase and in solution, compared with keto form.[47] Curcumin have been identified by Food and Drug administration as food additive with its E-number being E 100.[4] Curcumin and analogue is well known to exert radical scavenging, anti-inflammatory, antibacterial, antiviral, antifungal, hypolipidemic, antidiarrhoeal, hepatoprotective, antiasthmatic, and anticancer actions with wide usage as cosmetics. Moreover, curcumin is reported to supress the drug resistance via upregulation of P-glycoprotein and its mRNA induced by Adriamycin. Despite a vast range of therapeutic effects, the health utility of curcumin has been limited due to extremely low solubility (in water, oil of medium chain triglycerides, and in edible/pharmaceutical grade of oil is reported as 0.6–7.4 μg/mL, 2.90 ± 0.15 mg/g, and 0.41–0.53 mg/g, respectively[87]), poor gastrointestinal absorption, low oral bioavailability, and instability in solution form. To overcome such complications curcumin has been targeted for neurodegenerative disorders via nose to brain delivery using novel drug delivery technology including solid lipid nanoparticles, vesicular drug delivery, nasal implant film, microneedles, etc.[73]

13.3.13 *LANTANA CAMARA*

The verbena family (Verbenaceae) includes the flowering plant species *L. camara*, which is indigenous to the tropics of North America. Big-sage, tick berry, wild-sage, white-sage, red-sage, and West Indian lantana are some of the other popular names for *L. camara*. *L. camara* is used as an attractive plant and is thought to enhance the quality of agricultural soil in addition to having insecticide, antifungal, and herbicide properties. Given its efficacy and safety, a diversity of pharmacological activities in the medicinal plant *L. camara* make it a good candidate for use in a range of medical procedures. The plant included a variety of compounds, including tannins, anthraquinone alkaloids, glycosides, steroids, saponins, glycosides, flavonoids, carbohydrates, proteins, coumarins, phytosteroids, fixed oils, hydroxy anthraquinones, lipids, and triterpenoids.[40] A range of chemical substances with leishmanicidal, antibacterial, anticancer, antiulcer, and anti-inflammatory actions are present in the essential oil of the plant's flowers and leaves. These species can, however, be harmful to some animals in excessive concentrations. The dried flowers of *L. camara* are notable for their essential oil, which is a powerful AChE enzyme inhibitor. The synergistic interactions between the various chemical components could have drawn attention to this inhibitory potential. It has been discovered that synergistic chemicals have an inhibitory potential. As an illustration, interactions between 1,8-cineole/-pinene and 1,8-cineole/caryophyllene oxide have been shown to increase decrease of acetylcholinesterase activity; other compounds can also have this effect. There are various ways to use essential oils in therapies, but aromatherapy is by far the most popular.[48] Aromatherapy allowed researchers to see improvements in the cognitive abilities of AD. Essential oils have a positive impact on health and well-being through acting on the central nervous system, notably when treating neurodegenerative disorders like AD and PD. Despite being regarded as a weed, *L. camara* offers a number of biological advantages, including being a prospective source of a potent natural oil that inhibits the enzyme AChE. The creation of novel drugs to treat neurodegenerative illnesses may use this essential oil. Additionally, it is effective against pathogenic germs that harm people; hence, it is recommended as a different antibiotic.[22]

13.3.14 *RAUWOLFIA VOMITORIA*

The Apocynaceae shrub *R. vomitoria,* often known as serpent wood or swizzler stick, is used locally to treat fever, several neurological diseases, and snake bites. Numerous alkaloids, including ajmaline, ajmalicine, reserpine, serpentine, serpentinine, and yohimbine, are said to be present in the root bark, which is widely utilized. According to reports, *R. vomitoria* works well as an analgesic, an anticonvulsant, and an antipsychotic. On the other hand, Ekong et al. observed no negative impacts on behavioral and physiological indicators; yet, this plant has been linked to negative consequences. It impairs motor behavior, triggers Parkinson's syndrome and depression, and activates neurodegenerative characteristics in the cerebellum and cerebral cortex cyto-architectures.[72] It is said to be hepatotoxic and cardiotoxic in fetal tissues, as well as stimulating femur osteoblast and osteoclast hypertrophy and hyperplasia, wood, African serpent and/or African snakeroot, Swizzle stick are a few of its common names. This plant has anti-hyperglycemic, anticonvulsant, antipyretic, analgesic, antioxidant, antipsychotic, and sedative characteristics that are used to treat a variety of human health ailments, including jaundice, mental illness, gastrointestinal diseases, dysentery, cerebral cramps, and hypertension. Secondary metabolites, which can cause certain physiological reactions in the human body, are linked to these qualities. Reducing sugars, glycosides, polyphenols, and alkaloids are some of this plant's main secondary metabolites.[71] Although studies have demonstrated that phenolic components, particularly flavonoids, significantly contribute to the neuroprotective benefits of medicinal plants, alkaloid contents of this plant were formerly thought to be responsible for its biological activities. The idea explaining the use of alcohol by traditional healers in the extraction of *R. vomitoria* leaf, however, and the efficacy of the phenolic components of *R. vomitoria* leaf in the management and therapy of neurodegenerative disorders, are not well known scientifically. Thus, the phenolic components of the *R. vomitoria* leaf were isolated, and the effects of the aqueous and methanolic extracts on free radicals, Fe^{2+}

induced lipid peroxidation, and essential enzymes linked to neurodegeneration in the rat brain in vitro were investigated. Analgesic, antioxidant, and antidiabetic qualities are only a few of the medical benefits of *R. vomitoria*. Both a depressive and a brain stimulant, *R. vomitoria* also has been shown to have neurotoxic effects.[100] Despite the fact that this plant serves many beneficial purposes, its negative effects often exceed them. This herb may have a higher neuroprotective impact when combined with other effective herbs, according to certain theories. It is possible to investigate the advantages of this combination for managing health, including the prevention of neurodegenerative illnesses.[5]

13.3.15 KHAYA SENEGALENSIS

Senegal mahogany or dry zone are frequent names for *K. senegalensis,* often planted as a roadside and decorative shade tree in its native range. In the human brain, glutamate plays a part in a number of physiological processes such as memory, learning, neuronal plasticity, and central excitatory neurotransmission. However, excessive glutamate can stimulate the NMDA receptor, which causes a high Ca^{2+} influx, ROS, mitochondrial function to be impaired, neurotoxicity, and subsequently the death of neuronal cells.[90] A curative strategy for treating neurodegenerative illness has been neuroprotection against glutamate-induced neurotoxicity. Furthermore, neuropathological and neuropsychiatric conditions including brain injury, stroke, and a number of other neurodegenerative conditions have been linked to damage to neuronal cells brought on by too much glutamate. The limonoids are among the plant secondary metabolites of significant value. They are mostly found in the Meliaceae and Rutaceae (citrus) families and are found less frequently in the Simaroubaceae and Cneoraceae families. In addition to their abundance, limonoids found in the family Meliaceae, also known as meliacins, are of particular importance since they differ structurally from those found in other families and are very powerful with significant biological functions.[39] It is interesting to note that the family Meliaceae's genus Khaya, also known as African Mahogany, is well recognized for a number of biological functions that are related to limonoids found in various plant sections of various species. Limonoids are attracting more and more study attention due to their wide variety of biological effects, which include antimalarial, anticancer, anti-inflammatory, and anti-feedant properties among others. The name "limonoid" was first used by scientists more than a century ago when they identified limonin, a significant bitter component, in citrus seeds. Limonoids are a class of highly oxygenated modified triterpenoids that are most frequently found in the Meliaceae and Rutaceae plant families. They are less frequently found in the Simaroubaceae and Cneoraceae plant families.[67] Important secondary metabolites known as limonoids are produced when a side chain of a triterpene, such as apoeuphane or apotirucallane, loses four carbon atoms. This process results in the formation of a 17-furan ring following cyclization. However, limonoids have sometimes been found in a few species of the Flacourtiaceae, Boraginaceae, Burseraceae, and Euphorbiaceae families. They are classified into those with an unbroken ring structure and those with one of the four rings, and are also known as tetranortriterpenoids (A, B, C, or D) oxidized. Due to the limited number of plant families where they are found and their diverse spectrum of biological functions to support health and ward off disease, limonoids are of significant interest to scientists.[95]

13.3.16 AGERATUM CONYZOIDS

Ageratum conyzoides Linn. (AC) is an herbaceous plant that grows annually and member of the Asteraceae family. It has a long history of usage in conventional medicine, including as an anti-inflammatory, febrifuge, and therapy for ulcers, analgesic, colic, and other conditions. Additionally, the herb is used to heal infectious and mental diseases in various African nations. Scientific evidence also supports Ageratum conyzoides' anti-inflammatory, antioxidant, gastroprotective, hypoglycemic, and antihyperglycemic properties. The secondary metabolites of A. conzyoide, which include cumarins, flavonoids, essential oils, alkaloids, and tannins, are very variable. Numerous of these have biological activity. Ageratum conyzoides has 21 polyoxygenated flavonoids in total, making it a polyoxygenated flavonoid-rich plant. Quercetin, kaempferol, and their glycosides are polyhydroxyflavones.[70] Along with the triterpene friedelin, the two primary common sterols, sitosterol and stigmasterol, as well as a minor sterol, were identified. Sesamine, fumaric acid, caffeic acid, phytol, and long-chain hydrocarbons are further frequent compounds. Plants rich in antioxidants and anti-inflammatory compounds exhibit a protective effect against cognitive impairments. Therefore, using both exteroceptive and interoceptive behavioral models in mice, the current investigation was carried out to examine the impact of AC in memory deficits-associated dementia of AD and whole brain AchE activity.[28]

13.3.17 WITHANIA SOMNIFERA

The ayurvedic herb *W. Somnifera*, a member of the Solanaceae family commonly recognized as Indian winter cherry and Indian ginseng, has been utilized for thousands of years in India for its numerous health advantages. Another of the most important herbs in the more than 3000-year-old practise of Ayurveda is WS. It is used to boost energy, enhance cognitive health, and lower cortisol, inflammation, blood sugar levels, control stress, anxiety, and depression.[19] The plant is an evergreen shrub with short stems, upright, grayish, oblong, petiolate leaves, and bisexual flowers, greenish axillary. It also has long tuberous roots. There are 29 common metabolites formed from the leaf and root extracts that have therapeutic use for the leaves, roots, stems, and flowers. To date, it has been discovered that this medicinal plant also has palliative effects like analgesic, rejuvenating, regenerating, and growth-promoting properties in addition to anti-inflammatory, antidepressant, antiepileptic, anticoagulant, antiarthritic, antidiabetic, antioxidant, and antipyretic efficacies. Solanaceae is the family to which *W. somnifera* belongs. It has soothing effects on stress and prevented memory loss (500 mg/d). In a previous investigation, *W. somnifera's* cholinergic activity was reported. Because it may raise the amount of acetylcholine in the brain, *W. somnifera* has memory-improving and cognition-improving properties. In human neuroblastoma cells, *W. somnifera* has been shown to have time- and dose-dependent neurotic outgrowth action. Dendrite and axon regeneration are improved by *W. somnifera*. According to a study on molecular modeling, withanamides A and C bind to A and prevent the production of fibrils.[24]

13.3.18 PANAX QUINQUEFOLIUS, L.

Phytochemicals have been used for generations to safeguard human health and treat a variety of ailments. According to reports, these plant-derived compounds have anticancer, antibacterial, and antidiabetic properties. Additionally, they were said to lower the risk of a number of illnesses, including cardiovascular and neurological diseases.[37] An example of a plant abundant in bioactive phytochemicals is *P. quinquefolium* L. (American Ginseng, AG). Its key ingredients, known as ginsenosides, have been demonstrated to have a range of biological effects, including hypoglycemic, anti-inflammatory, cardioprotective, and antitumor properties. It has also been hypothesized that AG may have therapeutic promise for treating chronic obstructive pulmonary disease. Additionally, it has the ability to lessen uncomfortable menopausal symptoms.[45] Ginseng Panax A member of the Araliaceae family, Meyer is a perennial plant. Ginseng has gained worldwide popularity more lately. Its roots have been used for centuries to energize the body and mind, improve physical strength, delay ageing, and boost energy. Ginsenosides, which are triterpenoid dammarane derivatives, are the primary pharmacologically active substances in *P. ginseng*. From raw and processed *P. ginseng*, more than 31 ginsenosides have been identified, and more ginsenosides are still being discovered. All ginsenosides have a four-ring, steroid-like structure that is hydrophobic and has linked sugar moieties. The variety of the sugar components, as well as the quantity and arrangement of the sugar moieties, may affect the unique activity of each ginsenoside.[54] A single ginsenoside might have various actions in the same tissue, while different ginsenosides have diverse pharmacological effects. A novel pharmacological concept of *P. ginseng* has been developed by Asian and Western researchers, with a variety of activities on various bodily systems. Ginsenosides have recently been demonstrated to have a variety of advantageous effects on the neurological system. *P. ginseng* and its pharmacologically active constituents, ginsenosides, have recently been shown to have positive benefits in both *in vitro* and *in vivo* models of PD.[52]

13.4 NANOMEDICINE IN TREATMENT OF NEUROLOGICAL DISORDERS

The merging of nanotechnology, biology, and medicine is known as nanomedicine. It is a new discipline that exploits nanoscale phenomena for healthcare applications (e.g., nanoparticles or nanomaterials, see-through bioprinting, quantum dots, nano-biotechnology). Nanomedicine is particularly useful in the treatment of neurological disorders such as Alzheimer's, Parkinson's, and ALS. Nanomedicine is a multidisciplinary field that relies on nanoscale technologies. Nanotechnology is the process of developing gadgets and materials that are a billionth of a meter in size, or far smaller than the size of a cell. This size reduction enables materials to have properties that differ greatly from those found at the macroscale. Transport, delivery, and toxicity are the three most critical qualities of importance in biological applications. Nanomedicine is particularly useful in the treatment of neurological disorders such as AD, PD, and ALS. Because of their biocompatibility, biodegradability, and ability to be functionalized with a range of therapeutic agents, nanoparticles are frequently used in the field of nanomedicine. Nanoparticles can be employed for tailored drug delivery systems, allowing them to be used to treat neurological illnesses. Because of their capacity to pass the BBB and their tiny size, solid lipid nanoparticles can be employed for medication delivery to the brain. Polymeric micelles can be employed for targeted medication delivery. Because of their small size, vesicular drug delivery systems can be employed for targeted drug delivery and can cross the BBB.

13.4.1 LIPOSOMES

"Liposomes are colloidal vesicles generated by introducing phospholipids to the aqueous phase". They encourage the loading of hydrophilic drugs into the aqueous interior of liposomes, protecting them against first pass effect, acid degradation, and delayed renal clearance. Poorly water-soluble medications can also be delivered with the help of liposomes. Numerous nanotechnology techniques, including different active loading methods and passive loading methods comprising of ethanol injection, ether injection, thin-film hydration, can be used to create these drug-loaded liposomes.[69] Due to their inability to penetrate the BBB, the majority of these natural chemicals currently have limited therapeutic use. The ability to traverse the BBB after systemic administration should be a need for any novel antioxidant compounds intended as possible neuroprotective treatments for acute or chronic neurological diseases.[18] For instance, a combination of vitamins C and E is effective in treating both AD and cognitive impairments, although they are not up to par because of its poor ability to cross the BBB.[88] Similar to other powerful antioxidants, flavonoids are confined to the BBB due to highly polar nature and abundance of phenolic groups. Liposomes allow these potentially active substances to get to the brain. Future research should therefore take into account these issues since a balance between a molecule's antioxidant effects and BBB-crossing ability is required.

13.4.2 NANOPARTICLES

Nanoparticles contain polymers, metal, or lipids. Nanoparticles lacking any transport boosting or targeting moiety to direct their transport are referred to as conventional nanoparticles.

13.4.2.1 POLYMERIC NANOPARTICLES

Engineered nanoparticles coupled with therapeutic moieties and imaging agents with dimensions ranging from 1 to 100 nm have the potential to improve efficacy, cellular uptake, selective transport, and delivery of specific molecules to the brain due to their changed physicochemical properties. Polymeric nanoparticles are created from biodegradable and biocompatible polymers, providing an alternative for regulated medication delivery for pharmaceuticals in the treatment of neurodegenerative diseases. Polymeric nanoparticles are colloidal structures that function as vectors to control medication release, aiming it toward specified regions. Polymeric nanoparticles may improve the absorption of the active ingredients and decrease the therapeutic dose as compared to conventional formulations.

13.4.2.2 CHITOSAN NANOPARTICLES

Chitosan is a linear polyamine polymer with reactive amine and hydroxyl surface groups that is biocompatible, biodegradable, and nontoxic. It can possess a variety of variable properties, which include adjustable drug-loading capacity, pH sensitivity, HLB value, targetability, and controlled drug release. Additionally, chitosan is incorporated to improve the brain-to-blood ratio of medications whose capacity to cross the BBB is subpar.[18]

13.4.2.3 PLGA NANOPARTICLES

Poly lactic-co-glycolic acid (PLGA) and polymer NPs are biocompatible and so have significant potential for reducing neuro-inflammation in a mouse AD model. It is capable of crossing the BBB. Transgenic AD mice reacted favorably to therapy, with increased spatial memory and "new-object recognition" abilities.[35] Co-administration of PLGA NPs with phytol and selenium has also been shown to suppress amyloid formation in multiple AD models.[80] However, various parameters, including surface chemistry, hydrophobicity, shape, size, and charge, must be considered before they may be used. An ideal NP should have biocompatibility, low toxicity, and the ability to bind and deliver drugs or therapies. As long as it does not deteriorate quickly in vivo, it can penetrate the BBB and regulate drug release for longer periods of time. All of these traits combine to produce NPs that are highly effective at penetrating the BBB.

13.4.3 POLYMERIC MICELLES

Polymeric micelles are among the most promising nanomedicine delivery technologies. This system is made up of a lipophilic core and a shell made up of hydrophilic polymer blocks. The inclusion of hydrophobic active components is the system's key advantage. The polymeric micelles range in size from 10 to 100 nanometers. A micelle nano-Cur system was found to be safe and effective in ALS patients. As an additional treatment, the system boosted the likelihood of survival in ALS patients, particularly those with bulbar symptoms.[3] Curcumin encapsulated in chitosanalginate-sodium tripolyphosphate nanoparticles increased Cur bioavailability and half-life in a MS animal model.[32]

13.4.4 CELLULAR MEDIATED DELIVERY OF CARRIERS TO THE BRAIN

Drug delivery to the brain via cells can be used to treat neurological problems. Cells that can pass the BBB are used as drug carriers in this strategy to treat neurological illnesses. Glial and brain progenitor cells are examples of cells that can be employed for cellular-mediated medication delivery. Modified proteins have the potential to be used in the therapy of neurological illnesses. Nanoparticles can be used to modify these proteins so that they can bind to brain cells.[33]

13.4.5 NANOGELS

Because of their small size, nanogels can be used for targeted drug delivery. Nanogels are strongly crosslinked nano-sized hydrogel systems composed of nonionic or ionic monomers or copolymers. The nanogels range in size from 20 to 200 nanometers. This system has a medication loading capacity of 40–60%. Amyloid beta-protein (Abeta) fibril production is regarded as a crucial stage in the pathophysiology of AD. A promising strategy for treating AD is to prevent Abeta aggregation. The relevance of electrostatic interactions between CHPNH and Abeta is suggested by the fact that nanogels made of amino-group-modified CHP with positive charges had a stronger inhibitory impact than CHP-nanogels. Additionally, nanogels shielded PC12 cells against the toxicity of Abeta.[36]

13.5 CONCLUSIONS AND FUTURE PERSPECTIVE

For herbal pharmaceuticals, nanosized drug delivery techniques have the potential to enhance biological activity and address problems with effective treatment for neurogenerative diseases. The introduction of clinically effective drugs in this field still faces significant challenges, nevertheless. One of the main challenges to turning these technologies into medications is testing creative techniques to control how nanomaterials interact with biological systems. The feasibility of scale-up approaches that quickly introduce novel treatment procedures to the market and the potential for creating multifunctional systems to satisfy diverse biological and therapeutic requirements are the main challenges in the development of nanotechnology-based drug delivery systems. It is also important to highlight that nanotechnology can contribute to significant developments in basic and clinical neuroscience when integrated with other interdisciplinary fields like nano-informatics, biomedicine, and phytochemistry, among others.

KEYWORDS

- **neurodegenerative disorders**
- **Alzheimer's**
- **epilepsy**
- **Parkinson's**
- **natural product**

REFERENCES

1. Abdul Manap, A. S.; Vijayabalan, S.; Madhavan, P.; Chia, Y. Y.; Arya, A.; Wong, E. H.; Rizwan, F.; Bindal, U.; Koshy, S. Bacopa Monnieri, a Neuroprotective Lead in Alzheimer Disease: A Review on its Properties, Mechanisms of Action, and Preclinical and Clinical Studies. *Drug Target Insights* **2019,** *13,* 1177392819866412.
2. Agarwa, P.; Sharma, B.; Fatima, A.; Jain, S. K. An Update on Ayurvedic Herb Convolvulus Pluricaulis Choisy. *Asian Pac. J. Trop. Biomed.* **2014,** *4* (3), 245–252. https://doi.org/10.1016/s2221-1691(14)60240-9
3. Ahmadi, M.; Agah, E.; Nafissi, S.; Jaafari, M. R.; Harirchian, M. H.; Sarraf, P.; Faghihi-Kashani, S.; Hosseini, S. J.; Ghoreishi, A.; Aghamollaii, V.; Hosseini, M.; Tafakhori, A. Safety and Efficacy of Nanocurcumin as Add-On Therapy to Riluzole in Patients with

Amyotrophic Lateral Sclerosis: A Pilot Randomized Clinical Trial. *Neurotherapeutics* **2018,** *15* (2), 430–438. https://doi.org/10.1007/s13311-018-0606-7

4. Akram, M.; Shahab-Uddin, A. A.; Usmanghani, K.; Hannan, A.; Mohiuddin, E.; Asif, M. Curcuma Longa and Curcumin: A Review Article. *Rom. J. Biol. Plant Biol.* **2010,** *55* (2), 65–70.
5. Aryal, B.; Raut, B. K.; Bhattarai, S.; Bhandari, S.; Tandan, P.; Gyawali, K.; Sharma, K.; Ranabhat, D.; Thapa, R.; Aryal, D. Potential Therapeutic Applications of Plant-Derived Alkaloids against Inflammatory and Neurodegenerative Diseases. *Evid.-Based Complementary Altern. Med.* **2022,** *2022.*
6. Baspinar, Y.; Üstündas, M.; Bayraktar, O.; Sezgin, C. Curcumin and Piperine Loaded Zein-Chitosan Nanoparticles: Development and In-Vitro Characterisation. *Saudi Pharm. J.* **2018,** *26* (3), 323–334.
7. Bathaie, S. Z.; Farajzade, A.; Hoshyar, R. A Review of the Chemistry and Uses of Crocins and Crocetin, the Carotenoid Natural Dyes in Saffron, with Particular Emphasis on Applications as Colorants Including Their Use as Biological Stains. *Biotech. Histochem.* **2014,** *89* (6), 401–411.
8. Bordoni, M.; Rey, F.; Fantini, V.; Pansarasa, O.; Di Giulio, A. M.; Carelli, S.; Cereda, C. From Neuronal Differentiation of iPSCs to 3D Neuro-organoids: Modelling and Therapy of Neurodegenerative Diseases. *Int. J. Mol. Sci.* **2018,** *19* (12), 3972.
9. Boskabady, M. H.; Farkhondeh, T. Antiinflammatory, Antioxidant, and Immunomodulatory Effects of Crocus Sativus L. and its Main Constituents. *Phytother. Res.* **2016,** *30* (7), 1072–1094.
10. Brimson, J. M.; Brimson, S.; Prasanth, M. I.; Thitilertdecha, P.; Malar, D. S.; Tencomnao, T. The Effectiveness of Bacopa Monnieri (Linn.) Wettst. as a Nootropic, Neuroprotective, or Antidepressant Supplement: Analysis of the Available Clinical Data. *Sci. Rep.* **2021,** *11* (1), 1–11.
11. Bukhari, S. I.; Manzoor, M.; Dhar, M. A Comprehensive Review of the Pharmacological Potential of Crocus Sativus and its Bioactive Apocarotenoids. *Biomed. Pharmacother.* **2018,** *98,* 733–745.
12. Cai, J.; Yang, J.; Jones, D. Mitochondrial Control of Apoptosis: The Role of Cytochrome c. *Biochim. Biophys. Acta (BBA)-Bioenerget.* **1998,** *1366* (1–2), 139–149.
13. Chaudhari, K. S.; Tiwari, N. R.; Tiwari, R. R.; Sharma, R. S. Neurocognitive Effect of Nootropic Drug Brahmi (Bacopa Monnieri) in Alzheimer's Disease. *Ann. Neurosci.* **2017,** *24* (2), 111–122.
14. Chaudhary, B.; Bist, R. Protective Manifestation of Bacoside A and Bromelain in Terms of Cholinesterases, Gamma-amino Butyric Acid, Serotonin Level and Stress Proteins in the Brain of Dichlorvos-Intoxicated Mice. *Cell Stress Chaperones* **2017,** *22* (3), 371–376.
15. Chittasupho, C.; Tadtong, S.; Vorarat, S.; Imaram, W.; Athikomkulchai, S.; Samee, W.; Sareedenchai, V.; Thongnopkoon, T.; Okonogi, S.; Kamkaen, N. Development of Jelly Loaded with Nanogel Containing Natural L-Dopa from Mucuna pruriens Seed Extract for Neuroprotection in Parkinson's Disease. *Pharmaceutics* **2022,** *14* (5), 1079.
16. Corona, J. C. Natural Compounds for the Management of Parkinson's Disease and Attention-Deficit/Hyperactivity Disorder. *Biomed. Res. Int.* **2018,** *2018.*
17. D'Onofrio, G.; Nabavi, S. M.; Sancarlo, D.; Greco, A.; Pieretti, S. Crocus Sativus L. (Saffron) in Alzheimer's Disease Treatment: Bioactive Effects on Cognitive Impairment. *Curr. Neuropharmacol.* **2021,** *19* (9), 1606.

18. Dan, S.; Sharma, D.; Rastogi, K.; Ojha, H.; Pathak, M.; Singhal, R.; Shaloo. Therapeutic and Diagnostic Applications of Nanocomposites in the Treatment Alzheimer's Disease Studies. *Biointerface Res. Appl. Chem.* **2021,** *12,* 940–960. https://doi.org/10.33263/BRIAC121.940960
19. Dar, N. J. Neurodegenerative Diseases and Withania Somnifera (L.): An Update. *J. Ethnopharmacol.* **2020,** *256,* 112769.
20. Dong, X.-X.; Wang, Y.; Qin, Z.-H. Molecular Mechanisms of Excitotoxicity and Their Relevance to Pathogenesis of Neurodegenerative Diseases. *Acta Pharmacol. Sin.* **2009,** *30* (4), 379–387.
21. Dongjie, S.; Rajendran, R. S.; Xia, Q.; She, G.; Tu, P.; Zhang, Y.; Liu, K. Neuroprotective Effects of Tongtian Oral Liquid, a Traditional Chinese Medicine in the Parkinson's Disease-induced Zebrafish Model. *Biomed. Pharmacother.* **2022,** *148,* 112706.
22. Dos Santos, R. C.; De Melo Filho, A. A.; Chagas, E. A.; Fernández, I. M.; Takahashi, J. A.; Ferraz, V. P. Influence of Diurnal Variation in the Chemical Composition and Bioactivities of the Essential Oil From Fresh and Dried Leaves of Lantana Camara. *J. Essential Oil Res.* **2019,** *31* (3), 228–234.
23. Dubey, S. K.; Singhvi, G.; Krishna, K. V.; Agnihotri, T.; Saha, R. N.; Gupta, G. Herbal Medicines in Neurodegenerative Disorders: An Evolutionary Approach Through Novel Drug Delivery System. *J. Environ. Pathol., Toxicol. Oncol.* **2018,** *37* (3).
24. Duyu, T.; Khanal, P.; Dey, Y. N.; Jha, S. K. Network Pharmacology of Withania Somnifera Against Stress Associated Neurodegenerative Diseases. *Adv. Trad. Med.* **2021,** *21* (3), 565–578.
25. Dyer, L. A.; Palmer, A. D. *Piper: A Model Genus for Studies of Phytochemistry, Ecology, and Evolution*; Springer, 2004.
26. Elbaz, A.; Bower, J. H.; Maraganore, D. M.; McDonnell, S. K.; Peterson, B. J.; Ahlskog, J. E.; Schaid, D. J.; Rocca, W. A. Risk Tables for Parkinsonism and Parkinson's Disease. *J. Clin. Epidemiol.* **2002,** *55* (1), 2531.
27. Ferri, C. P.; Prince, M.; Brayne, C.; Brodaty, H.; Fratiglioni, L.; Ganguli, M.; Hall, K.; Hasegawa, K.; Hendrie, H.; Huang, Y. Global Prevalence of Dementia: A Delphi Consensus Study. *Lancet* **2005,** *366* (9503), 2112–2117.
28. Gogoi, R.; Sarma, N.; Begum, T.; Pandey, S. K.; Lal, M. North-East Indian Chromolaena Odorata (L. King Robinson) Aerial Part Essential Oil Chemical Composition, Pharmacological Activities-Neurodegenerative Inhibitory and Toxicity Study. *J. Essent. Oil Bear. Plants* **2020,** *23* (6), 1173–1191.
29. Gorman, A. M. Neuronal Cell Death in Neurodegenerative Diseases: Recurring Themes Around Protein Handling. *J. Cell. Mol. Med.* **2008,** *12* (6a), 2263–2280.
30. Gregory, J.; Vengalasetti, Y. V.; Bredesen, D. E.; Rao, R. V. Neuroprotective Herbs for the Management of Alzheimer's Disease. *Biomolecules* **2021,** *11* (4), 543.
31. Gupta, P.; Siripurapu, K. B.; Ahmad, A.; Palit, G.; Arora, A.; Maurya, R. Anti-stress Constituents of Evolvulus Alsinoides: An Ayurvedic Crude Drug. *Chem. Pharmaceut. Bull.* **2007,** *55* (5), 771–775.
32. Hashemian, M.; Anissian, D.; Ghasemi-Kasman, M.; Akbari, A.; Khalili-Fomeshi, M.; Ghasemi, S.; Ahmadi, F.; Moghadamnia, A. A.; Ebrahimpour, A. Curcumin-loaded Chitosan-alginate-STPP Nanoparticles Ameliorate Memory Deficits and Reduce Glial Activation in Pentylenetetrazol-Induced Kindling Model of Epilepsy. *Prog. Neuropsychopharmacol. Biol. Psychiatry* **2017,** *79* (Pt B), 462–471. https://doi.org/10.1016/j.pnpbp.2017.07.025

33. He, X.; Yang, S.; Zhang, R.; Hou, L.; Xu, J.; Hu, Y.; Xu, R.; Wang, H.; Zhang, Y. Smilagenin Protects Dopaminergic Neurons in Chronic MPTP/Probenecid—Lesioned Parkinson's Disease Models [Original Research]. *Front. Cell. Neurosci.* **2019,** *13.* https://doi.org/10.3389/fncel.2019.00018
34. Hingorani, L.; Patel, S.; Ebersole, B. Sustained Cognitive Effects and Safety of HPLC-standardized Bacopa Monnieri Extract: A Randomized, Placebo Controlled Clinical Trial. *Planta Med.* **2012,** *78* (11), PH22.
35. Huang, N.; Lu, S.; Liu, X. G.; Zhu, J.; Wang, Y. J.; Liu, R. T. PLGA Nanoparticles Modified with a BBB-penetrating Peptide Co-delivering Aβ Generation Inhibitor and Curcumin Attenuate Memory Deficits and Neuropathology in Alzheimer's Disease Mice. *Oncotarget* **2017,** *8* (46), 81001–81013. https://doi.org/10.18632/oncotarget.20944
36. Ikeda, K.; Okada, T.; Sawada, S.-I.; Akiyoshi, K.; Matsuzaki, K. Inhibition of the Formation of Amyloid β-protein Fibrils Using Biocompatible Nanogels as Artificial Chaperones. *FEBS Lett.* **2006,** *580* (28), 6587–6595. https://doi.org/https://doi.org/10.1016/j.febslet.2006.11.009
37. Jakaria, M.; Kim, J.; Karthivashan, G.; Park, S.-Y.; Ganesan, P.; Choi, D.-K. Emerging Signals Modulating Potential of Ginseng and its Active Compounds Focusing On Neurodegenerative Diseases. *J. Ginseng Res.* **2019,** *43* (2), 163–171.
38. Kamkaen, N.; Chittasupho, C.; Vorarat, S.; Tadtong, S.; Phrompittayarat, W.; Okonogi, S.; Kwankhao, P. Mucuna Pruriens Seed Aqueous Extract Improved Neuroprotective and Acetylcholinesterase Inhibitory Effects Compared with Synthetic L-Dopa. *Molecules* **2022,** *27* (10), 3131.
39. Kandeda, A. K.; Lewale, S.; Djeuzong, E.; Kouamouo, J.; Dimo, T. An Aqueous Extract of Khaya Senegalensis (Desv.) A. Juss. (Meliaceae) Prevents Seizures and Reduces Anxiety in Kainate-Treated Rats: Modulation of GABA Neurotransmission, Oxidative Stress, and Neuronal Loss in the Hippocampus. *Heliyon*, **2022,** e09549.
40. Kandeda, A. K.; Mabou, S. T.; Moutchida, C. An Aqueous Extract of Lantana Camara Attenuates Seizures, Memory Impairment, and Anxiety in Kainate-Treated Mice: Evidence of GABA Level, Oxidative Stress, Immune and Neuronal Loss Modulation. *Epilepsy Behav.* **2022,** *129,* 108611.
41. Kasai, T. Preparing for Population Ageing in the Western Pacific Region. *Lancet Reg. Health West Pac.* **2021,** *6.*
42. Kaur, N.; Dhiman, M.; Perez-Polo, J. R.; Mantha, A. K. Ginkgolide B Revamps Neuro-protective Role of Apurinic/Apyrimidinic Endonuclease 1 and Mitochondrial Oxidative Phosphorylation Against Aβ25-35 -Induced Neurotoxicity in Human Neuroblastoma Cells. *J. Neurosci. Res.* **2015,** *93* (6), 938–947. https://doi.org/10.1002/jnr.23565
43. Khalil, A. T.; Ovais, M.; Ullah, I.; Ali, M.; Jan, S. A.; Shinwari, Z. K.; Maaza, M. Bioinspired Synthesis of Pure Massicot Phase Lead Oxide Nanoparticles and Assessment of Their Biocompatibility, Cytotoxicity and In-Vitro Biological Properties. *Arabian J. Chem.* **2020,** *13* (1), 916–931.
44. Khalili-Fomeshi, M.; Azizi, M. G.; Esmaeili, M. R.; Gol, M.; Kazemi, S.; Ashrafpour, M.; Moghadamnia, A. A.; Hosseinzadeh, S. Piperine Restores Streptozotocin-Induced Cognitive Impairments: Insights into Oxidative Balance in Cerebrospinal Fluid and Hippocampus. *Behav. Brain Res.* **2018,** *337,* 131–138.
45. Kim, K. H.; Lee, D.; Lee, H. L.; Kim, C.-E.; Jung, K.; Kang, K. S. Beneficial Effects of Panax Ginseng for the Treatment and Prevention of Neurodegenerative Diseases: Past Findings and Future Directions. *J. Ginseng Res.* **2018,** *42* (3), 239–247.

46. Kim, M.; Cho, K.-H.; Shin, M.-S.; Lee, J.-M.; Cho, H.-S.; Kim, C.-J.; Shin, D.-H.; Yang, H. J. Berberine Prevents Nigrostriatal Dopaminergic Neuronal Loss and Suppresses Hippocampal Apoptosis in Mice with Parkinson's Disease. *Int. J. Mol. Med.* **2014,** *33* (4), 870–878.
47. Kongpol, K.; Chaihao, P.; Shuapan, P.; Kongduk, P.; Chunglok, W.; Yusakul, G. Therapeutic Hydrophobic Deep Eutectic Solvents of Menthol and Fatty Acid for Enhancing Anti-inflammation Effects of Curcuminoids and Curcumin on RAW264. 7 Murine Macrophage Cells. *RSC Adv.* **2022,** *12* (27), 17443–17453.
48. Kumar, S.; Singh, B.; Yadav, A. Ethanobotany and Phytochemistry of Lantana Camara L. (Verbenaceae). In *Botanical Leads for Drug Discovery*; Springer, 2020; pp 389–404.
49. Lamptey, R. N.; Chaulagain, B.; Trivedi, R.; Gothwal, A.; Layek, B.; Singh, J. A Review of the Common Neurodegenerative Disorders: Current Therapeutic Approaches and the Potential Role of Nanotherapeutics. *Int. J. Mol. Sci.* **2022,** *23* (3), 1851.
50. Liang, C.-P.; She, H.-C.; Huang, L.-Y.; Chou, W.-C.; Chen, S.-C.; Jung, T.-P. Human Brain Dynamics Reflect the Correctness and Presentation Modality of Physics Concept Memory Retrieval. *Front. Hum. Neurosci.* **2020,** *14,* 331.
51. Liu, S.; An, J.; Qi, F.; Yang, L.; Tian, Z.; Zhao, M. Neuroprotective Effects of Asiaticoside. *Neural Regen. Res.* **2014,** *9,* 1275–1282.
52. Lu, J.; Wang, X.; Wu, A.; Cao, Y.; Dai, X.; Liang, Y.; Li, X. Ginsenosides in Central Nervous System Diseases: Pharmacological Actions, Mechanisms, and Therapeutics. *Phytother. Res.* **2022,** *36* (4), 1523–1544.
53. Luca, S. V.; Gaweł-Bęben, K.; Strzępek-Gomółka, M.; Czech, K.; Trifan, A.; Zengin, G.; Korona-Glowniak, I.; Minceva, M.; Gertsch, J.; Skalicka-Woźniak, K. Insights into the Phytochemical and Multifunctional Biological Profile of Spices from the Genus Piper. *Antioxidants* **2021,** *10* (10), 1642.
54. Mahalanobish, S.; Ghosh, N.; Sil, P. C. Panax quinquefolium (American Ginseng) and Physostigma venenosum (Calabar Bean). In *Herbs, Shrubs, and Trees of Potential Medicinal Benefits*; CRC Press, 2022; pp 179–202.
55. Mahapatra, S. K.; Roy, S. Phytopharmacological Approach of Free Radical Scavenging and Anti-oxidative Potential of Eugenol and Ocimum Gratissimum Linn. *Asian Pac. J. Trop. Med.* **2014a,** *7* (S1), S391–S397. https://doi.org/10.1016/S1995-7645(14)60264-9
56. Mahapatra, S. K.; Roy, S. Phytopharmacological Approach of Free Radical Scavenging and Anti-oxidative Potential of Eugenol and Ocimum Gratissimum Linn. *Asian Pac. J. Trop. Med.* **2014b,** *7,* S391–S397.
57. Malik, J.; Karan, M.; Vasisht, K. Nootropic, Anxiolytic and CNS-depressant Studies on Different Plant Sources of Shankhpushpi. *Pharm. Biol.* **2011,** *49* (12), 1234–1242. https://doi.org/10.3109/13880209.2011.584539
58. Manikandaselvi, S.; Vadivel, V.; Brindha, P. Studies on Physicochemical and Nutritional Properties of Aerial Parts of Cassia Occidentalis L. *J. Food Drug Anal.* **2016,** *24* (3), 508–515. https://doi.org/https://doi.org/10.1016/j.jfda.2016.02.003
59. Martinez, R.; Morsch, P.; Soliz, P.; Hommes, C.; Ordunez, P.; Vega, E. Life Expectancy, Healthy Life Expectancy, and Burden of Disease in Older People in the Americas, 1990–2019: A Population-based Study. *Rev. Panamericana Salud Pública* **2021,** *45.*
60. McAlary, L.; Plotkin, S. S.; Yerbury, J. J.; Cashman, N. R. Prion-like Propagation of Protein Misfolding and Aggregation in Amyotrophic Lateral Sclerosis. *Front Mol. Neurosci.* **2019,** *262.*

61. Mehla, J.; Pahuja, M.; Dethe, S. M.; Agarwal, A.; Gupta, Y. K. Amelioration of Intracerebroventricular Streptozotocin Induced Cognitive Impairment by Evolvulus Alsinoides in rats: In vitro and In Vivo Evidence. *Neurochem. Int.* **2012,** *61* (7), 1052–1064.
62. Mettupalayam Kaliyannan Sundaramoorthy, P.; Kilavan Packiam, K. In vitro Enzyme Inhibitory and Cytotoxic Studies with Evolvulus Alsinoides (Linn.) Linn. Leaf Extract: A Plant From Ayurveda Recognized as Dasapushpam for the Management of Alzheimer's Disease and Diabetes Mellitus. *BMC Complementary Med. Ther.* **2020,** *20* (1), 1–12.
63. Milatovic, D.; Zaja-Milatovic, S.; Gupta, R. C. Oxidative stress and excitotoxicity: antioxidants from nutraceuticals. In *Nutraceuticals*; Elsevier, 2016; pp 401–413.
64. Morgan, S.; Orrell, R. W. Pathogenesis of Amyotrophic Lateral Sclerosis. *Br. Med. Bull.* **2016,** *119* (1), 87–97.
65. Morvaridzadeh, M.; Agah, S.; Dulce Estêvão, M.; Hosseini, A. S.; Heydari, H.; Toupchian, O.; Abdollahi, S.; Persad, E.; Abu-Zaid, A.; Rezamand, G. Effect of Saffron Supplementation on Oxidative Stress Parameters: A Systematic Review and Meta-analysis of Randomized Placebo-controlled Trials. *Food Sci. Nutr.* **2021,** *9* (10), 5809–5819.
66. Moujalled, D.; Strasser, A.; Liddell, J. R. Molecular Mechanisms of Cell Death in Neurological Diseases. *Cell Death Different.* **2021,** *28* (7), 2029–2044.
67. Mounkoro, P. P.; Togola, A.; de Jong, J.; Diallo, D.; Paulsen, B. S.; van't Klooster, C. Ethnobotanical Survey of Plants Used by Traditional Health Practitioners for Treatment of Schizophrenia Spectrum Disorders in Bandiagara, Mali, West Africa. *J. Herbal Med.* **2020,** *24,* 100402.
68. Mukherjee, P. K.; Kumar, V.; Kumar, N. S.; Heinrich, M. The Ayurvedic Medicine Clitoria Ternatea—From Traditional use to Scientific Assessment. *J. Ethnopharmacol.* **2008,** *120* (3), 291–301.
69. Mulvihill, J. J.; Cunnane, E. M.; Ross, A. M.; Duskey, J. T.; Tosi, G.; Grabrucker, A. M. Drug Delivery Across the Blood-brain Barrier: Recent Advances in the use of Nanocarriers. *Nanomedicine (Lond)* **2020,** *15* (2), 205–214. https://doi.org/10.2217/nnm-2019-0367
70. Ngoungoure, V. L.; Mfotie Njoya, E.; Ngamli Fewou, S.; Ella, A. F.; McGaw, L. J.; Moundipa, P. F. Acetylcholinesterase Inhibitory, Anti-inflammatory and Antioxidant Properties of Some Cameroonian Medicinal Plants Used to Treat Some Neurological Disorders. *Investig. Med. Chem. Pharmacol.* **2019,** *2* (2), 1–13.
71. Oboh, G.; Adebayo, A. A.; Ademosun, A. O. HPLC Phenolic Fingerprinting, Antioxidant and Anti-phosphodiesterase-5 Properties of Rauwolfia Vomitoria Extract. *J. Basic Clin. Physiol. Pharmacol.* **2019,** *30* (5).
72. Oyeniran, O. H.; Ademiluyi, A. O.; Oboh, G. Phenolic Constituents and Inhibitory Effects of the Leaf of Rauvolfia Vomitoria Afzel on Free Radicals, Cholinergic and Monoaminergic Enzymes in Rat's Brain in Vitro. *J. Basic Clin. Physiol. Pharmacol.* **2021,** *32* (5), 987–994.
73. Patel, R.; Singh, S.; Singh, S.; Sheth, N.; Gendle, R. Development and Characterization of Curcumin Loaded Transfersome for Transdermal Delivery. *J. Pharmaceut. Sci. Res.* **2009,** *1* (4), 71.
74. RajaSankar, S.; Manivasagam, T.; Sankar, V.; Prakash, S.; Muthusamy, R.; Krishnamurti, A.; Surendran, S. Withania Somnifera Root Extract Improves Catecholamines and Physiological Abnormalities Seen in a Parkinson's Disease Model Mouse. *J. Ethnopharmacol.* **2009,** *125* (3), 369–373.

75. Rameshrad, M.; Razavi, B. M.; Hosseinzadeh, H. Saffron and its Derivatives, Crocin, Crocetin and Safranal: A Patent Review. *Expert Opin. Ther. Patents* **2018,** *28* (2), 147–165.
76. Rao, B. R. R.; Kothari, S. K.; Rajput, D. K.; Patel, R. P.; Darokar, M. P. Chemical and Biological Diversity in Fourteen Selections of Four Ocimum Species. *Nat. Prod. Commun.* **2011,** *6* (11), 1934578X1100601134.
77. Rinwa, P.; Kumar, A. Quercetin Along with Piperine Prevents Cognitive Dysfunction, Oxidative Stress and Neuro-inflammation Associated with Mouse Model of Chronic Unpredictable Stress. *Arch. Pharm. Res.* **2017,** *40* (10), 1166–1175.
78. Ross, C. A.; Poirier, M. A. Protein Aggregation and Neurodegenerative Disease. *Nat. Med.* **2004,** *10* (7), S10–S17.
79. Samii, A.; Nutt, J. G.; Ransom, B. R. Parkinson's Disease. *Lancet* **2004,** *363* (9423), 1783–1793.
80. Sathya, S.; Shanmuganathan, B.; Balasubramaniam, B.; Balamurugan, K.; Devi, K. P. Phytol Loaded PLGA Nanoparticles Regulate the Expression of Alzheimer's Related Genes and Neuronal Apoptosis Against Amyloid-β Induced Toxicity in Neuro-2a Cells and Transgenic Caenorhabditis Elegans. *Food Chem. Toxicol.* **2020,** *136,* 110962. https://doi.org/10.1016/j.fct.2019.110962
81. Shinomol, G. K. Bacopa Monnieri Modulates Endogenous Cytoplasmic and Mitochondrial Oxidative Markers in Prepubertal Mice Brain. *Phytomedicine* **2011,** *18* (4), 317–326.
82. Singh, S. K.; Srivastav, S.; Castellani, R. J.; Plascencia-Villa, G.; Perry, G. Neuroprotective and Antioxidant Effect of Ginkgo Biloba Extract Against AD and Other Neurological Disorders. *Neurotherapeutics* **2019,** *16* (3), 666–674. https://doi.org/10.1007/s13311-019-00767-8
83. Singh, V.; Kahol, A.; Singh, I. P.; Saraf, I.; Shri, R. Evaluation of Anti-amnesic Effect of Extracts of Selected Ocimum Species Using In-Vitro and In-Vivo Models. *J. Ethnopharmacol.* **2016,** *193,* 490–499.
84. Soto, C. Unfolding the Role of Protein Misfolding in Neurodegenerative Diseases. *Nat. Rev. Neurosci.* **2003,** *4* (1), 49–60.
85. Soto, C.; Pritzkow, S. Protein Misfolding, Aggregation, and Conformational Strains in Neurodegenerative Diseases. *Nat. Neurosci.* **2018,** *21* (10), 1332–1340.
86. Srinivasan, E.; Chandrasekhar, G.; Chandrasekar, P.; Anbarasu, K.; Vickram, A.; Karunakaran, R.; Rajasekaran, R.; Srikumar, P. Alpha-synuclein Aggregation in Parkinson's Disease. *Front. Med.* **2021,** *8.*
87. Supaweera, N.; Chulrik, W.; Jansakun, C.; Bhoopong, P.; Yusakul, G.; Chunglok, W. Therapeutic Deep Eutectic Solvent-Based Microemulsion Enhances Anti-Inflammatory Efficacy of Curcuminoids and Aromatic-Turmerone Extracted From Curcuma Longa L. *RSC Adv.* **2022,** *12* (40), 25912–25922. https://doi.org/10.1039/D2RA03656H
88. Traber, M. G.; Stevens, J. F. Vitamins C and E: Beneficial Effects from a Mechanistic Perspective. *Free Radic Biol. Med.* **2011,** *51* (5), 1000–1013. https://doi.org/10.1016/j.freeradbiomed.2011.05.017
89. Tulisiak, C. T.; Mercado, G.; Peelaerts, W.; Brundin, L.; Brundin, P. Can Infections Trigger Alpha-Synucleinopathies? *Progress Mol. Biol. Transl. Sci.* **2019,** *168,* 299–322.
90. Ukekpe, U.; Okpashi, V. Phytochemical Screening and Antioxidant Properties of Stem Bark of Khaya Senegalensis (Dry-zone Mahogany). *J. Chem. Soc. Nigeria* **2019,** *44* (7).
91. Ullah, A.; Prottoy, N. I.; Araf, Y.; Hossain, S.; Sarkar, B.; Saha, A. Molecular Docking and Pharmacological Property Analysis of Phytochemicals From Clitoria Ternatea as

Potent Inhibitors of Cell Cycle Checkpoint Proteins in the Cyclin/CDK Pathway in Cancer Cells. *Comput. Mol. Biosci.* **2019,** *9* (03), 81.

92. Verkhratsky, A. J.; Petersen, O. H. Neuronal Calcium Stores. *Cell Calcium* **1998,** *24* (5–6), 333–343.
93. Verma, M.; Lizama, B. N.; Chu, C. T. Excitotoxicity, Calcium and Mitochondria: A Triad in Synaptic Neurodegeneration. *Transl. Neurodegenerat.* **2022,** *11* (1), 1–14.
94. Wankhede, N. L.; Kale, M. B.; Upaganlawar, A. B.; Taksande, B. G.; Umekar, M. J.; Behl, T.; Abdellatif, A. A.; Bhaskaran, P. M.; Dachani, S. R.; Sehgal, A. Involvement of Molecular Chaperone in Protein-misfolding Brain Diseases. *Biomed. Pharmacother.* **2022,** *147,* 112647.
95. Wu, S.; Liao, X.; Zhu, Z.; Huang, R.; Chen, M.; Huang, A.; Zhang, J.; Wu, Q.; Wang, J.; Ding, Y. Antioxidant and Anti-inflammation Effects of Dietary Phytochemicals: The Nrf2/NF-κB Signaling Pathway and Upstream Factors of Nrf2. *Phytochemistry* **2022,** 113429.
96. Yadav, J.; Arya, V.; Yadav, S.; Panghal, M.; Kumar, S.; Dhankhar, S. Cassia Occidentalis L.: A Review on its Ethnobotany, Phytochemical and Pharmacological Profile. *Fitoterapia* **2010,** *81* (4), 223–230.
97. Yakovlev, A. G.; Faden, A. I. Mechanisms of Neural Cell Death: Implications for Development of Neuroprotective Treatment Strategies. *NeuroRx* **2004,** *1* (1), 5–16.
98. Zandi, N.; Pazoki, B.; Roudsari, N. M.; Lashgari, N.-A.; Jamshidi, V.; Momtaz, S.; Abdolghaffari, A. H.; Akhondzadeh, S. Prospects of Saffron and its Derivatives in Alzheimer's Disease. *Arch. Iranian Med.* **2021,** *24* (3), 233.
99. Zeinali, M.; Zirak, M. R.; Rezaee, S. A.; Karimi, G.; Hosseinzadeh, H. Immunoregulatory and Anti-Inflammatory Properties of Crocus Sativus (Saffron) and its Main Active Constituents: A Review. *Iranian J. Basic Med. Sci.* **2019,** *22* (4), 334.
100. Zhan, G.; Miao, R.; Zhang, F.; Chang, G.; Zhang, L.; Zhang, X.; Zhang, H.; Guo, Z. Monoterpene Indole Alkaloids with Acetylcholinesterase Inhibitory Activity from the Leaves of Rauvolfia Vomitoria. *Bioorg. Chem.* **2020,** *102,* 104136.
101. Zhao, Y.; Xiong, S.; Liu, P.; Liu, W.; Wang, Q.; Liu, Y.; Tan, H.; Chen, X.; Shi, X.; Wang, Q. Polymeric Nanoparticles-Based Brain Delivery with Improved Therapeutic Efficacy of Ginkgolide B in Parkinson's Disease. *Int. J. Nanomed.* **2020,** *15,* 10453.
102. Zhuang, Z.; Yang, R.; Wang, W.; Qi, L.; Huang, T. Associations Between Gut Microbiota and Alzheimer's Disease, Major Depressive Disorder, and Schizophrenia. *J. Neuroinflam.* **2020,** *17* (1), 1–9.

CHAPTER 14

Medical Laboratory Diagnosis of Neurodegenerative Diseases Toward Adequate Treatment in Nanomedicine

UCHEJESO MARK OBETA, AMAECHI EZE ODONO, NKEREUWEM SUNDAY ETUKUDOH, and OBIORA REGINALD EJINAKA

Department of Medical Laboratory Management, Federal School of Medical Laboratory Science, Jos, Nigeria

ABSTRACT

Medical laboratory science is an autonomous profession that entails the examination of human, animal, and environmental samples for accurate diagnosis and illness treatment that is efficient and effective. This field has been overlooked in neurodegenerative (ND) illnesses in the past neurodegenerative diseases (NDDs). NDDs are progressive ND illnesses that primarily affect the central nervous system, particularly the neurons of the brain. NDDs are most often represented by a-synucleinopathies, Huntington's disease (HD), amyloidoses, prion disease, amyotrophic lateral sclerosis (ALS), tauopathies, Alzheimer's disease (AD), Parkinson's disease (PD), and ALS are all neurological disorders with TDP-43 proteinopathies. Currently, cerebrospinal fluid (CSF) and blood are among the top common diagnostic samples for NDDs based on the related biomarkers and nanoparticles (NPs). Although different forms of diagnosis and symptoms are utilized to diagnose NDDs, each NDD has a unique and particular medical laboratory diagnostic that is used to identify the many NDDs of public health significance. Efficient use of medical laboratory diagnostics

Nanomedicine for Neurodegenerative Disorders: Selective Treatment Strategies. Rishabha Malviya, Kamla Pathak, & Swati Verma (Eds.)

in nanomedicine for ND illnesses would be a significant advancement in the field.

14.1 INTRODUCTION

Neurons are the brain cell type, and in most cases, they cannot multiply or replace themselves. Neurodegenerative diseases (NDDs) are chronic conditions that deteriorate nerve cells in the brain and spinal cord over time (primarily neurons in the brain). The incidence rises as people become older. The most prevalent of them include a-synucleinopathies, Huntington's disease (HD), amyloidoses, Alzheimer's disease (AD), tauopathies, Parkinson's disease (PD), amyotrophic lateral sclerosis (ALS), prion disease, and TDP-43 proteinopathies. The illnesses, which are fatal and cause cognitive decline and dyskinesia, are defined by the slow and progressive death and loss of particularly susceptible groups of neurons.[1,2,4,5] The most common classification of the diseases based on their clinical manifestations are cognitive or behavioral disorders and extrapyramidal and pyramidal movement disorders. While some affected individuals have what could be termed "pure syndromes", the majority have combined clinical features.[2] They are mainly caused by genetic mutations. Other causes may include apoptosis, protein misfolding, mitochondrial dysfunction, DNA damage, and necrosis. Neurodegeneration (ND) may be brought on by a number of different things, including genetic mutations, brain protein buildup, and cognitive decline creation of neurotoxic chemicals brought on by the loss of mitochondrial activities.[5] There may be more than one NDD process in one person and the protein misfolding and pathophysiological processes that characterize NDDs may be present a long time prior to the appearance of clinical features.[2,3] The progressive death and loss of neurons cause problems with ataxias and dementias. It is crucial to get a proper diagnosis as soon as possible so that appropriate treatment can be adminisstered.[4]

NDDs provide evidence of neuronal loss of structures or neuronal death as seen in AD (Figure 14.1-Figure 14.2) due to tangles of neurones.

Medical laboratory testing and diagnostics contribute immensely to the clinical and medical cases available towards the detection of diseases and monitoring of treatments. Studies have shown that medical laboratories contribute up to 70% of decisions taken on any clinical case. It also contributes up to 70% of the income generated by any health care establishment.[6,7] Though medical laboratory science may differ in nomenclature in various countries,[8] their services remain the same across the globe.

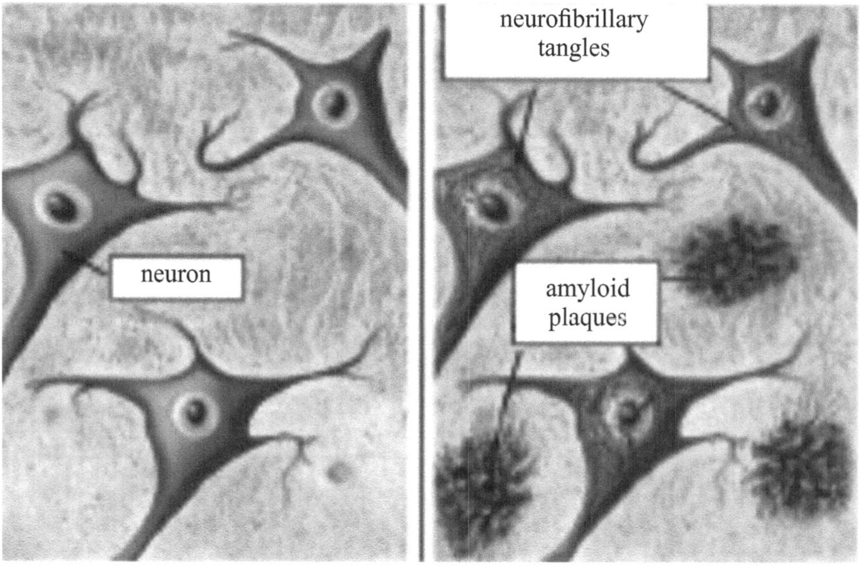

FIGURE 14.1 Neurodegenerative (Alzheimer's) disease when compared with normal neurones.

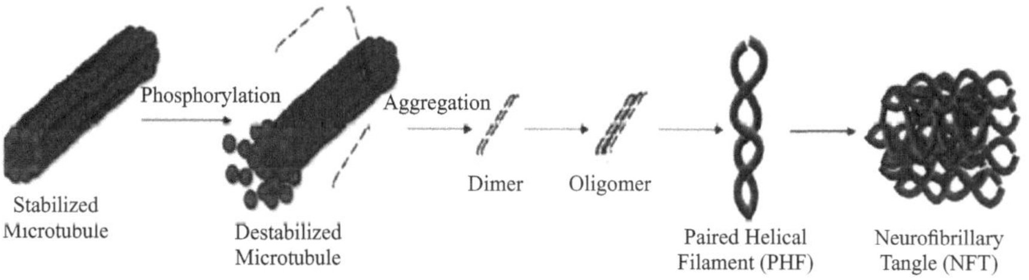

FIGURE 14.2 Stages of neuronal disease development.

The contribution of medical laboratory science in disease management and treatment gives impetus to this chapter to provide a literature towards the contribution of the medical laboratory in NDD diagnosis and therapy in general medical practice including nanomedicine.

This chapter provides a short review, summary, and discussion of ND disorders and their laboratory diagnostics for successful treatment in nanotechnology-based nanomedicine.

Nanobiotechnology is a contemporary scientific discipline that has the potential to enhance medical practice and might have significant participation in the study and treatment of impairments in nerve cell function called disorders of the nervous system NDDs. It may be used in NDD diagnosis, medicine delivery, and treatment.[1,9]

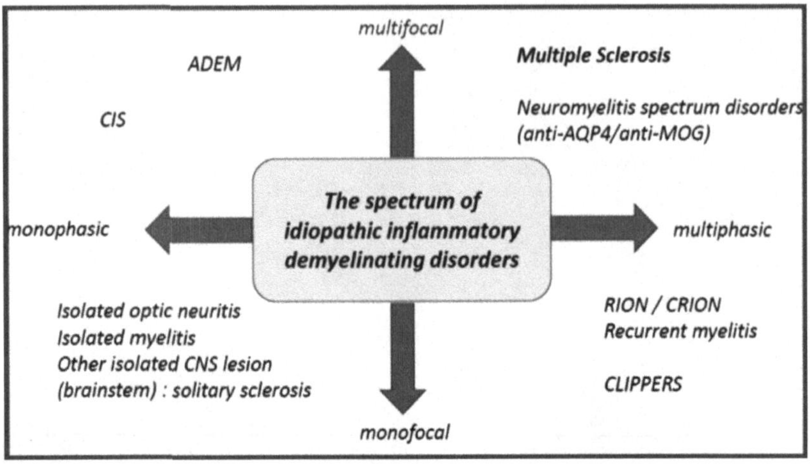

FIGURE 14.3 Nueroinflammatory or neurodegenerative disorders.

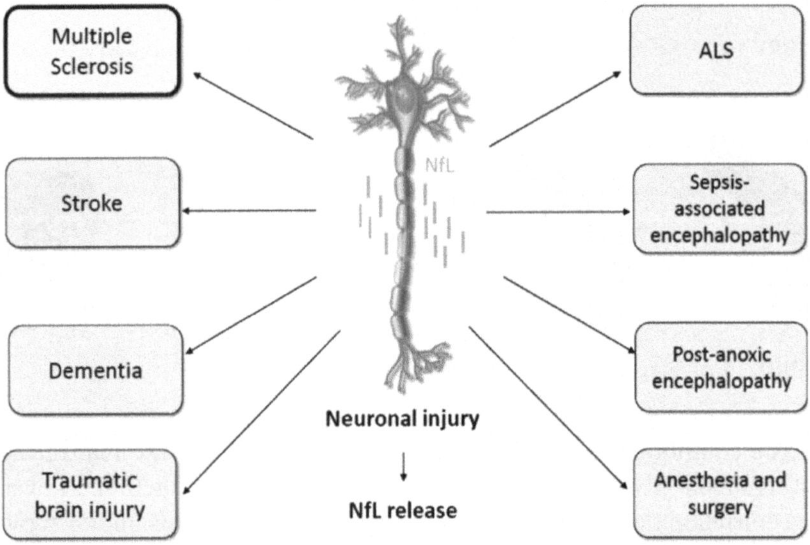

FIGURE 14.4 Various Neuronal damages leading to neurofilament release with various biomarkers.

14.2 MEDICAL DIAGNOSIS OF NDDS-NEURODEGENERATIVE DISEASES

There has been detailed information gathered from a successful thorough examination of NDDs, especially in histology, there are still limitations on the early diagnoses and treatment of the NDDs from a routine medical laboratory perspective. This is attributable to the fact that the majority of drugs and agents that effectively treat the disorders cannot pass via the vascular system of the brain (BBB).[1,9]

Autopsy and examination of neuropathologic findings after a patient's death remain the gold standard for diagnosing ND illness at this time. There is a paucity of information on the available diagnostic biomarkers for the illnesses, except in rare instances when a genetic mutation is established to be the cause of the disease.[2,10] There is a significant societal cost associated with diagnosing and treating NDDs; as a result, advances in the medical laboratory are desperately needed. To a large extent, a differential diagnosis of NDDs is based on the observation of clinical symptoms. However, ND illnesses cannot be diagnosed just by clinical physical examination. Hence, economical, specific, and sensitive biomarkers are recommended[4] and this chapter shall provide insight.

Diagnosis of NDDs may involve stepwise processes (Figure 14.5) like taking the patient's medical history, necropsy testing, neuroimaging techniques, and estimation of blood and/or cerebrospinal fluid (CSF) biomarkers (CSF Aβ42, CSF Tau,).[11]

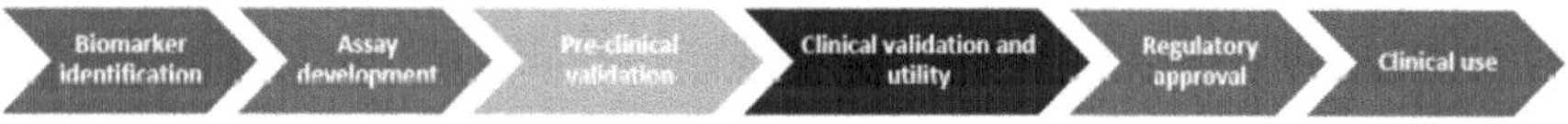
Biomarker identification
Assay development
Pre-clinical validation
Clinical validation and utility
Regulatory approval
Clinical use

FIGURE 14.5 Steps for clinical use of neurofilaments in neurological disease management.

14.3 BIOMARKERS OF NEURODEGENERATIVE DISEASES

Biomarkers, are defined as "biological molecules found in blood or other body fluids or tissues that indicate the sign of normalcy," or abnormal processes in normal or diseased conditions". A biomarker can be referred to as a nanomolecule or nanoparticle and has helped in detecting how the normal or diseased body responds to various normal or disease conditions.[12]

Nanoparticles (NPs) with sizes of about 1–100 nm can provide an innovative approach towards solving issues associated with ND diseases. The small sizes of NPs make them able to cross the BBB and can interact with biological and biochemical systems at cellular levels. Thus, their biochemical and physical properties can be exploited for diagnosis, therapy, tissue regeneration, and drug administration.[1]

Biomarkers are used in nanomedicine and general medical practice for disease management and are not an exception in NDDs. Such biomarkers are mostly used in medical laboratory science, imaging technologies and advanced medical and diagnostic techniques. The biomarkers have a relation with proteinopathies/proteopathies especially when it involves NDDs[13,14] no wonder the biomarkers of NDDs are mostly proteins (Figure 14.6). (Tables 14.1- 14.2) present biomarkers based on samples or types of NDDs involved.

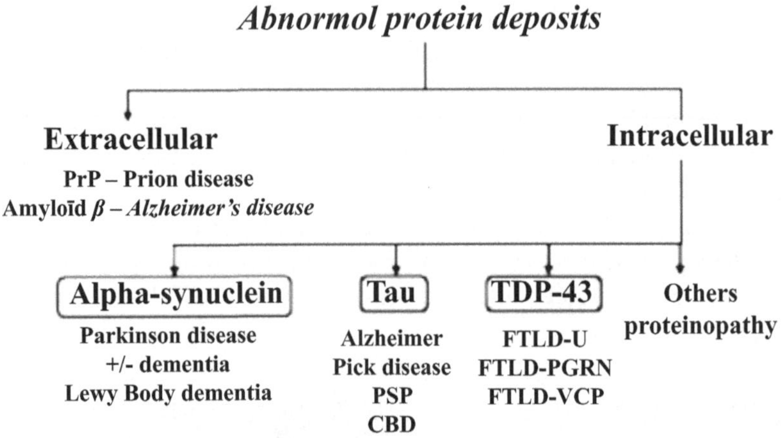

FIGURE 14.6 Some Abnormal proteins involved in NDDs.

TABLE 14.1 Some Biomarkers in Medical Laboratory Samples.

S.No.	Samples	Biomarkers
1	**Blood**	Aß, Tau, NFl, GPAP, SNAP-25, Neurogranin
2	**CSF**	Tau, Aß-42

TABLE 14.2 Biomarkers Present in some NDDs.

S.No.	NDDs	Biomarkers
1	Alzheimer's disease	Aß, Tau, APP, GASR1ά, PSEN1
2	Amyotrophic lateral sclerosis	Neurofilament
3	Frontotemporal dementia	Tau
4	Huntington's disease	Huntington
5	Parkinson's disease	ά-synaclein
6	Prick's disease	Tau
7	Prion disease	PrP, TSE

For successful treatment, the therapeutic process has to be initiated at the point between the asymptomatic and mildly symptomatic stages of the disease. However, the clinical diagnosis does not give accurate results at these stages. The detection of the earliest signs of NDD is very vital. This is because it allows early treatment which could be effective in halting the development of the NDD in question.[10,12] There have been concerted efforts by different research groups to develop criteria that define the diseases at prodromal or preclinical stages, using biomarkers that characterize features of pathophysiological changes.[3]

Fluid biomarkers may be very useful to detect patients who are in the course of the disease already among those at risk for developing ND disorders.

The biomarkers in blood that could be estimated/analysed to diagnose NDDs include Aβ Peptides, T-Tau, P-Tau181, P-tau Alternative Isoforms, and Nfl.[3] Biomarkers in CSF and/or blood (Figure 14.7) and imaging techniques are useful when determining the best course of treatment for NDDs, this aid is especially useful during the diagnostic process, particularly during the phases of early and differential diagnosis.[4] Biomarkers can be determined or measured using advanced imaging techniques like nuclear magnetic resonance spectroscopy, positron emission tomography, and magnetic resonance imaging.[6]

14.4 MEDICAL LABORATORY DIAGNOSIS OF NDDS

Clinical course, diagnosis, disease progression monitoring, and patient recruitment for targeted therapy[14] all require the validation and use of large panels of biomarkers that reflect specific pathophysiological mechanisms such as synaptic dysfunction, accumulation of misfolded proteins, neuro-inflammation, neuronal injury, genetic expression and regulation. Current AD-specific pathophysiological biomarkers for ND illnesses are costly to acquire and/or entail intrusive sampling of bodily fluids, making them unsuitable for application in broad populations. The ideal screening tests would have a high NPV, low false positive rates, and be simple to apply. If you need a sample that fits these requirements, blood is your best bet. Nonetheless, other types of samples, such as olfactory mucosa, retina, and saliva, are currently being tested for their usefulness. Protein misfolding cyclic amplification (PMCA) tests and CSF biomarkers may also be used to characterize NDDs.[3]

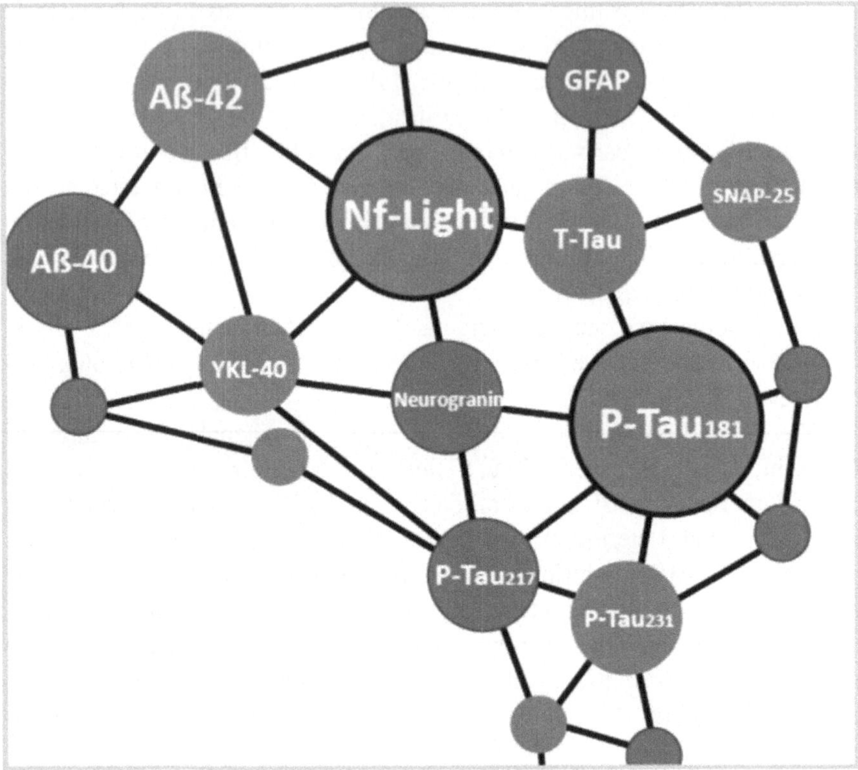

FIGURE 14.7 Biomarkers found in blood for diagnosis of NDDs.

PMCA assays are among the most accurate diagnostic tests for prion diseases. They play a significant role in the in vivo analysis of protein accumulation abnormalities and misfolding. They are essential in NDDs due to their ability to identify and quantify misfolded proteins, as well as to perform amplification tests. The RT-QuIC and the PMCA are the two most important tests created so far. They are useful for detecting low levels of misfolded proteins because, in theory, these proteins will cause the nearby unfolded proteins to also misfold.[3]

Both techniques involve the fragmentation step, detection and quantitation of the misfolded proteins.[14]

Utilizing mechanical shaking, RT-QuIC detects and quantifies misfolded proteins in real time by using a fluorescent dye that generates a signal upon interacting with fibrils. Misfolded proteins increase the signal's strength.[3]

In PMCA, the fragmentation is done by a sonication process. Quantification of the misfolded proteins is not done in real time during the reaction.

Rather, it occurs after the amplification phase. Conventional immunoassays such as western blotting are coupled to PMCA reaction process to enhance the quantification of misfolded proteins.[3]

The medical laboratory diagnosis of NDDs has grown from manual/ELISA (Figure 14.8) to automation (Figure 14.9) and advanced techniques such as fully automated systems as the case of SIMOA technology (Figure 14.10).

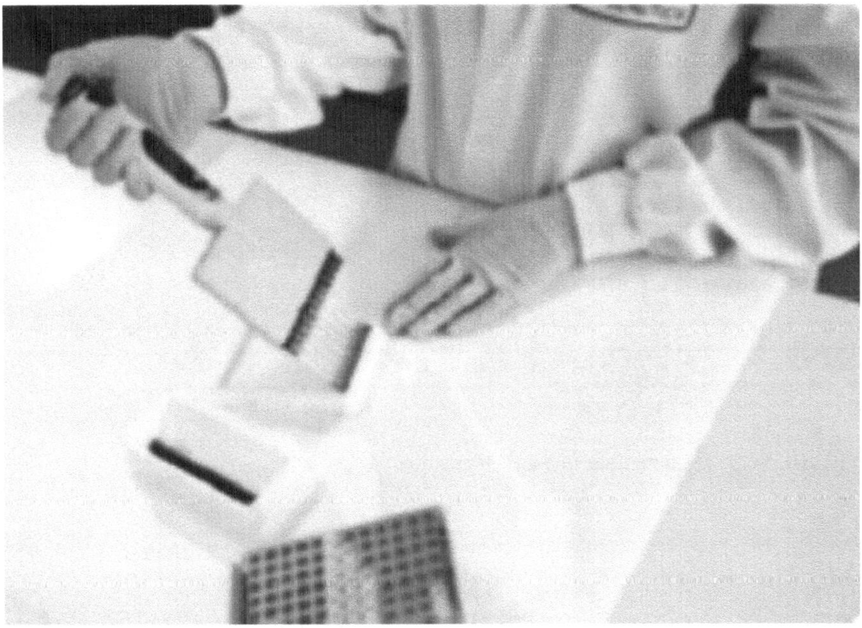

FIGURE 14.8 Manual/ELISA methods of NDDs Biomarkers Testing.

The methodologies and procedures employed are based on the NDDs of interest or the diagnostic method adopted which may be manual, semi-automated or fully automated. The methodology also has to follow the manufacturers' instructions and procedures.

Recombinant protein is incubated with the biological sample containing the misfolded protein to be quantified for a given time duration at a specific temperature. This promotes further misfolding of recombinant protein and the elongation of the fibrils (nucleation).

In most cases, the sample undergoes a sonication PMCA or shaking RT-QuIC to promote fragmentation of the fibrils and amplification of the protein species, thereby promoting further misfolding and amplification.

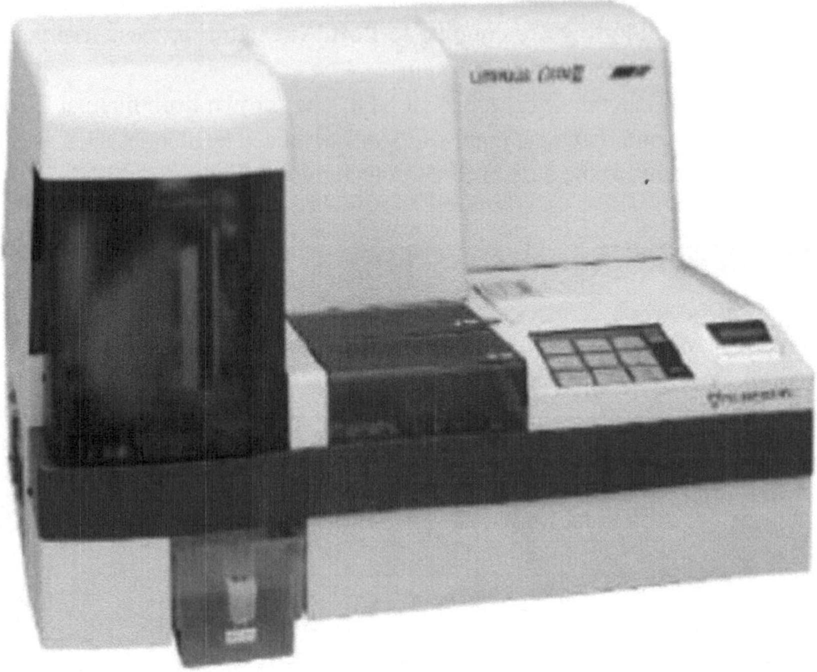

FIGURE 14.9 Automations in NDDs biomarker assays.

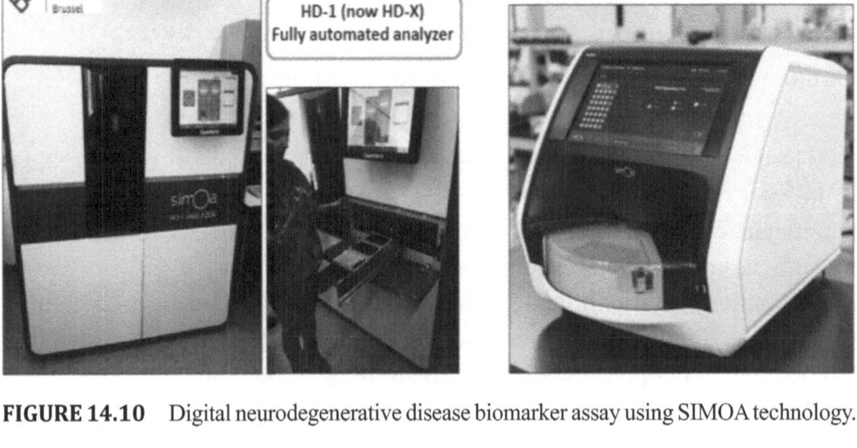

FIGURE 14.10 Digital neurodegenerative disease biomarker assay using SIMOA technology.

The incubation-sonication/shaking cycles are repeated several times, enabling the amplification of small amounts of misfolded proteins.[3]

14.5 DISCUSSION ON MEDICAL LABORATORY DIAGNOSIS OF SPECIFIC NDDS

14.5.1 DEMENTIA ALZHEIMER'S (AD)

The incidence of AD is the highest among all the major neurological NDD, responsible for 60–70% of dementia cases. It is characterized by the presence of protein tangles (tau) within neurons and the presence outside brain cells, characterized by the protein fragment beta-amyloid (plaques). Simply put, death results from the destruction of neurons necessary for basic somatic processes like walking and swallowing. Patients must be identified and treated for the illness in the preclinical stages if they are to experience any relief from the symptoms.

To diagnose AD effectively, it is necessary to observe signs/symptoms of AD with at least one biomarker. The core biomarkers include Aβ42, t-tau, and p-tau18.

The NIA-AA proposed the "A/T/N" framework to classify AD biomarkers into three groups based on three brain pathological changes linked to AD.[5]

When referring to biomarkers for -amyloid, "A" refers to A42 in CSF or other similar substances. When referring to biomarkers for -amyloid, "A" refers to A42 in CSF or other similar substances. "T" represents p-tau in CSF. p tau181 reflects the level of NDand the decrease in cognitive ability. The uniqueness of p-tau increases and the development of AD.

"N" represents neurodegeneration.[4]

If you want an accurate diagnosis of AD, nothing beats neuropathology analysis performed on a deceased patient AD. Evaluating using magnetic resonance (MR) or computed tomography (CT) imaging is helpful, and PET and single-photon emission CT can help distinguish AD from other forms of dementia. CSF samples are often employed in clinical labs for biomarker detection. The levels of cortisol, pancreatic polypeptide, protein 2 microglobule, insulin-like growth factor binding protein 2, and vascular cell adhesion molecule one are elevated in the plasma. Apolipoprotein E, epidermal growth factor receptor, haemoglobin, calcium, zinc, interleukin 17, and albumin are all decreased, while CD40, carcinoembryonic antigen, matrix metalloprotein 2, macrophage inflammatory protein 1, superoxide dismutase, and homocysteine are all increased. We found that this panel of plasma biomarkers allowed for reliable differentiation between AD patients and cognitively healthy controls.[15]

Mutations in genes that code for proteins like presenilin 1 (PSEN1), presenilin 2 (PSEN2), and amyloid precursor protein (APP) are major contributors to ADAPP. Amyloid- (A) as senile plaques and aggregation of hyperphosphorylated tau-mediated neurofibrillary tangles (NFTs) in the brain can be used to diagnose AD in the CSF.[14,15]

14.5.2 PRION DISEASE

Transmissible spongiform encephalopathies (TSEs) is another name for prion disease. Conformational alterations in cellular prion proteins (PrPc) lead to the accumulation of pathogenic prion proteins (PrPsc), which are responsible for the disease. Diseases that are susceptible to protease variations include Creutzfeldt-Jakob disease (CJD), kuru, fatal familial insomnia, Gerstmann-Sträussler-Scheinker disease, and variably protease-sensitive prionopathy, are all examples of human illnesses. The most prevalentCJD is the name for prion disease. 0.85% of all CJD cases are caused by sporadic instances.

Proteins 14-3-3, tau, NSE (Neuron-specific enolase), and S100B are all indicators of prion disease.

It has been discovered that 14-3-3, an acidic soluble protein with extensive evolutionary conservation, is present in a broad range of eukaryotic cells. Neuronal injury, prion disease, and other neurological illnesses may be indicated by its detection at elevated levels in CSF. Patients with CJDalso have an abnormally high concentration of the protein tau in their CSF.[14]

For example, NSE is an enolase that helps in the glycolytic process. The brain is where it is most active. NDDs are triggered by abnormal NSE, which is seen in the CSF of CJD patients.

A higher concentration of S100B, a protein found in astrocytes, is associated with an uptick in astrocyte activity.

It's possible that a more precise and accurate diagnosis might be made by combining test findings from several biomarkers. Protein 14-3-3 and protein tau in CJD patients might have a specificity and sensitivity of a low ratio of phosphorylated tau to total protein tau (96:84) is associated with a reduced risk of developing AD. combined 14-3-3 test has a specificity and sensitivity of 96% and 79%, respectively. These tests are now the gold standard for diagnosing CJD. They have not yet been implemented outside of the lab.[4]

Diagnosis can be accomplished via a variety of imaging modalities, including electroencephalography (EEG), CT, magnetic resonance imaging (MRI), and positron emission tomography (PET) prion disease because of the damage they may detect to nerves and eyes. CSF has been primarily obtained by spinal taps for medical study for quite some time. The increased levels of 14-3-3 protein, S-100, and neuronal-specific enolase (NSE) in the CSF are encouraging. The disease causing PrP isoform may be measured by utilizing a technique called conformation-dependent immunoassay (CDI), which examines both the protease-resistant and protease-sensitive forms of PrPSc.

14.5.3 PARKINSON'S DISEASE (PD)

The worldwide incidence rate for Parkinson's Disease (PD) is around 3.0×10^{-3}, making it the second most frequent NDD. Muscular stiffness, rest tremor, and bradykinesia are typical clinical manifestations. Over 80-year olds have a higher incidence rate. Dopaminergic neuron loss in the substantia nigra pars compacta (SNpc) at an early stage and aberrant accumulations of -synuclein protein, known as Lewy bodies and Lewy neurites, are the predominant clinical characteristics.

At present, PD does not have specific CSF or other laboratory tests to detect it. However, some biomarkers in blood and CSF are potential markers for early detection and differential diagnosis of PD. These include DJ-1, αsynuclein, glial fibrillary acidic protein (GFAP) and coenzyme Q10. However, their specificity and sensitivity are not reliable.[14]

When it comes to diagnosing PD, imaging biomarkers fare the best. Dopamine transporter single-photon emission computed tomography scans (DAT SPECT), MRI, transcranial sonography, and fluorodopa positron emission tomography (F-DOPA PET) are all examples. Dopamine depletion in the nigro-striatum may be shown on DAT SPECT. Regular use of MRI in the diagnosis of PD is now the gold standard for ruling out any confounding factors.[4]

Using a variety of methods of neuroimaging may improve the accuracy of diagnosing complex NDDs. Imaging techniques such as PET, SPECT, MRI, CT, and other imaging techniques like CT scans all belongs to CT. Brain physiology and biochemistry may be studied using several MR techniques, such as perfusion SPECT and MRI, magnetization transfer MRI, MRS on the 1H and 31P nuclear spins, as well as MRS imaging (MRSI). Methods such as these might be used to learn how certain brain processes contribute to the onset of disease.[12,16]

Human, cell, and animal model studies have shown that the nanotheranostics method offers revolutionary promise for treating a variety of ND illnesses.[5]

Through the use of design materials and technologies that interact with biological systems on a molecular level to trigger, respond to, and intermix with target locations to promote biological responses while decreasing side effects, nanotechnology may be employed in the medical industry to better control NDDs. The BBB poses a significant challenge to the delivery of pharmaceuticals for the diagnosis, targeting, and treatment of NDDs.[5] Drugs administered in these ways often fail to treat NDDs because they are unable to cross the BBB.

The translational usefulness and safety of nanotheranostic techniques is a major worry, even though research is assuring their evolution from animal to human models. This needs an in-depth knowledge of how various bodily systems interact with nanomaterials. For both the diagnosis and therapy of these NDDs, numerous nano bioactive substances derived from plants be useful.[5]

Imaging techniques such as computed tomography, MRI, positron emission tomography, and SPECT have all proven useful in diagnosing PD, but pinpointing the precise alterations has proven more difficult. Microscopical postmortem research in the medical laboratory or pathology has uncovered a characteristic of cell death linked to PD: the presence of widespread Lewy bodies. Having Lewy-type -synucleinopathy in the submandibular glands is indicative of PD at autopsy.[14,16]

14.6 NANO-MEDICINE AND MEDICAL LABORATORY DIAGNOSTICS OF NDDS

Nanotheranostics is the practice of injecting NPs for diagnostic purposes via different drug particles. Once the medicine has reached its destination, the outer coating will begin to breakdown, allowing the active ingredients to seep out. This helps narrow down the potential causes of the disease to certain substances or neurons. It's tailored specifically to each patient's illness and needs, and it ultimately helps the field as a whole to advance (personalized medicine).

Confirmation of the diagnosis helps with early detection and medical counselling, which directs individual patients toward therapy. Because of this, we can learn more about the causes of NDDs and how to treat them.[5,8,12,17]

Improvements in nanomedicine may help treat diseases for which there are now few treatment options thanks to recent findings in polymer science and cell-based delivery methods. The development of effective and safe therapeutic and diagnostic methods is hampered by the difficulty of low molecular weight chemicals and biomacromolecules (such as imaging contrast agents, medicines, nucleic acids, and proteins) accessing the brain.[12] Since exosomes may traverse the BBB unhindered, they are also being exploited as nanomaterials for therapies and medication delivery in ND disorders.[2]

14.7 CONCLUSION

There is a general growth in the medical laboratory testing for NDDs using various samples and techniques for detecting biomarkers. Automation in neurochemistry allows for better standardization and faster turnaround time for more accessible biomarkers in the diagnosis of NDDs. Blood-based biomarkers provide an easier and cheaper tool for the diagnosis, treatment and follow-up of different neurological disorders. However, there are still some limitations which make CSF OCB detection remain the gold standard in NDDs in addition to autopsy because of the detection of intrathecal IgG synthesis in neuroinflammatory disorders. The application of nanotechnology in medicine is a promising field in the diagnosis using various samples and nanocompliant products and management of neurodegenerative diseases with the aid of nanomedicine of which medical laboratory components shall not be ignored.

The practices involving NPs work efficiently under automated medical laboratory facilities which are currently lacking in very low-income/developing countries. Such facilities need to be established in poor countries for optimum usage especially in the nanodiagnosis of NDDs and better practices for quality public health medical laboratory services.

KEYWORDS

- **medical laboratory diagnosis**
- **neurodegenerative diseases**
- **nanomedicine**

REFERENCES

1. Rai, M.; Yadav, A. *Nanobiotechnology in Neurodegenerative Diseases*; Springer Nature: Switzerland AG, 2019. https://doi.org/10.1007/978-3-030-30930-5
2. Dugger, B. N.; Dickson, D. W. Pathology of Neurodegenerative Diseases. *Cold Spring Harb. Perspect. Biol.* **2016,** *9*, a028035. https://doi.org/10.1101/cshperspect.a028035
3. Giampietri, L.; Belli, E.; Beatino, M. F.; Giannoni, S.; Palermo, G.; Campese, N.; Tognoni, G.; Siciliano, G.; Ceravolo, R.; De Luca, C.; Baldacci, F. Fluid Biomarkers in Alzheimer's Disease and Other Neurodegenerative Disorders: Toward Integrative Diagnostic Frameworks and Tailored Treatments. *Diagnostics* **2022,** *12*, 796. https://doi.org/10.3390/diagnostics12040796
4. Li, Y.; Zhang, Z.; Xu, C.; Gan, J.; Yao, Y. For Early Diagnosis of Neurodegenerative Diseases: Acting of Biomarkers. *Am. J. Biomed. Sci. Res.* **2020,** *11* (3). AJBSR.MS.ID.001628. https://doi.org/10.34297/AJBSR.2020.11.001628.
5. Kumar, A.; Chaudhary, R. K.; Singh, R.; Singh, S. P.; Wang S-Y, Hoe Z-Y, Pan C-T, Shiue Y-L, Wei D-Q, Kaushik, A. C.; Dai, X. Nanotheranostic Applications for Detection and Targeting Neurodegenerative Diseases. *Front. Neurosci.* **2020,** *14*, 305. (2020) https://doi.org/10.3389/fnins.2020.0030
6. Etukudoh, N. S.; Nelson, A. B.; Obeta, M. U.; Ejinaka, O. R.; Ibanga, I. E.; Nwapi, L. L.; Samuel, P. Health care delivery business and the role of Medical Laboratory Scientists. *IAR J. Med. Sci.* **2021,** *2* (4), 76–80.
7. Obeta, M. U.; Maduka, K. M.; Ofor, I. B.; Ofojekwu, N. M. Improving Quality and Cost Diminution in Modern Healthcare Delivery: The Role of the Medical Laboratory Scientists in Nigeria. *Int. J. Busi. Manag. Invent.* **2019,** *08* (03), 8–19.
8. Obeta, M. U.; Maduka, M. K.; Ejinaka, O. R. Medical Laboratory Science; the Distortion of Nomenclature Across the Globe. *NZ J. Med. Lab. Sci.* **2020,** 52.
9. Ngowi, E. E.; Wang, Y. Z.; Qian, L.; Helmy YASH, Anyomi, B.; Li, T.; Zheng, M.; Jiang E-S, Duan, S. F.; Wei, J. S.; Wu, D. D.; Ji, X. Y. The Application of Nanotechnology for the Diagnosis and Treatment of Brain Diseases and Disorders. *Front. Bioeng. Biotechnol.* **2021,** *9*, 629832. https://doi.org/10.3389/fbioe.2021.629832
10. Agrawal, M.; Biswas, A. Molecular Diagnostics of Neurodegenerative Disorders. *Front. Mol. Biosci.* **2015,** *2*, 54. https://doi.org/10.3389/fmolb.2015.00054
11. van Pesch, V.; Bayart, J. L. *Diagnosis of Neurodegenerative Diseases: Current Tools and New Trends in Laboratory Medicine*; RBSLM 2020 Meeting, 2020.
12. Kabanov, A. V.; Gendelman, H. E. Nanomedicine in the Diagnosis and Therapy of Neurodegenerative Disorders. *Prog. Polym. Sci.* **2007,** *32* (8–9), 1054–1082. https://doi.org/10.1016/j.progpolymsci.2007.05.014.
13. Obeta, M. U.; Nkereuwem, S. E.; Okoli, C. C. Nigerian Medical Laboratory Diagnosis of COVID-19; from Grass to Grace as Chapter 5. In: *Intelligent Computing Applications for COVID-19: Predictions, Diagnosis, and Prevention*; Saba, T., Khan, A. R., Eds.; CRC Press Tailor and Francis Group, 2021; pp 84–93. http://dx.doi.org/10.1201/9781003141105-5
14. Ohanube AKG, Obeta, M. U.; Ikeagwulonu, R. C. Protein Detection in Clinical Diagnosis and Management of Prevalent Neurodegenerative Diseases and Metabolic Disorders A Chapter. In: *Protein Detection*; Tutar, Y., Ed.; IntechOpen, 2021; pp 33–56. http://dx.doi.org/10.5772/intechopen.101051

15. Waldemar, G.; Dubois, B.; Emre, M.; Georges, J.; McKeith, I. G.; Rossor, M. et al. Ecommendations for the Diagnosis and Management of Alzheimer's Disease and Other Disorders Associated with Dementia: EFNS Guideline. *Eur. J. Neurol.* **2007,** *14* (1), e1–e26.
16. Sanabria-Castro, A.; Alvarado-Echeverría, I.; Monge-Bonilla, C. Molecular Pathogenesis of Alzheimer's Disease: An Update. *Ann. Neurosci.* **2017,** *24* (1), 46–54.
17. Adler, C. H.; Dugger, B. N.; Hinni, M. L.; Lott, D. G.; Driver-Dunckley, E.; Hidalgo, J. et al. Submandibular gland needle biopsy for the diagnosis of Parkinson disease. *Neurology* **2014,** *82* (10), 858–864.

CHAPTER 15

Role of Biomarkers in Detection, Diagnosis, and Prognosis of Neurodegenerative Disorders

RUCHI SINGH[1], ANKITA MOHARANA[2], SRISHTI TIWARI[3], SOUBHIK BHATTACHARYYA[2], GARIMA TRIPATHI[3], and DHANALEKSHMI UNNIKRISHNAN MEENAKSHI[4]

[1]*Swaminarayan University, Shree Swaminarayan College of Pharmacy, Saij Kalol, Gandhinagar, Gujarat, India*

[2]*Department of Pharmacy, Arka Jain University, Tata Jamshedpur, India*

[3]*Narayan Institute of Pharmacy, Jamuhar, Sasaram, Bihar, India*

[4]*College of Pharmacy, National University of Science and Technology, Muscat, Oman*

ABSTRACT

Over the last 20 years, there has been a dramatic change in our understanding of neurodegenerative illnesses (NDs). Previously, these disorders were thought to be well-delineated entities with recognizable clinical presentations. NDs are notoriously difficult to diagnose without the use of invasive procedures like lumbar punctures to check cerebrospinal fluid levels or functional brain imaging. Biomarkers showing proteinopathy that is present in the cerebral fluid as well as the blood serum have been the primary focus of novel biological approaches and research efforts, particularly in vivo. However, diagnosing particular proteinopathies is very challenging and certainly not totally correct because there are so many clinical studies that overlap and because the neurodegenerative processes that affect the central nervous system

Nanomedicine for Neurodegenerative Disorders: Selective Treatment Strategies. Rishabha Malviya, Kamla Pathak, & Swati Verma (Eds.)

are so complex and diverse categories. As a result, there is a pressing need to establish reliable laboratory techniques for finding specific biomarkers, for understanding the molecular basis of NDs, and for classifying the quantitative and widely available instruments that might speed up attempts to apply this information into disease prevention and treatment—therapeutic adjustments that aid in differential diagnosis make monitoring illness development easier, and provide more reliable estimates of prognosis and treatment outcomes. This chapter's goal is to provide a concise review of NDs.

15.1 INTRODUCTION

Neurodegenerative diseases (NDs) include a broad category of incapacitating disorders; neurodegenerative disorders are those that cause gradual decline in neuronal neurons' form, behavior, or even complete demise. Neurological disorders are quite frequent, with neurodegenerative processes being the root cause of conditions like (AD), (PD), (ALS), (LBD), (MS), (FTD), and (HD). As the illness progresses, cognitive impairments (dementia) and movement issues (ataxias) are the most common outcomes. The most prevalent ND and the main reason for dementia is Alzheimer's disease (AD). 5.8 million Americans currently have AD, according to the latest recent statistics (Alzheimer's Association, 2020). Thirty percent of those over the age of 85 have AD. About 1 million individuals in the United States are living with PD, making it second only to schizophrenia as the most common neurological illness. The NDs are growing more common as the population ages, placing a significant financial and emotional strain on households. Unfortunately, effective treatments for AD and PD that have been tested in clinical trials are still a long way off. Possible causes include tardy diagnosis and inadequate treatment.[1]

In the clinic, NDs often display a wide variety of symptoms that have several possible causes. Thus, biomarkers that are early detection of a disease require a high degree of specificity and sensitivity. Identification and treatment for these conditions: AD, PD, ALS, and HD are the four most prevalent forms of neurodegeneration. For risk assessment, diagnosis, and prognosis, genetic biomarkers are highly accurate for the familial versions of these illnesses, which start in early age. In sporadic variants of the illnesses, which often present at a later age, symptoms emerge gradually over decades. Although there is currently no treatment for NDs, they may be prevented and managed with the use of accurate biomarkers for each disease subtype and stage.[2] Current molecular diagnostics based on genetics, biochemistry, and neuroimaging for the sporadic form of the disorders provide minimal insight into the outlook and development of an illness.

To get the most out of current treatments and to start on modified therapy for illnesses, prompt and precise diagnosis is essential. Current treatments for AD are only helpful for mild cases of the disease and do nothing for moderate or severe cases. The discovery of protein biomarkers in bodily fluids (particularly cerebrospinal fluid (CSF) or blood) that reflect illness state is now one of the most appealing parts of ND research.[3] Cerebral amyloidosis mediated by amyloid- (A), tauopathy mediated by tau proteins, alpha-synuclein mediated by alpha-synuclein, prion protein mediated by PrP, transactive response disorders mediated by PrP, and many other conditions can be categorized by the main cytopathologically linked proteins that cause them. Likewise, in the diseases of synaptic degeneration, neuroinflammation, and cerebrospinal fluid molecules interacting with DNA-binding protein-43 (TDP-43) or blood serve as important indicators of NDs. Neuropathological studies have shown that these protein indicators often coexist, making them vague.[4] The two most prevalent types of ND are vascular dementia and Alzheimer's disease as well as corticobasal degeneration, PD dementia, and FTD. Changes in total tau levels in CSF were also seen in certain dementias other than AD (LBD, PDD, FTD). Therefore, identifying highly specific biomarkers in CSF or blood that may diagnose ND illness while it is still early is crucial. Disease-related glycoproteins have promise as ND biomarkers. It is known that protein glycosylation occurs posttranslationally in all eukaryotic organisms. Through multiple glycoenzyme reactions, glycans are attached to protein substrates during the non-template-driven enzymatic process of glycosylation. In contrast to O-glycosylation, which involves the attachment of a glycan to a protein by a glycosidic link with a Thr, Ser, or sporadically a Tyr side chain, N-glycosylation involves the formation of an amide bond with an Asn side chain. An embryonic protein with the consensus sequence Asn-X-Thr/Ser (X is any amino acid other than proline) transports oligosaccharides from the Asn donor to the Asn acceptor.[5] O-GlcNAcylation, which involves adding N-acetylglucosamine (GlcNAc) to Thr/Ser, and mucin-type glycosylation, which involves adding N-acetylgalactosamine (GalNAc) to Thr/Ser/Tyr, are two common O-glycosylation processes. A few of the numerous biological processes that glycoproteins control include cell adhesion, intracellular transport, and the quality of protein synthesis. Aberrant protein glycosylation has been linked to a variety of conditions, including NDs, prostate cancer, viral propagation, and cardiovascular hypertrophy. Neuronal processes, including development, migration, and regeneration, rely on a wide variety of brain glycoproteins. Similarly, numerous NDs were shown to have dysregulated glycans.[6] The production of N-glycosylated tau protein compared to people without AD, and tau O-GlcNAcylation may inhibit hyperphosphorylation in this disease. Most proteins in human biofluids are released from the cell surface; hence, there are many glycoproteins present. During the biosynthetic secretion process in the endoplasmic reticulum, O- and N-linked glycans are responsible for glycosylation of these proteins before being transported to the Golgi apparatus. Biofluids including CSF and plasma have a high concentration of glycoproteins, making them a promising source for the identification of glycoprotein biomarkers. After introducing the existing limits of ND biomarkers, the first part of this study provides a concise summary of the current findings about glycoprotein biomarkers for diseases that affect the nervous system, such as Parkinson's and Alzheimer's. The methodology of quantitative glycomics, which uses a solid-phase chemoenzymatic approach to examine glycans and identify site-specific glycosylation, was then described as a follow-up. Additionally, we offered the most recent mass spectrometry-based techniques for locating and describing glycoprotein biomarkers.[7]

The nervous system is affected by a wide variety of disorders collectively known as neurodegeneration. The disease's pathophysiology and clinical presentation are both defined by a preferential involvement of the neural subset of cells. Overproduction of precursor protein is often linked to the creation of an abnormal protein with an unstable structure, which is very important to the development of NDs. The accumulation of this abnormal protein, both within and outside cells, has been linked to cause the death of neurons in the area of the brain that is injured. We refer to these groups of data as biomarkers. There is a lot of focus right now on trying to find indicators that can be used to diagnose NDs. Biomarkers are quantifiable, impartial indicators of healthy biological functioning, pathological functioning, pharmacological reactions to therapeutic intervention, among others.[8] Use of a biomarker is primarily intended to improve clinical diagnosis via enhanced differential diagnosis. Biomarkers need to be able to indicate the frequency with which a disease responds to treatment and the pace at which it progresses. There are qualitative distinctions in biomarkers' sensitivity and specificity. In scientific terms, a test's sensitivity is defined as its accuracy to identify the existence of the circumstances under study. A measure to be specific is to be able to discern between situations in which the characteristics being studied do not appear. Depending on their function, biomarkers may be classified into several categories.[9] In the first category are biomarkers used in diagnosis. These may be further clinical biomarkers that can be identified and used to distinguish between patients with seemingly identical symptoms and diseases; neurological disease can be detected before any noticeable symptoms appear thanks to prodromal indicators and preclinical biomarkers. Biomarkers used to predict a patient's prognosis fall into the second category that can be used to predict the severity of an illness or its prognosis forecast how quickly an existing condition will worsen. The third class consists of biomarkers that may be used to gauge how far a disease process is. In the fourth category, we find therapeutic biomarkers, which are used to track the effects of treatment. Clinical symptoms, neuroimaging methods, genetics, biochemical signs in serum, cerebrospinal fluid, or specific tissues, as well as neurophysiology, are all used in the present understanding of NDs as possible biomarkers.[10] Besides traditional gene analysis, there are now a plethora of methods for detecting gene expression. Examining how different molecules perform their functions (proteins and neurotransmitter metabolites) that may be implicated in neurodegenerative processes is the focus of other scientific fields, including proteomics and metabolomics. The primary goal is to identify a set of biomarkers that are unique to a particular clinical setting or cluster of illnesses with comparable characteristics (a "characteristic profile"). Because of its close relationship to the brain's extracellular space, CSF is a very important source of biomarkers. We think that the CSF reflects all metabolic changes occur in the brain. Neurodegeneration biomarker detection in CSF has been used in clinical practice, while others are currently being worked on to standardize analytic methodologies. Furthermore, it is anticipated that the relevance of additional biomarkers will be validated in future investigations.[11] Pathologically changed proteins are associated with neurodegenerative processes, and their classification into proteinopathies reflects the disease subtypes to which they are most closely linked. All of these processes entail dysfunctions in several physiological pathways, such as loss of the activation of glia can cause problems with oxidative stress, inflammatory response cells, and mitochondrial or lysosomal function all contribute to the death of neurons. Neurodegeneration is thought to include these pathways in varying degrees, notwithstanding their universality across disease units.[12] CSF biomarkers may be differentiated in a similar fashion. Amyloid- (A), phosphorylated tau protein (p-tau), transactive response (TAR) DNA-binding protein 43, and alpha-synuclein (-syn) and prion protein (PrP) are all examples of biomarkers that indicate the presence of a specific kind of accumulating pathogenic protein (PrPSc). Two of the most researched nonspecific markers for tau degeneration are neurofilament light chains (NFL) and total tau protein (t-tau) CSF indicators for axonal injury and degeneration, respectively. Nonspecific indicators include indicators of glial activation, synaptic, lysosomal, and mitochondrial dysfunction markers, as well as proteins necessary for the synthesis of intracellular proteins, as well as for the breakdown and elimination of misfolded or otherwise abnormal proteins (Table 15.1). In addition, the diagnostic value of a panel of biomarkers may exceed that of a single biomarker. Some of the biomarkers discussed in this chapter have been implemented into clinical practice for certain types of NDs; others are currently being examined as potential biomarkers for future studies.[13]

The following table provides a review of the most critical cerebrospinal fluid indicators for the various classes of neurodegenerative diseases; the "#" sign indicates practical unique ND markers that either uniquely identify an illness or help distinguish between diseases. If a biomarker is not represented by a symbol, it is not routinely used in clinical diagnostics for that condition. Total alpha-synuclein (t-a-syn), alpha-synuclein in total oligomeric (o-a-syn), and phosphorylated (p-a-syn) forms of alpha-synuclein, as well as total tau (t-tau) and phosphorylated tau (p-tau) proteins, are among the key biomarkers assessed. Additionally, hyperphosphorylated amyloid beta isoforms 42 and 40 are denoted by the acronyms Aß42 and Aß40, respectively. Hyperphosphorylated amyloid beta isoforms 42 and 40 are denoted by the acronyms Aß42 and Aß40, respectively. Light chains in the neurofilaments (NFL) and heavy chains (NFH) DOPAC stand for dihydroxyphenyl acetate; TDP-43 stands for TAR DNA-binding protein 43; (pTDP43); (UCH-L1); (GBA); chitinase-3-like protein 1, DJ-1, SNAP25, VILIP-1, TREM-2, YKL-40, BACE1, and VILIP-1 abbreviations include homovanillic acid (HVA), miRNA, GFAP, and MCP-1.

15.2 MOLECULAR DIAGNOSIS FOR NDS: A POSSIBLE IMPROVEMENT OVER THE CURRENT PRACTICE OF RELYING ON BEHAVIORAL SYMPTOMS

NDs may be preemptively diagnosed using behavioral signs. The most fundamental shortcoming of a behavioral symptom-based diagnosis is that it cannot identify people at an early stage in the course of their illness, when pharmaceutical intervention may considerably halt the progression of the condition. For example, patients with modest symptoms may have false-negative findings from the ADAS-Cog, the "gold standard" for AD diagnosis. The current neuropathologic approaches have been integrated with molecular biology tools, leading to a better knowledge of NDs and new, biologically

TABLE 15.1 The Presence of Disease-Specific Biomarkers in Cerebrospinal Fluid

CSF Biomarkers	α-Synucleinopathies					Tauopathies					Prion Diseases
	AD	Lewy Body Diseases			MSA	"Primary Tauopathies" FTLD-Tau				Non-Tau FTLD	
		DLB	PD	PDD		CBD	FTD	Pick's Disease	PSP	TDP-43 Proteinopathies	
o-α-syn		#		#	#	#		#		#	#
p-α-syn		#		#			#		#		
α-synuclein (t-α-syn)		#									#
o-α-syn/t-α-syn		#		#	#		#			#	
tau protein (t-tau)	#	#	#					#	#		#
p-tau	#	#	#				#		#	#	
t-tau/p-tau								#	#		#
t-tau/α-synuclein										#	
Aβ42	#	#	#	#				#	#		#
Aβ40	#				#		#		#	#	#
Aβ42/Aβ40	#		#	#			#	#	#		#
t-tau/Aβ42	#				#			#			#
p-tau/Aβ42	#			#		#		#		#	
NFL	#	#							#		#
NFH				#					#	#	
14-3-3 protein						#		#			#
t-tau/14-3-3 protein				#				#		#	#
TDP-43					#	#					#
pTDP-43							#	#			

TABLE 15.1 *(Continued)*

CSF Biomarkers	α-Synucleinopathies					Tauopathies					Prion Diseases
	AD	Lewy Body Diseases			MSA	"Primary Tauopathies" FTLD-Tau				Non-Tau FTLD	
		DLB	PD	PDD		CBD	FTD	Pick's Disease	PSP	TDP-43 Proteinopathies	
dopamine/DOPAC	#				#			#			#
UCH-L1		#			#			#		#	
GBA		#		#							#
YKL-40		#									#
VILIP-1	#	#		#		#		#	#		#
TREM2	#				#				#	#	#
DJ-1	#				#	#		#	#		
SNAP25	#	#		#						#	#
BACE1	#							#		#	
neurogranin	#				#						#
chromatogranin A	#			#			#	#	#	#	
cystatin C		#				#					
Clusterin	#		#	#	#		#		#	#	
Progranulin	#	#			#	#	#	#		#	
DPRs											
GFAP											
MCP-1	#	#			#	#		#	#	#	
miRNA	#						#				
HVA		#			#	#	#		#	#	

Source: Adapted from Ref.[70]

based classifications of these diseases, which has allowed clinicians to overcome the diagnostic hurdles.[16]

In many neurological disorders, molecular diagnostics has emerged as a significant tool for diagnosis. Many hereditary NDs, for instance, have been defined and classified with the use of disease-causing gene mutation analysis. Alterations in patient pathologies, biochemistries, and genetics may provide us with in-depth knowledge on the nature of a disease. However, genetic counselling and careful thought are required before molecular testing is conducted. The following sections give a rundown of the most typical neurological disease, as well as the scope and potential of molecular diagnostics in identifying and treating them.[17,18]

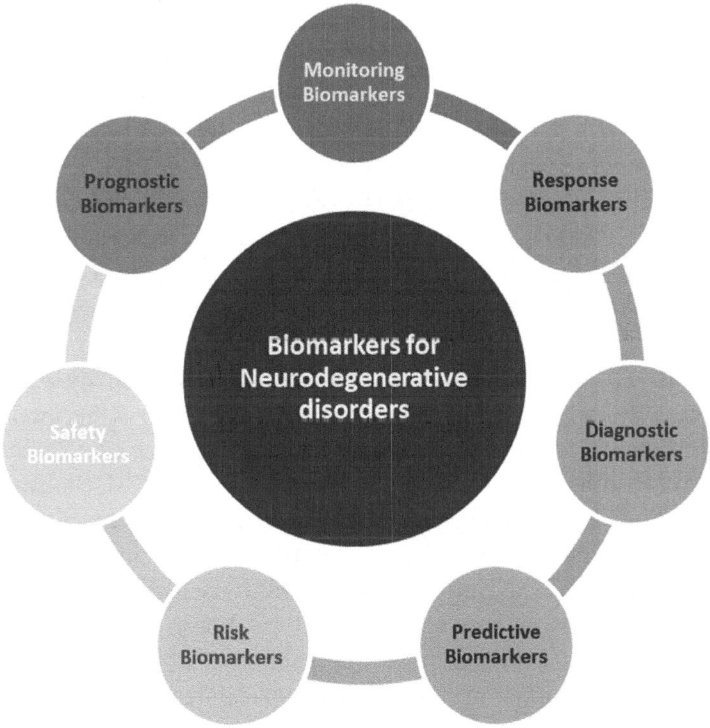

FIGURE 15.1 Biomarkers are categorized according to the primary clinical use for which they were developed.

15.3 ALZHEIMER'S DISEASE

Most cases of dementia are caused by AD. Clinically, it manifests mostly as episodic memory impairment and a slow, steady decline in mental capacity.

There are two main causes of dementia: amyloid (Alzheimer's plaques) and tau protein neurofibrillary tangles (NFT) provide morphological foundation. The present model differentiates between the "preclinical," "prodromal," and "clinical" phases of AD. Although Aβ deposits in the brain are to be anticipated at the preclinical stage, none of the typical clinical symptoms have yet been shown. When the onset of a cognitive problem does not yet demonstrate moderate cognitive impairment (MCI) with significant deficits in episodic memory, the condition does not meet the diagnostic criteria for dementia but also does not warrant a dementia diagnosis. While in the clinic, the symptoms of cognitive dysfunction become severe enough to impair the afflicted person's ability to carry out even the most basic daily tasks.[19] For treatments that have the potential to alter the disease's course, such as those under research and testing in clinical stages or those that need to be implemented at the right time, this idea is of paramount importance. The current national institute on aging-association (NIA-AA) Alzheimer's criteria advocate the use of many biomarkers, including hippocampus volumetry, FDG-PET, amyloid PET, and CSF biomarkers for the diagnosis and prediction of late-onset AD and separating MCI-AD from normal aging.[20] These biomarkers can aid in advancing the clinical diagnosis of AD to the initial stages of the illness. The major AD biomarkers are tau, specifically hyperphosphorylated tau-42, tau, and p-tau (especially phosphorylated form at position 181: p-tau181). Cortical amyloid deposition is reflected by Aβ-42, the severity of the neurodegenerative process by t-tau, and the intensity of neurofibrillary alterations by p-tau. Alzheimer's disease is diagnosed when cerebrospinal fluid (CSF) A42 levels are low and CSF t-tau and p-tau levels are high.[21] Taken as a whole, they can serve as a clinical biomarker to make a diagnosis before the onset of classic dementia symptoms including memory loss and disorientation. It is also recommended to look at the relationship between t-tau and A-42 or p-tau and A-42. These signs may help doctors distinguish AD from other illnesses that gradually decrease cognitive function, such as corticobasal degeneration (CBD) and progressive supranuclear palsy (PSP), as well as from depression, which can mirror cognitive impairment.[22] Protein levels in the CSF are consistent with normal standards for the pertinent clinical circumstances. The protein p-tau has been proposed as a diagnostic biomarker to distinguish between lysosomal storage disorder, frontotemporal dementia, and Alzheimer's disease (LSD). A differential diagnosis based on CSFA-40 is also advised. Despite A-40 being the most common type of A, there are no discernible changes in CSF levels between AD patients and healthy individuals. The A-42/A-40 ratio may be more helpful than A-42 alone in differentiating AD from non-AD dementias, such as PDD, DLB, and vascular dementia, due to the higher levels of A-40 detected in CSF in AD compared to PDD and DLB.[23]

AD is a gradual, degenerative sickness that destroys the neurons of the brain, resulting in forgetfulness, difficulty thinking and speaking, and behavioral abnormalities, and is the most prevalent NDs across most countries. As the illness progresses, a large number of neurons in the brain deteriorate, including those that use the neurotransmitter acetylcholine to interact with one another.[24] Although a lack of acetylcholine is the most obvious and common sign, changes in AChE and BuChE are also characteristic of the illness Alzheimer's. Plaques of extracellular senility (A peptides) and intracellular tau tangles are two forms of brain lesions observed in people with Alzheimer's disease NFTs (NFTs, composed of tau protein). The secretase produces the amyloid precursor protein; enzyme cleaves it (APP). Damage to axons carrying synaptic information results in synaptic degeneration or atrophy, and this is mediated by NFTs.[25] In NFTs, tau protein is hyperphosphorylated and insoluble, forming paired helical filaments (PHF). Diseases like Alzheimer's can be diagnosed and treated with the help of clinical observations and cognitive testing, such as neuropsychological evaluations, which impact emotional regulation, cognitive processing, and behavioral norms. A battery of neuropsychological tests, including tests of attention, memory, language, the ability to plan and reason, the ability to modify behavior, and others, can help the doctor and the family better understand neuropsychological tests, such as those that evaluate the effects of a disorder on a patient's day-to-day functioning and tests of personality and emotional stability. Brain amyloid plaques and neurofibrillary tangles provide conclusive postmortem evidence of the illness.[26] However, the illness process itself is a persistent phenomenon that causes major harm to the brain long before clinical signs arise. As a result, researchers from a variety of fields, including molecular biology, biomedicine, and biotechnology, are collaborating to create cutting-edge diagnostic molecular markers for AD that could one day be used for the identification of AD at an early stage and objective evaluation of treatment outcomes. The detection and diagnosis of AD have been aided by a number of genetic and biochemical diagnostic indicators.[27]

15.4 GENETIC MARKERS

Rarely, PD follows any familial trait that follows the autosomal-dominant or autosomal-recessive patterns described by Mendelian genetics. Patients with early-onset disease had mutations in parkin (PARK2), ubiquitin carboxy-terminal hydrolase L1 (UCH-L1), PTEN-induced putative kinase 1 (PINK1), and oncogene DJ, whereas those with late-onset disease had mutations in -synuclein (SNCA) and leucine-rich repeat kinase 2 (LRRK2). The alpha-synuclein gene on chromosome 4 is the site of the majority of cases of PD, including the incredibly rare early-onset familial variant.[28] These mutations can be either single mutations, duplications, or triplications. The single-gene autosomal-dominant PD variations' features have helped identify the disease's causal genes and associated by-products. Mitochondrial malfunction, oxidative stress, and poor control of faulty or aberrant gene product forms are all present in several mutant gene products in autosomal-dominant forms (such as oligomeric α-synuclein). There are approximately 70 variants in the major parkin gene that have been linked to early-onset PD in adults. About half of families with juvenile onset autosomal-recessive Parkinsonism likely contain a disease-causing mutation in the parkin gene. UCH-L1 is a ubiquitin carboxy-terminal hydrolase that is encoded by a gene on chromosome 4 deubiquitinating enzyme.[29] UCH-L1, which makes up about 1% of brain protein, is thought to hydrolyze ubiquitinated peptides to recycle ubiquitin. In the absence of this enzyme, damaged proteins might accumulate in hazardous amounts inside the cell. Additionally, specifically, two PINK1 homozygous mutations were discovered in families from Spain and Italy. With this discovery, the link between PINK1 mutations and PARK6 was strengthened even more. PARK7 is linked to DJ-1 gene mutations.[30] There is growing evidence linking the DJ-1 protein to neurodegeneration and oxidative stress. Parkinsonism DJ-1 is distinguished by a gradual onset of symptoms and a durable response to levodopa therapy. Discovering how these genes function in the body might provide light on the processes that keep neurons healthy in the brain.[31]

15.5 BIOCHEMICAL MARKERS

Two other significant biomarkers have been used to identify PD. Two of them are: (1) the presence of a protein called α-synuclein in the Lewy body lesions and (2) the loss of a protein called PET imaging of the dopamine transporter (DAT) Electrogenically, via Na+ and Cl- transport coupling,[32] DAT mediates dopamine (DA) absorption into dopaminergic neurons. It is anticipated that DA and cocaine (uptake blockers) will bind to the transporter's common and specific domains due to the transporter's sensitivity to cations. DAT's role in toxin absorption is important when it comes to Parkinson's illness. The detection of DAT concentration in the striatum has been theorized, and more specifically the putamen is the most accurate molecular diagnostic marker and the most sensitive method for the PD's early diagnosis. The hallmark brain lesions of Parkinson's disease (PD) and dementia, Lewy bodies and Lewy neuritis, were first identified following the discovery of two mutations in the -synuclein gene.[33] Due to its presence in other synucleinopathies, -synuclein should be used in concert with other diagnostic techniques to increase its specificity and sensitivity for PD. Single-photon emission computed tomography (SPECT) using [123I] and positron emission tomography (PET) with the [18F]-Dopa tracer -CIT are two imaging methods that have been used to diagnose PD.[34] Since PET only requires injecting small amounts of radioactive tracers or isotopes intravenously, it is the most efficient method for diagnosing PD. The amount of 18F-Dopa absorbed by the striatum of the brain in PD patients is around 40% less than that of controls. 18F-Dopa distribution is typically normal in patients with PD who are taking medication for the condition. In contrast to the very restricted clinical availability of the tracer [18F]-Dopa, the SPECT tracer ioflupane iodine-123 (DatSCAN) is frequently used to resemble the presynaptic DaT system of dopamine receptors. Unlike PET, which uses off-site storage for radioactive isotopes with lengthy half-lives, SPECT may keep such isotopes on-site.[35] Six age-matched healthy controls and 16 PD patients (9 men and 7 women) were involved in a recent SPECT imaging study using 99mTc-TRODAT-1 (4 men; 2 women; Shinto et al., 2014). Images were taken 3 h after the intravenous tracer was administered. 99mTc-specific TRODAT-1's striatal uptake was 3.77 ng/mL in healthy controls, 2.56 ng/mL in stage I Parkinson's disease patients, 1.57 ng/mL in stage II PD patients, and 0.63 ng/mL in stage III PD patients (P 0.05). To evaluate DAT activity, 99mTc-TRODAT-1 is reliable and readily accessible. Although these methods have the potential to enhance PD differential diagnosis, the issue of cost-effectiveness remains.[36] Biological fluids are a great place to seek biomarkers as they are convenient and inexpensive. Additionally, the proximity of biological fluids to cells accurately reflects their biological status. The potential for developing circulating biomarkers for PD is promising in light of rising recognition of miRNA's value in biofluids. People with Parkinson's disease (PD) have decreased peripheral blood levels of miR-1, miR-22-5p, and miR-29 compared to healthy individuals, whereas patients receiving treatment for

PD had greater levels of miR-16- 2-3p, miR-26a-2-3p, and miR30a. In a recent study using next-generation sequencing for whole blood leukocytes, 16 miRNAs, including miR-16, miR-20a, and miR-320, were reported to be significantly altered in PD patients compared to healthy controls.[37] There is not currently a single trustworthy test for diagnosing PD. There is not a definitive "biological marker" (test, scan, or blood sample) that researchers can utilize at the moment. A sophisticated brain scan that assesses the dopamine system and brain metabolism serves as the most objective test for Parkinson's disease. However, these exams are very costly and can only be done in dedicated imaging facilities.[38]

Biomarkers of the molecular interactions that characterize NDs may be located in both cerebrospinal fluid and blood. A biomarker that is sensitive to disease yet unique to brain alterations would be ideal for early diagnosis brought on by aging rather than the disease itself. Peripheral markers appear to be helpful alterations in brain function and cognitive ability in this setting, as well as remedies to diagnostic restrictions.[39] Brain tissue biochemical activities are immediately reflected in CSF, making it perhaps the most priceless of all bodily fluids. Creating the early preclinical detection of disease is made easier with the use of a central nerve system biological signature. On the other hand, blood plasma or serum monitoring of NDs is a less invasive and more easily accessible method.[40] Glymphatic system, lymphatic veins, and the hematoencephalic barrier-allow blood to interact with the brain. The analysis of blood, however, presents a number of challenges. For example, if the concentration of a biomarker from the brain or spinal cord is found in cerebrospinal fluid (CSF), its concentration will be substantially lower than if it were found with blood. When compared to the robust biological background created outside the CNS, the CNS contribution may be reduced if the biomarker is not CNS-specific but expressed in the peripheral organs and vice versa if the biomarker is not expressed in the peripheral tissues.[41]

15.6 BIOMARKER ANALYSIS

A variety of difficulties arise when trying to detect biomarkers of NDs in the blood, making it necessary to use assays that are both sensitive and specific. The central nervous system (CNS) and blood compartments are separated by the selective hematoencephalic barrier, which alters the blood's chemical composition. The cerebrospinal fluid (CSF) volume ration in blood contains significantly lower concentrations of CNS-derived proteins than CSF. Noninvasive and low-cost tests like biomarker analysis could be used in the first stage of a multi-step diagnosis process to distinguish between NDs. Early diagnosis and successful medical procedures and treatments are hampered by the diversity of NDs.[42] Differentiating between NDs subtypes based on shared molecular characteristics is facilitated by omics approaches, which also facilitate a deeper comprehension of the underlying chemical mechanisms driving disease progression. Methods including genomic sequencing, transcriptome and noncoding RNA profiling, epigenomics, proteomics, and metabolomics have all been developed to better understand illnesses (metabolomics). The pathogenesis of most human illnesses, including NDs, involves many molecular abnormalities that work simultaneously or synergistically. Omics studies are restricted in their diagnostic and therapeutic use since they can only identify markers along a single route.[43] They may simultaneously optimize accessible information, raise the likelihood of identifying the primary causes of the illness, and discover molecular abnormalities at many levels (genes, transcripts, protein production, and posttranslational mutations, cellular metabolic activity, etc). Using multi-omics investigations and omics profile characterizations, NDs may be examined in greater detail which provides a more holistic view of multifactorial disorders and lends credence to the creation of targeted and individualized therapeutics.[44] If the prerequisites for reproducibility and repeatability are met, they will reveal the most effective biomarkers for tracking the development of illness and the effectiveness of treatments designed to slow or stop its spread. Measuring proteins in exosomes might be a useful peripheral technique for identifying neuron-derived indicators. Compared to traditional methods of studying the CNS proteome, this method is less intrusive since it allows for the measurement of nucleic acid and protein levels in extracellular vesicles. Unfortunately, the ELISA technique lacks the sensitivity necessary to accurately detect and quantify CNS biomarker concentrations in plasma or serum. Highly sensitive and cutting-edge approaches, technology advancements, such as RNA sequencing (RNA-Seq) microarrays and the single molecule array (SIMOA) method, have substantially improved the identification of peripheral biomarkers, paving the path for the eventual development of blood biomarkers. They have the potential to be both a dependable indicator of treatment efficacy and a measure of target engagement.[45]

15.7 DIAGNOSTIC AND PROGNOSTIC BIOMARKERS FOR NDS

Glycoproteins as AD biomarkers include Aβ peptides (especially Aβ42) in the CSF, -tau or, p-tau, neurogranin (NRGN), neurofilament light chain protein (NEFL), myeloid-derived triggering receptor (TREM2) expressed on APP-cleaving enzyme 1 (BACE1), and chitinase (GAP-43).[46] Glycosylated proteins have been shown to constitute the majority of these biomarkers. BACE1 is a four-N-glycosite β-secretase that causes toxic APP cleavage and elevated amounts to draw a line in the middle of GlcNAc between AD's phases. Excessive O-GalNAcylation of APP has been shown to reduce Aβ synthesis, and N-glycans, O-GlcNAc, and O-GalNAc of the mucin type have all been found to have an effect on the APP protein. An increase in the O-glycosylation of certain Tyr residues was found in CSF Aβ peptides from AD patients compared to non-AD patients by mass spectrometry. The improved kinase substrate properties of N-glycosylated tau compared to the native form suggest that it may be useful for treating tau-related disorders to enhance hyperphosphorylation, which begins before N-glycosylation in the AD brain.[47] In addition, tau N-glycans have been shown to be crucial in maintaining the helical shape of tau filaments (PHF). Reduced tau phosphorylation and O-GlcNAcylation resulted from this cross-talk in the AD brain. The protein's stability is compromised by elevated O-GlcNAcylation of tau aggregation, according to in vitro studies. As a result, researchers have come up with a new way to treat tau disease by inhibiting the enzyme responsible for removing O-GlcNAc.[48] MK-8719, a new selective OGA inhibitor, has only recently entered phase 1 clinical trials. Recent studies have detailed the N-glycan profile in AD patients' cerebrospinal fluid, using MS as a model system. Patients, especially women, exhibit more fucosylated and bisected GlcNAc structures and less high-mannose N-glycans than healthy controls. Bisected GlcNAc patients with higher levels were observed in individuals with mild cognitive impairment and Alzheimer's disease.[49] Additionally, it was discovered that CSF N-glycans may be used to identify AD pathology early in all MCI patients who developed AD during clinical follow-up. This supports earlier research's findings that highly branched glycoforms and bisected N-glycans were more prevalent in AD patients' CSF and blood serum. The lower concentrations of sialylated N-glycans observed in serum and postmortem brains of Alzheimer's disease patients may be explained by decreased sialyltransferase activity. Alzheimer's disease (AD) patients' cerebrospinal fluid (CSF) was shown to have differing levels of N-glycosylation of C1-inhibitor (CI) and -1-acid glycoprotein (AGP) than healthy controls (AGP). The levels of p-tau and t-tau in AD CSF were found to be correlated with the amounts of N-glycans containing bisecting GlcNAc in the CSF of the SCI patient group, according to MS-based glycomics. The levels of A peptide and p-tau in cerebral fluid were also significantly higher in

AD patients compared to a control group, and these results were obtained using DNA sequencer-assisted, fluorophore-assisted carbohydrate electrophoresis (CSF) which are likewise directly related to NA2F (DSA-FACE).[50] The focus of traditional PD diagnosis is on symptom evaluation, which can delay the identification of underlying pathophysiological problems. For this reason, it is crucial to identify accurate biomarkers for Parkinson's disease that can aid in diagnosis and prognosis. Biomarkers in plasma and spinal fluid include alpha-synuclein, lysosomal enzymes, A peptides, tau, and neuron-specific fMRI ligand (NEFL), have been hypothesized to be especially useful for diagnosis.[51] In comparison to healthy controls, people with Parkinson's disease had lower amounts of total -synuclein in their CSF. However, PD patients are more likely to have phosphorylated and oligomeric alpha-synuclein. Patients with PD had elevated amounts of oligomeric alpha-synuclein in their serum and red blood cells. Cerebrospinal fluid (CSF) lysosomal enzyme activity was decreased in PD patients. Prognostic evaluation for PD may be enhanced by combining the use of conventional AD biomarkers (such as CSF A42, t-tau, and p-tau) with other assays. Increased levels of the axonal protein NEFL are linked to several NDs, including AD, ALS, and FTD. It has been suggested that the concentration of NEFL in the plasma can be utilized as a biomarker of PD severity and progression, and that it can also be used to reliably differentiate CSF samples of PD and atypical parkinsonian syndromes (APSs) O-GlcNAcylation of -synuclein which has been demonstrated using proteomics analysis. In vivo toxicity, aggregation tendency, and stability of the A non-A component (NAC) are all influenced by the presence of many O-glycosides. O-GlcNAcylation at Tyr72 and Ser87 of -synuclein may inhibit the protein's ability to form aggregates. Alpha-synuclein aggregation is associated with O-GlcNAcylation of Tyr72 and Ser87, which prevents calpain-mediated cleavage.[53] Next-generation biomarkers of chronic illnesses may include N-glycosylated IgG even when comparing N-glycosylation patterns between healthy controls and AD patients, there is no obvious difference. However, when IgG N-glycans in the plasma of PD patients were examined using ultra-performance liquid chromatography, a statistically significant difference between PD cases and healthy controls was found for seven N-glycan peaks and 11 derived characteristics (UPLC). Through capillary electrophoresis-twin-quadrupole mass spectrometry, other researchers found that sialylation was decreased on tri-antennary glycans containing 2, 3-linked sialic acids, while fucosylation was increased in the serum N-glycans of PD patients.[54]

15.8 BIOMARKERS FOR OTHER NDS

Despite extensive research, no effective treatments exist for HD, a progressive ND that affects progressively more people over time. Mutant Huntingtin (mHTT) proteins and immune-related indicators such IL-6, IL-8, proteins like NEFL, t-tau/p-tau, and CHI3L1 are considered promising biomarkers for this condition. Bioinformatic predictions indicate that these proteins are glycosylated or may be glycosylated.[55] It was shown that inhibiting reduced toxicity of the mutant mHTT protein is achieved through O-induction GlcNAcylation's of autophagy and suppression of mHTT aggregation in neural cells. This result is in line with that of a mouse model that demonstrated the pathophysiology of HD is significantly influenced by the control of O-GlcNAc expression. By analyzing glycans using mass spectrometry, it was discovered that HD transgenic mice had more compared to non-HD transgenic mice; they had more core-fucosylated N-glycans, sialylated biantennary N-glycans, and bisected GlcNAc N-glycans in their brains.[56] Dyskinesia may be one of the symptoms of ALS, a fast-developing non-demyelinating ND. There is currently no treatment for this fatal illness. TDP-43 protein and NEFL protein are biofluid indicators for ALS. Reduced OGlcNAc levels have been shown that a mutation in the glycosyltransferase GLT8D1 hinders the normal O-GlcNAc synthesis in the transgenic mice model of ALS group, addition to proteins is necessary for axonal and synaptic function. Patients with ALS had a higher concentration of sialylated glycans and a lower concentration of core-fucosylated glycans in their blood, according to an analysis of N-glycan profiles.[57] Biomarkers for ALS (ALS-IgG) include the IgG-derived glycan specifically, A2BG2 (N-linked oligosaccharides at Asn 297 of IgG Fc sections), which has been related to neuronal damage. The Gal-index, a measure of galactosylation structures, was considerably greater among patients with ALS versus non-ALS subjects after further analysis of CSF IgG N-glycans. Demyelination, inflammation, and neurodegeneration are hallmarks of MS, a disease that disproportionately affects young individuals. Another recognized sign is oligoclonal bands (OCB) IgG and lipid-specific IgM are generated in the cerebrospinal fluid (CSF) and blood.[58] A number of additional proteins, including nuclear envelope-localized (NEFL) protein and glial fibrillary acidic protein (GFAP), CHI3L1 protein, soluble CD163 (sCD163) protein, and the CSF IgG index, are also used. In order to track the development of MS, an N-glucosylated peptide probe called CSF114(Glc) may prove to be an invaluable tool. Analysis of IgG Fc glycosylation in MS patients has shown that there is a shift in the pattern of glycosylation on IgG1 in the cerebrospinal fluid, but not in the blood. Disease severity is associated with the glycocalyx (GLX), which may represent a novel group of biomarkers for MS.[59]

15.9 LIMITATIONS OF EXISTING BIOMARKERS

A biomarker is a physiologically meaningful signature with potential applications in illness screening, diagnosis, prognosis, staging, and therapy response monitoring. The best biomarkers would not only be very sensitive and specific but also easy to get from patients with little discomfort. Significant search for a potential ND biofluid has advanced indicators during the last several decades. These biomarkers were found using blood and CSF samples. Due to their proximity to the brain and spinal cord, biomarkers identified in CSF frequently have higher sensitivity and specificity.[60] The most thoroughly investigated biofluid biomarkers for AD which have undergone the most rigorous clinical trial validation are CSF A42, t-tau, and p-tau. Nonetheless, compared to blood, CSF is not easily accessible for samples. It is more efficient financially and time-wise to use blood biomarkers than CSF biomarkers. However, due to the absence of particular biomarkers that may yield consistent findings in various labs, valid blood biomarkers are still being created[61] for the diagnosis of ND. High blood levels of albumin and IgG could confound analysis of the target proteins. Brain alterations could not be reflected in blood because brain proteins are constantly being broken down and digested. Important biological proteins associated with NDs are prime candidates for use as diagnostic biomarkers. It is challenging to depend on a single biomarker for an accurate diagnosis of ND due to the variability of ND pathophysiology. Therefore, it is important to find new indicators that may shed light on the pathophysiology of ND.[62] Using a panel of biomarkers looks more viable for future clinical applications due to the potential for increased sensitivity, specificity, and predictive values, which may be limited by using a single biomarker alone. Current biomarkers may not be illness-specific because of the common disease pathophysiology across NDs. Both tau pathology and increased levels of CSF tau are seen in various forms of dementia that are not caused by AD. After the damage to neurons or axons, the concentration of the NEFL protein, which is found in the axonal cytoskeletons, rises.[63] Due to its lack of specificity, NEFL has been investigated for a wide variety of NDs (including FTD, PD, ALS, and MS), all of which lack a universally accepted biomarker categorization scheme. Therefore, it is crucial to identify novel targeted disease biomarkers that can differentiate among ND subtypes. The structural examination of already-established disease-specific glycoforms together with a high level of glycosides and bisected GlcNAc, proteins are examples of biomarkers may potentially lead to improved predictive values. As far as we are aware, there are no biofluid indicators that are currently accepted for use in the regular clinical diagnosis of NDs. A new generation of biomarkers (NGBs) is desperately needed for early and precise diagnosis. These biomarkers may be found in glycoproteins. Most proteins in human biofluids are glycosylated, according to the literature.[64] This is notably true for extracellular matrix and membrane proteins. The functions of immunological molecules, enzymes, hormones, transporters, and receptors are all influenced by these ubiquitous glycoproteins. Illness-specific glycosylation and the development of disease are both possible. Additionally, it was shown that patients' blood plasma had higher levels of N-glycan branching and sialylation than healthy controls did. Additionally, the disease's development and prognosis were both correlated with the glycan changes that occurred. Similarly, a disease's distinctive glycosylation may provide a panel of putative biomarkers that, when paired with machine learning techniques, might significantly enhance both diagnosis and prognosis. Extracellular vesicles (EVs), of which exosomes are a subtype, have emerged as a potentially fruitful new route for identifying ND biomarkers. These tiny vesicles carry disease-causing molecules and facilitate cell-to-cell communication. The future of NGB discovery may lie in the analysis of exosome content (particularly glycoproteins) extracted from common biofluids (blood or CSF).[53]

Motor neuron disease, or amyotrophic lateral sclerosis (ALS), is a deadly ND that comes in a wide variety of forms, the causes of which are still poorly understood. Upper motor neuron (UMN) and/or lower motor neuron (LMN) degeneration in the primary motor cortex, brain stem, and spinal cord characterize this disorder. ALS has long been thought of being a neurodegenerative disorder that attacks motor neurons and causes weakness and atrophy in affected individuals.[54] However, there is mounting evidence that suggests it is a multisystem disorder that affects not only motor but also extramotor areas; it causes a variety of cognitive, behavioral, and dysautonomic symptoms. Even though 10% of ALS cases have familial ties and 90% of ALS cases occur sporadically, the presence of a family history of the condition is surprisingly common. In certain prospective studies where genealogies have been thoroughly examined, the prevalence of familial history climbs to 17–23%.[57] Around 60% of instances in families had the underlying mutation identified. The C9ORF72 expansion is the most prevalent genetic change in European populations, subsequent to shifts in SOD1, TARDBP, and FUS. However, among families with a history of sporadic ALS, mutations in genes involved in the disease have been discovered. It is likely that ALS results from a confluence of several different pathogenic pathways, some of which we do not yet understand. The pathobiology of ALS is influenced by a multitude of molecular processes, such as oxidative stress, mitochondrial dysfunction, excitotoxicity, protein aggregation, decreased axonal transport, neuroinflammation, and dysregulated RNA signaling.[48] Histopathologically, ALS is characterized by the loss of motor neurons in the spinal cord and motor cortex as well as the degeneration of the corticospinal tract. The precentral gyrus atrophy, corticospinal tract atrophy, sclerosis, and pallor and atrophy of the hypoglossal nerve and the ventral roots of the spinal cord are the three most obvious gross degenerative abnormalities in the neurological system. Motor cortex big pyramidal neurons and spinal cord motor neurons are lost, and the remaining motor neurons become atrophic and basophilic. A wide range of astrocytosis in the motor cortex's gray matter and underlying subcortical white matter indicates varied levels of astrocyte activation and proliferation, suggesting complex cellular responses within these regions. The hallmarks of ALS include muscle wasting, exhaustion, and eventually death from respiratory failure,[22] which often presents itself initially in the extremities or bulbar musculature. Even while 2–3 years is the average survival time after the onset of symptoms, it can vary greatly. As a result, the beginning site of the disease (bulbar vs. spinal), the relative mix of UMN and LMN involvement, the rate of disease progression, the age at which symptoms first appear, and the presence of extra-motor symptoms all have a role in the vast range of phenotypic presentation and prognosis of ALS. UMN symptoms predominate over LMN symptoms to variable degrees in illnesses such as primary lateral sclerosis (PLS) and progressive muscular atrophy (PMA). It is still possible to diagnose ALS by eliminating clinical and electrophysiological LMN signs and by eliminating ALS mimics.[61] Patients are placed into one of three certainty categories (definite, probable, or potential) based on the number of afflicted regions (bulbar, cervical, dorsal, or lumbar) and current diagnostic criteria (the revised El Escorial criteria or the more recent Awaji criteria). Specificity of these criteria is high, but their sensitivity is low due to the fact that they are meant to be used in research and clinical trials rather than ordinary treatment. Both the clinical variability of ALS and the lack of a reliable UMN biomarker[46] contribute to a lengthy diagnosis delay (of up to 12 months in incomplete morphologies), delaying the start of potentially neuroprotective therapy. Clinical studies have many difficulties, such as trouble finding participants and analyzing the data. Therefore, ALS biomarkers (particularly those from the University of Minnesota) are essential for both clinical use and research. Misdiagnoses of amyotrophic lateral sclerosis would decrease with the use of the most efficient UMN biomarkers (ALS). They should aid in our understanding of the processes behind the progression and signs of amyotrophic lateral sclerosis. They should also be helpful as biological markers for assessing the effectiveness of novel medicines in the clinic and the laboratory, as well as prognostic indicators for patients.[46]

15.10 BIOMARKERS IN IMAGING: AN OVERVIEW

When it comes to magnetic resonance (MR), radiologists typically rely on imaging findings generated from specialized tests performed in specific clinical circumstances in accordance with precise protocols designed to emphasize the predicted signs of the disease; qualitative integration and appraisal of these data. Due to the MR signal's and image reconstructions' digital nature obtained, we can use them to extract quantitative information about the picture's properties, such as parameters of biological models, such as gray matter iron deposits, and descriptions of texture or shape. Quantitative imaging biomarkers cannot be used in the clinic without first being processed through the radiomic pipeline and then having structured reports generated. Data collection, image analysis, VIO delineation, data extraction, statistical analysis, and result presentation are all part of the process.[65] Relevant data amounts and extraction requirements are defined with the help of computational medical imaging tools. This branch of radiology analyzes digitally acquired images to describe imaging facts pertinent to the patient, studying characteristics and actions of tissues. The information obtained must be reliable and honest.[66] The radiomic high-dimensional information retrieved from images may be mined for descriptive, predictive, and prognostic models. The estimated values are considered biomarkers if they can be tested reliably and serve as indications of regular biological processes, pathological alterations, or drug reactions. Information of a quantitative nature, such as the location and strength of an event, can be used to show feature, can be retrieved from medical pictures using subrogated features and parameters will thus be known as imaging biomarkers.[55] The computational images are spatially (via parametric analysis) and temporally (via voxelization) resolved (as a longitudinal evaluation). The main areas of research interest include susceptibility and risk factors for disease, accurate diagnosis and differential diagnosis of suspected diseases, individualized grading of lesions, disease classification and staging, lesion phenotyping, patient prognosis and expected natural history, best treatment options, assessment of potentially image-guided interventions, and treatment effects.[23] Patient outcomes (including survival, QoL, and symptom alleviation) and disease severity condition are the primary clinical objectives against which the validity of the specified biomarkers may be assessed (lesion phenotype and progression). Contrary to multimodality imaging, which combines two modalities to overcome the limits of single-parameter analysis, multiparametric imaging tackles the radiomic parameters voxel-by-voxel, the shortcomings of each, while maximizing their individual benefits, as in PET/CT. Clinical use precludes the resolution of variability.[44] Test–retest data sets can be used to attribute variation among patients to acquisition mistakes and bio/physiological changes, whereas independent data sets can be utilized to evaluate the effects of different MR acquisition methodologies, scanner manufacturers, and healthcare institutions. Expected precision values provide a measure of these reproducibility and repeatability doubts. Signals from many different structures and components are combined to form the voxel's reconstructed image attributes, which may lead to flaws in repeatability. As a result, a measurement based on an image must have a direct and unmistakable connection to the process it purports to quantify equivalent to the underlying physical reality.[67] Biases must be managed during data collection as well as in post-processing steps for reliable results. Variations in image acquisition (from different places, vendors, procedures, and patient preparation) and image processing can impact the accuracy of the measurements (computational model, social dynamics). Reliability of a biomarker, however, requires both phantom calibration (relative error to synthetic ground truth) and pathological truth (relative error to current gold standards, such as biopsy). There are two main ways in which clinical endpoints can be evaluated: prospectively (using their ability to diagnose and treat lesions and diseases) and retrospectively (using their ability to predict patients' outcomes).[68] Before being used in a clinical setting, imaging biomarkers should have at least one validation study demonstrating their precision, accuracy, and utility in that setting. The application of artificial intelligence through the use of machine learning technologies will have an impact on automatic segmentation, identifying tissue changes and trends, and categorizing patients (such as neural networks, deep learning, random forests, and support vector machines). Models for early patient stratification and prediction based on macroscopic MR imaging features can be constructed, trained, and validated with the help of machine learning. These techniques are not restricted to MR imaging alone; instead, they can be utilized in tandem with a wide variety of other imaging approaches as well as clinical, molecular, and genetic indicators to provide a more complete picture of the pathology at hand.[52]

15.11 CONCLUSION

The relevance of biomarkers in identifying NDs is a particularly fascinating and researched issue. To effectively treat proteinopathies, researchers must first identify an accurate biomarker that might be used to help distinguish between clinical-diagnostic units or differentiate illness presentations across a wider range of proteinopathies, including their course and treatments. Currently, diagnostic procedures rely on a variety of biomarkers that have either been identified and are being investigated, or whether biochemical indicators are found by standard testing. Blood samples are examined for the presence of biomarkers exhibiting the major characteristics of neurodegenerative disorders (NDs), with a particular focus on their concentrations in the cerebral spinal fluid, thus establishing significant correlations for diagnostic purposes. Even in the absence of disease-modifying medicines, early and precise diagnosis is essential for the therapy of NDs. Clinical trials of novel therapeutics for altering the course of the disease and the eventual administration of these medications to correct diagnosis are crucial in identifying people in need of cognitive rehabilitation before irreversible neuronal injury and loss create cognitive deficiencies. Standard clinical practice stands to benefit greatly from the discovery of new biomarkers using novel and sensitive state-of-the-art technology. Dementias caused by neurodegenerative diseases: new algorithms for detection, diagnosis, and monitoring cannot be created without further research verifying the current findings.

KEYWORDS

- **neurodegeneration**
- **cerebrospinal fluid**
- **biological markers**
- **biomarkers**
- **blood-based biomarkers**
- **neurodegenerative diseases**
- **Alzheimer's disease**
- **Parkinson's disease**

REFERENCES

1. Koníčková, D.; Menšíková, K.; Tučková, L.; Hényková, E.; Strnad, M.; Friedecký, D.; Stejskal, D.; Matěj, R.; Kǎnovský, P. Biomarkers of Neurodegenerative Diseases: Biology, Taxonomy, Clinical Relevance, and Current Research Status. *Biomedicines* **2022,** *10*, 1760. https://doi.org/ 10.3390/biomedicines10071760.
2. Basha, F. H.; Waseem, M.; Srinivasan, H. Cellular and Molecular Mechanism in Neurodegeneration: Possible Role of Neuroprotectants. *Cell Biochem. Funct.* **2021,** *39*, 613–622.
3. Cova, I.; Priori, A. Diagnostic Biomarkers for Parkinson's Disease at a Glance: Where Are We? *J. Neural Transm.* **2018,** *125*, 1417–1432.
4. He, R.; Yan, X.; Guo, J.; Xu, Q.; Tang, B.; Sun, Q. Recent Advances in Biomarkers for Parkinson's disease. *Front. Aging Neurosci.* **2018,** *10*, 305.
5. Blennow, K.; Zetterberg, H. The Past and Future of Alzheimer's Disease Fluid Biomarkers. *J. Alzehimers Dis.* **2018,** *62*, 1125–1140.
6. Zou, K.; Abdullah, M.; Michikawa, M. Current Biomarkers for Alzheimer's Disease: From CSF to Blood. *J. Pers. Med.* **2020,** *10*, 85.
7. Agosta, F.; Spinelli, E. G.; and Filippi, M. Neuroimaging in Amyotrophic Lateral Sclerosis: Current and Emerging Uses. *Expert Rev. Neurother.* **2018,** *18*, 395–406. DOI: 10.1080/14737175.2018.1463160.
8. Lee, J. M.; Blennow, K.; Andreasen, N.; Laterza, O.; Modur, V.; Olader, J.; Gao, F.; Ohlendorf, M.; Landenson, J. H. The brain injury biomarker VLP-1 Is Increased in the Cerebrospinal Fluid of Alzheimer Disease Patients. *Clin. Chem.* **2008,** *54*, 1617–1623; Hansson, O. Biomarkers for Neurodegenerative Diseases. *Nat. Med.* **2021,** *27*, 954–963.
9. Dharmadasa, T.; Huynh, W.; Tsugawa, J.; Shimatani, Y.; Ma, Y.; Kiernan, M. C. Implications of Structural and Functional Brain Changes in Amyotrophic Lateral Sclerosis. *Expert Rev. Neurother.* **2018,** *18*, 407–419. DOI: 10.1080/14737175.2018.1464912
10. Hermann, P.; Appleby, B.; Brandel, J. P.; Caoughey, B.; Collins, S.; Geschwind, M. D.; Green, A.; Haïk, S.; Kovacs, G. G.; Ladogana, A. et al. Biomarkers and Diagnostic Guidelines for Sporadic Creutzfeldt-Jakob Disease. *Lancet Neurol.* **2021,** *20*, 235–246.
11. Donatelli, G.; Ceravolo, R.; Frosini, D.; Tosetti, M.; Bonuccelli, U.; Cosottini, M. Present and Future of Ultra-High Field MRI in Neurodegenerative Disorders. *Curr. Neurol. Neurosci. Rep.* **2018,** *18*, 31. DOI: 10.1007/ s11910-018-0841-7
12. Rusina, R.; Matěj, R.; Cséfalvay, Z.; Keller, J.; Franková, V.; Vyhnálek, M. Frontotemporální demence. *Cesk. Slov. Neurol. N* **2021,** *84* (117), 9–29.
13. Donatelli, G.; Retico, A.; Caldarazzo Ienco, E.; Cecchi, P.; Costagli, M.; Frosini, D. et al. Semiautomated Evaluation of the Primary Motor Cortex in Patients with Amyotrophic Lateral Sclerosis at 3T. *Am. J. Neuroradiol.*, **2018,** *39*, 63–69. DOI: 10.3174/ajnr.A5423
14. Martinez-Murcia, F. J.; Gorriz, J. M.; Ramirez, J.; Ortiz, A. Convolutional Neural Networks for Neuroimaging in Parkinson's Disease: Is Preprocessing Needed? *Int. J. Neural Syst.* **2018**. DOI: 10.1142/S0129065718500351
15. Vázquez-Costa, J. F.; Martínez-Molina, M.; Fernández-Polo, M.; Fornés-Ferrer, V.; Frasquet-Carrera, M.; Sevilla-Mantecón, T. Analysis of the Pathway and Diagnostic Delay of Amyotrophic Lateral Sclerosis in Valencian Community. *Neurologia* **2018.**
16. Vázquez-Costa, J. F.; Mazón, M.; Carreres-Polo, J.; Hervás, D.; Pérez-Tur, J.; Martí Bonmatí, L. et al. Brain Signal Intensity Changes as Biomarkers in Amyotrophic Lateral Sclerosis. *Acta Neurol. Scand.* **2018,** *137*, 262–271. DOI: 10.1111/ ane.12863

17. Yamashita, R.; Nishio, M.; Do, R. K. G.; Togashi, K. Convolutional Neural Networks: An Overview and Application in Radiology. *Insights Imaging* **2018**. DOI: 10.1007/s13244-018-0639-9.
18. Bruzová, M.; Rusina, R.; Stejskalová, Z.; Matěj, R. Autopsy–Diagnosed Neurodegenerative Dementia Cases Support the Use of Cerebrospinal Fluid Protein Biomarkers in Diagnostic Work–Up. *Sci. Rep.* **2021,** *11*, 10837.
19. Saijo, E.; Metrick, M. A.; Koga, S.; Parchi, P.; Litvan, I.; Spina, S.; Boxer, A.; Rojas, J. C.; Galasko, D.; Kraus, A. et al. 4–Repeat Tau Seeds and Templating Subtypes as Brain and CSF Biomarkers of Frontotemporal Lobar Degeneration. *Acta Neuropathol.* **2020,** *139*, 63–77.
20. Metrick, M. A.; Ferreira, N. d. C.; Saijo, E.; Kraus, A.; Newell, K.; Zanusso, G.; Vendruscolo, M.; Ghetti, B.; Caughey, B. A. single ultrasensitive assay for detection and discrimination of tau aggregates of Alzheimer and Pick diseases. *Acta Neuropathol. Commun.* **2020,** *8*, 22.
21. Baiardi, S.; Rizzi, R.; Capellari, S.; Bartoletti-Stella, A.; Zangrandi, A.; Gasparini, F.; Ghidoni, E.; Parchi, P. Gerstmann–Sträussler–Scheinker disease (PRNP p.D202N) Presenting with Atypical Parkinsonism. *Neurol. Genet.* **2020,** *6*, e400.
22. Chelliah, S. S.; Bhuvanendran, S.; Magalingam, K. B.; Kamarudin, M. N. A.; Radharkrishnan, A. K. Identification of Blood–Based Biomarkers for Diagnosis and Prognosis of Parkinson's Disease: A Systematic Review of Proteomics Studies. *Aging Res. Rev.* **2022,** *73*, 101514.
23. Lawton, M.; Baig, F.; Toulson, G.; Morovat, A.; Evetts, S. G.; Ben-Shlomo, Y.; Hu, M. T. Blood Biomarkers with Parkinson's Disease Clusters and Prognosis: The Oxford Discovery Cohort. *Mov. Disord.* **2020,** *35*, 279–287.
24. Altuna-Azkargorta, M.; Mendioroz-Iriarte, M. Blood Biomarkers in Alzheimer's Disease. *Neurologia* **2021,** *36*, 704–710.
25. Toombs, J.; Zetterberg, H. In the Blood: Biomarkers for Amyloid Pathology and Neurodegeneration in Alzheimer's Disease. *Brain Commun.* **2020,** *2*, fcaa054.
26. Lopez, O. L.; Klunk, W. E.; Mathis, C. A.; Snitz, B. E.; Chang, Y.; Tracy, R. P.; Kuller, L. H. Relationship of Amyloid–β1–42 in Blood and Brain Amyloid: Ginkgo Evaluation of Memory Study. *Brain Commun.* **2020,** *2*, fcz038.
27. Zvěřová, M. Přehled známých fluidních biomarkerů neurodegenerativních změn v mozku u Alzheimerovy choroby a možnosti jejich využití. *Ces A Slov. Psychiat.* **2019,** *115*, 77–80.
28. Barkovits, K.; Kruse, N.; Linden, A.; Tönges, L.; Pfeiffer, K.; Mollenhauer, B.; Marcus, K. Blood Contamination in CSF and Its Impact on Quantitative Analysis of Alpha–Synuclein. *Cells* **2020,** *9*, 370.
29. Gaetani, L.; Paoletti, F. P.; Bellomo, G.; Mancini, A.; Simoni, S.; Di Filipo, M.; Parnetti, L. CSF and Blood Biomarkers in Neuroinflammatory and Neurodegenerative Diseases: Implications for Treatment. *Trend Pharmacol. Sci.* **2020,** *41*, 1023–1037.
30. Zetterberg, H.; Blennow, K. From Cerebrospinal Fluid to Blood: The Third Wave of Fluid Biomarkers of Alzheimer's Disease. *J. Alzheimers Dis.* **2018,** *64*, 271–279.
31. Zetterberg, H.; Burnham, S. C. Blood–Based Molecular Biomarkers for Alzheimer's Disease. *Mol. Brain* **2019,** *12*, 26.
32. Congata, V. L.; Morello, G.; Cavallaro, S. Omics Data and Their Integrative Analysis to Support Stratified Medicine in Neurodegenerative Diseases. *Int. Mol. Sci.* **2021,** *22*, 4820.
33. Baldacci, F.; Mazzucchi, S.; Vecchia, A. D.; Giampietri, L.; Giannini, N.; Koronyo-Hamaoui, M.; Ceravolo, R.; Siciliano, G.; Boniccelli, U.; Elahi, F. M. et al. The Path to

Biomarker–Based Diagnostic Criteria for the Spectrum of Neurodegenerative Diseases. *Expert Rev. Mol. Diagn.* **2020,** *20*, 421–441.

34. Obrocki, P.; Khatun, A.; Ness, D.; Senkevich, K.; Hanrieder, J.; Capraro, F.; Mattsson, N.; Andreasson, U.; Portelius, E.; Ashton, N. J. et al. Perspectives in Fluid Biomarkers in Neurodegeneration from the 2019 Biomarkers in Neurodegenerative Diseases Course—A Joint PhD Student Course at University College London and University of Gothenburg. *Alzheimers Res. Ther.* **2020,** *12*, 20.
35. Yu, H.; Sun, T.; An, J.; Wen, L.; Liu, F.; Bu, Z.; Cui, Y.; Feng, J. Potential Roles of Exosomes in Parkinson's Disease: From Pathogenesis, Diagnosis, and Treatment to Prognosis. *Front. Cell Dev. Biol.* **2020,** *8*, 86.
36. Wang, X.; Zhou, Y.; Gao, Q.; Ping, D.; Wang, Y.; Wu, W.; Lin, X.; Fang, Y.; Zhang, J.; Shao, A. The Role of Exosomal microRNAs and Oxidative Stress in Neurodegenerative Diseases. *Oxidative Med. Cell. Longev.* **2020,** *2020*, 3232869.
37. Kitamura, Y.; Kojima, M.; Kurosawa, T.; Sasaki, R.; Ichihara, S.; Hiraku, Y.; Tomimoto, H.; Murata, M.; Oikawa, S. Proteomic Profiling of Exosomal Proteins for Blood–Based Biomarkers in Parkinson's Disease. *Neuroscience* **2018,** *392*, 121–128.
38. Console, L.; Scalise, M.; Indiveri, C. Exosomes in Inflammation and Role as Biomarkers. *Clin. Chim. Acta* **2019,** *488*, 165–171. [CrossRef] 47. Meldolesi, J. News About the Role of Fluid and Imaging Biomarkers in Neurodegenerative Diseases. *Biomedicines* **2021,** *9*, 252.
39. Gagliardi, D.; Bresolin, N.; Comi, G. P.; Corti, S. Extracellular Vesicles and Amyotrophic Lateral Sclerosis: From Misfolded Protein Vehicles to Promising Clinical Biomarkers. *Cell Mol. Life Sci.* **2021,** *78*, 561–572.
40. Htike, T. T.; Mishra, S.; Kumar, S.; Padmanabhan, P.; Gulyás, B. Peripheral Biomarkers for Early Detection of Alzheimer's and Parkinson's Diseases. *Mol. Neurobiol.* **2019,** *56*, 2256–2277. [CrossRef] 50. Shao, Y.; Le, W. Recent Advances and Perspectives of Metabolomics–Based Investigations in Parkinson's Disease. *Mol. Neurodegener.* **2019,** *14*, 3.
41. Angelopoulou, E.; Paudel, Y. N., Piperi, C. miR–124 and Parkinson's Disease: A Biomarker with Therapeutic Potential. *Pharm. Res.* **2019,** *150*, 104515.
42. Jiang, C.; Hopfner, F.; Katsikoudi, A.; Hein, R.; Catli, C.; Evetts, S.; Huang, Y.; Wang, H.; Ryder, J. W.; Kuhlenbaeumer, G. et al. Serum Neuronal Exosomes Predict and Differentiate Parkinson's Disease from Atypical Parkinsonism. *J. Neurol. Neurosurg. Psychiatry* **2020,** *91*, 720–729.
43. Lin, Y. S.; Lee, W. J.; Wang, S. J.; Fuh, J. L. Levels of Plasma Neurofilament Light Chain and Cognitive Function in Patients with Alzheimer or Parkinson Disease. *Sci. Rep.* **2018,** *8*, 17368.
44. Parnetti, L.; Gaetani, L.; Eusebi, P.; Paciotti, S.; Hansson, O.; El-Agnaf, O.; Mollenhauer, B.; Blennow, K.; Calabresi, P. CSF and Blood Biomarkers for Parkinson's Disease. *Lancet Neurol.* **2019,** *18*, 573–586.
45. Pilotto, A.; Imarisio, A.; Conforti, F.; Scalvini, A.; Masciocchi, S.; Nocivelli, S.; Turrone, R.; Gipponi, S.; Cottini, E.; Borroni, B. et al. Plasma NfL, Clinical Subtypes and Motor Progression in Parkinson's Disease. *Parkinsonism Relat. Disord.* **2021,** *87*, 41–47.
46. Pinell, J. R.; Cui, M.; Tieu, K. Exosomes in Parkinson Disease. *J. Neurochem.* **2021,** *157*, 413–428.
47. Karikari, T. K.; Pascoal, T. A.; Ashton, N. J.; Janelidze, S.; Benedet, A. L.; Rodriguez, J. L.; Chamoun, M.; Savard, M.; Kang, M. S.; Therriault, J. et al. Blood Phosphorylated

Tau 181 as a Biomarker for Alzheimer's Disease: A Diagnostic Performance and Prediction Modelling Study Using Data from Four Prospective Cohorts. *Lancet Neurol.* **2020,** *19*, 422–433.

48. Palmquist, S.; Tideman, P.; Cullen, N.; Zetterber, H.; Blennow, K.; Dage, J. L.; Stomrud, E.; Janelidze, S.; Mattsson-Calgren, N.; Hansson, O. Prediction of future Alzheimer's Disease Dementia Using Plasma Phospho–Tau Combined with Other Accessible Measures. *Nat. Med.* **2021,** *27*, 1034–1042.
49. Karikari, T. K.; Benedet, A. L.; Ashton, N. J.; Rodriguez, J. L.; Snellman, A.; Suárez-Calvet, M.; Saha-Chaudhuri, P.; Lussier, F.; Kvatsberg, H.; Rial, A. M. et al. Diagnostic Performance and Prediction of Clinical Progression of Plasma Phospho–tau181 in the Alzheimer's Disease Neuroimaging Initiative. *Mol. Psychiatry* **2021,** *26*, 429–442.
50. Moscoso, A.; Grothe, M. J.; Ashton, N. J.; Karikari, T. K.; Rodriguez, J. L.; Snallman, A.; Suárez-Calvet, M.; Zetterberg, H.; Blennow, K.; Schöll, M. et al. Time Course of Phosphorylated–tau181 in Blood Across the Alzheimer's Disease Spectrum. *Brain* **2021,** *144*, 325–339.
51. Mattsson-Carlgren, N.; Janelidze, S.; Palmquist, S.; Cullen, N.; Svenningsson, A. L.; Strandberg, O.; Mengel.; D.; Walsh, D. M.; Stomrud, E.; Dage, J. L. et al. Longitudinal Plasma p–tau217 Increased in Early Stages of Alzheimer's Disease. *Brain* **2020,** *143*, 3234–3241.
52. Doxakis, E. Insights into the Multifaceted Role of Circular RNAs: Implications for Parkinson's Disease Pathogenesis and Diagnosis. *NPJ Parkinsons Dis.* **2022,** *8*, 7.
53. van den Berg, M. M. J.; Krauskopf, J.; Ramaekers, J. G.; Kleinjans, J. C. S.; Prickaerts, J.; Briedé, J. J. Circulating microRNA as Potential Biomarkers for Psychiatric and Neurodegenerative Disorders. *Prog. Neurobiol.* **2020,** *185*, 101732.
54. Siedlecki-Wullich, D.; Miñano-Molina, A. J.; Rodríguez-Álvarez, J. microRNAs as Early Biomarkers of Alzheimer's Disease: A Synaptic Perspective. *Cells* **2021,** *10*, 113.
55. Wu, Q.; Kong, W.; Wang, S. Peripheral Blood Biomarkers CXCL12 and TNFRSF13C Associate with Cerebrospinal Fluid Biomarkers and Infiltrating Immune Cells in Alzheimer Disease. *J. Mol. Neurosci.* **2021,** *71*, 1485–1494.
56. Abdullah, M.; Kimura, N.; Akatsu, H.; Hashizume, Y.; Ferdous, T.; Tachita, T.; Iida, S.; Zou, K.; Matsubara, E.; Michikawa, M. Flotillin Is a Novel Diagnostic Blood Marker of Alzheimer's Disease. *J. Alzheimers Dis.* **2019,** *72*, 1165–1176.
57. Varma, V. R.; Oommen, A. M.; Varma, S.; Casanova, R.; An, Y.; Andrews, R. M.; O'Brien, R.; Pletnikova, O.; Troncoso, J. C.; Toledo, J. et al. Brain and Blood Metabolite Signatures of Pathology and Progression in Alzheimer Disease: A Target Metabolomics Study. *PLoS Med.* **2018,** *15*, e1002482.
58. Leuzy, A.; Mattsson-Carlgren, N.; Palqvist, S.; Janelidze, S.; Dage, J. L.; Hansson, O. Blood–Based Biomarkers for Alzheimer's Disease. *EMBO Mol. Med.* **2021,** *14*, e14408.
59. Xiong, Y. I.; Meng, T.; Luo, J.; Zhang, H. The Potential of Neurofilament Light as a Biomarker in Alzheimer's Disease. *Eur. Neurol.* **2021,** *84*, 6–15.
60. Moscoso, A.; Grothe, M. J.; Ashton, N. J.; Karikari, T. K.; Rodríguez, J. L.; Snellman, A.; Suárez-Calvet, M.; Blennow, K.; Zetterberg, H.; Schöll, M. Longitudinal Associations of Blood Phosphorylated Tau181 and Neurofilament Light Chain with Neurodegeneration in Alzheimer Disease. *JAMA Neurol.* **2020,** *78*, 396–406.
61. Mattsson, N.; Cullen, N. C.; Andreasson, U.; Zetterberg, H.; Blennow, K. Association Between Longitudinal Plasma Neurofilament Light and Neurodegeneration in Patients with Alzheimer Disease. *JAMA Neurol.* **2019,** *76*, 791–799.

62. Menšíková, K.; Tučková, L.; Kolăriková, K.; Bartoníková, T.; Vodička, R.; Ehrmann, J.; Vrtěl, R.; Procházka, M.; Kănovský, P.; Kovacs, G. G. Atypical Parkinsonism of Progressive Supranuclear Palsy–Parkinsonism (PSP–P) Phenotype with Rare Variants in FBXO7 and VPS35 Genes Associated with Lewy Body Pathology. *Acta Neuropathol.* **2019,** *137*, 171–173.
63. Mazón M, Vázquez Costa JF, Ten-Esteve A and Martí-Bonmatí L, Imaging Biomarkers for the Diagnosis and Prognosis of Neurodegenerative Diseases. The Example of Amyotrophic Lateral Sclerosis. *Front. Neurosci.* **2018,** *12*, 784.
64. Nättinen, J. Towards Personalized Ocular Surface Diagnosis and Treatment with Tear Fluid Proteomics and Bioinformatics. 2019.
65. Herbert, M. K.; Eeftens, J. M.; Aerts, M. B.; Esselink, R. A. J.; Bloem, B. R.; Kuiperij, H. B.; Verbeek, M. M. CSF Levels of DJ–1 and Tau Distinguish MSA Patients from PD Patients and Controls. *Parkinsonism Relat. Disord.* **2014,** *20*, 112–115.
66. Vranová, H.; Hényková, E.; Kaiserová, M.; Menšíková, K.; Vaštík, M.; Mareš, J.; Hluštík, P.; Zapletalová, J.; Strnad, M.; Stejskal, D. et al. Tau protein, Beta-Amyloid42 and Clusterin CSF Levels in the Differential Diagnosis of Parkinsonian Syndrome with Dementia. *J. Neurol. Sci.* **2014,** *343*, 120–124.
67. Zerr, I.; Kallenberg, K.; Summers, D. M.; Romero, C.; Taratuto, A.; Heinemann, U.; Breithaupt, M.; Vargers, D.; Meissner, B.; Ladogana, A. et al. Updated Clinical Diagnostic Criteria for Sporadic Creutzfeldt–Jakob Disease. *Brain* **2009,** *132*, 2659–2668.
68. Saijo, E.; Ghetti, B.; Zanusso, G.; Oblak, A.; Furman, J. L.; Diamond, M. I.; Kraus, A.; Caughey, B. Ultrasensitive and Selective Detection of 3–Repeat Tau Seeding Activity in Pick Disease Brain and Cerebrospinal Fluid. *Acta Neuropathol.* **2017,** *133*, 751–765.
69. Garc´ıa-Gutie´rrez MS, Navarrete F, Sala F, Gasparyan A, Austrich-Olivares A and Manzanares J (2020) Biomarkers in Psychiatry: Concept, Definition, Types and Relevance to the Clinical Reality. Front. Psychiatry 11:432. doi: 10.3389/fpsyt.2020.00432
70. Koníčková D, Menšíková K, Tučková L, Hényková E, Strnad M, Friedecký D, Stejskal D, Matěj R, Kaňovský P. Biomarkers of Neurodegenerative Diseases: Biology, Taxonomy, Clinical Relevance, and Current Research Status. Biomedicines. 2022 Jul 21;10(7):1760. doi: 10.3390/biomedicines10071760. PMID: 35885064; PMCID: PMC9313182.

CHAPTER 16

Use of Nano-Formulations in the Treatment of Neurodegenerative Disorders

UJJWAL GUPTA, SURYAWANSHI AJAY, FARHAN MAZAHIR, and A. K. YADAV

Department of Pharmaceutics, National Institute of Pharmaceutical Education and Research, Raebareli, Uttar Pradesh, India

ABSTRACT

Alzheimer's disease (AD), Parkinson's disease (PD), Huntington's disease (HD), amyotrophic lateral sclerosis (ALS), and other various disorders are categorized as neurodegenerative disorders (NDOs). Further, NDOs are the clinical features of protein misfolding, change in confirmation of protein, and prevent the degradation of misfolded proteins. Neurodegenerative disorders are characterized by progressive loss of neurons. The efficacy, neuronal uptake, and transport of therapeutic agents/imaging/diagnostic agents to the brain are challenging due to the presence "blood–brain barrier" (BBB), that is, tight junctions (TJs) of epithelial cells surrounding the blood capillaries. Thus, BBB allows the selective permeation of molecules to the brain and is responsible for no or less permeation of therapeutics/imaging/diagnostic agents to the brain. Recent advances in nanotechnology can be helpful to overcome these limitations in the management of disorders. The nanomaterials due to their unique physicochemical properties and easy modification of their surface allow them to travel across the BBB. The dimension or size of nanomaterials ranges from 1 to 100 nm. These nanomaterials can act as nanocarriers for the delivery of biomedical agents to the brain by different mechanisms.

Nanomedicine for Neurodegenerative Disorders: Selective Treatment Strategies. Rishabha Malviya, Kamla Pathak, & Swati Verma (Eds.)

Thus, nanoformulations may help to achieve higher concentrations of biomedical agents in the brain in comparison with conventional dosage forms. Nanomaterials have been used as nanomedicine in various forms such as nanoparticles (NPs) (polymeric and lipidic), vesicular systems (liposomes and niosomes), metal NPs, and carbon nanomaterials have been used to treat NDOs. This chapter describes the role and efficacy of nanomaterial-based nanoformulations in the management of NDOs.

16.1 INTRODUCTION

According to the World Health Organization (WHO), neurodegenerative disorders (NDOs) will be the biggest public health concern in the 21st century. The most severe, incurable neurological disorders of this group include Alzheimer's and Parkinson's diseases (PDs), amyotrophic lateral sclerosis (ALS), Huntington's disease (HD), and Prion disease. Nanotechnology is being studied and developed as a potential therapeutic strategy for the diagnosis and treatment of neurodegenerative diseases. This therapeutic approach aims to reverse neurodegenerative diseases such as Alzheimer's disease (AD). One of the most prevalent types of impaired brain function, AD results in several grave consequences. The methods of treatment used now simply address symptoms. However, nanotechnology methods can lower nerve cell death, lower inflammation, and enhance medicine transport to the brain.[1]

Although the blood–brain barrier (BBB) exists in the central nervous system (CNS), nanotechnology is a rapidly expanding area of the pharmaceutical business. The BBB has a tight junction (TJ), which causes resistance to the standard dosage forms since they have low BBB diffusion. This is the cause of the restriction. The brain has several efflux systems that shield it from different xenobiotic substances. Endothelial cells from the brain's microvessels and capillaries, which are closely connected and gap-free, make up the majority of the BBB. Unsuitably, over 98% of active medications are unable to penetrate BBBs, which presents a potential problem for treating the complicated neurological illnesses outlined above.[2] New methods for creating medications for the CNS have been developed as a result of the past 30 years' worth of research (CNS). They have not, however, been fully put into practice. This chapter examines seven BBB characteristics that were recently discovered as well as possible drug delivery applications. Efflux transporters have a big impact on how drugs are distributed. The main difference is that they stop ligand accumulation in the CNS. However, there are other implications, some of which are demonstrated by P-glycoprotein (P-gP). P-GP has different pharmacological affinities for the transporter, and many of them are not only competing for ligands but also activity or expression regulators.[3] Small, winding channels that cut through gaps in the intercellular junctional complex constitute the paracellular transport pathway in peripheral, continuous capillaries. Only molecules with a diameter of 5–10 nm or smaller can diffuse via these "paracellular channels." Endothelial BBB cells. Adherent junctions (AJs) and TJs, which exhibit an incredibly high level of continuity and stringently restrict paracellular diffusion of solutes and water between the blood and the brain, make up its extraordinarily complex junctional complex[1–3] In comparison to when it would if it relied on extracellular or membrane diffusion, an administered ligand typically crosses the BBB 10–100 times more quickly. Thus, the adoption of a transporter can significantly improve the augmentation of therapeutic effects at the level of the brain. Transporters are used in the drug distribution process to transfer endogenous ligands. Few medications are now used for CNS effects. Ligands make use of saturable systems, which may be found by chance or by high-throughput in vitro testing. Monolayer models might be more favorable when transported ligands are absent. Transporters for biologicals do, nevertheless, offer the potential for their exploitation, especially those that are water-soluble.[4] The energy dependence determines the direction of the transport and may transport in either direction, whereas the direction of energy-independent transportation depends on the concentration gradient. For instance, the molecular flux of Na1 and K1 ions at the BBB is controlled by luminal Na1/K1/2Cl2 cotransporters and abluminal Na1/K1 ATPases.[5]

Through the BBB transport mechanisms, endogenous amino acids reach the brain. One attractive method for delivering drugs to the brain utilizes the conjugation of various compounds such as amino acids and other numerous compounds that have shown the capacity to cross through the BBB and let large amounts of systemically ingested substances get chemotherapeutics to the brain.[6]

An efficient way to transfer medications into the brain is intranasal. In this method, medicines directly reach the brain without passing through the BBB via the olfactory pathway. Due to the first-pass impact and restricted BBB permeability, most drugs are used to treat the human immunodeficiency virus (HIV). The BBB is a dynamic physical and biological barrier that separates the CNS from blood flow (CNS) Brain capillary endothelial cells, which block transcellular transit, and excessively complicated tight adhesion junctions between cells, which block paracellular flux and are primarily responsible for the BBB functional complexity. There have been several attempts to break through the BBB, ranging from invasive methods to chemical medication changes and in silico methods to create molecules with improved permeability. Additionally, the "Trojan horse" technique, in which a drug that does not cross the BBB is paired with one that does, has been used. Additionally, efforts have been made to find ways around the BBB, such as intranasal or via the olfactory bulb.[7]

Location-specific delivery has the potential to reduce drug dosage, boost bioavailability at the target site, and lessen side effects in other areas. Due to this, numerous researchers have concentrated their work recently on developing and using poly(glycolic acid) PGA, polylactic acid (PLA), and poly(lactic-co-glycolic acid) (PLGA) nanoparticles (NPs) that can penetrate the BBB and deliver medications to treat neurological disorders. The surface of NPs can be changed during synthesis to improve the interaction with various BBB components. By preloading PLA-NPs with the flavonoid breviscapine, Liu et al. demonstrated that these PLA-NPs could cross the BBB in a size-dependent method, with greater particles (300 nm) transporting more concentrations of the drug to the brain than smaller particles (200 nm). In another instance, the PLA-NPs' surface-associated transactivating transcriptor (TAT) peptide increased the transport of identical NPs through the BBB by avoiding efflux transporters. Polysorbate 80 and poloxamer 188 surface-coated PLGA-NPs demonstrated increased CNS penetration. Once more, the BBB was improved by paclitaxel-loaded PLGA-NPs with glutathione at the surface.[7,8]

One of the progressive NDOs known as AD affects more than 24 million individuals globally and is marked by memory and cognitive problems. Intraneural neurofibrillary tangles are comprised of paired helical filaments of hyperphosphorylated tau protein and extracellular plaques made of amyloid peptide, a 39–43 amino acid fragments of amyloid precursor protein (APP), which are the neuropathological hallmarks of AD. The major culprits for the synapse loss and memory deficits in AD are now thought to be due to small aggregates of amyloid-derived diffusible ligands (ADDLs).[9]

PD is the result of the loss of dopaminergic neurons in the substantia nigra, a degenerative neurological disorder that affects 1–2% of people over the age of 65 and affects the regulation of movements. The cytoplasmic inclusions called Lewy's bodies, which are made up of 50–700-nm long filaments of the protein -synuclein, are the pathological signature in the brains of PD patients. It is believed that a variety of physiological processes, including endoplasmic reticulum (ER) stress, proteasomal malfunction, and mitochondrial dysfunction, contribute to neuronal death in PD.[10] A fatal NDO that affects 1–2/10,0000 people a year is ALS. Selective motor neuron loss in the brain and spinal cord, which results in the paralysis of voluntary muscles, is the hallmark of the illness. Riluzole-loaded NPs for the treatment of ALS showed a remarkable ability to transport riluzole to the brain and a reduction in discriminate biodistribution in rats.[11] Hence, it could be said that nanotechnology has emerged as a very versatile tool in the biomedical field. Usually, nanotechnology refers to a material with particle sizes ranging from 1 to 100 nm. We use numerous NPs in the treatment of various disorders such as neurological disorders. Nanotechnology has a great advantage over the traditional method.[12] The movement of drugs across BBB using NPs can be achieved with ease for the treatment of various brain-related disorders. The size and shape of the NPs can alter the change in the physicochemical properties and toxicity. To increase the efficacy of NPS, we can conjugate them with different biologically active moieties with amines and thiols. In Figure 16.1, the various neurodegenerative diseases and the neurons they affect are stated. These provide great penetration and drug release at the tumor site giving great therapeutic effects. Nanotechnology has valuable effects on the enhancement of sensorymotor and cognitive functions in stroke, Parkinson's disorder (PD), HD, AD, ALS, and spinal muscular atrophy (SMA).[13]

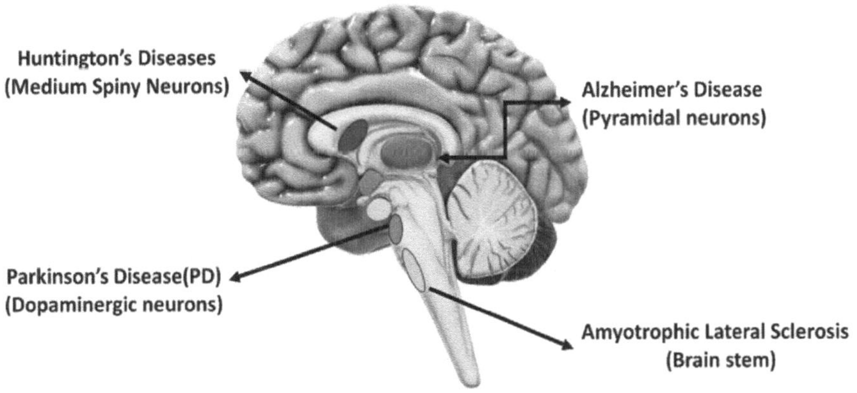

FIGURE 16.1 Neurodegenerative diseases and the neurons they affect.

Because NDOs target various parts of the brain and exhibit unique symptoms, they are typically regarded as discrete clinical entities. Nevertheless, they have some similar genetic, cellular, or molecular characteristics (e.g., initial vascular dysfunction, the spread, and aggregation of misfolded proteins, activation of immune responses as well as selective vulnerability of particular neurons). Protein misfolding buildup is another feature of NDOs. Figure 16.1 shows the various NDOs and the neurons they affect. The mechanism of protein misfolding and aggregation, which causes cellular malfunction, synaptic loss, and ultimately brain injury, is very similar even though the proteins are frequently different for each NDO. Additionally, these proteins frequently self-replicate via seeding, disseminating the pathogenic deviations between cells and tissues.[10,13] The causes of NDs and potential treatments have been the subject of numerous investigations, however, there are now only a few medicines available that merely deal with the symptoms and not the mechanisms underlying the disorder. The therapy of these disorders encounters numerous issues. The BBB's permeability, which prevents medications from being administered from reaching therapeutic levels in the brain, is one of the key issues. Therefore, it is necessary to create bioactive substances that can penetrate the BBB. Gene therapy is a promising method to enhance intracerebral drug delivery. Modulation of the expression of specific genes with the help of adeno-associated viral vectors using nanocarriers may alter the pathogenesis of NDOs.

In-depth research has been done with NPs for tumor imaging and diagnosis. However, little study has concentrated on CNS brain imaging, potentially as a result of the BBB's difficulty, technological advancements in imaging, particularly in the quality of MRI and CT scans have improved the management and forecasting of neurological disorders.

This chapter explores new nanotechnology methods such as nanocarriers and their role in the delivery of drugs to BBB.

16.2 TRANSPORT MECHANISM THROUGH THE BLOOD-BRAIN BARRIER

Paracellular and transcellular pathways can be used to transport chemicals via endothelial cells, respectively. Molecules are transported via the intracellular space between cells using the paracellular route. Hormones, alcohol, and gases (CO_2 and O_2) are examples of small, lipid-soluble substances with low molecular weight (400 Da) that can passively permeate through the plasma membrane of endothelial cells. Figure 16.2 shows the passing of nanocarriers across BBB. Although paracellular channels are frequently used for transport in peripheral capillaries, TJs in the BBB cause most of the transport to occur through transcellular pathways, severely restricting their use. PLGA NPs have been combined with a glyco-heptapeptide to facilitate the delivery of loperamide and rhodamine-123 inside the brain. The various pathways of transport across BBB are shown in Figure 16.2. These NPs were discovered to be able to effortlessly cross the BBB because of the glyco-heptapeptide coating on their surface, which mimics the actions of opioid peptides through absorption-mediated endocytosis.[7]

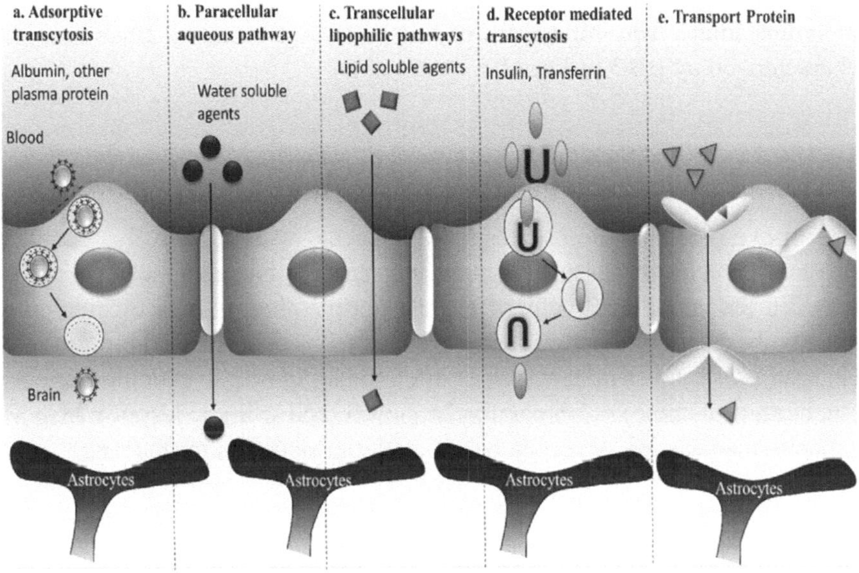

FIGURE 16.2 Schematic illustration of transport mechanism through BBB.

16.2.1 CARRIER-MEDIATED TRANSCYTOSIS

Nutrient and efflux transporter proteins are the names of the transporter protein carriers that are found on the basolateral sides of the endothelial cells and luminal, respectively. Proteins called nutrient transporters are specialized for solutes such as amino acids, hormones, and glucose. These solutes cause reversible conformational changes when they bind to their respective transporter proteins. The solutes are transferred to the basolateral side of the cell after being taken up by it and follow a gradient of high to low solute concentration.[14]

16.2.2 RECEPTOR-MEDIATED TRANSCYTOSIS

Highly specific macromolecule receptors including hormones, plasma protein, and enzymes are expressed by cerebral endothelial cells. Insulin, transferrin (Tf), and low-density lipoprotein (LDL) cholesterol have all been extensively researched ligands crucial for BBB transit. These ligands attach to the endothelial cells' respective insulin, Tf, and LDL receptors. The production of uncoated vesicles is a caveolin-dependent process, which is activated by caveolin protein, is only used by a select few compounds, including folate. The importance of this pathway for neurological diseases characterized by BBB leakage.[14]

16.2.3 ADSORPTIVE-MEDIATED TRANSCYTOSIS

Adsorptive-mediated transcytosis can occur with positively charged substances such as drugs or substrates. It is set off by electrostatic interactions between the endothelial cells of the plasma membrane surface containing negatively charged heparin sulfate proteoglycans found and the positively charged substrate surface, which is often made up of polycationic proteins (such as protamine). Comparatively slower and with a lesser transport capacity than carrier- or receptor-mediated transport, this mechanism.[15]

16.3 NANOMATERIAL AND NEURODEGENERATION

Various materials have been used for the synthesis of nanocarriers and have been evaluated for their efficacy in the management of NDOs. Refer to Figure 16.3 for the schematic presentation of different nanocarriers.

16.4 CARBON BASED NANOMATERIALS

A developing field of research, integrating nanotechnology, biotechnology, and medicine has been used in several areas, most notably the prevention, treatment, and detection of numerous disorders, including Alzheimer's. The creation of nanomedicine has been the subject of extensive study up to this point, necessitating knowledge of or comprehension of the cellular response to NPs' different cell lines or specific cell lines. Chemical vapor deposition (CVD) and exfoliation processes have recently been used to create carbon nanostructure-based materials such as carbon nanotubes (CNTs), carbon nanofibers (CNFs), graphene, and their derivatives. These carbon-based nanomaterials are readily used in drug delivery, agriculture, water remediation, and wound dressing. The figure shows various types of nanocarriers.[16]

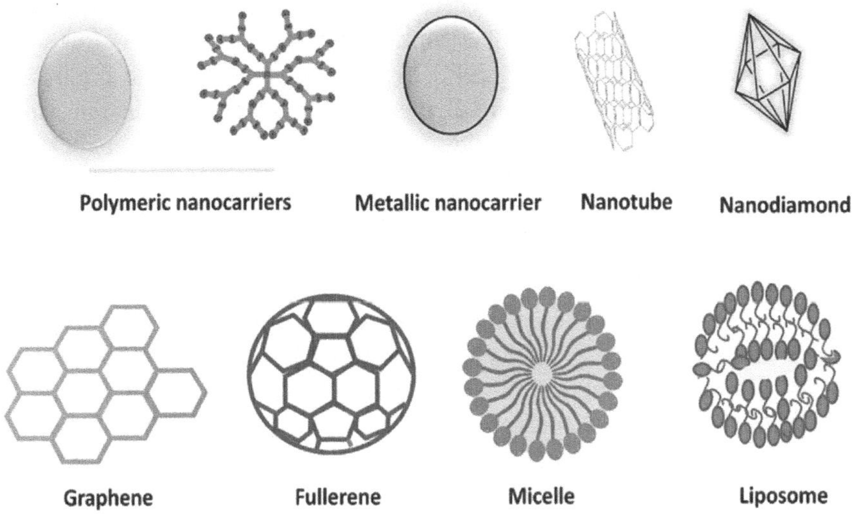

FIGURE 16.3 Schematic illustration of different kind of nanocarriers.

16.4.1 *CARBON NANOTUBES*

Iijima was the first to identify CNTs, a novel class of extremely inventive nanomaterials that are currently being researched for their potential in medicine. Carbon atoms are arranged in a network in large tensile strength and strong electrical and thermal conductivity are both present at the nanoscale scale. CNTs are regarded as the best nanomaterials for a variety of applications which include field emission displays and very strong fibers most recently, CNTs sparked a lot of interest in the field of medicine, where appropriately engineered CNTs can various systems, such as protein transporters or vaccine delivery systems.[17] CNTs have excellent thermal and electrical properties, that is, thermal conductivity, low thermal expansion coefficients, and lesser electromigration tendency in comparison with other materials. They also have a larger current carrying capacity. At that scale, common materials such as copper, tungsten, and aluminum are used in it. Furthermore, CNTs have outstanding mechanical and electrical properties, which will perhaps be used as prospective future lab-on-chip application solutions.[18] A sizable portion of the global population is afflicted with a wide variety of ailments known as neurological disorders. Neurological research is anticipated to be significantly impacted by developments in nanomedicine, advancing our knowledge of the CNS and fostering the creation of new methods of treatment for neurological interventions. The most appealing method for neurological applications is the utilization of carbon-based nanostructures, such as CNT. Many components of the brain (ion channels, signaling proteins, and elements) share structural characteristics and size with CNTs. These qualities could provide an additional benefit by improving molecular interactions and, as a result, improved control over the CNS. These materials can be easily functionalized with different functional groups as well as with different types of proteins such as albumin, lactoferrin (Lf), and Tf.[17,18]

CNTs may now be chemically functionalized to regulate chemical characteristics, such as toxicity and solubility. CNTs may be used in a variety of biological applications, with medication transport standing out as one in particular. The modification of CNTs has been investigated using a variety of functionalization techniques. Strong acids can be used to oxidize CNTs, which shortens them while generating carboxylic groups that make them more dispersible in aqueous solutions. In contrast to multi-walled CNTs, which feature several concentric graphene tubes, pure single-walled CNTs (SWCNTs) are very hydrophobic hexagonal carbon tubes (graphene). According to several research, the hydrophobicity and propensity for aggregation of CNTs render them toxic to cultured live cells. The length of CNTs can be in micrometer ranges, and diameter in the nonmetric range.[19]

The solubility of CNTs has been addressed through the use of several techniques. End-groups and sidewalls of CNTs have undergone organic functionalization, resulting in covalent changes. Starch or oligomers such as poly(vinylpyrrolidone) (PVP) can wrap and transport SWCNTs into aqueous buffers by forming water-soluble nanohybrids. Strong acids introduced to oxidized CNTs form hydroxyl and carboxyl groups at their ends, which facilitate coupling to a range of biomolecules and improve dispersion in aqueous solutions. Prion disorders are also called transmissible spongiform encephalopathies (TSEs). These are a group of uncommon, slowly progressing neurodegenerative illnesses that can affect both animals and people. PrP, an aberrant, transmissible agent that may cause abnormal cellular prion proteins folding in the brain, is thought to be the cause of TSEs and is responsible for the disorder's recognizable signs and symptoms as well as brain damage. Designing medications and delivery methods that can not only pass the BBB but also deliver sufficient amounts of treatment to the tumor location are recent approaches to combating brain tumors. Therefore, a dual-targeted line of action is now required. Receptor targeting is one such strategy that can preferentially reach the tumor location. According to reports, the BBB and brain tumors both have an excessive expression of the LDL receptor-related protein (LRP) receptor. Doxorubicin is dual targeted against brain glioma using PEGylated oxidized MWCNTs.[20]

Activating the innate immune system may be a viable tactic in conquering the local immunosuppressive milieu of the brain tumor. Since it has been shown that brain cancers have created their mechanism for evading the body's immune system. Numerous studies on biomolecules and macro-molecules in brain tumors have been conducted. It has been discovered that these biomolecules frequently have a role in controlling the immune response while treating brain cancers. In brain microglia, Toll-like receptors and tumor-associated macrophages are overexpressed (TAMs).[21]

16.4.2 FULLERENE

As can be seen, fullerenes are closed, hollow cages filled with carbon atoms that have undergone sp^2 hybridization. However, the structure cannot be produced only from hexagonal rings to produce the spherical cage. It is feasible to demonstrate, using Euler's theorem, that a spherical surface must have precisely 12 pentagons. The class of closed-cage carbon compounds known as fullerenes is denoted by the symbol C_n, where n denotes the total number of carbon atoms that make up the 12 pentagons and a variable number of hexagons. Different-sized fullerenes can be produced depending on how many hexagons are present. The reactivity of fullerenes is also influenced by their dimension. The reduction of stress on the cage structure, which enables the restoration of sp^3 hybridization, is another significant driving factor. When fullerenes grow in size, their chemical reactivity rises, leading to a decreased curvature and strain toward a flat surface that resembles graphite more.[22] The chemical characteristics of C_{60}, which has an external diameter of 0.71 nm, are extremely comparable with that of molecules. The C_{60} molecule may be less aromatic than usual because of the pentagon's presence, in which carbon atoms commonly prevent the formation of the double bond. The C_{60} fullerene molecule will undergo a straightforward reduction, it has been shown in the literature, and due to the surface's curvature, fullerene hybridization takes place between the sp^2 and sp^3 areas. This explains the exceptional electron-receiving abilities of C_{60} along with topology. C_{60} and C_{70} fullerenes were mixed with an aqueous solution including nitric and sulfuric acids at a temperature of 85–115 °C. The fullerenes were subjected to acid-induced oxidation, which led to the average grafting of 15 hydroxyl groups per fullerene. If tetrabutylammonium hydroxide is present and functioning as a catalyst, adding strongly basic NaOH to C_{60} benzene solutions can also result in the formation of OH-functionalized fullerenes.[23]

Numerous scientists predicted various possibilities for these molecules in the realm of biology due to their distinctive physical and chemical characteristics. However, the biological uses have been limited as a result of the insolubility in polar solvents and the aggregation characteristics. The most prevalent hydrophobic compounds, fullerenes, are soluble in benzenes, naphthalenes, and alkanes. The lowest unoccupied molecular orbital (LUMO) of fullerenes is energetically low-lying, threefold-degenerate, and can easily accept up to six electrons, assaulting by radical species more likely. This is the basis for fullerene's antioxidant function. As a result of their reaction with superoxide, hydroxyl, and peroxyl radicals, fullerenes and their derivatives can harm biomolecules as well as other macromolecules that would otherwise cause cell death. This interaction prevents the chain reaction of lipid peroxidation.[24]

Numerous neurological conditions, including ischemia and neurodegenerative illnesses, are influenced by oxidative stress. These conditions are linked to progressively worsening mitochondrial dysfunction, an increase in oxidative damage, and altered antioxidant defense system activities. New neuroprotective drugs are being developed to lessen the oxidative stress associated with brain damage. Materials made of fullerene have been used for their outstanding antioxidant properties, giving them a wide range of neuroprotective properties. In numerous animal models, carboxy fullerenes are the most capable and intensively researched family of water-soluble derivatives of fullerene and have neuroprotective properties. Research using cortical cell cultures showed apoptotic and excitotoxic conditions and found that C_{60} is the derivative of malonic acid, $(C_{63}((COOH)_2)_3$, and N-methyl-D-aspartate (NMDA) reduced excitotoxic neuronal death in cortical neurons exposed to oxygen–glucose deprivation, amino-3-hydroxy-5-methyl-4-isoxazole propionic acid (AMPA), or NMDA. Interesting in vivo results from a transgenic mouse model of familial ALS showed that the administration of carboxy fullerenes delayed the onset of symptoms and mortality.[25]

It is important to note that these carboxy fullerenes' protective benefits were also linked to unfavorable behavioral alterations, suggesting that these fullerene derivatives may have unfavorable side effects when used in vivo. This study raises concerns about the toxicity of C_{60} and its application in nanomedicine. In reality, studies done in vitro support the idea that depending on the concentration utilized, fullerene derivatives have two different effects. According to this study, water-soluble polyhydroxy fullerene dramatically enhanced hippocampus neuronal viability at low concentrations and shielded neurons from oxidative damage, however at high concentrations, this fullerene-derivative lowered hippocampal neuron viability and triggered apoptosis. The unique family of chemicals known as water-soluble buckminsterfullerene (C_{60}) derivatives possesses strong antioxidant capabilities. Studies on one family of these chemicals, the malonic acid C_{60} derivatives (carboxy fullerenes), showed that they were efficient lipid peroxidation inhibitors as well as superoxide anion and H_2O_2 removers. In cortical cell cultures, carboxy fullerenes showed strong neuroprotection against excitotoxic, apoptotic, and metabolic insults. Additionally, they were able to protect mesencephalic dopaminergic neurons against degeneration brought on by MPP1 and 6-hydroxydopamine.[23,24]

TABLE 16.1 CNTs for the Treatment of Diseases: Potential Uses and Problems.

Type of carbon nanotubes (CNTs)	Type of disease	The potential efficacy of treatment	References
CNTs	Mold infection	In vitro—extremely high. Extremely high in vitro. Problem with very high toxicity level for in vivo applications, potentially high in vivo	[26]
SWCNTs	*Staphylococcus aureus*, *Escherichia coli*, Mycobacterium	In vitro—extremely high. Additional in vitro experiments are necessary to determine the toxicity of the potential in vivo model	[27]
SWCNTs	Hepatitis C virus (HCV)	Very high in vitro. Potentially significant toxicity issues in vivo	[28]
CNTs, single-walled SWCNTs	Prions	Potentially high in vitro. Additional in vitro and in vivo models are necessary, as well as for toxicity research	[29]
f-CNTs (siRNA, antisense)	Cancer	Potentially high in vitro. Basic animal models are necessary to have an initial idea of the potential	[30]
Functionalized CNTs (f-CNTs) (maleimido-derivatized water soluble)	Foot-and-mouth disease virus (FMDV)	Preliminary research is quite encouraging and has potential. Additional in vitro and in vivo studies are needed to determine the efficacy and toxicity.	[31]

16.4.3 GRAPHENE

The distinctive electrochemical, mechanical, thermal, and optical characteristics of graphene-based materials (GBMs) make them desirable candidates for a variety of biological applications. GBMs have been at the vanguard of biomedical research since the discovery of graphene, providing creative treatments for a variety of illnesses, including neurological ailments [nanodiamonds (NDs)]. Reviews on the synthesis and functionalization of GBMs may be found anywhere. However, this review mainly focuses on the most recent developments in GBM research for NDs, particularly in the areas of sensing and therapeutic applications. Following a brief explanation of the primary characteristics of NDs, special emphasis is placed on functionalization techniques used to enhance the biomedical capabilities of GBMs, as well as recent applications for multiple sclerosis (MS), ALS, PD, and AD.[32] With its exceptional electrochemical, mechanical, and optical characteristics, graphene, a single sheet of atoms organized in a honeycomb lattice, is well suited for use in a variety of biomedical applications. Additionally, physicochemical changes (e.g., oxidation and reduction) lead to the derivative GBMs known as reduced graphene oxide (GO) (rGO). Each of these items displays a distinct quality and can be used as per their applications. For instance, the superb GBMs are appropriate because of their mechanical rigidity, electrical conductivity, and engineering of bone and neural tissue, while their superior optical qualities make them suitable for optical applications.[33]

Additionally, GBM is helpful in drug/gene delivery and biosensing applications due to its vast surface area and capacity to adsorb different aromatic biomolecules (such as DNA or RNA) through stacking and/or electrostatic interactions. The excellent biocompatibility of GBMs is another quality that makes them a promising choice for biological applications. Excellent mechanical, thermal, and electrical characteristics may be found in graphene. However, due to its huge surface area and powerful van der Waals pressures, it aggregates and cannot be further dispersed. Additionally, even though graphene has demonstrated a therapeutic component in numerous disorders (including cancer), its biological compatibility has been proven debated. Consequently, to increase the biological and colloidal stability compatibility with graphene and a variety of functionalization techniques have been put forth. Amyloid plaques (amyloid hypothesis) and tau protein misfolding, which results in neurofibrillary tangles, are two features of AD. Consequently, finding A monomers and tau protein concentration can offer crucial details regarding the severity of the illness and available therapeutic alternatives. Due to the GBMs' superior electrical characteristics, they have been successfully used as electrochemical detectors of the aforementioned biomarkers examined in recent years.[33,34]

Only a small number of research have explored graphene-based nanotechnologies (GBMs) as a treatment strategy, despite the numerous published studies on its use for AD diagnosis. GO-coated, GO quantum dots (GOQDs), and plain GO nanoflakes. Some of these methods include electrospun nanofibrous scaffolds and graphene-based nanocomposites such as GO/graphitic carbon nitride (GO/g-C3N4) and GO/iron oxide (GOIO). Even though all of these methods aim to treat AD by dissociating. Each of the amyloid fibrils has a unique trajectory. One of the main pathways for protein degradation is autophagy. It is recognized that AD patients experience disruptions in aggregate clearance. Consequently, autophagy regulation is a popular strategy with intriguing promise for healing. Since there are currently no particular tests or procedures for the diagnosis of PD, the majority of individuals go untreated for many years until their symptoms become obvious. PD worsens over time as an ND, leading to a stage where the drug is taken and fails to handle the signs. Therefore, developing methods to identify PD in its early stages is crucial for treating it and enhancing the sufferers' standard of living. Because graphene and its derivative have good electrical characteristics and a huge surface area many graphene-based nanocomposites have been made from various investigated as possible diagnostic instruments. Despite this, graphene is a great sensor material for the electrochemical detection of several biomarkers, including dopamine, levodopa, and homophilic acid), its purest form is insensitive and insensitive to selection.[32,35]

16.4.4 NANODIAMONDS

The diamond structure of a family of carbon nanomaterials known as NDs is present at the nanoscale. Similar to CNTs and fullerene C60, Nanodiamonds have special optoelectronic, mechanical, biological, and thermal properties for a range of significant uses such as nanomedicine. Scientists in the former USSR made the incredible discovery nearly 40 years ago that ultrafine diamond particles are created when oxygen-deficient explosives (such as TNT or hexogen) are detonated in an inert medium. Due to the inadequate burning of explosives that act as energy as well as carbon sources and the absence of oxygen during the detonation process, soot that contains 80% microscopic diamond crystallites with size ranges from 4 to 5 nm can be found.[35] On the contrary, the smaller, nonfluorescent denotation NDs can only be used for imaging after being loaded with imaging probes, such as radiotracers for PET, fluorescent stain molecules for fluorescent imaging, and bioluminescent proteins for imaging in the field of luminescence. It is essential to thoroughly investigate and analyze the surface chemistry of NDs inside living animals to do this. A few other critical concerns that must be referred to include biodistribution, tumor extravasation in the case of tumor targeting, circulation time, therapy, and probe dissociation from the NP.

Nanodiamonds are a useful tool for bioimaging. Although nonfluorescent denotation NDs (NFNDs) may also be used for imaging, they must first be loaded with imaging probes such as radiotracers for PET, and bioluminescent proteins for bioluminescence imaging, or fluorescent dye molecules for fluorescent imaging to be utilized imaging. To do this, rigorous research and examination of the surface chemistry of NDs within living animals are required.[35] A few other critical concerns that must be included are biodistribution, probe dissociation, tumor extravasation, circulation time in the treatment, and tumor targeting. There is a wealth of research describing how the reticuloendothelial system (RES) prevents NPs from reaching their destinations. It has been noted that surface modification, such as PEGylation, can lessen the uptake of RES and/or the accumulation and/or aggregation of small particles.

Nanodiamonds interact with biomolecules and can be employed in a variety of biological uses, involving bioassays (using lab-on-a-chip devices,), targeted drug administration, and particular cell labeling. For example, instance, several teams have successfully used amide linkages, ester bridges, or the considerably more reliable direct C–C bonds to covalently attach DNA molecules to diamond surfaces for sensor chip applications. In addition to fluorescent tagging, Nanodiamonds synthesized with biomolecules have been applied for medical administration.[36]

NDs have also been utilized for protein immobilization, purification, and bioseparation, all of which are somewhat linked to drug delivery. For instance, Bondar et al. showed how to physically absorb recombinant proteins (such as luciferase and apoobelin) from *E. coli* using denotation NDs. After cell lysis, these scientists first included NDs in the recombinant protein solution. The modification and imbalance of different neurotransmitters and proteases describe the majority of CNS disorders. It has recently been demonstrated that NDs can change how quickly neurotransmitters are taken in and stored. The neurotransmitters glutamate and GABA may be taken up by nerve terminals and their initial absorption and accumulation can be decreased by NDs. To better understand the neurotransmitter processes in numerous CNS illnesses involving aberrant neurotransmissions, such as epilepsy, schizophrenia, ADD, AML, and PD, the study showed the neuroactive features of NDs that may be utilized.[37]

The BBB shields the CNS neurons. Therefore, it is essential that the drug carriers themselves are biocompatible with the neural machinery and do not conflict with the therapeutic purpose if drug delivery methods are to be used to boost therapeutic efficacy. Even though in vivo tests revealed a dose-dependent reduction in neurite length, by contrasting these outcomes with those of prior research in which neurite length rises. Numerous NPs that are utilized as medication carriers are neurotoxic. In addition, the CNS interactions and biocompatibility of NDs may potentially be problematic. NDs are reportedly biocompatible with neurons, according to recent studies. Although this technology is costly and not practical for large-scale manufacturing, NDs made using the CVD method exhibit the least level of cytotoxicity and are ideal scaffolds for the differentiation and proliferation of neural stem cells (NSCs).[37]

16.5 METAL-BASED NANOMATERIALS

16.5.1 GOLD NANOPARTICLES

Gold has traditionally been thought of as a sign of royalty, and many people have been drawn to it because of its brilliant golden aspect. Gold has high molecular recognition abilities, ductility, and biocompatibility. Gold is now employed in several industries. once gold particles can be many nanometers in size, and their chemical and physical characteristics depend on dimensions in nanometers. A nanoscale gold surface's surface area has a unique impact. Consequently, gold can cause a variety of biological activities both directly and indirectly. A metallic gold nanoparticle (Au NP) is used in the treatment as well as in the bioimaging of neurological disorders.[46]

The BBB, which enables certain chemicals to flow through but prohibits others from doing so, is semi-permeable. Endothelial cells in the brain are closely packed together, making it impossible for chemicals to pass outside of the blood arteries. Brain disorders are extremely challenging to treat. Numerous studies have demonstrated that NPs may easily pass through the BBB.

Gold tetra-chloric acid is reduced by citrate, which is inexpensive and carried out in a moderate preparation environment, and is the most widely

TABLE 16.2 Nanocarriers/Nanoformulations and Their Application in NDOs.

Nano Vehicle	Diseases	Applications	References
Gold NP-Polyvinylpyrrolidone (PVP)	AD	Dissolve the generated aggregates and prevent $A\beta_{1-16}$ aggregation.	[38]
PLGA (poly D, L-lactic-co-glycolic acid)	AD	The proliferation and differentiation of brain cells are improved, and memory and learning disabilities are recovered.	[39]
Curcumin-loaded chitosan-alginate-sodium tripolyphosphate NPs (CS-ALGSTPP NPs)	MS	Increased cur bioavailability, durability, and circulation; decreased demyelination Maintain myelinated axons by improving	[40]
Polysorbate 80-modified cerasome	PD	Pharmacokinetic profile improvement	[41]
Lf NPs	Neuroprotection activity, brain Targeting	More intracellular medication absorption and improved neuroprotective qualities	[42]
Cationic solid lipid NPs (CSLNPs)	HD	Reduction of lipid peroxidation, protein carbonyls, reactive oxygen species (ROS), and swelling of the mitochondria.	[43, 44]
Nanomicelle	MS	STAT1, NF-B, and AP-1 miRNA expression are suppressed, while STAT5 mRNA expression is increased	[44]
Micelle	ALS	Enhanced chance of surviving	[45]

used technique for creating gold NPs. Other preparation techniques include chemical reduction, sonoelectrochemical synthesis, laser ablation, seed-mediated growth, photochemical synthesis utilizing ultraviolet (UV) light, sonochemical synthesis, and sonochemical synthesis. Because of their unique optical and thermal characteristics and the simplicity of surface functionalization, gold NPs in particular have drawn significant attention as promising biomaterials in bio-nanotechnology and related fields. This enables the targeted delivery of various biological assays, proteins, and genes, as well as drugs. The localized surface plasmon resonance (LSPR), which absorbs and emits different hues of light depending on the size, structure, local reflective index, and aggregation state of NPs, is primarily responsible for the optical characteristic.[47]

Gold nanoshells and nanocages have recently been produced for use in high-resolution imaging methods such as magnetic resonance imaging (MRI). Gold NPs are currently in development for CNS illnesses. Long-term cytotoxicity, however, is a significant issue that must be addressed in the future. In many scientific studies, it is found that the gold NPs can penetrate through the BBB as it is the most important criterion for drug delivery in neurological disorders. Earlier studies have shown that the nanogold (Au NPs) properties inhibit the degradation of Aβ aggregates and accumulation of Aβ peptides. Au NPs also exhibited inhibition of acetylcholinesterase and butyrylcholinesterase, contributing to an anti-AD result.[46,47]

16.5.2 SILVER NANOPARTICLE

Noble metal NPs have generated a great deal of attention as a cutting-edge platform for nanobiotechnology and biomedicine because of their vivid and interesting hues. Due to practical surface bioconjugation with molecular probes and outstanding optical features associated with localized plasmon resonance, the applications of nanotechnology have expanded. Silver has been used as a metal since far before the Neolithic revolution. Silver's use as a medicine was first noted by Moyer in the eighth century. The adaptable photophysical properties of silver nanoparticles (Ag NPs), their effective optical and spectroscopic addressability, and recent advances in NP synthesis and fabrication have propelled these NPs to the forefront of nanotechnology research aimed at fields such as photonics and biomedicine.[48] Because of their interesting physicochemical properties, which include their large surface area, simple synthesis method, and adaptability, as well as their capacity to cross the BBB and elicit an immune reaction in the brain, Ag NPs are capable nanosystems used for the treatment of nanodiamonds. While Ag NPs reduce trans endothelial electrical resistance by blocking TJ proteins of BBB as a result of cell death brought on by ROS, they do not cause the release of inflammatory cytokines. However, it is important to note that silver ions can do so. On the contrary, the induction of the APP gene expression, as well as expression of neurodegenerative gene and activation of inflammation was discovered in research whose authors analyze the effect of Ag NPs *in vivo*.[49]

The chemical approach is the one used the most frequently to create Ag NPs. It begins by applying a reduction agent to reduce the metallic ion in a non-aqueous or aqueous solution. The NMNPs with high surface energy acquired after this stage make it difficult to create a stable colloidal solution, necessitating a stabilization step. The reducing agents used to produce Ag NPs include hydrogen and saturated alcohols. hydroxylamine, unsaturated alcohols, formaldehyde, and amine boranes.[48,50] When compared to chemical approaches, physical ones offer the benefit of producing uniform NP dispersion and avoiding solvent contamination of thin films. Evaporation–condensation and laser ablation are the two most significant physical techniques. The effectiveness of the laser ablation process for bulk metallic materials depends on laser characteristics including wavelength, pulse width, fluence, and ablation time. The presence or absence of surfactants and an efficient liquid medium are additional aspects that affect the synthesis process. The evaporation–condensation process involves heating the materials to cause them to evaporate under an inert environment, then combining them with a cold gas to lower the temperature. The lack of chemicals in the laser ablation approach is a significant benefit over the other methods described.[48,50]

16.5.3 IRON NANOPARTICLES

Fe and other transition metals are necessary for nearly all living things to properly carry out their crucial metabolic functions. Several crucial nervous system processes involve metals, including Fe is necessary for the brain's rapid respiratory rate, myelination, gene expression, and the creation of neurotransmitters. In several cases of neurodegenerative illnesses, it has contributed to neuronal damage. Alzheimer's (AD), ALS, Parkinson's (PD), and Huntington's (HD), are among the NDOs linked to the alteration of brain metal homeostasis. Metals may have a role in neurodegenerative illnesses since it has been discovered that individuals with these conditions collect metals in their nervous systems. Under specific circumstances, iron (Fe) homeostasis is commonly disturbed in NDOs; due to its high availability, this metal is the most effective pro-oxidant.[51]

In AD, patients Fe is present in the postmortem brain of neurofibrillary tangles as well as senile plaques suggesting that it is implicated in the pathogenesis of the disorder. Through the Fenton reaction, which produces the extremely reactive hydroxyl radical, Fe has been linked to the production of free radicals. It is important to note that the hydroxyl radical appears to provide beta aggregation by enhancing covalent binding between peptide monomers, in addition to having an impact on cell components such as membrane lipids, proteins, and nucleic acids.[51] Higher spinal cord Fe levels associated with ALS may contribute to oxidative damage via the Fenton reaction. Since Lf is elevated in motoneurons afflicted by ALS, it has been hypothesized that Fe buildup may be caused by increased absorption of this metal. Just before the illness reaches its terminal stage, ferritin levels in SOD1-G93A mice are elevated, which suggests enhanced Fe deposition. Additionally, CSF ferric-reducing capacity is diminished in ALS patients, although the level of oxidized proteins is raised in both the CSF and plasma. Transferrin receptors (TfRs), ferritin, and Ireg-1 levels are all affected by SOD activity. HD patients have been found to accumulate Fe in their basal ganglia. Total Fe levels were found to be higher in the caudate and putamen nuclei (by 44 and 56%, respectively) after postmortem metal levels in brain tissue from Huntington's patients were examined by Dexter et al. These same brain regions also displayed significant pathological disturbances as a result of the disorder. Ferritin levels were the same in all of the brain areas analyzed between HD patients and control participants in the same research. Other investigators, however, have discovered elevated ferritin levels in HD brains; these disparities may be caused by problems with the experiments.[52,53]

16.6 BIOPOLYMERS

A polymer that degrades under physiological conditions is referred to as being biodegradable. These biopolymers may self-assemble into nanometric structures with sizes between 1 and 100 nm when appropriate circumstances are met, earning them the moniker "nanobiopolymers." Because they offer several benefits, including the administration of non-water-soluble medications and the preservation of unstable substances from deterioration, biopolymer NPs have been extensively exploited as drug delivery systems (DDSs). NPs can be drug-loaded by encapsulation, dispersion within the polymer matrix, or adsorption.[53] One of the most capable approaches for controlled-release systems is the utilization of biodegradable NPs as molecular carriers. A biomaterial must be biocompatible or have the capacity to be digested without causing any negative consequences, to be utilized in this way. These kinds of systems must be capable of ensuring qualities such as the ability to pass through anatomical barriers in the body, most commonly the BBB or the ophthalmic barrier, releasing the active molecule at the site of action, and controlling the drug's concentration over time.[54]

16.6.1 POLYMERIC NANOPARTICLES

Numerous monomers can be used to create PNPs, which can then be polymerized using a variety of methods, and their characteristics can be tailored for diverse uses. In this segment, we first go over the most prevalent types of PNP systems that have been used to target the brain, namely synthetic, natural-based, and hybrid NPs. They are made of organic or synthetic polymers, whether the medication is loaded in a solid form or a solution. An approach for administering medications to the CNS uses PNPs. They aid in the active molecule's delivery to the target site and shield the medication from enzymatic breakdown. Polyalkyl cyanoacrylate (PACA) is employed in NPs for medication delivery to the CNS and is one of the most widely used polymers. PACA has been employed to treat tumors. Doxorubicin, an anticancer medication, is coated on a PACA NP and has a high tolerance against cancers that are resistant to it. The best alternative medication delivery method is via PNPs because of their characteristic biodegradability and nontoxicity.[55] The enhanced stability, higher concentration delivered, and ease of incorporation of PNPs are major advantages. Due to their natural origins and similarity to the BBB membrane, lipid-based nanocarriers are advised. The polymeric nanostructured-based system is the greatest solution for medication administration to the CNS since PNPs still have a large capacity and can readily have their surface modified by targeting molecules.[56]

Applications of NPs in the therapeutic field have grown in recent years. Given the prevalence of neurodegenerative illnesses, including AD and PD, in the general population, researchers' focus has switched to the investigation of functionalized NPs for these conditions. In these circumstances, NPs are created with a twofold functionalization in that the medicine being evaluated is placed onto them, and they are coated with precise BBB targets. Many studies in the scientific literature suggest new NP formulations with various medication combinations and BBB targets. For the treatment of AD, a PEGylated PLA-NPs-based activated NP DDS was created in a study by Zhang et al.[57] PNPs have a large drug loading capacity, an average size of 10–100 nm, and a positive or negative surface charge depending on the polymeric matrix. Their component matrices can be either synthetic [(such as polycaprolactone (PCL)] or natural (such as gelatin or chitosan). They can be formed of non-biodegradable polymers, such as polyurethane, or biodegradable polymers, for example, PLGA, and cyanoacrylate. The U.S. Food and Drug Administration (FDA), and the European Medical Agency (EMA) approved several biodegradable polymers for their use in various biomedical purposes. These polymers are biocompatible, non-toxic, and can be removed from the body via physiological processes.[58]

16.6.1.1 CHITOSAN

Drug transport to the brain has been thoroughly investigated with chitosan. The benefits of using chitosan-prepared NPs to encapsulate drugs have been demonstrated, including protection from enzyme degradation, controlled release, and improved bioavailability. Chitosan is the only naturally occurring alkaline polysaccharide with good biocompatibility and biodegradability. In addition, chitosan can alter the TJ, which increases medication permeability across the BBB. Chitosan NPs, which have a positive charge, can bind to negatively charged cell membranes, prolonging their stay there and improving medication delivery from the nasal cavity to the brain. Chitosan NPs were particularly well suited for brain administration due to all these characteristics.[59] Chitosan may be a suitable polymer for drug delivery purposes, due to several reasons, that is, chitosan NPs can be formed in the aqueous environment without the use of any toxic reagents, modulation of release of therapeutic agents, presence of the free amino groups, which can be utilized for bio-conjugation and crosslinking purposes, cationic nature may help to interact with anionic substances/materials, cell surfaces, and mucous membrane. Thus, an increase in residual time can be enhanced due to an increase in residence time at the site.[60]

Tzeyung et al. in a study RNPs were created, improved, and tested effectively. For nose-to-brain administration, the requisite particle size, PDI, and entrapment efficiency were attained. RNPs may have a longer nasal residency time and a slower mucociliary clearance from the nasal cavity due to their smaller particle size, positive zeta potential, and mucoadhesion ability. The cross-linking between chitosan and TPP, into which rotigotine was successfully entrapped, was shown by the Fourier transform infrared spectroscopy FTIR and X-ray diffraction (XRD) examination of NPs. Data from in vitro release kinetics showed that the medication was released continuously from the formulation. Histopathological analysis of the nasal mucosa revealed no signs of toxicity or structural damage. To determine the potential of rotigotine-loaded chitosan NPs, preclinical and clinical investigations, as well as studies using an in vitro cell line, are necessarily done for the delivery of the drug.[61] Shuangwen et al. Recent advancements in chitosan DDSs for the treatment of brain diseases have been emphasized in this review. Researchers have focused their efforts on enhancing medication concentrations in the brain region due to the BBB's presence. The amount of drug loaded into chitosan NPs is often lower for lipophilic compounds than for hydrophilic molecules because chitosan NPs are generated in a hydrophilic environment. The drug carriers constructed of chitosan stabilize the therapeutic molecules and increase the concentration in the brain. Hence, chitosan-based NPs seem great carriers for the treatment of neurological diseases.[62,63]

16.6.1.2 ALBUMIN

Human serum albumin (HSA) is a globular protein that is mostly present in the circulatory system and has up to about 585 amino acids or 66 kDa in molecular weight. HSA is made up of three main units: I, II, and III, each of which also includes subunits A and B. The Sudlow's sites I and II, obtained in subunits IIA and IIIA, respectively, are the HSA's two primary binding sites. The HSA is a well-known transporter of other compounds and an enhancer of hydrophobic molecule solubility in blood. HSA is employed to deliver various chemicals to particular biological tissues because of these benefits, studies on protein binding and applications for targeted drug delivery frequently employ bovine and HSAs.[64] HSA can interact non-covalently with numerous medications and peptide substances to bind to them. Covalent ligand binding and surface modification are made easier by reactive groups, including amino, thiol, and carboxyl, that are present on the surface of NPs. Known for its superior ligand-binding abilities, HSA can be used to load several medications for distribution through the circulatory system. For loading medicinal medicines in high concentrations, HSA has strong binding affinity sites as well as high stability.[65] Seven long-chain fatty acids can be bound by HSA at a variety of binding sites with varying affinities. Depending on the circumstances surrounding their creation, HSA NPs can have a variety of properties, including size and polydispersity. Additionally, it was confirmed that albumin NPs demonstrated mucosal adherence and did not exhibit toxicity in vivo. Albumin NPs have been suggested as an effective vehicle for delivering antibodies.[66]

16.6.1.3 GELATIN

Gelatin has a long history of safe use in food, cosmetic, and pharmaceutical goods. One of the most versatile naturally occurring biopolymers is this one. FDA-certified gelatin is generally recognized as safe (GRAS) because of its non-toxic and biodegradable nature. The functional groups of the gelatin polymer are open to chemical reactivity. The insoluble animal collagen is frequently transformed into gelatin through alkaline or partial acid hydrolysis. Collagen, which makes up about 25–35% of the body's total protein content, is one of the crucial structural proteins. Although collagen is mostly found in connective tissues such as skin, tendons, and ligaments, it is also present in blood, corneas, bones, and cartilage.[67]

Many diseases of the CNS, including AD, PD, MS, strokes, and brain tumors, remain incurable as a result of the BBB's low permeability. Glial processes, basal lamina, and endothelial cell TJs make up the BBB, a specific region of the vascular system that blocks the passage of more than 98% of CNS disease-candidate drugs into the brain from the bloodstream.[68] Drugs can be delivered to the lesion site via nanoparticulate systems, which allows them to be more effective. Combining long-circulating NPs with brain-targeting ligands appears to be a potential strategy to augment or encourage movement across the BBB. In a work by Tian et al., they created Tat-PEG-GS NPs, which are double-coated gelatin-siloxane nanoparticulate delivery systems for targeting the brain. The in vivo image and TEM analysis demonstrated that Tat-PEG-GS NPs escaped the RES, permeated BBB, and reached the brain. Additionally, Tat-PEG-GS NPs were able to meaningfully elicit more fluorescence signals in the brain than PEG-GS NPs did in the liver.[69]

16.6.1.4 POLY(LACTIC-CO-GLYCOLIC ACID) (PLGA)

The benefits of PLGA NPs include better cellular uptake, increased targeting efficiency, and protection against enzymatic digestion. In addition to being non-toxic and biocompatible, PLGA NPs have some other benefits. This study will give a summary of the most current discoveries and advancements in the NPs -based PLGA approach to treating neurodegenerative diseases such as AD, PD, and ALS. The field of PLGA NPs is flourishing, particularly in the creation of NDOs treatments. PLGA, a synthetic copolymer made from lactic acid and glycolic acid that is sold commercially, has received approval from both the EMA and the FDA. In South Korea, India, and Indonesia, paclitaxel-loaded PEG-PLA micelles have been commercialized so far; they are not based on PLGA but rather a PLA.[70] The literature lists a variety of PLGA NP preparation techniques, such as spray drying, nanoprecipitation, coacervation, single and double emulsion solvent evaporation, and so on. Depending on the technique, medications may be hydrophobic, amphiphilic, or hydrophilic and the NP core is loaded with them, entangled in the polymer chains, or adsorbed on the NP. There is space for improvement by adjusting the molecular weight or the poly(D, L-lactic acid) (PLA) or poly(D, L-glycolic acid) (PGA) ratio even though PLGA NPs have a low encapsulation efficiency, particularly for hydrophilic drugs.[71] As a result of the BBB's lack of drug-specific transport systems, many neuroprotective medications are unable to reach the brain. Nitrogen and ROS are produced by mitochondrial complexes and monoamine oxidase B (MAO-B), which is found within the mitochondria. One aspect of neuro-inflammation in AD, PD, and MS is the malfunctioning of these pathways. A defense system called neuro-inflammation initially guards the brain by eradicating or suppressing various infections. In the case of NDO, neuro-inflammation involves a large number of activated microglia that prevent amyloid-beta (Aβ) phagocytosis and cause plaque to build up. For the treatment of protein aggregation illnesses (proteinopathies), such as AD, PD, HD, and ALS, these pathways are the preferred targets. Meng et al. developed PLGA NPs loaded with Huperzine Aco-conjugated through Lf to improve nose-to-brain transport and also N-trimethyl chitosan (TMC) for simpler mucoadhesion were created as an intranasal DDS. HupA has neuroprotective properties, especially when used to treat AD. However, it exhibits poor brain selectivity, leading to several adverse effects (such as nausea, diarrhea, vomiting, etc.), supporting the need for a more focused DDS.[72] To optimize their brain delivery, many active compounds with neuroprotective properties still need to be studied for the PLGA NP method. Some of them, such as trehalose, boast a variety of qualities, from anti-inflammatory to antioxidant that may be used for current applications for the treatment of NDDs. Trehalose is an excellent protein stabilizer, keeping the structural integrity of proteins intact, and an mTOR-independent autophagy inducer, thus, may help to clear mutant proteins.

Animal models of NDDs such as AD, PD, and HD showed improved behavioral symptoms and lifespan when treated with trehalose, which also decreased the number of harmful protein aggregates.[73]

16.6.1.5 POLY(ALKYL CYANOACRYLATE)

Superglues, also known as PACAs, are frequently employed as suture materials. Couvreur et al. in 1972 PACA NPs were created for the first time. These have minimum toxicity and are metabolized by serum esterase in the blood or esterase from pancreatic juice in the intestinal system (when taken orally). By adjusting the length of the alkyl side chain, the degradation time, which is on the order of hours, may be managed. PACA NPs can be made by either interfacial emulsion polymerization or polymerization in an aqueous acidic phase. Various polymerization techniques such as free radical, anionic, and zwitterionic polymerization techniques can be utilized for the synthesis of PACA.[74] Hydrophilic or less aqueous soluble compounds, proteins, peptides, and nucleic acid can be loaded via either encapsulation or adsorption. PACA NPs can be altered for the distribution to the brain, either with polyethylene glycol to escape RES or polysorbate 80 to increase BBB penetration. In a different study, the anti-A1-42 antibody was used to coat PACA NPs and improved cognition in a mouse model of AD may be due to more penetration into the brain.[75] Mitoxantrone and doxorubicin-loaded PACA NPs have been evaluated for their promising efficacy in patients with hepatocellular carcinoma or resistant solid tumors. The phase II study depicted substantial acute respiratory distress episodes. Also, the phase III trial indicated no significant improvement in life expectancy. The variable drug entrapment and lack of precise drug release may be the reasons for the failure of clinical translation.[76]

16.6.1.6 POLY-ϵ-CAPROLACTONE

PCL, a biodegradable polyester that has FDA approval, has been used in a wide range of goods, including implants, contraceptive devices, medication delivery systems, and sutures (monocryl). The body can hydrolyze PCL to create 6-hydroxy caproic acid, which can subsequently be converted to adipate and catalyzed to CO. Hexanoate repeating units make up PCL chemically.[77]

ACKNOWLEDGMENT

The authors are thankful to the National Institute of Pharmaceutical Education and Research, Raebareli, Ministry of Chemicals and Fertilizers, Government of India, for their support in writing the chapter.

CONFLICT OF INTEREST

The authors declare no conflict of Interest.

KEYWORDS

- **nanoformulations**
- **neurodegenerative disorder**
- **drug delivery**
- **nanomedicine**
- **brain targeting**
- **nanoparticles**

REFERENCES

1. Re, F.; Gregori, M.; Masserini, M. Nanotechnology for Neurodegenerative Disorders. *Maturitas* **2012,** *73* (1), 45–51.
2. Ul Islam, S.; Shehzad, A.; Bilal Ahmed, M.; Lee, Y. S. Intranasal Delivery of Nanoformulations: A Potential Way of Treatment for Neurological Disorders. *Molecules* **2020,** *25* (8), 1929.
3. Waris, A.; Ali, A.; Khan, A. U.; Asim, M.; Zamel, D.; Fatima, K. et al. Applications of Various Types of Nanomaterials for the Treatment of Neurological Disorders. *Nanomaterials* **2022,** *12* (13), 2140.
4. Banks, W. A. Drug Transport into the Central Nervous System: Using Newer Findings About the Blood–Brain Barriers. *Drug Deliv. Transl. Res.* **2012,** *2* (3), 152–159.
5. Tajes, M.; Ramos-Fernández, E.; Weng-Jiang, X.; Bosch-Morató, M.; Guivernau, B.; Eraso-Pichot, A. et al. The Blood–Brain Barrier: Structure, Function and Therapeutic Approaches to Cross It. *Mol. Membr. Biol. Informa Healthcare* **2014,** *31*, 152–167.
6. Kadry, H.; Noorani, B.; Cucullo, L. A Blood–Brain Barrier Overview on Structure, Function, Impairment, and Biomarkers of Integrity. *Fluids Barriers CNS*, **2020,** *17* (1), 69.
7. Zhang, W.; Mehta, A.; Tong, Z.; Esser, L.; Voelcker, N. H. Development of Polymeric Nanoparticles for Blood–Brain Barrier Transfer—Strategies and Challenges. *Adv. Sci. (Weinh).* **2021,** *8* (10), 2003937.
8. Agrawal, M.; Dethe, M. R.; Ahmed, H.; Yadav, A.; Gupta, U. et al. Nose-to-Brain Drug Delivery for the Treatment of Alzheimer's Disease: Current Advancements and Challenges. *Expert Opin. Drug Deliv.* **2022,** *19* (1), 87–102.
9. Khan, N. H.; Mir, M.; Ngowi, E. E.; Zafar, U.; Khakwani MMAK, Khattak, S. et al. Nanomedicine: A Promising Way to Manage Alzheimer's Disease. *Front. Bioeng. Biotechnol.* **2021,** *9*, 630055.

10. Jagaran, K.; Singh, M. Nanomedicine for Neurodegenerative Disorders: Focus on Alzheimer's and Parkinson's Diseases. *Int. J. Mol. Sci.* **2021,** *22* (16), 9082.
11. Dhasmana, S.; Dhasmana, A.; Narula, A. S.; Jaggi, M.; Yallapu, M. M.; Chauhan, S. C. The Panoramic View of Amyotrophic Lateral Sclerosis: A Fatal Intricate Neurological Disorder. *Life Sci.* **2022,** *288*, 120156.
12. Nikolova, M.; Slavchov, R.; Nikolova, G. Nanotechnology in Medicine. In: *Drug Discovery and Evaluation: Methods in Clinical Pharmacology*; Springer: Cham, 2020; pp 533–546.
13. Xiao, M.; Xiao, Z. J.; Yang, B.; Lan, Z.; Fang, F. Blood–Brain Barrier: More Contributor to Disruption of Central Nervous System Homeostasis Than Victim in Neurological Disorders. *Front Neurosci.* **2020,** 14.
14. Pardridge, W. M. CSF, Blood–Brain Barrier, and Brain Drug Delivery. *Expert Opin. Drug Deliv.* **2016,** *13*, 963–975.
15. Profaci, C. P.; Munji, R. N.; Pulido, R. S.; Daneman, R. The Blood–Brain Barrier in Health and Disease: Important Unanswered Questions. *J. Exp. Med.* **2020,** *217*.
16. Rosen, Y.; Elman, N. M. Carbon Nanotubes in Drug Delivery: Focus on Infectious Diseases. *Expert Opin. Drug Deliv.* **2009,** *6*, 517–530.
17. Meher, J. G.; Kesharwani, P.; Chaurasia, M.; Singh, A.; Chourasia, M. K. Carbon Nanotubes (CNTs). In: *Nanotechnology-Based Targeted Drug Delivery Systems for Brain Tumors*; Elsevier; 2018; pp 375–396.
18. Norizan, M. N.; Moklis, M. H.; Ngah Demon, S. Z.; Halim, N. A.; Samsuri, A.; Mohamad, I. S. et al. Carbon Nanotubes: Functionalisation and Their Application in Chemical Sensors. *RSC Adv.* **2020,** *10* (71), 43704–43732.
19. Prajapati, S. K.; Malaiya, A.; Kesharwani, P.; Soni, D.; Jain, A. Biomedical Applications and Toxicities of Carbon Nanotubes. *Drug Chem. Toxicol.* **2022,** *45* (1), 435–450.
20. Henna, T. K.; Raphey, V. R.; Sankar, R.; Ameena Shirin, V. K.; Gangadharappa, H. V.; Pramod, K. Carbon Nanostructures: The Drug and the Delivery System for Brain Disorders. *Int. J. Pharm.* **2020,** *587*, 119701.
21. Costa, P. M.; Bourgognon, M.; Wang JTW, Al-Jamal, K. T. Functionalised Carbon Nanotubes: From Intracellular Uptake and Cell-Related Toxicity to Systemic Brain Delivery. *J. Controll. Release* **2016,** *241*, 200–219.
22. Dugan, L. L.; Lovett, E. G.; Quick, K. L.; Lotharius, J.; Lin, T. T.; O'malley, K. L. Fullerene-Based Antioxidants and Neurodegenerative Disorders. *Parkinsonism Relat. Disord.* **2001,** *7* (3), 243–246.
23. Lemos, V. S.; Aires, R. D.; Ladeira, M.; Guatimosim, S. Fullerene-Derivatives as Therapeutic Agents in Respiratory System and Neurodegenerative Disorders. In: 2016; pp 71–84.
24. Yan, W.; Seifermann, S. M.; Pierrat, P.; Bräse, S. Synthesis of Highly Functionalized C60 Fullerene Derivatives and Their Applications in Material and Life Sciences. *Org. Biomol. Chem.* **2015,** *13*, 25–54.
25. Speranza, G. Carbon Nanomaterials: Synthesis, Functionalization and Sensing Applications. *Nanomaterials (Basel)* **2021,** *11* (4), 967.
26. Matthews, L.; Kanwar, R. K.; Zhou, S.; Punj, V.; Kanwar, J. R. Applications of Nanomedicine in Antibacterial Medical Therapeutics and Diagnostics Overview and Perspectives. *Nano Today* *9* (4), 478–498.
27. Wu, W.; Wieckowski, S.; Pastorin, G.; Benincasa, M.; Klumpp, C.; Briand, J. P. et al. Targeted Delivery of amphotericin B to Cells by Using Functionalized Carbon Nanotubes. *Angew. Chem. Int. Ed.* **2005,** *44* (39), 6358–6362.

28. Chevalier, C.; Saulnier, A.; Benureau, Y.; Fléchet, D.; Delgrange, D.; Colbère-Garapin, F. et al. Inhibition of Hepatitis C Virus Infection in Cell Culture by Small Interfering RNAs. *Mol. Therapy*. **2007,** *15* (8), 1452–1462.
29. Prato, M.; Kostarelos, K.; Bianco, A. Functionalized Carbon Nanotubes in Drug Design and Discovery. *Acc. Chem. Res*. **2008,** *41* (1), 60–68.
30. Bennett, J. E.; Dolin, R.; Blaser, M. J. Mandell, Douglas, and Bennett's Principles and Practice of Infectious Diseases. In: *Mandell, Douglas, and Bennett's Principles and Practice of Infectious Diseases*, Vol. 1–2; Elsevier Inc., 2014; pp 1–3697.
31. Pantarotto, D.; Partidos, C. D.; Hoebeke, J.; Brown, F.; Kramer, E.; Briand, J. P. et al. Immunization with Peptide-Functionalized Carbon Nanotubes Enhances Virus-Specific Neutralizing Antibody Responses to Prepare the bis-FMDV Peptide-Carbon Nanotube. *Chem. Biol.* **2003,** *10* (10), 961–966.
32. Tapeinos, C. Graphene-Based Nanotechnology in Neurodegenerative Disorders. *Maturitas* **2012,** *73* (1), 45–51.
33. Bai, R. G.; Tuvikene, R. Biomedical Applications of Graphene. In: *Handbook of Carbon-Based Nanomaterials*; Elsevier, 2021; pp 551–571.
34. Kulakova, I. I.; Lisichkin, G. V. Chemical Modification of Graphene. *Russ. J. Gen Chem.* **2020,** *90* (10), 1921–1943.
35. Saraf, J.; Kalia, K.; Bhattacharya, P.; Tekade, R. K. Growing Synergy of Nanodiamonds in Neurodegenerative Interventions. *Drug Discov. Today* **2019,** *24*, 584–594.
36. Say, J. M.; van Vreden, C.; Reilly, D. J.; Brown, L. J.; Rabeau, J. R.; King, N. Luminescent Nanodiamonds for Biomedical Applications. *Biophys. Rev.* **2011,** *3* (4), 171–184.
37. Bhogale, D.; Mazahir, F.; Yadav, A. K. Recent Synergy of Nanodiamonds: Role in Brain-Targeted Drug Delivery for the Management of Neurological Disorders. *Mol. Neurobiol.* **2022,** *59* (8), 4806–4824.
38. Brahmkhatri, V. P.; Sharma, N.; Sunanda, P.; D'Souza, A.; Raghothama, S.; Atreya, H. S. Curcumin Nanoconjugate Inhibits Aggregation of *N*-Terminal Region (Aβ-16) of an Amyloid Beta Peptide. *New J. Chem.* **2018,** *42* (24), 19881–19892.
39. Tiwari, S. K.; Agarwal, S.; Seth, B.; Yadav, A.; Nair, S.; Bhatnagar, P. et al. Curcumin-Loaded Nanoparticles Potently Induce Adult Neurogenesis and Reverse Cognitive Deficits in Alzheimer's Disease Model *via* Canonical Wnt/β-Catenin Pathway. *ACS Nano*. **2014,** *8* (1), 76–103.
40. Naeimi, R.; Safarpour, F.; Hashemian, M.; Tashakorian, H.; Ahmadian, S. R.; Ashrafpour, M. et al. Curcumin-Loaded Nanoparticles Ameliorate Glial Activation and Improve Myelin Repair in Lyolecithin-Induced Focal Demyelination Model of Rat Corpus Callosum. *Neurosci. Lett.* **2018,** *674*, 1–10.
41. Zhang, N.; Yan, F.; Liang, X.; Wu, M.; Shen, Y.; Chen, M. et al. Localized Delivery of Curcumin into Brain with Polysorbate 80-Modified Cerasomes by Ultrasound-Targeted Microbubble Destruction for Improved Parkinson's Disease Therapy. *Theranostics* **2018,** *8* (8), 2264–77.
42. Bollimpelli, V. S.; Kumar, P.; Kumari, S.; Kondapi, A. K. Neuroprotective Effect of Curcumin-Loaded Lactoferrin Nano Particles Against Rotenone Induced Neurotoxicity. *Neurochem. Int.* **2016,** *95*, 37–45.
43. Sandhir, R.; Yadav, A.; Mehrotra, A.; Sunkaria, A.; Singh, A.; Sharma, S. Curcumin Nanoparticles Attenuate Neurochemical and Neurobehavioral Deficits in Experimental Model of Huntington's Disease. *NeuroMol. Med.* **2014,** *16* (1), 106–118.

44. Dolati, S.; Ahmadi, M.; Aghebti-Maleki, L.; Nikmaram, A.; Marofi, F.; Rikhtegar, R. et al. Nanocurcumin Is a Potential Novel Therapy for Multiple Sclerosis by Influencing Inflammatory Mediators. *Pharmacol. Rep.* **2018,** *70* (6), 1158–1167.
45. Ahmadi, M.; Agah, E.; Nafissi, S.; Jaafari, M. R.; Harirchian, M. H.; Sarraf, P. et al. Safety and Efficacy of Nanocurcumin as Add-On Therapy to Riluzole in Patients with Amyotrophic Lateral Sclerosis: A Pilot Randomized Clinical Trial. *Neurotherapeutics* **2018,** *15* (2), 430–438.
46. Kang, Y. J.; Cutler, E. G.; Cho, H. Therapeutic Nanoplatforms and Delivery Strategies for Neurological Disorders. *Nano Convergence* **2018,** *5* (1), 35.
47. Ko, W. C.; Wang, S. J.; Hsiao, C. Y.; Hung, C. T.; Hsu, Y. J.; Chang, D. C. et al. Pharmacological Role of Functionalized Gold Nanoparticles in Disease Applications. *Molecules* **2022,** *27* (5), 1551.
48. Khaydarov, R. R.; Khaydarov, R. A.; Estrin, Y.; Scheper, T.; Endres, C.; Cho, S. Y. SILVER NANOPARTICLES Environmental and Human Health Impacts *Int. J. Mol. Sci.* **2020,** 2375.
49. Ravindran, A.; Chandran, P.; Khan, S. S. Biofunctionalized silver nanoparticles: Advances and Prospects. *Colloids Surfaces B: Biointerfaces* **2013,** *105*, pp 342–352.
50. Huang, C. L.; Hsiao, I. L.; Lin, H. C.; Wang, C. F.; Huang, Y. J.; Chuang, C. Y. Silver Nanoparticles Affect on Gene Expression of Inflammatory and Neurodegenerative Responses in Mouse Brain Neural Cells. *Environ Res.* **2015,** *136*, 253–263.
51. Rivera-Mancía, S.; Pérez-Neri, I.; Ríos, C.; Tristán-López, L.; Rivera-Espinosa, L.; Montes, S. The Transition Metals Copper and Iron in Neurodegenerative Diseases. *Chem.Biol. Interactions* **2010,** *186*, 184–199.
52. Cano, A.; Sánchez-López, E.; Ettcheto, M.; López-Machado, A.; Espina, M.; Souto, E. B. et al. Current Advances in the Development of Novel Polymeric Nanoparticles for the Treatment of Neurodegenerative Diseases. *Nanomedicine* **2020,** *15*, 1239–61.
53. Calzoni, E.; Cesaretti, A.; Polchi, A.; di Michele, A.; Tancini, B.; Emiliani, C. Biocompatible Polymer Nanoparticles for Drug Delivery Applications in Cancer and Neurodegenerative Disorder Therapies. *J. Funct. Biomater.* **2019,** *10* (1), 4.
54. Jacob, J.; Haponiuk, J. T.; Thomas, S.; Gopi, S. Biopolymer Based Nanomaterials in Drug Delivery Systems: A Review. *Mater. Today Chem.* **2018,** *9*, 43–55.
55. Pepe, G.; Calce, E.; Verdoliva, V.; Saviano, M.; Maglione, V.; di Pardo, A. et al. Curcumin-Loaded Nanoparticles Based on Amphiphilic Hyaluronan-Conjugate Explored as Targeting Delivery System for Neurodegenerative Disorders. *Int. J. Mol. Sci.* **2020,** *21* (22), 1–13.
56. Sim, T. M.; Tarini, D.; Dheen, S. T.; Bay, B. H.; Srinivasan, D. K. Nanoparticle-Based Technology Approaches to the Management of Neurological Disorders. *Int. J. Mol. Sci.* **2020,** *21* (17), 6070.
57. Mohi-ud-din, R.; Mir, R. H.; Wani, T. U.; Shah, A. J.; Mohi-Ud-Din, I.; Dar, M. A. et al. Novel Drug Delivery System for Curcumin: Implementation to Improve Therapeutic Efficacy against Neurological Disorders. *Comb. Chem. High Throughput Screen* **2022,** *25* (4), 607–615.
58. Rabiee, N.; Ahmadi, S.; Afshari, R.; Khalaji, S.; Rabiee, M.; Bagherzadeh, M. et al. Polymeric Nanoparticles for Nasal Drug Delivery to the Brain: Relevance to Alzheimer's Disease. *Adv. Ther. (Weinh)*. **2021,** *4* (3), 2000076.
59. Nabi, B.; Rehman, S.; Fazil, M.; Khan, S.; Baboota, S.; Ali, J. Riluzole-Loaded Nanoparticles to Alleviate the Symptoms of Neurological Disorders by Attenuating Oxidative Stress. *Drug Dev. Ind. Pharm.* **2020,** *46* (3), 471–483.

60. Wechsler, M. E.; Vela Ramirez, J. E.; Peppas, N. A. 110th Anniversary: Nanoparticle Mediated Drug Delivery for the Treatment of Alzheimer's Disease: Crossing the Blood–Brain Barrier. *Ind. Eng. Chem. Res.* **2019,** *58*, 15079–15087.
61. Yu, S.; Xu, X.; Feng, J.; Liu, M.; Hu, K. Chitosan and Chitosan Coating Nanoparticles for the Treatment of Brain Disease. *Int. J. Pharm.* **2019,** *560*, 282–293.
62. Manek, E.; Darvas, F.; Petroianu, G. A. Use of Biodegradable, Chitosan-Based Nanoparticles in the Treatment of Alzheimer's Disease. *Molecules* **2020,** *25*.
63. Tzeyung, A. S.; Md, S.; Bhattamisra, S. K.; Madheswaran, T.; Alhakamy, N. A.; Aldawsari, H. M. et al. Fabrication, Optimization, and Evaluation of Rotigotine-Loaded Chitosan Nanoparticles for Nose-to-Brain Delivery. *Pharmaceutics*. **2019,** *11* (1).
64. Wong, L. R.; Ho, P. C. Role of Serum Albumin as a Nanoparticulate Carrier for Nose-to-Brain Delivery of R-flurbiprofen: Implications for the Treatment of Alzheimer's Disease. *J. Pharm. Pharmacol.* **2018,** *70* (1), 59–69.
65. Hong, S.; Choi, D. W.; Kim, H. N.; Park, C. G.; Lee, W.; Park, H. H. Protein-Based Nanoparticles as Drug Delivery Systems. *Pharmaceutics 12* (7), 604, 1–28.
66. Rai, G.; Yadav, A. K.; Jain, N. K.; Agrawal, G. P. Eudragit-Coated Dextran Microspheres of 5-Fluorouracil for Site-Specific Delivery to Colon. *Drug Deliv.* **2016,** *23* (1), 328–337.
67. Mahmoudi Saber, M. Strategies for Surface Modification of Gelatin-Based Nanoparticles. *Colloids Surf B Biointerfaces*. **2019,** *183*, 110407.
68. Shakeri, S.; Ashrafizadeh, M.; Zarrabi, A.; Roghanian, R.; Afshar, E. G.; Pardakhty, A. et al. Multifunctional Polymeric Nanoplatforms for Brain Diseases Diagnosis, Therapy and Theranostics. *Biomedicines*. **2020,** *8* (1), 13.
69. Hekmatimoghaddam, S.; Iman, M.; Shahdadi Sardo, H.; Jebali, A. Gelatin Hydrogel Containing Cerium Oxide Nanoparticles Covered by Interleukin-17 Aptamar as an Anti- Inflammatory Agent for Brain Inflammation. *J. Neuroimmunol.* **2019,** *326*, 79–83.
70. Cunha, A.; Gaubert, A.; Latxague, L.; Dehay, B. PLGA-Based Nanoparticles for Neuroprotective Drug Delivery in Neurodegenerative Diseases. *Pharmaceutics* **2021,** *13* (7), 1042.
71. Xu, R.; Wang, J.; Xu, J. et al. Rhynchophylline Loaded-mPEG-PLGA Nanoparticles Coated with Tween-80 for Preliminary Study in Alzheimer's Disease. *Int. J. Nanomed.* **2020,** *15*, 1149–1160.
72. Rigon, L.; Salvalaio, M.; Pederzoli, F.; Legnini, E.; Duskey, J. T.; D'Avanzo, F. et al. Targeting Brain Disease in MPSII: Preclinical Evaluation of IDS-Loaded PLGA Nanoparticles. *Int. J. Mol. Sci.* **2019,** *20* (8), 2014.
73. Hoyos-Ceballos, G. P.; Ruozi, B.; Ottonelli, I.; da Ros, F.; Vandelli, M. A.; Forni, F. et al. PLGA-PEG-ANG-2 Nanoparticles for Blood–Brain Barrier Crossing: Proof-of-Concept Study. *Pharmaceutics* **2020,** *12* (1), 72.
74. Shakeri, S.; Ashrafizadeh, M.; Zarrabi, A.; Roghanian, R.; Afshar, E. G.; Pardakhty, A. et al. Multifunctional Polymeric Nanoplatforms for Brain Diseases Diagnosis, Therapy and Theranostics. *Biomedicines* **2020,** *8* (1), 13.
75. Mydin RBSMN, Moshawih, S. Nanoparticles in Nanomedicine Application: Lipid-Based Nanoparticles and Their Safety Concerns. In: *Nanotechnology: Applications in Energy, Drug and Food*; Springer: Cham, 2019; pp 227–232.
76. Mura, S.; Fattal, E.; Nicolas, J. From Poly (Alkyl Cyanoacrylate) to Squalene as Core Material for the Design of Nanomedicines. *J. Drug Target.* **2019,** *27* (5–6), 470–501.
77. Lahkar, S.; Das, M. K. Surface-Modified Polycaprolactone Nanoparticles for the Brain-Targeted Delivery of Nevirapine. *J. Nanopart. Res.* **2020,** *22* (5), 109.

CHAPTER 17

Nanostructured Drug Carriers for Nose-to-Brain Drug Delivery in the Treatment of Neurological Disorders

NOOPUR SRIVASTAVA[1], PAWAN UPADHYAY[1], ALKA SRIVASTAVA[1], SHIBU DAS[1], and SUDHANSHU MISHRA[2]

[1]*School of Pharmaceutical Sciences, Maharishi University of Information Technology, Lucknow, India*

[2]*Department of Pharmaceutical Science & Technology, Madan Mohan Malaviya University of Technology, Gorakhpur, India*

ABSTRACT

The advancement in the field of neuroscience results in the development of alternative therapies that can easily cross blood–brain barrier (BBB). Intranasal drug delivery or nose-to-brain (NTB) drug delivery is one of the efficient routes. NTB drug delivery offers a wide range of medicinal breakthroughs for the treatment of many neurological disorders because of attractive physiological characteristics such as a highly vascularized mucosa, a large surface area, and a porous endothelium membrane. Alzheimer's disease (AD), Parkinson's disease (PD), amyotrophic lateral sclerosis (ALS), Huntington's disease (HD), and Prion illnesses are examples of neurological disorders. Nasal drug delivery can be achieved via the olfactory or trigeminal nerve pathway which originates from the brain to the respiratory epithelium. This pathway offers the advantage of bypassing the hepatic first-pass metabolism. This approach is more appealing for the direct distribution of small molecules, proteins, and peptides to the brain because of its site-specific delivery and noninvasiveness. This delivery strategy offers rapid onset of

Nanomedicine for Neurodegenerative Disorders: Selective Treatment Strategies. Rishabha Malviya, Kamla Pathak, & Swati Verma (Eds.)

action, improved BBB permeations, increased bioavailability lesser systemic side effects. Nanostructured carriers have shown promising outcomes for precise delivery to the brain by overcoming physical and chemical barriers. Various nanostructured carriers have been evaluated for their efficacy in delivering drugs to the brain. These include nanoparticles, liposomes, exosomes, nanospheres, nanogels, and nanoemulsions. This chapter includes details about various nanostructured carried developed for nasal drug delivery related to neurological disorders.

17.1 INTRODUCTION

The central nervous system's (CNS's) high sensitivity and delicate neuronal structures require a constant flow of gases and nutrients to conduct electrical signals correctly and effectively. The fluids that surround and bathe the brain, neurons, and related cells not only offer the most practical ionic and nutritional milieu, supplying all necessary materials and eliminating trash while protecting against mechanical disruption. Therefore, rigorous regulation of the amount, content, and alteration of these fluids is essential to preserving the optimum milieu for the nervous system. Several cellular and acellular barriers work together to safeguard the brain tissues from changes in blood composition, which is how this is accomplished The BBB, which successfully divides blood from the brain's interstitial fluid, is created by highly specialized endothelial cells and is the strictest and most complicated barrier in the brain.[1]

Despite the existence of intrinsic defense systems, there are more than 600 known medical conditions that can affect the neurological system and cause impairment. Conditions Neurodegenerative illnesses need to receive extra attention. The treatment options for various neurodegenerative diseases such as Alzheimer's disease (AD), and PD include restricted, simply planning to address the symptoms. At this time, none of the existing medications can halt or postpone the ongoing death of neurons. Despite the existence of some possible therapeutic agents, the creation of new, practical substitutes continues to be one of the primary issues, as the greatest obstacle to their achievement is the CNS is surrounded by defenses.[2]

The olfactory or trigeminal nerve pathways, which run from the brain to the respiratory epithelium, can be used to administer medications through the nose. The benefit of avoiding hepatic first-pass metabolism is provided by this pathway. Due to its site-specific delivery and noninvasive nature, this method is more desirable for the direct administration of tiny molecules, proteins, and peptides to the brain. This method of distribution provides a quick start to action, better BBB permeations, greater bioavailability, and fewer systemic side effects. To precisely transport drugs to the brain, nanostructured carriers have demonstrated promising results by bypassing physical and chemical barriers. The effectiveness of several nanostructured carriers in delivering medications to the brain has been tested. Nanoparticles, liposomes, exosomes, nanospheres, nanogels, and nanoemulsions are some of these.[3]

Neurodegenerative problems can be managed with the use of drug-loaded nanosystems. Specifically, lipid-based compositions including lipid nanoparticles and liposomes [solid lipid nanoparticles (SLNs) and nanostructured lipid carriers (NLCs)], whether microemulsions or nanoemulsions, have been widely used to target the CNS through media and get around obstacles by medicinal drug delivery across the BBB. These nanostructures offer many benefits that make them very appealing colloidal compared to other nanocarriers, carriers for brain delivery. These methods have been a key focus in CNS nanotechnology research due to their capacity to evade spontaneously penetrating the capillary endothelial cells of the brain via phagocytosis by the reticuloendothelial system (RES) (BCECs). Additionally, it is possible to create lipid nanocarriers that interact with particular molecules or cell receptors found in the BBB through surface modification and coating. This not only improves the ability to target the brain but also increases the bioavailability and CNS concentration of some drugs that cannot normally cross the BBB. Nasal delivery became more popular, especially in the developing field of nose-to-brain (NTB) delivery. Unlike systemic delivery, NTB delivery offers a promising substitute that enables the transfer of therapeutic medications to the CNS while avoiding the blood–brain barrier (BBB). NTB delivery is a noninvasive alternative to traditional drug delivery methods that allows for direct CNS access via the trigeminal or olfactory nerves. Systems that each drug formulation favors from the nasal cavity to the higher brain areas, including intracellular and extracellular pathways. The impact of absorption into the cerebral fluids, lymphatic systems, and blood circulation must be taken into account while developing pharmacological formulations. There are already specific and effective therapeutic proteins for some CNS illnesses, but for others, novel biologics must be produced. Opportunity to improve therapeutic outcomes and minimize toxic effects when compared to systemic medications that are currently approved or when compared to the systemic doses required if delivery to the site of action is improved.[4]

The purpose of this study is to aims to highlight the developments and problems of the potential approach nanoformulations for the control of neurodegenerative disorders. As a beginning point, a succinct explanation of the BBB's anatomy and physiology, and is provided for the BBB transport systems. After that, a description of the key neurodegenerative conditions and associated licensed pharmacological treatments are provided.

17.2 BLOOD–BRAIN BARRIER

The concept of the BBB is used to refer to the distinct characteristics of the CNS's microvasculature. The BBB is a dynamic biological and physical barrier that separates blood flow from the CNS. Brain capillaries make up the BBB. Endothelial cells are tightly packed in a layer on the blood capillary walls, which inhibits the passage of harmful substances into the brain. Tight and adherent junctions connect the endothelial cells. Particularly, this kind of connection restricts paracellular flow inside the CNS. The BBB protects the majority of drug molecules and imaging agents from entering the brain and causes negative effects on the periphery.[5]

17.3 INTRANASAL PATHWAY

For centuries, intranasal drug delivery has been the most promising drug delivery option. In 1991, the use of nasal pathways for drug delivery to the CNS was established. This pathway enables the drug to bypass the BBB. It is a type of noninvasive technique of drug delivery.[6] The nose is one of the organs among the five senses used for olfaction. Nostrils to the nasopharynx are included in the nasal cavity. It consists of three functional regions, that is, the vestibular region, the respiratory region, and the olfactory region. Further, the nasal cavity extends toward the paranasal sinuses. The olfactory region is a key area that directs the passage of drugs from the nose to the brain. The olfactory region is made up of the olfactory epithelium, the uppermost part of the nasal cavity. It is also known as the olfactory cleft. The olfactory receptor neurons (ORNs) are found in this portion of the nasal cavity. The axons of these neurons are covered by neural fibroblast cells. These neurons connect the olfactory epithelium and the olfactory bulb in the brain.[7]

The intranasal drug delivery mechanism has been patented by William Frey II in 1991. NTB drug delivery has been proven effective in the treatment of many neurological disorders. Intranasal drug delivery includes the olfactory nerve and trigeminal nerve pathways via intracellular, paracellular, and transcellular mechanisms. It utilizes the process of endocytosis in which the drug is transported to the brain. The drugs are transported via the ORN axons. The drug reaches the cerebrum and pons regions and is distributed throughout the brain. The drug may also reach the brain via the olfactory epithelium. The substance will be absorbed into the lamina propia and then enter the brain by the gaps present around the olfactory nerve tract.[8]

17.3.1 PATHWAYS

When one opts for the intranasal pathway, there are two ways by which a drug can reach the brain. The direct pathways opt for the olfactory nerve pathway and the trigeminal nerve pathway. While comparing both routes, the olfactory pathway has been reported for faster brain drug delivery.[9]

When the drug opts for the olfactory pathway, it goes through various encampments. Its encampments include olfactory epithelium, olfactory nucleus, olfactory tract, amygdala, hypothalamus, and piriform cortex. The olfactory pathway includes the first cranial nerve, that is, the olfactory nerve. It originates in the nasal epithelium and proceeds toward the brain by the cribriform plate of the ethmoid bone. Further, it reaches the olfactory bulb. The NTB delivery via the olfactory pathway utilizes either intraneuronal transport or extraneuronal transport. Ultimately the drug reaches the parts of the brain, that is, the cerebrum or the cerebellum. The transport via the intraneuronal pathway occurs by the axons of the olfactory nerve. This mechanism requires more time ranging from several hours to some days. Another transport mechanism is the extraneuronal pathway. It is a much faster mechanism of brain drug delivery. It includes the paracellular or transcellular mechanism. Paracellular stands for the fact that nanostructure carriers are absorbed by the gaps present between cells of the nasal epithelium. While, when the formulation is absorbed by the cells of the nasal epithelium, it is termed transcellular. A transcellular mechanism is effective for the lipophilic formulations while the paracellular mechanism supports the absorption of the hydrophilic formulations.[10]

Another cranial nerve, that is trigeminal nerve (V) has also been targeted in the intranasal pathway. This nerve is the largest never among the 12 cranial nerves. Through this pathway, the delivery can be achieved within a few minutes. This transport pathway includes axonal transport and endocytic transport. The olfactory region and the respiratory both are innervated by the trigeminal nerve. The ultimate destination of the trigeminal nerve pathway is the brainstem. It has three branches, that is, the mandibular branch, the ophthalmic branch, and the maxillary branch. The formulation is absorbed via the respiratory epithelium and reaches the brainstem. When the formulation is absorbed by the olfactory region it reaches the caudal and rostral parts of the brain.[11]

17.3.2 ADVANTAGES OF INTRANASAL PATHWAY

The NTB drug delivery offers various advantages over the other techniques employed for drug delivery into the brain. It helps in easily bypassing the BBB. The delivery occurs via the olfactory mucosa, olfactory nerve axons, and connective tissue that surround the olfactory nerve bundle. Firstly, this pathway offers the increased bioavailability of the drug in the brain. As the bioavailability increases, the affectivity of the pathway increases by itself. The drug delivery via the intranasal pathway has been reported to show rapid absorption and onset of action. It is a noninvasive technique, that is, no instrument is needed for the delivery. This offers the reduction in the systemic adverse effects of the medication by the method of targeted drug delivery.[12]

17.4 TYPES OF NANOSTRUCTURED CARRIERS

According to colloidal, chemical, or biological features, the noninvasive approaches use endogenous cellular mechanisms to make it easier for Nanoparticulate-based systems to cross the BBB through the transcellular pathway. Using invasive procedures, a system based on nanoparticles is administered directly into the brain tissue. Other techniques include intraventricular, intrathecal, or interstitial injections. The BBB is also disrupted via motic, ultrasonic, chemical, or magnetic approaches. It has been shown that nanoformulations enhance medication permeability and absorption, as well as their entry and accumulation into the CNS and uptake in the olfactory region.[13]

Lipid-based nanoparticles have received a lot of attention as potential medication delivery agents. These NPs can transport both hydrophilic and hydrophobic components in a single particle because they are amphiphilic. Lipid-based carriers are created using lipids that are biocompatible and biodegradable and are similar to those found in cell membranes. These characteristics enable them to efficiently enter the cells while reducing their toxicity.

Liposomes, micelle-based nanoemulsions, SLN, and NLCs are the most widely utilized lipid-based NP formulations.[14] A liposome typically contains one or more phospholipid bilayers, frequently along with additional lipids such as cholesterol or phosphatidylcholine. The size and surface charge of the liposome membranes can be altered by using different kinds of lipids. For instance, hydrophilic (within their aqueous core) and hydrophobic (inside the lipid membrane) active substances can both be present in neutral or slightly negatively charged liposomes. On the contrary, the negatively charged nucleic acid cannot form multiplexes with positively charged liposomes.[15] The most recent generation of lipid-based nanocarriers, known as SLNs, are lipid emulsions in which a solid lipid has taken the place of the liquid lipid. They typically form a solid lipid matrix and range in size from 100 to 300 nm. They frequently contain aqueous surfactants or physiological lipids in water. For drug delivery, SLNs provide a number of benefits, including the capacity to be made without the use of organic solvents, a high level of physical stability, and increased, controlled release of loaded medicines. Due to their rigid form, SLNs have a low drug loading efficiency (particularly for hydrophilic molecules), and unwanted particle development by agglomeration, which may result in the drug's burst release.[16]

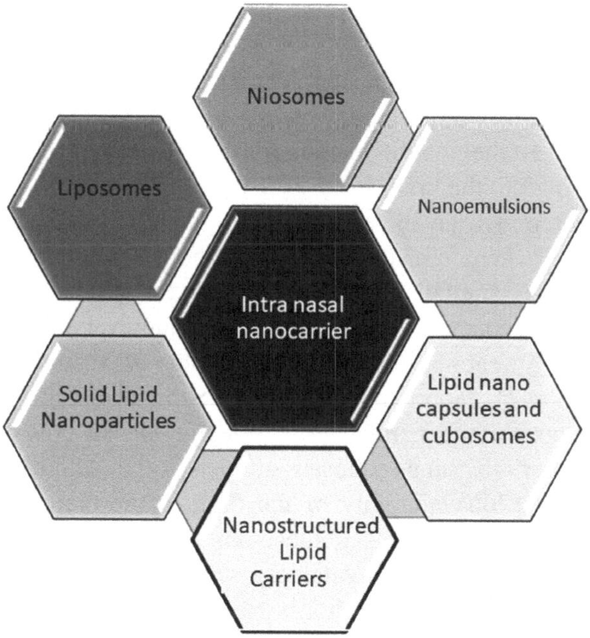

FIGURE 17.1 Type of nanocarriers used in NTB drug delivery for neurological disorders.

17.5 NANOSTRUCTURED CARRIERS IN TREATMENT OF ND

17.5.1 PARKINSON'S DISEASE (PD)

The second most problematic neurological condition in the world is PD. Inflammation, oxidative stress, and the buildup of misfolded proteins are all factors involved in the development of these neurological disorders. In the nasal cavity, the hydrogels are responsible for the transformation of the solution state to a gel state depending on the temperature. Glycyrrhizic acid–zinc alginate nanogel, (GA-NG) has been reported for sustained drug release. The hydrogen bonding between sodium alginate and glycyrrhizic acid was responsible for the sustained release. This hydrogel reported improved drug loading. Fluorescently labeled AL-GA-NGTH (albiflorin and glycyrrhizic acid encapsulated nanogel thermosensitive gel was intranasally delivered to mice and effectively enriched in the brain region administered via an intranasal pathway. The nanogel-encased thermosensitive hydrogel adhered to the nasal cavity for a prolonged period and was shown to have improved olfactory epithelium absorption. The results of the neurotransmitter assay revealed that the content of dopamine, and homovanillic in the substantia nigra of mouse brains were considerably reversed by AL-GA-NGTH administration via intranasal pathway. Following the intranasal administration of AL-GA-NGTH to the PD mice model, the protein level of a-syn was dramatically reduced. PD model mice showed significant therapeutic benefits from the upgraded AL-GA-NGTH system, which proved an efficient therapeutic method for the effective, nontoxic, and drug delivery method into the brain.[17]

Rao et al. reported an increased AUC_{brain}/AUC_{Plasma} ratio of ropinirole-loaded nasal gel when compared with intravenous administration. Pluronic F127 and hydroxy methyl propyl cellulose were responsible for gelling activity in the preparation of ropinirole thermoreversible nasal gels.[18] Rotigotine is the treatment drug for PD. It acts as a dopamine receptor agonist. Wang et al. reported improved CNS bioavailability of the drug when loaded on polymeric micelles.[19] Selegine-loaded poloxamers made up of poloxamer 407 and chitosan intranasal the administration have reported escalated bioavailability of the drug in the brain. According to behavioral research, the animals' photoactometer scores improved, and their level of motor impairment (the catalepsy score) decreased.[20] Rasagiline, a monoamine oxidase (MAO) inhibitor is used in the PD treatment. Chitosan-coated PLGA NPs were used to encapsulate the rasagiline for increased brain concentrations. The NPs were administered via the intranasal pathway.

Mucoadhesive polymers (carbopol 934 P and chitosan) with poloxamer 407 and poloxamer 188 are combined to create a thermosensitive gel loaded with rasagiline mesylate. This formulation showed increased drug levels in the brain.[21] Another PD treatment drug, pramipexole hydrochloride encapsulated into the chitosan NPs. The treatment regimen showed improved locomotor activity and catalepsy in animals.[22]

Bromocriptine and glutathione are therapeutically long-term treatments of PD. Both drugs possess low absorption and high first-pass metabolism. Ashhar et al. formulated bromocriptine and glutathione nanoemulsion using a high-energy ultrasonication process. In vitro drug release studies demonstrated prolonged action. Nanoemulsion formulation enhanced absorption of drugs via nasal mucosa. Toxicity studies showed that nanoemulsion was safe and nontoxic for transport to the brain. According to behavioral tests, administering an intranasal BRM and GSH-loaded nanoemulsion to rats that had been exposed to haloperidol had favorable results and nearly neutralized the drug's effects.[23]

17.5.2 EPILEPSY

Chitosan-PLGA NPs loaded with antiepileptic thyrotropin-releasing hormone (TRH) analogs were used for epilepsy treatment. The treatment was administered via the intranasal route. In vitro studies have quantified prolonged drug release due to chitosan coating. These NPs effectively controlled the epileptic seizures in the animals.[24] Catechin hydrate-loaded chitosan-coated PLGA nanoparticles have shown better efficacy in epilepsy treatment. The nanoparticles administered intranasally greatly increased the bioavailability of the drug in the brain. PAMAM dendrimers encapsulated carbamazepine increased the drug solubility. This formulation has reported the controlled drug release.[25] To enhance the brain absorption of clonazepam for the treatment of seizure disorder, Abbas et al. investigated poloxamer 407 and sodium alginate in situ gel on epilepsy animal models. The animals were administered in situ gels of NLCs loaded with clonazepam and displayed a protracted start period for their first clonic seizure. Additionally, superparamagnetic iron oxide nanoparticles have been incorporated into the clonazepam-loaded NLCs that extended the start period of the first clonic seizure by 7.5 times. These findings imply that the intranasal route combined with nanoparticles is a potentially effective treatment for epileptic episodes.[26]

Pires et al. worked on different fosphenytoin nanoformulations for effective epilepsy treatment. They developed in situ nanoemulsion hydrogel and nanoemulsion for drug encapsulation. The nanoformulations reported sustained drug release in a controlled manner. Fosphenytoin nanoemulsion showed fast release and can be used for acute pain episode treatment. Fosphenytoin-loaded nanoemulsion hydrogel displayed an extended drug release.[27] The nanostructured spherical molecules consisting of the hydrophobic core and the hydrophilic shell have been proven effective in drug delivery in the brain for the treatment of neurological disorders. These molecules are termed as the polymeric micelles. Nour et al. reported good encapsulation of clonazepam into the polymeric micelles. Clonazepam has been used for the epilepsy treatment. Pluronic P123:Pluronic L121 has been used for the micelles formations. This nanostructured drug delivery method has been reported to increase the brain bioavailability of the drug. It has been shown to prevent seizures for a long period.[28]

17.5.3 ALZHEIMER'S DISEASE (AD)

The rabbits were given thiolated chitosan hydrogel loaded with donepezil. When drugs are delivered intravenously, in vivo studies have shown higher drug concentrations.[29] Donepezil is an AChE inhibitor used to treat AD, and Kaur et al. produced nanoemulsions of 65 nm particle sizes for delivery via an intranasal pathway. The controlled donepezil release from the nanoemulsions has been reported by the in vitro drug release studies. The formulation showed substantial levels of drug absorption into the brain and without any toxic effects.[30]

Rajput et al. researchers examined changes in the levels of resveratrol in the brain and plasma when rats were administered gellan gum in situ gel intranasally. This formulation was used for Alzheimer's disease treatment. Outcomes demonstrated that intranasal resveratrol-loaded NLC in situ gel increases the brain/blood ratio by 2.5 times compared to oral suspension.[31] Jojo et al. formulated NLCs loaded with pioglitazone for Alzheimer's treatment. Clinical trial failure of pioglitazone has been linked to low BBB penetration and side effects in the periphery. Animal studies demonstrated that administering the NLC-leaded drug increased the drug absorption into the brain. Rivastigmine, an AChE inhibitor, has low BBB penetration and high first-pass metabolism. Rivastigmine hydrogen tartrate-loaded NLC was created by Anand et al. to treat AD dementia. When compared to a rivastigmine solution, drug-loaded NLC showed enhanced drug concentration in the brain reported by the aldicarb assay. Rivastigmine-loaded NLC may be a viable novel treatment for dementia caused by AD, as evidenced by in vivo experiments that showed considerable memory enhancement, escape latency, and transfer latency.[32]

Quercetin has been reported to reduce neuronal cell death, lipid peroxidation, protein oxidation, and Aβ protein aggregation in AD patients. To boost quercetin's brain bioavailability, Pinheiro et al. formulated SLN and NLC and encapsulated quercetin into them. To aid in the transit across the BBB, transferrin was used to functionalize SLN and NLC. The geraniol-ursodeoxycholic acid complex is a prodrug used for AD dementia treatment. The SLN showed enhanced drug encapsulation and increased drug concentration in rat brains.

In several literatures, Alzheimer's disease has been designated as type III diabetes. The in vivo studies have demonstrated the protective role of insulin in AD treatment. Picone et al. formulated insulin-attached poly(N-vinyl pyrrolidone) nanogels for brain absorption. They prepared the formulation by electron-beam irradiation. They reported the escalated brain absorption of insulin. The formulation has nonimmunogenic properties, complete clearance from the body, and enhances biocompatibility with good BBB crossing ability.[33]

17.5.4 PSYCHOSIS

Psychosis stands for hallucinations and delusions; it has been observed in patients with Alzheimer's disease. The clinicians also target treating psychosis in Alzheimer's patients. An in vivo study demonstrated the easy delivery of the antipsychotic drug resperidone into the brain via the nanostructured dosage form. They encapsulated the drug into the mucoadhesive nanoemulsion. The dosage form has been reported for increased absorption via the nasal mucosa and increased bioavailability.[34]

Another nanostructure formulation, that is, the polymeric nanoparticle has also been demonstrated to increase the brain drug delivery in the cases of psychosis. Piazza et al. formulated haloperidol loaded onto the nanoparticles. These nanoparticles were formulated by the poly(ethylene glycol)-b-poly(D,L)-lactic-co-glycolic acid (PEG-PLGA), and the surface of the formulation was modified by the *Solanum tuberosum* coating. The formulation showed a reduction in the catalepsy in animal models and increased brain absorption.[35]

17.5.5 MIGRAINE

Migraines are a type of headache illness that causes moderate to severe pain. Because nausea and vomiting cause poor gastrointestinal absorption of medications, oral drug administration is not suitable for treating migraines. Therefore, the most effective drug delivery methods for treating migraines are parenteral and nasal. Rizatriptan, 5HT 1B/1D receptor agonist, is used for migraine treatment. There have been studies done on approaches for administering rizatriptan intranasally to increase the drug's absorption and brain tissue deposition. Studies on rizatriptan's intranasal delivery methods have been conducted to enhance the medication's absorption and brain tissue deposition. Zolmitriptan-loaded nanoemulsion was formulated for intranasal delivery. The formulation showed high permeation through the nasal mucosa.[36]

17.5.6 MULTIPLE SCLEROSIS (MS)

Multiple sclerosis is a complex neurodegenerative condition that presents with a variety of clinical symptoms, including vision issues, sensory alterations, muscle weakness, and issues with coordination and speed of movement. Patients with multiple sclerosis have been tested on NE formulations that have received FDA approval, such as Camptosar and Fluosol.[36] One of the first-line treatments for MS is interferon (IFN). To transport IFN into the brain via intranasal pathway, Gonzalez et al. created IFN-NPs, which are chitosan/sulfobutylether-cyclodextrin nanoparticles loaded with IFN. Subsequent nasal delivery of fluorescent probe-loaded NPs, biodistribution analysis revealed a quick and intense fluorescence in the brain. A possible, efficient, noninvasive, and inexpensive treatment for MS is represented by inIFN-NPs.[37]

17.5.7 AMYOTROPHIC LATERAL SCLEROSIS (ALS)

The medication riluzole is authorized to treat ALS. Riluzole is a substrate of P-glycoprotein that's why it cannot cross the blood-brain barrier to be absorbed into the brain. This problem was resolved by the formation of riluzole-loaded NEs. The phase titration approach was used to create riluzole-loaded NEs. When riluzole NEs were administered intravenously rather than orally, the drug's brain absorption was considerably higher.

Riluzole nanoemulsion administered intranasal could be a promising method for treating ALS.[38]

17.5.8 DEPRESSION

In the current world scenario, depression is the main hurdle in the life of an individual. The development of depression includes a deficiency in the induction of the neuronal pathway activity. The antidepressant medication shows high adverse effects due to the accumulation of the drug in nontargeted tissues. This problem can be overcome via targeted drug delivery methods. Many researchers have utilized the polymeric nanoparticles for the encapsulation of the anti-depressant medication. This delivery methods offer a great advantage over the drug given in solution form. Desvenlafaxine has been encapsulated in chitosan-modified poly(D,L-lactic-cglycolic acid) (PLGA) NPs of approximately173 nm size. The treatment by the formulation has been reported to effectively reduce depressive symptoms and increase the level of various monoamines in the rat brain.[39] Selegiline encapsulated in polymeric nanoparticles has been also administered in rats. The animal study has demonstrated promising results.[40]

17.6 CONCLUSION

Memory problems can be brought on by neurodegenerative conditions such as AD, migraine, schizophrenia, PD, and brain injury. Traditional oral approaches only provide surface-level medication, while invasive administration methods have negative cardiac and extrapyramidal side effects. As a result, the noninvasive, efficient, safe, and focused delivery of neurotherapeutics has made the intranasal route of administration an important alternative. To control AD, using the nasal route instead of parenteral and oral medication administration is a viable alternative. To increase drug absorption, several methods have been researched. Nanosystems that are lipid based, such as nanoemulsions and NLC, with or without in situ-forming hydrogel matrices, NTB delivery is a noninvasive, practical, and patient-friendly method of administration that bypasses the BBB to swiftly reach the brain while also exhibiting accurate drug targeting, a rapid commencement of action, and less systemic adverse effects [124]. Based on the various research, We find that the intra-nasal route combined with the utilization of lipid-based nanocarriers, such as NLCs, SLNs, and NEs, is favorable for delivering medications to the

TABLE 17.1 Nanoformulations Administered via an Intranasal Pathway in ND.

Disease	Drug	Nanoformulation	Route
PD	Albiflorin and glycyrrhizic acid	Glycyrrhizic acid-zinc alginate nanogel (hydrogel)	Intranasal
PD	Ropinirle	Pluronic F127 and hydroxy methyl propyl cellulose nasal gel	Intranasal
PD	Rotigotine	Polymeric micelles	Intranasal
PD	Rasagiline mesylate	Poloxamer 407, poloxamer 188,carbopol 934 P and chitosan thermosensitive gel	Intranasal
PD	Rasagiline	Nanoparticle	Intranasal
PD	Selegiline	Poloxamer 407 and chitosan poloxamers	Intranasal
PD	Pramipexole hydrochloride	Chitosan Nanoparticles	Intranasal
PD	Naringenin	Vitamin E-loaded nanoemulsion	Intranasal
PD	Bromocriptine and glutathione	Nanoemulsion	Intranasal
Epilepsy	TRH analogs	Chitosan-PLGA nanoparticles	Intranasal
Epilepsy	Catechin hydrate	Chitosan-coated PLGA nanoparticles	Intranasal
Epilepsy	Carbamazepine	PAMAM dendrimers	Intranasal
Epilepsy	Clonazepam	Poloxamer 407 and sodium alginate in situ gel	Intranasal
Epilepsy	Clonazepam	NLC's	Intranasal
Epilepsy	Clonazepam	Superparamagnetic iron oxide nanoparticles	Intranasal
Epilepsy	Clonazepam	Polymeric micelles pluronic P123:Pluronic L121	Intranasal
Epilepsy	Fosphenytoin	Nanoemulsion	Intranasal
Epilepsy	Fosphenytoin	In situ nanoemulsion hydrogel	Intranasal
Alzheimer's disease	Donepezile	Thiolated chitosan hydrogel	Intranasal
Alzheimer's disease	Donepezile	Nanoemulsions	Intranasal
Alzheimer's disease	Resveratrol	In situ gel of gellan gum with NLC's	Intranasal

TABLE 17.1 *(Continued)*

Disease	**Drug**	**Nanoformulation**	**Route**
Alzheimer's disease	Pioglitazone	NLC's	Intranasal
Alzheimer's disease	Rivastigmine	Hydrogen tartrate loaded NLC	Intranasal
Alzheimer's disease	Quercetin	Solid lipid nanoparticles	Intranasal
Alzheimer's disease	Quercetin	NLC's	Intranasal
Alzheimer's disease	Geraniol-ursodeoxycholic acid	SLN	Intranasal
Alzheimer's disease	Insulin	Poly(N-vinyl pyrrolidone) nanogels	Intranasal
Psychosis	Resperidone	Mucoadhesive nanoemulsion	Intranasal
Psychosis	Haloperidol	Poly(ethylene glycol)-b-poly(D,L)-lactic-co-glycolic acid (PEG-PLGA) polymeric nanoparticles	Intranasal
Migraines	Rizatriptan	Nanoformulation	Intranasal
Migraines	Zolmitriptan	Nanoemulsion	Intranasal
Multiple sclerosis	IFN	Chitosan/sulfobutylether-cyclodextrin nanoparticles	Intranasal
Depression	Desvenlafaxine	chitosan modified poly(D, L-lactic-cglycolic acid) (PLGA) Nanoparticles	Intranasal
Depression	Selegiline	Polymeric nanoparticles	Intranasal
ALS	Riluzole	Nanoemulsion	Intranasal

brain. In comparison to alternative routes of administration or administering free drugs through the nose as liquids or suspensions, these methods have shown superior efficacy upon NTB transport. To ensure that the drug reaches the brain with the fewest possible losses due to mucociliary elimination and enzymatic breakdown, or systemic circulation absorption, it is crucial to recognize the elements that affect the nasal absorption of the drug when developing a lipid-based nanocarrier formulation.

KEYWORDS

- **neurological disorders**
- **nanostricture carriers**
- **intranasal drug delivery**
- **nose-to-brain drug delivery**

REFERENCES

1. Correia, A. C.; Monteiro, A. R.; Silva, R.; Moreira, J. N.; Sousa Lobo, J. M.; Silva, A. C. Lipid Nanoparticles Strategies to Modify Pharmacokinetics of Central Nervous System Targeting Drugs: Crossing or Circumventing the Blood–Brain Barrier (BBB) to Manage Neurological Disorders. *Adv. Drug Deliv. Rev.* **2022,** *189*, 114485. https://linkinghub.elsevier.com/retrieve/pii/S0169409X22003751
2. Vassilopoulos, A.; Mohammad, S.; Dure, L.; Kozlowska, K.; Fobian, A. D. Treatment Approaches for Functional Neurological Disorders in Children. *Curr. Treat Options Neurol.* **2022,** *24* (2), 77–97. https://link.springer.com/10.1007/s11940-022-00708-5
3. Lochhead, J. J.; Kumar, N. N.; Nehra, G.; Stenslik, M. J.; Bradley, L. H.; Thorne, R. G. Intranasal Drug Delivery to the Brain. In: 2022; pp 461–500. https://link.springer.com/10.1007/978-3-030-88773-5_15
4. Lombardo, R.; Musumeci, T.; Carbone, C.; Pignatello, R. Nanotechnologies for Intranasal Drug Delivery: An Update of Literature. *Pharm. Dev. Technol.* 2021, *26* (8), 824–845. https://www.tandfonline.com/doi/full/10.1080/10837450.2021.1950186
5. Hajal, C.; Le Roi, B.; Kamm, R. D.; Maoz, B. M. Biology and Models of the Blood-Brain Barrier. *Annu. Rev. Biomed. Eng.* **2021,** *23*, 359–384.
6. Keller L-A, Merkel, O.; Popp, A. Intranasal Drug Delivery: Opportunities and Toxicologic Challenges During Drug Development. *Drug Deliv. Transl. Res.* **2022,** *12* (4), 735–757. https://link.springer.com/10.1007/s13346-020-00891-5
7. Alfertshofer, M. G.; Frank, K.; Ehrl, D.; Freytag, D. L.; Moellhoff, N.; Gotkin, R. H.; et al. The Layered Anatomy of the Nose: An Ultrasound-Based Investigation. *Aesthetic Surg J.* **2022,** *42* (4), 349–357. https://academic.oup.com/asj/article/42/4/349/6345378

8. Crowe, T. P.; Greenlee MHW, Kanthasamy, A. G.; Hsu, W. H. Mechanism of Intranasal Drug Delivery Directly to the Brain. *Life Sci.* **2018,** *195*, 44–52. https://linkinghub.elsevier.com/retrieve/pii/S002432051730663X
9. Gänger, S.; Schindowski, K. Tailoring Formulations for Intranasal Nose-to-Brain Delivery: A Review on Architecture, Physico-Chemical Characteristics and Mucociliary Clearance of the Nasal Olfactory Mucosa. *Pharmaceutics*. **2018,** *10* (3):116. http://www.mdpi.com/1999-4923/10/3/116
10. Liu, Q.; Zhang, Q. Nanoparticle Systems for Nose-to-Brain Delivery. In: *Brain Targeted Drug Delivery System*; Elsevier, 2019; pp 219–239. https://linkinghub.elsevier.com/retrieve/pii/B978012814001700010X
11. Li, Y.; Wang, C.; Zong, S.; Qi, J.; Dong, X.; Zhao, W.; et al. The Trigeminal Pathway Dominates the Nose-to-Brain Transportation of Intact Polymeric Nanoparticles: Evidence from Aggregation-Caused Quenching Probes. *J. Biomed. Nanotechnol.* **2019,** *15* (4), 686–702. https://www.ingentaconnect.com/content/10.1166/jbn.2019.2724
12. Xie, J.; Shen, Z.; Anraku, Y.; Kataoka, K.; Chen, X. Nanomaterial-Based Blood-Brain-Barrier (BBB) Crossing Strategies. *Biomaterials*. **2019,** *224*, 119491. https://doi.org/10.1016/j.biomaterials.2019.119491
13. Islam, S. U.; Shehzad, A.; Ahmed, M. B.; Lee, Y. S. Intranasal Delivery of Nanoformulations: A Potential Way of Treatment for Neurological Disorders. *Molecules* **2020,** *25* (8), 1929. https://www.mdpi.com/1420-3049/25/8/1929
14. Estapé Senti, M.; de Jongh, C. A.; Dijkxhoorn, K.; Verhoef JJF, Szebeni, J.; Storm, G.; et al. Anti-PEG Antibodies Compromise the Integrity of PEGylated Lipid-Based Nanoparticles via Complement. *J. Control Release*. **2022,** *341*, 475–486. https://linkinghub.elsevier.com/retrieve/pii/S0168365921006374
15. van der Koog, L.; Gandek, T. B.; Nagelkerke, A. Liposomes and Extracellular Vesicles as Drug Delivery Systems: A Comparison of Composition, Pharmacokinetics, and Functionalization. *Adv. Healthc. Mater*. **2022,** *11* (5), 2100639. https://onlinelibrary.wiley.com/doi/10.1002/adhm.202100639
16. Nguyen T-T-L, Maeng H J. Pharmacokinetics and Pharmacodynamics of Intranasal Solid Lipid Nanoparticles and Nanostructured Lipid Carriers for Nose-to-Brain Delivery. *Pharmaceutics* **2022,** *14* (3), 572. https://www.mdpi.com/1999-4923/14/3/572
17. Chen, Y. B.; Qiao, T.; Wang, Y. Q.; Cui, Y. L.; Wang, Q. S. Hydrogen Bond-Enhanced Nanogel Delivery System for Potential Intranasal Therapy of Parkinson's Disease. *Mater Des*. **2022,** *219*, 110741. https://doi.org/10.1016/j.matdes.2022.110741
18. Rao, M.; Agrawal, D. K.; Shirsath, C. Thermoreversible Mucoadhesive In Situ Nasal Gel for Treatment of Parkinson's Disease. *Drug Dev Ind Pharm*. **2017,** *43* (1), 142–150. https://www.tandfonline.com/doi/full/10.1080/03639045.2016.1225754
19. Wang, F.; Yang, Z.; Liu, M.; Tao, Y.; Li, Z.; Wu, Z. et al. Facile Nose-to-Brain Delivery of Rotigotine-Loaded Polymer Micelles Thermosensitive Hydrogels: In Vitro Characterization and In Vivo Behavior Study. *Int. J. Pharm.*. 2020;577(January):119046. https://doi.org/10.1016/j.ijpharm.2020.119046
20. Sridhar, V.; Wairkar, S.; Gaud, R.; Bajaj, A.; Meshram, P. Brain Targeted Delivery of Mucoadhesive Thermosensitive Nasal Gel of Selegiline Hydrochloride for Treatment of Parkinson's Disease. *J. Drug Target*. **2018,** *26* (2), 150–161. https://www.tandfonline.com/doi/full/10.1080/1061186X.2017.1350858
21. Awad, R.; Avital, A.; Sosnik, A. Polymeric Nanocarriers for Nose-to-Brain Drug Delivery in Neurodegenerative Diseases and Neurodevelopmental Disorders. Acta Pharm Sin B. **2022**. https://doi.org/10.1016/j.apsb.2022.07.003

22. Raj, R.; Wairkar, S.; Sridhar, V.; Gaud, R. Pramipexole Dihydrochloride Loaded Chitosan Nanoparticles for Nose to Brain Delivery: Development, Characterization and In Vivo Anti-Parkinson Activity. *Int. J. Biol. Macromol.* **2018,** *109*, 27–35. https://linkinghub.elsevier.com/retrieve/pii/S0141813017336978
23. Ashhar, M. U.; Kumar, S.; Ali, J.; Baboota, S. CCRD based development of Bromocriptine and Glutathione Nanoemulsion Tailored Ultrasonically for the Combined Anti-Parkinson Effect. *Chem. Phys. Lipids.* **2021,** *235*, 105035. https://doi.org/10.1016/j.chemphyslip.2020.105035
24. Kaur, S.; Manhas, P.; Swami, A.; Bhandari, R.; Sharma, K. K.; Jain, R.; et al. Bioengineered PLGA-Chitosan Nanoparticles for Brain Targeted Intranasal Delivery of Antiepileptic TRH Analogues. *Chem. Eng. J.* **2018,** *346*, 630–639. https://linkinghub.elsevier.com/retrieve/pii/S1385894718305345
25. Igartúa, D. E.; Martinez, C. S.; Temprana, C. F.; Alonso S del, V., Prieto, M. J. PAMAM Dendrimers as a Carbamazepine Delivery System for Neurodegenerative Diseases: A Biophysical and Nanotoxicological Characterization. *Int. J. Pharm.*. **2018,** *544* (1), 191–202. https://linkinghub.elsevier.com/retrieve/pii/S0378517318302497
26. Abbas, H.; Refai, H.; El Sayed, N. Superparamagnetic Iron Oxide–Loaded Lipid Nanocarriers Incorporated in Thermosensitive In Situ Gel for Magnetic Brain Targeting of Clonazepam. *J. Pharm. Sci.* **2018,** *107* (8), 2119–2127. https://linkinghub.elsevier.com/retrieve/pii/S0022354918302107
27. Pires, P. C.; Peixoto, D.; Teixeira, I.; Rodrigues, M.; Alves, G.; Santos, A. O. Nanoemulsions and Thermosensitive Nanoemulgels of Phenytoin and Fosphenytoin for Intranasal Administration: Formulation Development and In Vitro Characterization. *Eur. J. Pharm. Sci.* **2020,** *141*, 105099. https://linkinghub.elsevier.com/retrieve/pii/S0928098719303720
28. Nour, S. A.; Abdelmalak, N. S.; Naguib, M. J.; Rashed, H. M.; Ibrahim, A. B. Intranasal Brain-Targeted Clonazepam Polymeric Micelles for Immediate Control of Status Epilepticus: In Vitro Optimization, Ex Vivo Determination of Cytotoxicity, In Vivo Biodistribution and Pharmacodynamics Studies. *Drug Deliv.* **2016,** *23* (9), 3681–3695. https://www.tandfonline.com/doi/full/10.1080/10717544.2016.1223216
29. Al Harthi, S.; Alavi, S. E.; Radwan, M. A.; El Khatib, M. M.; AlSarra, I. A. Nasal Delivery of Donepezil HCl-Loaded Hydrogels for the Treatment of Alzheimer's Disease. *Sci. Rep.*. **2019,** *9* (1), 9563. http://www.nature.com/articles/s41598-019-46032-y
30. Kaur, A.; Nigam, K.; Bhatnagar, I.; Sukhpal, H.; Awasthy, S.; Shankar, S., et al. Treatment of Alzheimer's Diseases Using Donepezil Nanoemulsion: An Intranasal Approach. *Drug Deliv. Transl. Res.* **2020,** *10* (6), 1862–1875. https://link.springer.com/10.1007/s13346-020-00754-z
31. Rajput, A. P.; Butani, S. B. Resveratrol Anchored Nanostructured Lipid Carrier Loaded in Situ Gel via Nasal Route: Formulation, Optimization and In Vivo Characterization. *J. Drug Deliv. Sci. Technol.* **2019,** *51*, 214–223. https://linkinghub.elsevier.com/retrieve/pii/S1773224718310049
32. Anand, A.; Arya, M.; Kaithwas, G.; Singh, G.; Saraf, S. A. Sucrose Stearate as a Biosurfactant for Development of Rivastigmine Containing Nanostructured Lipid Carriers and Assessment of Its Activity Against Dementia in, *C. elegans* Model. *J. Drug Deliv. Sci. Technol.* **2019,** *49*, 219–226. https://linkinghub.elsevier.com/retrieve/pii/S1773224718302120
33. Picone, P.; Sabatino, M. A.; Ditta, L. A.; Amato, A.; San Biagio, P. L.; Mulè, F.; et al. Nose-to-Brain Delivery of Insulin Enhanced by a Nanogel Carrier. *J. Control Release.* **2018,** *270*, 23–36. http://dx.doi.org/10.1016/j.jconrel.2017.11.040

34. Kumar, M.; Pathak, K.; Misra, A. Formulation and Characterization of Nanoemulsion-Based Drug Delivery System of Risperidone. *Drug Dev. Ind. Pharm.* **2009,** *35* (4), 387–395. http://www.tandfonline.com/doi/full/10.1080/03639040802363704
35. Piazza, J.; Hoare, T.; Molinaro, L.; Terpstra, K.; Bhandari, J.; Selvaganapathy, P. R.; et al. Haloperidol-Loaded Intranasally Administered Lectin Functionalized Poly(Ethylene Glycol)–Block-Poly(d,l)-Lactic-Co-Glycolic Acid (PEG–PLGA) Nanoparticles for the Treatment of Schizophrenia. *Eur. J. Pharm. Biopharm.* **2014,** *87* (1), 30–39. https://linkinghub.elsevier.com/retrieve/pii/S0939641114000526
36. Bahadur, S.; Pardhi, D. M.; Rautio, J.; Rosenholm, J. M.; Pathak, K. Intranasal Nanoemulsions for Direct Nose-to-Brain Delivery of Actives for CNS Disorders. *Pharmaceutics* **2020,** *12* (12), 1–27.
37. González, L. F.; Acuña, E.; Arellano, G.; Morales, P.; Sotomayor, P.; Oyarzun-Ampuero, F. et al. Intranasal Delivery of Interferon-β-Loaded Nanoparticles Induces Control of Neuroinflammation in a Preclinical Model of Multiple Sclerosis: A Promising Simple, Effective, Non-Invasive, and Low-Cost Therapy. *J. Control Release.* **2021,** *331,* 443–459. https://linkinghub.elsevier.com/retrieve/pii/S0168365920306684
38. Parikh, H. R.; Patel, J. R. Nanoemulsions for Intranasal Delivery of Riluzole to Improve Brain Bioavailability: Formulation Development and Pharmacokinetic Studies. *Curr. Drug Deliv.* **2016,** *13* (7), 1130–1143. http://www.eurekaselect.com/openurl/content.php?genre=article&issn=1567-2018&volume=13&issue=7&spage=1130
39. Tong G-F, Qin, N.; Sun L-W. Development and Evaluation of Desvenlafaxine Loaded PLGA-Chitosan Nanoparticles for Brain Delivery. *Saudi Pharm J.* **2017,** *25* (6), 844–851. https://linkinghub.elsevier.com/retrieve/pii/S1319016416301372
40. Singh, D.; Rashid, M.; Hallan, S. S.; Mehra, N. K.; Prakash, A.; Mishra, N. Pharmacological Evaluation of Nasal Delivery of Selegiline Hydrochloride-Loaded Thiolated Chitosan Nanoparticles for the Treatment of Depression. *Artif. Cells Nanomedicine, Biotechnol.* **2015,** 1–13. http://www.tandfonline.com/doi/full/10.3109/21691401.2014.998824

Index

C

O

P

Q

R

S

T

U

V